Obesity

Prevention
and Treatment

Obesity

Prevention and Treatment

Edited by
James M. Rippe, MD
Theodore J. Angelopoulos, PhD, MPH

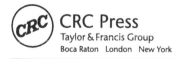

CRC Press
Taylor & Francis Group
Boca Raton   London   New York

CRC Press is an imprint of the
Taylor & Francis Group, an **Informa** business

CRC Press
Taylor & Francis Group
6000 Broken Sound Parkway NW, Suite 300
Boca Raton, FL 33487-2742

First issued in paperback 2016

© 2012 by Taylor & Francis Group, LLC
CRC Press is an imprint of Taylor & Francis Group, an Informa business

No claim to original U.S. Government works

Version Date: 20120417

ISBN 13: 978-1-138-19849-4 (pbk)
ISBN 13: 978-1-4398-3671-2 (hbk)

Library of Congress Cataloging-in-Publication Data

Obesity : prevention and treatment / editors, James M. Rippe and
    Theodore J. Angelopoulos.
        p. ; cm.
    Includes bibliographical references and index.
    ISBN 978-1-4398-3671-2 (hardcover : alk. paper)
    I. Rippe, James M. II. Angelopoulos, Theodore J.
    [DNLM: 1. Obesity--prevention & control. 2. Obesity--complications. 3.
Obesity--therapy. WD 210]

    616.3'98--dc23   2011050261

Visit the Taylor & Francis Web site at
http://www.taylorandfrancis.com

and the CRC Press Web site at
http://www.crcpress.com

To our families
Stephanie, Hart, Jaelin, Devon, and Jamie
and
Kristi, Zoe, and Sophia

Contents

PART I The Modern Management of Obesity

PART II   Obesity and Specific Medical Conditions

Preface

It is with great pleasure that we present our new book *Obesity: Prevention and Treatment*. This is a book for every health-care provider who wishes to understand both the basic science and the clinical applications behind the prevention and treatment of obesity and its associated conditions. Never has there been a time when these issues are more critical to address.

The prevalence of overweight and obesity in the United States and the rest of the industrialized world has skyrocketed in the past 20 years. Currently, over two-thirds of the adult population in the United States is either overweight or obese. Shockingly, the prevalence of obesity has grown 40% in the last decade, for which we have reliable data.

Obesity is associated with numerous significant medical conditions as follows:

- Obesity is strongly associated with diabetes (80%–85% of diabetic patients in the United States are obese).
- Obesity is strongly associated with hypertension (40%–70% of hypertension patients in the United States are obese).
- Obesity is strongly associated with dyslipidemia (40%–50% of dyslipidemia patients in the United States are obese).
- Obesity is strongly associated with the metabolic syndrome (the current prevalence of the metabolic syndrome in the adult population of the United States is estimated to be between 25% and 35%).
- Obesity is strongly associated with glucose intolerance (recent CDC estimates suggest that 35%–40% of the adult population in the United States has glucose intolerance).
- Obesity is the leading cause of osteoarthritis in women and the second leading cause of osteoarthritis in men.
- Obesity is one of the leading causes of cancer (second only to smoking), and the gap is closing rapidly.

In addition to these grim statistics on the prevalence of obesity among adults, an equally significant epidemic is the occurrence of obesity in children, which has tripled in the last 30 years in the United States. Associated with this increase are significant increases in diabetes, hypertension, lipid problems, and the metabolic syndrome in children.

This problem is neither unique to the United States nor to other developed countries. Less developed nations are also experiencing rapid growth in the prevalence of obesity, making this a worldwide epidemic. The World Health Organization estimates that there are now 1.5 billion people in the world who are obese.

Obesity is also causing enormous health-care expenditures in the United States and other countries. A government-sponsored report issued on July 28, 2009, estimates that obesity accounts for 9.1% of all health-care expenditures in the United States.

Over \$140 billion are currently being spent in the United States annually to treat obesity and obesity-related conditions. There can be no effective health-care reform unless the growing problem of obesity is resolved.

There is some good news in this otherwise grim picture. The Institute of Medicine has estimated that significant reduction in risk factors for various metabolic diseases occurs in overweight or obese individuals who lose as little as 5% of their body weight. The Diabetes Prevention Program Study showed that individuals with glucose intolerance who lost 5%–7% of their body weight by adopting some simple nutritional practices and increasing their physical activity reduce their risk of developing diabetes by 58%. The National Weight Control Registry (a registry of over 3000 individuals who have lost at least 30 lb and kept it off for at least one year) provides important data about how individuals can lose weight and keep it off.

To meet the challenge of providing a book that spans modern knowledge about obesity from its basic pathophysiology to its clinical treatment, we have been joined by an internationally distinguished group of scientists and clinicians. We have challenged all of our collaborating authors to blend state-of-the-art knowledge in basic science with a particular emphasis on clinical applications that will be relevant to the practicing physician and other health-care workers, and all of the authors have responded to this challenge admirably.

What has emerged is a state-of-the-art compendium of information about the modern understandings of obesity—both its prevention and treatment. We hope that this book will help guide physicians, nurses, nutritionists, exercise physiologists, and other health-care providers as well as students in these disciplines as they take steps to both prevent obesity and/or, if already present, treat it and its associated conditions.

The worldwide epidemic of obesity demands the best practices, information, and commitment on the part of health-care workers. We are proud to play a role in helping to combat this major worldwide epidemic with *Obesity: Prevention and Treatment*.

Acknowledgments

Numerous individuals have made significant contributions to all phases of editing and production of this textbook and deserve our recognition and gratitude.

First, we wish to acknowledge the outstanding work of every chapter author in the book. We set out to generate a book that would bridge the gap between basic science and clinical practice in the prevention and treatment of obesity. We challenged each of the authors to provide state-of-the-art knowledge in basic science while emphasizing its clinical applications, and all of them responded to this challenge admirably.

We would also like to acknowledge Dr. Rippe's managing editor, Elizabeth Grady. Beth coordinates multiple publications for health-care professionals, including four major textbooks, two academic journals, and numerous books and publications for the general public. She has an unparalleled work ethic and phenomenal organizational skills. She manages to meet deadlines, coordinates the work and contributions of literally hundreds of academic professionals, and coordinates seamlessly with multiple publishers, all the while maintaining a sense of calm and good humor. This book would not have been possible without Beth's superb efforts.

Our research staff at Rippe Health and the University of Central Florida have contributed greatly to our insights about obesity as have our academic colleagues and peers at the University of Central Florida and Tufts Medical School.

Dr. Rippe's executive assistants, Carol Moreau in Massachusetts and Noy Supaswud in Florida, and office assistant, Debra Adamonis, have helped us coordinate and manage our complex professional and personal lives and create the space for the substantial amount of time required to write and edit this book.

Our editors at Taylor & Francis Group/CRC Press, including Randy Brehm, senior editor, and Jennifer Ahringer, production coordinator, have been extraordinarily helpful and accommodating, supervising all phases of production in a professional and efficient manner. A special thanks to Ira Wolinsky, consultant in nutrition at CRC Press, who helped with the initial conceptual phase of this project.

Lastly, we are grateful to Joette Lynch, project editor, Taylor & Francis, Boca Raton, Florida; and Suganthi Thirunavukarasu, project manager, SPi Global, Pondicherry, India, for the production of this book.

Our families continue to support our efforts with unfailing encouragement and love. To them and the many others who have helped in ways too numerous to count, we are deeply grateful.

Editors

James M. Rippe, MD, is a graduate of Harvard College and Harvard Medical School with postgraduate training at Massachusetts General Hospital. He is currently the founder and director of the Rippe Lifestyle Institute (RLI), associate professor of medicine (cardiology) at Tufts University School of Medicine, and professor of biomedical sciences at the University of Central Florida, where he also serves as the chairman of the Center for Lifestyle Medicine.

Over the past 20 years, Dr. Rippe has established and run the largest research organization (RLI) in the world, exploring how daily habits and actions impact short- and long-term health and quality of life. This organization has published hundreds of papers that form the scientific basis for the fields of lifestyle medicine and high-performance health. RLI also conducts numerous studies every year on nutrition and healthy weight management.

A lifelong and avid athlete, Dr. Rippe maintains his personal fitness with a regular walk, jog, swimming, and weight training program. He holds a black belt in karate and is an avid wind surfer, skier, and tennis player. He lives outside of Boston with his wife, television news anchor Stephanie Hart, and their four children, Hart, Jaelin, Devon, and Jamie.

Theodore J. Angelopoulos, PhD, MPH, as a former scholar of Greece's National Secretary of Education, pursued training in exercise physiology and epidemiology at the University of Pittsburgh, Pittsburgh, Pennsylvania. He also completed a three-year postdoctoral training in metabolism at Washington University School of Medicine in St. Louis. He is currently a professor in the Department of Health Professions and director of the Laboratory of Applied Physiology at the University of Central Florida, Orlando, Florida, where he also served as research director of the Center for Lifestyle Medicine (2006–2010).

Dr. Angelopoulos' major research areas include metabolism and physiogenomics. He has developed a strong research partnership with the Exercise and Genetics Collaborative Research Group and has received funds from the National Institutes of Health and from industry sponsors. His work has been published in a number of high-impact journals.

Dr. Angelopoulos played water polo for the Nautical Club of Vouliagmeni in Greece. He maintains his personal fitness with running and weight training and enjoys snow skiing. He lives in Orlando, Florida, with his wife, Kristin, and their two daughters, Zoe and Sophia.

Contributors

Theodore J. Angelopoulos, PhD, MPH
Professor and Director
Laboratory of Applied Physiology
Department of Health Professions
University of Central Florida
Orlando, Florida

Caroline M. Apovian, MD, FACN, FACP
Professor of Medicine
and Pediatrics
Department of Medicine
Boston University School of
Medicine
and
Director
Center for Nutrition and Weight
Management
Boston Medical Center
Boston, Massachusetts

Raymond E. Bourey, MD
Interim Chief
Division of Endocrinology
and
Division of Pulmonary, Critical Care,
and Sleep Medicine
and
Center for Diabetes and Endocrine
Research
University of Toledo College
of Medicine
and
Medical Director
Regional Center for Sleep
Medicine
Toledo, Ohio

George A. Bray, MD
Boyd Professor
Chief, Division of Clinical Obesity
and Metabolism
Pennington Biomedical Research Center
Baton Rouge, Louisiana

Clarence H. Brown, III, MD
President and CEO
MD Anderson Cancer Center Orlando
and
Adjunct Professor
University of Texas MD Anderson
Cancer Center
and
Professor
University of Central Florida College
of Medicine
Orlando, Florida

Johanna Dwyer, DSc
Professor of Medicine and Community
Health
School of Medicine
and
Friedman School of Nutrition Science
and Policy
and
Senior Nutrition Scientist
Jean Mayer Human Nutrition Research
Center on Aging
Tufts University
Boston, Massachusetts

Ioannis G. Fatouros, PhD
Assistant Professor
Department of Physical Education
and Sport Sciences
Democritus University of Thrace
Komotini, Greece

John P. Foreyt, PhD
Professor
Department of Psychiatry
   and Behavioral Science
and
Director
Department of Medicine
Behavioral Medicine Research Center
Baylor College of Medicine
Houston, Texas

Peter W. Grandjean, PhD, FACSM
Associate Professor
Department of Health, Human
   Performance and Recreation
Baylor University
Waco, Texas

**Gregory W. Heath, DHSc, MPH,
   FACSM, FAHA**
Guerry Professor of Health and Human
   Performance
and
Professor of Medicine
College of Medicine
The University of Tennessee
   at Chattanooga
Chattanooga, Tennessee

Athanasios Z. Jamurtas, PhD
Associate Professor in Exercise
   Biochemistry
Department of Physical Education
   and Sports Science
University of Thessaly
and
Centre for Research and Technology,
   Thessaly
Institute of Human Performance
   & Rehabilitation
Trikala, Greece

Craig A. Johnston, PhD
Assistant Professor
Agricultural Research Service
United States Department of Agriculture
Children's Nutrition Research Center
and
Department of Medicine
and
Department of
   Pediatrics-Nutrition
Baylor College of Medicine
Houston, Texas

Nikita Kapur, MS, RD
Nutrition Science
Friedman School of Nutrition
   Science and Policy
Tufts University
Boston, Massachusetts

and

Clinical Nutrition
Department of Nutrition
University of California, Davis
Davis, California

Dong Wook Kim, MD
Instructor of Medicine and
   Pediatrics
Department of Medicine
Boston University School of
   Medicine
Boston, Massachusetts

George D. Kitas, MD, PhD
Consultant Rheumatologist
Department of Rheumatology
Dudley Group of Hospitals
NHS Foundation Trust
Russell's Hall Hospital
Dudley, United Kingdom

Yiannis Koutedakis, PhD
Professor in Exercise Physiology
Department of Physical Education
    and Sports Science
University of Thessaly
and
Centre for Research
    and Technology, Thessaly
Institute of Human Performance
    & Rehabilitation
Trikala, Greece

and

School of Sports, Performing Arts,
    and Leisure
University of Wolverhampton
Walsall, United Kingdom

Charles P. Lambert, PhD
Volunteer Clinical Assistant
    Professor
Division of Endocrinology,
    Diabetes, and Metabolism
Center for Diabetes and Endocrine
    Research
The University of Toledo School of
    Medicine
Toledo, Ohio

Joshua Lowndes, MA
Associate Director of Clinical
    Research
Rippe Lifestyle Institute
Celebration, Florida

Asimina Mitrakou, MD, PhD
Assistant Professor
Department of Clinical Therapeutics
Alexandra Hospital
Athens University Medical School
Athens, Greece

Jennette P. Moreno, PhD
Instructor
Agricultural Research Service
United States Department of
    Agriculture
Children's Nutrition Research Center
and
Department of Pediatrics-Nutrition
Baylor College of Medicine
Houston, Texas

James M. Rippe, MD
Professor of Biomedical Sciences
Burnett School of Biomedical Sciences
University of Central Florida
and
Founder and Director
Rippe Health Evaluation
Orlando, Florida

and

Associate Professor of Medicine
    (Cardiology)
Tufts University School of Medicine
Boston, Massachusetts

and

Founder and Director
Rippe Lifestyle Institute
Shrewsbury, Massachusetts

Richard L. Seip, PhD
Senior Physiologist
Genetics Research Center
Hartford Hospital
Hartford, Connecticut

and

Adjunct Professor
Department of Kinesiology
University of Connecticut
Storrs, Connecticut

Antonios Stavropoulos-Kalinoglou, PhD
Post-Doctoral Research Fellow
Department of Physical Education
   and Sports Science
University of Thessaly
and
Centre for Research and Technology,
   Thessaly
Institute of Human Performance
   & Rehabilitation
Trikala, Greece

Richard R. Suminski, PhD, MPH, FACSM
Associate Professor of Physiology
Department of Physiology
Kansas City University of Medicine
   and Biosciences
Kansas City, Missouri

Alan C. Utter, PhD, MPH, FACSM
Professor
Department of Health, Leisure,
   and Exercise Science
Appalachian State University
Boone, North Carolina

Part I

The Modern Management
of Obesity

1 Preventing and Managing Obesity
The Scope of the Problem

James M. Rippe, MD and
Theodore J. Angelopoulos, PhD, MPH

CONTENTS

Both childhood and adult obesity represent enormous global health problems both for developed and underdeveloped nations [1–4]. Obesity affects both genders and every ethnicity. In the United States, for example, the prevalence for obesity is currently 32.2% in adult men and 35.5% in adult women [5]. By any criteria, the obesity problem has reached epidemic proportions [6].

The most recent estimates from 2010 indicate that 33.8% of adults, over 66 million American adults, are obese (30 million men and 36 million women), while an additional 74 million (42 million men and 32 million women) are overweight. The prevalence of obesity has grown a shocking 40% in the last 30 years [7].

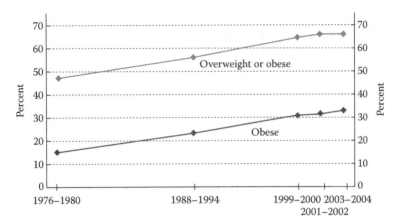

FIGURE 1.1   Trends in adult overweight and obesity ages 20–74 years. *Note*: Age adjusted by the direct method to the year 2000 U.S. Bureau of the Census estimates using the age groups 20–39, 40–59, and 60–74 years. Overweight defined as BMI ≥ 25. Obesity defined as BMI ≥ 30. (Courtesy of The National Center for Health Statistics, Hyattsville, MD.)

As depicted in Figure 1.1, the increase in both obese and overweight individuals has grown in a parallel, fairly linear fashion over the past 30 years.

While the rate of increase in obesity appears to have leveled off over the last 2 years [5], these are nonetheless sobering data that carry enormous health consequences. Moreover, the prevalence of severe obesity (BMI [body mass index] ≥ $40\,kg/m^2$) and very severe obesity (BMI ≥ $50\,kg/m^2$) has grown disproportionately rapidly during this period of time [8].

Nor are these increases and potential adverse health consequences confined only to adults. The prevalence of overweight and obese children in the United States has more than tripled over the last 30 years from approximately 6% to over 18%. As depicted in Figure 1.2, the prevalence of obesity has sharply increased in every childhood age group over the past 30 years [9].

Among American children aged 6–11 years old, an estimated 4.2 million (2.3 million boys and 1.9 million girls) are overweight, while among American adolescents 12–19 years old, 5.7 million (3.1 million boys and 2.6 million girls) are overweight (BMI > 95% percentile weight and gender-specific criteria based on 2000 CDC Growth Charts). As with adults, the percentage of severely obese children has grown even faster. If these same trends continue through the year 2015, 40% of adults and 25% of children will be obese [10]. If these same trends continue through 2030, 86% of the adult population in the United States will be either overweight or obese [10].

The obesity epidemic is truly global. In European countries, obesity ranges from 20% to 30% and is even higher in Australia, South America, and Polynesia. The World Health Organization estimates that there will be over 1.5 billion obese individuals worldwide by 2015 if current trends continue [11].

Obesity not only carries adverse health consequences in and of itself, but it is also associated with multiple other metabolic problems. For example, it is estimated that

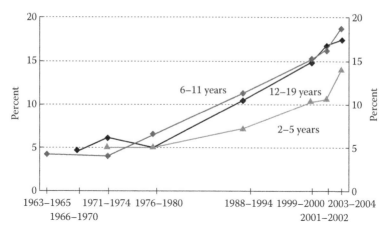

FIGURE 1.2 Trends in childhood overweight. *Note*: Overweight is defined as BMI greater than or equal to gender- and weight-specific 95th percentile from the 2000 CDC Growth Charts. *Source:* National Health Examination Surveys II (ages 6–11) and III (ages 12–17), National Health and Nutrition Examination Surveys I, II, III, and 1999–2004 NCHS, CDC. (Courtesy of National Center for Health Statistics, Hyattsville, MD.)

80%–85% of all type 2 diabetes is related to obesity [12]. Over 50% of all hypertension is associated with obesity [13], and approximately 50% of lipid abnormalities are associated with obesity [14]. It is currently estimated that 25%–35% of the adult population in the United States has the metabolic syndrome [15], which is strongly associated with obesity, while 35%–40% of the adult population has glucose intolerance, which is also associated with obesity [16].

Obesity is not only strongly and independently associated with coronary heart disease (CHD), the leading killer of both men and women in the United States [17], but it is also associated with a number of risk factors for CHD including hypertension, dyslipidemia, diabetes, physical inactivity, and poor nutrition [18–20]. It is estimated that obesity is associated with over 35% of cancers and will become the leading lifestyle-related risk factor associated with cancer within the next decade, surpassing even cigarette smoking [21–23].

In addition to the enormous health toll attributable to obesity, the obesity epidemic is also driving enormous costs. It is estimated that in the United States, for example, obesity may cost as much as $147 billion per year [24]. Roughly one-half of this total is paid by the government (i.e., taxpayers) and the other half is paid by private insurers; thus, taxes and employee premiums (paid by all employees regardless of weight) finance much of the cost of treating obesity or its related conditions [25]. It is estimated that an obese individual costs a health plan 47% more in healthcare expenditures and an overweight individual costs a health plan 16% more than a healthy weight individual [26]. For all of these reasons, multiple stakeholders including governments, employers, taxpayers, and employees all have significant motivation to restrain rising rates of obesity if only for its financial impact.

It is also abundantly clear that obesity is a complicated multifactorial problem with numerous external and internal influences impacting on the obese individual.

There is no question that in the United States and most of the Western world, we live in an obesogenic environment (some have even called it a "toxic" environment for weight gain). In addition to individual choices, there are significant impacts from family, culture, community, government, and world food policies [27]. In addition, there are clearly influences from genetics since some individuals are much more likely to gain weight than others and some ethnic groups (e.g., Black and Hispanic women) are more affected than others [28].

The recognition that obesity is an urgent national imperative has been articulated by numerous evidence-based documents. Perhaps most prominent of these are the Dietary Guidelines for Americans 2010 [29], which characterizes obesity as the leading nutritional health problem facing our country. The goal of limiting obesity to no more than 15% of the adult population in the United States, which was articulated in the Healthy People 2010 document [30], can now be seen, in retrospect, as wishful thinking. The United States is moving away from this goal rather than toward it. The same 15% goal for obesity prevalence has been incorporated in the Healthy People 2020 Guidelines [31].

Numerous private and governmental initiatives have been announced in an attempt to reduce the health impact of childhood obesity. For example, First Lady Michelle Obama's "Let's Move" campaign established the goal of ending childhood obesity within the next generation [32]. Other efforts such as the collaboration between the William J. Clinton Foundation and numerous health-care and commercial organizations in "The Partnership for a Healthy America" [33] have articulated similar goals and an increasing sense of urgency.

For all of these reasons, it is no longer a viable option for health-care professionals to stay on the sidelines both as individual practitioners and as community leaders when it comes to the urgent problem of both adult and childhood obesity. It is for this reason that we have assembled a world-class group of experts as contributors to this book to offer state-of-the-art knowledge, clinical information, and recommendations to all health-care providers in the areas of preventing and managing obesity. This is both our goal and the mission of this book.

BURDEN OF OVERWEIGHT AND OBESITY IN THE UNITED STATES

ADULTS

As will be utilized throughout this book, overweight and obesity are generally defined using BMI, which is a measure of weight related to height that is closely correlated with total body fat content. The National Heart, Lung, and Blood Institute defines healthy weight for adults as a BMI of $19–24.9\,kg/m^2$, overweight as a BMI of $25–29.9\,kg/m^2$, obesity $\geq 30\,kg/m^2$, and extreme obesity $\geq 40\,kg/m^2$ [34]. Body fat distribution also impacts on risk of chronic disease [35–38], and both waist circumference [35–38] and waist to hip ratio are added in some guidelines.

As a practical matter, however, most research linking weight to health relies on BMI. As depicted in Figure 1.1, there has been a steady and significant increase in the overweight and obese population in the United States over the last 30 years. The combined prevalence of overweight and obesity has increased from

47.4% to 66%—a relative increase of 39.2% since 1980 [39]. Of note, most of this increase is due to increases in the prevalence of obesity (BMI ≥ 30) while only minor increases have occurred in the prevalence of overweight (BMI 25–29.9). The prevalence of obesity increased from 15.1% to 32.1% (a relative increase of over 100%) in individuals between 20 and 74 years of age when comparing the 1976–1980 NHANES and the 2001–2004 NHANES data.

CHILDREN AND ADOLESCENTS

Several different criteria are utilized for the term "overweight" or "obese" for children and adolescents up to the age of 20. The Centers for Disease Control and Prevention (CDC) uses the term "overweight" for children and adolescents with BMI at or above the 95th percentile for sex-specific BMI for age values from the 2000 CDC Growth Charts [40]. The term "at risk" of overweight is utilized by the CDC for children and adolescents who are between a BMI of 85th and 95th percentiles. Other organizations such as the American Medical Association have recommended that the terminology be changed so that children and adolescents who are over the 85th percentile for BMI values be classified as "overweight" and over the 95th percentile classified as "obese" [41].

As depicted in Figure 1.2, the percentage of children who are "overweight" by the current CDC criteria has more than tripled since 1970 [9]. For children aged 6–11, the percentage of overweight increased from 4.2% to 18.8% (348% relative increase between 1963–1965 and 2003–2004). During the same period of time, percentages of those considered overweight, who are adolescents between the ages of 12 and 19 years of age, rose from 4.6% to 17.4% (278% relative increase) [39].

HEALTH EFFECTS OF OBESITY

ROLE OF ADIPOCYTES

It used to be thought that adipocytes were primarily storage sites for excess fat; however, research over the past two decades has clarified that adipocytes are in fact highly complicated inflammatory endocrine and metabolic cells. In a sense, adipose tissue thus serves as a complicated endocrine organ and a potent source of inflammatory molecules such as IL-6, tumor necrosis factor-α (TNF α), and many others [42–45]. The complex properties of adipocytes may underlie the strong relationship between obesity and chronic metabolic conditions such as CHD, diabetes, and the metabolic syndrome. These complex metabolic and inflammatory properties seem to be particularly prominent in adipocytes located in the abdominal region [35–38].

HEALTH EFFECTS IN ADULTS

As will be described in detail in numerous chapters throughout this book, the adverse health consequences of obesity are diverse and profound. Obesity is strongly associated with diabetes (see Chapter 13), the metabolic syndrome (see Chapter 14), CHD (see Chapter 12), some cancers (see Chapter 15), and osteoarthritis (see Chapter 16).

This list of adverse health consequences of obesity is by no means exhaustive. A more complete listing is found in Table 1.1.

The negative health consequences of obesity are so profound that it has been argued that, unless we can control the twin epidemics of obesity and diabetes, mortality from these two adverse health conditions could potentially wipe out all of the other gains in prevention in cardiovascular disease over the past 20 years [46]. According to an

TABLE 1.1

Medical Conditions Associated with Obesity

Metabolic Conditions
  Type 2 diabetes
  Metabolic syndrome
  Glucose intolerance
  Cardiovascular disease
  CHD
  Stroke
  Heart failure
  Deep venous thrombosis

CHD Risk Factors
  Dyslipidemia
  Hypertension
  Inflammation
  Hypercoagulability

Pulmonary Diseases
  Obstructive sleep apnea
  Hypoventilation syndrome
  Asthma

Cancers
  Colorectal
  Esophageal
  Endometrial
  Breast (postmenopausal)
  Kidney

Gastrointestinal Diseases
  Nonalcoholic fatty liver disease
  Gallstones cholecystitis
  Gastroesophageal reflux

Other Conditions
  Gout
  Kidney stones
  Osteoarthritis
  Psychological disorders
  Fertility and pregnancy complications
  Erectile dysfunction

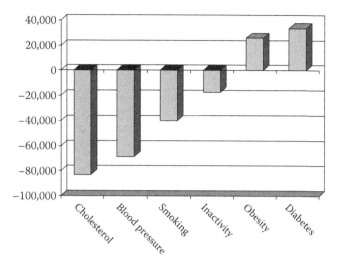

FIGURE 1.3 From 1980 to 2000, an estimated 149,635 fewer deaths occurred from CHD from decreased prevalence of some major risk factors and an estimated 59,370 more deaths from higher rates of two risk factors. (From Ford, E.S. et al., *N. Engl. J. Med.*, 256, 2388, July 2007.)

article by Ford et al., an estimated 149,635 fewer deaths from CVD occurred between 1980 and 2000 as a result of decreased prevalence of some major risk factors [47]. An estimated 59,370 more deaths, however, occurred from the higher rates of obesity and diabetes. These data are depicted graphically in Figure 1.3.

HEALTH EFFECTS IN CHILDREN

While the manifestations of many metabolic diseases occur in middle age or later years, increasing research now supports that events or conditions that occur in childhood [48] or even before birth [49] may significantly influence the risk of obesity, diabetes, and CHD. In addition, excess weight during childhood not only increases chronic disease morbidity and adverse psychosocial effects but also increases the risk of being obese as an adult [48]. It is now estimated that over half of new cases of diabetes found in children are type 2 diabetes, which used to be designed as "adult onset diabetes" but now is increasingly being found in the pediatric population [50]. Furthermore, obesity in adolescent years carries a significant increased risk of severe obesity in adulthood [51].

SEARCHING FOR SOLUTIONS

SOCIOECONOMIC FRAMEWORK

Given the complexity of interacting underlying causes for the obesity epidemic, it is doubtful that one single solution will resolve this problem. A comprehensive approach involving multiple levels of influencers and multiple areas of intervention appears most appropriate. One framework for approaching obesity and weight management has been proposed by the Dietary Guidelines Advisory Committee. Figure 1.4 depicts the socioeconomic framework offered by the DGAC for the Dietary Guidelines for

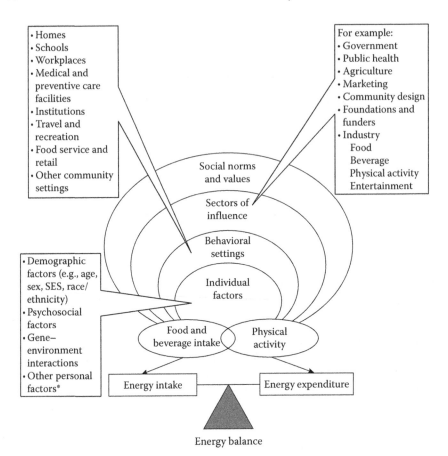

- Homes
- Schools
- Workplaces
- Medical and preventive care facilities
- Institutions
- Travel and recreation
- Food service and retail
- Other community settings

For example:
- Government
- Public health
- Agriculture
- Marketing
- Community design
- Foundations and funders
- Industry
  Food
  Beverage
  Physical activity
  Entertainment

- Demographic factors (e.g., age, sex, SES, race/ethnicity)
- Psychosocial factors
- Gene–environment interactions
- Other personal factors*

Social norms and values

Sectors of influence

Behavioral settings

Individual factors

Food and beverage intake   Physical activity

Energy intake   Energy expenditure

Energy balance

FIGURE 1.4 The socioeconomic framework impacting on energy balance. *Note*: Other relevant factors that influence obesity prevention interventions are culture and acculturation; biobehavioral interactions; and social, political, and historical contexts. (From Centers of Disease Control and Prevention, Division of Nutrition, Physical Activity, and Obesity, *State Nutrition, Physical Activity and Obesity Program: Technical Assistance Manual*, January 2008, available at: http://www.cdc.gov/obesity/downloads/TA_Manual_1_31_08.pdf-pg 41 of the document, accessed: August 31, 2011.)

Americans 2010 [52]. This framework stresses that the issues of maintaining proper energy balance are complex and factors that influence this issue are multiple and interconnected. While other frameworks have also been put forth, this one seems particularly appropriate for providing structure for potential comprehensive interventions for weight loss and weight management.

FOOD ENVIRONMENT

It will be impossible to solve the global obesity problem without a comprehensive approach to the modern food environment. For example, in the United States, the average caloric consumption has increased dramatically over the past 40 years.

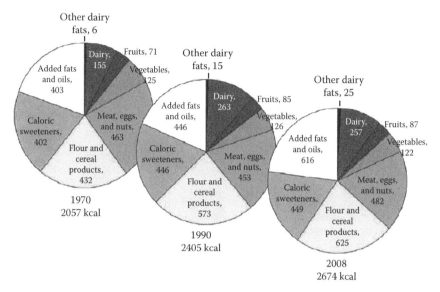

FIGURE 1.5 Average daily per capita calories from the U.S. food availability in 1970, 1990, and 2008, adjusted for spoilage and other waste. (From ERS Food Availability (Per Capita) Data System, http://www.ers.usda.gov/Data/FoodConsumption/.)

As depicted in Figure 1.5, the average daily caloric consumption in the United States has increased from 2057 kcal in 1970 to 2674 kcal in 2008 [53].

While there have been significant increases in virtually every category of food, the increases are particularly prominent in the areas of added fats and oils, flour, and cereal products [53].

The increase over 600 kcal daily on average for every man, woman, and child in the United States over the past 40 years constitutes almost the equivalent of an extra meal per day. It has been argued by Swinburne [54] and others that increased caloric consumption in the United States during the past four decades is more than sufficient to explain the U.S. epidemic of obesity. Other investigators, however, have disputed this notion and argue that issues related to diminished physical activity and other aspects of the environment also have made significant contributions to the obesity epidemic [55,56].

What is abundantly clear is that individuals in the United States are not following the guidance from various Dietary Guidelines. As Figure 1.6 shows, the American population is falling far short when it comes to vegetable, dairy, and fruit consumption compared to MyPyramid recommendations [57].

The number of meal occasions and the increase in portion sizes have also been argued to play significant roles in the obesity epidemic in the United States [58]. While the number of meal occasions has appeared to be stable over the last 25 years [59], the number of calories consumed in snacking has increased by approximately 25% during this period of time [58].

While there is some disagreement as to whether or not snacking per se constitutes a significant component of weight gain in the American population [58–61],

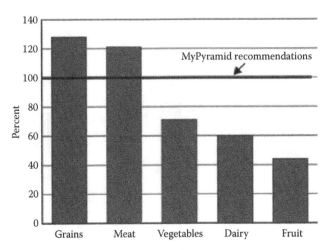

FIGURE 1.6 The loss-adjusted per capita food availability in comparison to MyPyramid recommendations for a 2000 calorie diet. Availability of grains (128%) and meat (121%) was above recommendations, while availability of vegetables (71%), dairy (60%), and fruit (44%) was below recommendations. *Note*: Based on a 2000 cal diet. (From USDA, Economic Research Service, Food Availability (Per Capita) Data System. Available at http://www.ers.usda.gov/AmberWaves/March10/PDF/TrackingACentury.pdf.)

TABLE 1.2
Changes over Time in the Average Portion Size of Selected Food Items Sold in the U.S. Marketplace

	Portion Size (Year)	Portion Size (Year)	Percent Increase
Beer, can	12 oz (1936)	8–24 oz (2002)	33%–100%
Beer, bottle	7 oz (1976)	7–40 oz (2002)	0%–471%
Chocolate bar, milk chocolate	0.6 oz (1908)	1.6–8 oz (2002)	167%–1233%
French fries	2.4 oz (1955)	2.4–7.1 oz (2002)	0%–196%
Hamburger	3.9 oz (1954)	4.4–12.6 oz (2002)	13%–223%
Soda, fountain	7 oz (1955)	12–42 oz (2002)	71%–500%
Soda, bottle, and can	6.5 oz (1916)	8–34 oz (2002)	23%–423%

Source: Report of the DGAC on the Dietary Guidelines for Americans, 2010; Young, L.R. and Nestle, M., *J. Am. Diet. Assoc.*, 103, 231, 2003.

increases in portion size appear to have made a significant contribution to the overall increase in caloric consumption. As depicted in Table 1.2, portion sizes of common foods sold in the United States have skyrocketed between 100% and 1000% over the past 50 years [62].

It is apparent from these data that the food environment does not support Americans in consuming a healthy eating pattern. Solutions to this issue, however, will require the participation of many stakeholders in the food system including farmers, the commercial food industry, supermarkets, and individuals themselves.

Consumer education will play a role, but comprehensive solutions will require changes at all levels in the overall food system.

PHYSICAL ACTIVITY

Unfortunately, the U.S. population has become an inactive one. The Dietary Guidelines for Americans 2010 [29] concluded that there was "strong, consistent evidence that physically active people are at reduced risk for becoming overweight or obese." Beyond the benefits in prevention of obesity and long-term weight maintenance, multiple other benefits accrue to physically active people. These benefits have been outlined in considerable detail in the evidence-based Physical Activity Guidelines for Americans 2008 [63].

GENETICS

There is no question that genetics plays an important role in the modern obesity epidemic. The so-called thrifty gene hypothesis posits that over many millennia those human beings survived who had a genetic makeup that allowed them to continue to survive during periods of low food supplies. In the modern food environment, however, this genetic makeup has become maladaptive since it may contribute to individuals storing excess calories as fat in a world where the food supply is abundant.

Twin studies and other lines of evidence suggest that there is a significant genetic component concerning why some individuals have more problems with weight gain than others. It has been estimated that up to 40% of obesity in both children and adults results from genetic factors [28,49,64]. Of course, this still leaves a large component of weight gain and obesity attributed to lifestyle habits and practices, making it all the more important that individuals who are susceptible to weight gain maintain particular vigilance over food and exercise choices.

Exploration of specific areas of the genome controlling food intake, physical activity, and weight gain is under active investigation. While some progress has been made in this area locating certain genes associated with obesity and type 2 diabetes [28], this work is far from ready for clinical application. Nonetheless, researchers anticipate a time when genetic research will yield important answers that will help make issues of weight control more individualized and precise.

CLOSING THE ENERGY GAP

A provocative article by Blackburn et al. [65] has suggested that health-care professionals should focus first on individuals with extreme obesity (BMI of $\geq 40 \, kg/m^2$) since this segment of the obese population is increasing at rates faster than any other class of obesity in the United States. These investigators have suggested that a useful construct in guiding interventions for individuals with severe obesity is the "energy gap."

By their estimates, an energy gap of approximately 400 kcal per day now exists, which was not present in the 1970s. These investigators argue that closing this excess energy gap should be the highest priority for treating individuals with severe obesity.

While surgery for extreme obesity has been demonstrated to be effective, it will certainly not be a solution for the large number and rapidly growing population of individuals with severe obesity. Blackburn et al. suggest a lifestyle approach involving improved dietary composition, calorie restriction, and increasing physical activity as key components of a synergistic lifestyle intervention to close this energy gap.

SMALL STEP APPROACH

A recent special task force report from the American Society of Nutrition has argued that current initiatives designed to combat obesity have not succeeded in reversing the obesity epidemic. This panel presented an alternative strategy of not focusing on weight loss but promoting small changes in physical activity and nutrition to initially prevent further weight gain [66]. Such approaches are supported by a variety of lines of evidence and appear to hold some promise to help combat the obesity epidemic.

NEED FOR HEALTH-CARE PROFESSIONAL INVOLVEMENT

Given the severity of the worldwide obesity epidemic and its potential adverse health consequences, it is critically important that health-care professionals become actively involved and knowledgeable in multiple aspects of this issue. This is the basic underlying premise for our book, *Obesity: Prevention and Treatment*. Our goal is to provide modern understandings of obesity as well as specific tools and practical applications for clinicians to use in their daily practices.

Our approach on the topic of preventing and treating obesity is divided into two major parts as follows:

PART I: THE MODERN MANAGEMENT OF OBESITY

In the first part of the book, we provide a summary of the modern understandings of obesity. Chapter 2 delves into the underlying pathophysiology of obesity including its genetics. This chapter summarizes modern understandings of the complex pathophysiology of obesity and provides the fundamentals of a science-based approach to guide its treatment.

Chapter 3 emphasizes that this is a worldwide problem that affects both genders and all ethnic groups. Chapter 4 provides an excellent framework for the individual clinician to identify, evaluate, and treat the overweight or obese individual.

The next three chapters in this part focus on specific management aspects of great relevance to clinicians treating obese individuals. Chapter 5 provides clinically oriented direction for accessing nutritional aspects of obesity. This chapter also provides the tools for assessing patients' nutritional habits and evaluates current popular diet books and programs.

Chapter 6 provides a framework for considering both exercise testing and management of obese individuals. This chapter focuses on developing a clear understanding for the purpose of both exercise testing and exercise prescription for each patient and makes recommendations based on the risk and benefits of exercise for obese individuals.

Chapter 7 reminds us that behavioral management is fundamental to all clinical programs designed to manage obesity.

Chapter 8 provides guidance for clinicians on the assessment of obesity in children as well as behavioral approaches to this issue involving both the child and the family.

Extensive Chapters 9 and 10 provide state-of-the-art information on these treatment modalities and their indications. The drug treatment chapter addresses not only on currently available agents but also work in progress to develop additional pharmaceutical agents to treat obesity. Chapter 10 provides a summary of available procedures and their indications and potential complications.

The first part of the book concludes with Chapter 11. This chapter reminds us that obesity is not just a problem for the individual but will require multiple approaches at many different levels including public policy.

PART II: OBESITY AND SPECIFIC MEDICAL CONDITIONS

The second part of our book focuses on the relationship with obesity and specific medical conditions. While not all medical conditions are covered, the chapters in this part are devoted to the key diseases and their metabolic links to obesity with detailed discussions and specific clinical recommendations.

The part opens with Chapter 12. The links between obesity and heart disease are multiple and profound. Not only does obesity represent a significant, independent risk factor for heart disease, but it is also linked to multiple other risk factors for heart disease. Moreover, it may be difficult to assess heart disease in obese patients. All of these issues are discussed in detail in this chapter.

Chapter 13 delineates the significant linkages between these two entities including their pathophysiology and treatment. Chapter 14 sorts through the complexities related to the metabolic syndrome and its significant relationship to obesity. Chapter 15 delves into the relationship between obesity and certain forms of cancer and reminds us that obesity is increasingly associated as an underlying cause of cancer.

Chapter 16 provides an extensive discussion of the linkages between obesity and osteoarthritis. This chapter also contains a part on the relationship of obesity to rheumatoid arthritis and provides clinical guidance for exercise and nutritional prescriptions for obese individuals with arthritis.

Chapter 17 summarizes the emerging evidence that fat deposition in obese individuals occurs not only in subcutaneous tissues but also in the liver, muscle, and other areas of the body, creating a diverse set of clinical challenges.

SUMMARY/CONCLUSIONS

There is no longer any serious doubt that obesity represents one of the great modern health challenges. Health-care professionals no longer have the luxury of sitting on the sidelines and either ignoring obesity or treating its multiple manifestations individually. It is time for us to attack the problem of obesity as an urgent priority. With this in mind, it is essential that clinicians understand the modern evidence and techniques both for preventing and managing obesity. This is the goal, challenge, and vision of *Obesity: Prevention and Treatment.*

REFERENCES

1. WHO/FAO. Expert consultation on diet, nutrition and the prevention of chronic diseases: Report of the joint WHO/FAO expert consultation. Geneva, Switzerland: World Health Organization, 2003.
2. Monteiro CA, Moura EC, Conde WL, Popkin BM. Socioeconomic status and obesity in adult populations of developing countries: A review. *Bull World Health Organ* 2004;82:940–946.
3. Monteiro CA, Conde WL, Lu B, Popkin BM. Obesity and inequities in health in the developing world. *Int J Obes Relat Metab Disord* 2004;28:1181–1186.
4. Popkin BM. Global nutrition dynamics: The world is shifting rapidly toward a diet linked with noncommunicable diseases. *Am J Clin Nutr* 2006;84:289–298.
5. Flegal KM, Carroll MD, Ogden CL, Curtin LR. Prevalence and trends in obesity among US adults, 1999–2008. *JAMA* 2010;303(3):235–241.
6. Rosamond W, Flegal K, Friday G, Furie K, Go A, Greenlund K, Haase N et al., American Heart Association Statistics Committee and Stroke Statistics Subcommittee. Heart disease and stroke statistics–2007 update: A report from the American Heart Association Statistics Committee and Stroke Statistics Subcommittee. *Circulation* 2007;115:e69–e171.
7. Center for Disease Control and Prevention (CDC). Overweight and Obesity: US Obesity Trends. Atlanta, GA: U.S. Department of Health and Human Services, Centers for Disease Control and Prevention, 2010. Available at: http://www.cdc.gov/obesity/data/trends.html. Accessed: September 19, 2011.
8. Sturm R. Increases in morbid obesity in the USA: 2000–2005. *Public Health* 2007;121:492–496.
9. National Center for Health Statistics. Available at: http://www.cdc.gov/nchs/products/pubs/pubd/hestats/overweight/overwght_child_03.htm. Accessed: August 30, 2011.
10. Wang Y, Beydoun MA. The obesity epidemic in the United States—Gender, age, socioeconomic, racial/ethnic, and geographic characteristics: A systematic review and meta-regression analysis. *Epidemiol Rev* 2007;29:6–28.
11. World Health Organization. *Risk Factor Projects. Overweight and Obesity.* 2005. Available at: http://www.who.int/chp/chronic_disease_report/part2_ch1/en/index16.html. Accessed: August 30, 2011.
12. Kelley DE. Managing obesity as first-line therapy for diabetes mellitus. *Nutr Clin Care* 1998;1(Suppl 1):38–43.
13. Heyka R. Obesity and hypertension. *Nutr Clin Care* 1998;1:30–37.
14. Ebbeling CB, Ockene IS. Obesity and dyslipidemia. *Nutr Clin Care* 1998;1:15–29.
15. Ford ES, Giles WH, Dietz WH. Prevalence of the metabolic syndrome among US adults: Findings from the third National Health and Nutrition Examination Survey. *JAMA* 2002;287(3):356–359.
16. Centers for Disease Control and Prevention. Prevalence of diabetes and impaired fasting glucose in adults—United States, 1999–2000. *MMWR Morb Mortal Wkly Rep* 2003;52:833–837.
17. Poirier P, Giles TD, Bray GA, Hong Y, Stern JS, Pi-Sunyer FX, Eckel RH. Obesity and cardiovascular disease: Pathophysiology, evaluation, and effect of weight loss. *Circulation* 2006;113:898–918.
18. Wilson PW, D'Agostino RB, Sullivan L, Parise H, Kannel WB. Overweight and obesity as determinants of cardiovascular risk: The Framingham experience. *Arch Intern Med* 2002;162:1867–1872.
19. Manson JE, Colditz GA, Stampfer MJ, Willett WC, Rosner B, Monson RR, Speizer FE, Hennekens CH. A prospective study of obesity and risk of coronary heart disease in women. *N Engl J Med* 1990;322:882–889.

20. Hubert HB, Feinleib M, McNamara PM, Castelli WP. Obesity as an independent risk factor for cardiovascular disease: A 26-year follow-up of participants in the Framingham Heart Study. *Circulation* 1983;67:968–977.
21. Polednak AP. Estimating the number of U.S. incident cancers attributable to obesity and the impact on temporal trends in incidence rates for obesity-related cancers. *Cancer Detect Prev* 2008;32:190–199.
22. Calle EE, Thun MJ. Obesity and cancer review. *Oncogene* 2004;23:6365–6378.
23. Vainio H, Kaaks R, Bianchini F. Weight control and physical activity in cancer prevention: International evaluation of the evidence. Review. *Eur J Cancer Prev* 2002;11(Suppl 2):94–100.
24. Finkelstein EA, Trogdon JG, Cohen JW, Dietz W. Annual medical spending attributable to obesity: Payer- and service-specific estimates. *Health Aff* 2009;28:w822–w831.
25. Finkelstein EA, Strombotne KL. The economics of obesity. *Am J Clin Nutr* 2010;91(Suppl):1520S–1524S.
26. Washington Business Group on Health (now National Business Group on Health). *Best Practices and Strategies for Weight Management: A Toolkit for Large Employers.* June 2003.
27. Report of the DGAC on the Dietary Guidelines for Americans, 2010. Available at: www.cnpp.usda.gov. Accessed: September 26, 2011.
28. McCarthy MI. Genomics, type 2 diabetes, and obesity. *N Engl J Med* 2010;363:24.
29. U.S. Department of Agriculture and U.S. Department of Health and Human Services. *Dietary Guidelines for Americans, 2010.* 7th edn., Washington, DC: U.S. Government Printing Office, December 2010.
30. Healthy People 2010. U.S. Department of Health and Human Services 200 Independence Avenue, S.W., Washington, DC 20201.
31. Healthy People 2020. U.S. Department of Health and Human Services 200 Independence Avenue, S.W., Washington, DC 20201.
32. Michelle Obama—Let's Move. Available at: http://www.letsmove.gov. Accessed: August 24, 2011.
33. Partnerships for a Healthy America. Available at: http://www.ahealthieramerica.org. Accessed: August 24, 2011.
34. National Institutes of Health. Clinical guidelines on the identification, evaluation, and treatment of overweight and obesity in adults—The evidence report. *Obes Res* 1998;6t(Suppl 2):51S–209S.
35. Despres JP. Dyslipidaemia and obesity. *Baillieres Clin Endocrinol Metab* 1994;8:629–660.
36. Despres JP. Abdominal obesity as important component of insulin-resistance syndrome. *Nutrition* 1993;4:452–459.
37. Prineas R, Folsom A, Kayes S. Central adiposity and increased risk of coronary artery mortality in older women. *Ann Epidemiol* 1993;3:35–41.
38. Terry R, Page W, Haskell W. Waist/hip ratio, body mass index and premature cardiovascular mortality in US Army veterans during a 23 year follow up study. *Int J Obes* 1992;16:417–423.
39. National Center for Health Statistics. Hyattsville, MD: Chartbook on Trends in the Health of Americans; 2006. Available at http://www.cdc.gov/nchs/data/hus/hus06.pdf. Accessed: August 24, 2011.
40. Kuczmarski RJ, Ogden CL, Grummer-Strawn LM, Flegal KM, Guo SS, Wei R, Mei Z, Curtin LR, Roche AF, Johnson CL. CDC growth charts: United States. *Adv Data* 2000;314:1–27.
41. Barlow SE. Expert committee recommendations regarding the prevention, assessment, and treatment of child and adolescent overweight and obesity (summary report). *Pediatrics* 2007;210(Suppl 4):S164–S192.

42. Wajchenberg BL. Subcutaneous and visceral adipose tissue: Their relation to the metabolic syndrome. *Endocr Rev* 2000;21:697–738.
43. Hotamisligil GS, Arner P, Caro JF, Atkinson RL, Spiegelman BM. Increased adipose tissue expression of tumor necrosis factor-alpha in human obesity and insulin resistance. *J Clin Invest* 1995;95:2409–2415.
44. Lundgren CH, Brown SL, Nordt TK, Sobel BE, Fujii S. Elaboration of type-1 plasminogen activator inhibitor from adipocytes: A potential pathogenetic link between obesity and cardiovascular disease. *Circulation* 1996;93:106–110.
45. Yudkin JS, Stehouwer CD, Emeis JJ, Coppack SW. C-reactive protein in healthy subjects: Associations with obesity, insulin resistance, and endothelial dysfunction: A potential role for cytokines originating from adipose tissue? *Arterioscler Thromb Vasc Biol* 1999;19:972–978.
46. William J. Clinton Foundation. Available at: http://www.clintonfoundation.org/. Accessed: August 24, 2011.
47. Ford ES, Ajani UA, Croft JB, Critchley JA, Labarthe DR, Kottke TE, Giles WH, Capewell S. Explaining the decrease in US deaths from coronary disease, 1980–2000. *N Engl J Med* 2007;256:2388–2398.
48. Biro FM, Wien M. Childhood obesity and adult morbidities. *Am J Clin Nutr* 2010;91:1499S–1505S.
49. Wardle J, Carnell S, Haworth C, Plomin R. Evidence for a strong genetic influence on childhood adiposity despite the force of the obesogenic environment. *Am J Clin Nutr* 2008;87:398–404.
50. Dietz WH, Robinson TN. Overweight children and adolescents. *N Engl J Med* 2005;352:2100–2109.
51. Daniels SR, Arnett DK, Eckel RH, Gidding SS, Hayman LL, Kumanyika S, Robinson TN, Scott BJ, St. Jeor S, Williams CL. AHA scientific statement, overweight in children and adolescents: Pathophysiology, consequences, prevention, and treatment. *Circulation* 2005;111:1999–2012.
52. Centers of Disease Control and Prevention. Division of Nutrition, Physical Activity, and Obesity. *State Nutrition, Physical Activity and Obesity Program: Technical Assistance Manual.* January 2008. Available at: http://www.cdc/gov/obesity/downloads/ TA_Manual_1_31_08.pdf—pg 36 of the document. Accessed: August 31, 2011.
53. ERS Food Availability (per capita) Data System. Available at: http://www.ers.usda.gov/ Data/FoodConsumption/. Accessed: September 26, 2011.
54. Swinburne B, Sacks G, Ravussin E. Increased food energy supply is more than sufficient to explain the US epidemic of obesity. *Am J Clin Nutr* 2009;90:1453–1456.
55. Booth FW, Gordon SE, Carlson CJ, Hamilton MT. Waging war on modern chronic disease: Primary prevention through exercise biology. *J Appl Physiol* 2000;88:774–787.
56. Booth FW, Laye MJ, Lees SJ. Rector RS, Thyfault JP. Reduced physical activity and risk of chronic disease: The biology behind the consequences. *Eur J Appl Physiol* 2008:102:381–390.
57. U.S. Department of Agriculture. Center for Nutrition Policy and Promotion. Available at: http://www.mypyramid.gov/ Accessed: September 26, 2011.
58. Kant AK, Graubard BI. Secular trends in patterns of self-reported food consumption of adult Americans: NHANES 1971–1975 to NHANES 1999–2002. *Am J Clin Nutr* 2006;84(5):1215–1223.
59. Piernas C, Popkin BM. Snacking increased among US adults between 1977 and 2006. *Am J Nutr* 2010;140:325–332.
60. Cleland VJ, Schmidt MD, Dwyer T, Venn AJ. Television viewing and abdominal obesity in young adults: Is the association mediated by food and beverage consumption during viewing time or reduced leisure-time physical activity? *Am J Clin Nutr* 2008;87:1148–1155.

61. Keast DR, Nicklas T, O'Neil C. Snacking is associated with reduced risk of over-weight and reduced abdominal obesity in adolescents: National Health and Nutrition Examination Survey (NHANES) 1999–2000. *Am J Clin Nutr* 2010;92:428–435.

62. Young LR, Nestle M. Expanding portion sizes in the US marketplace: Implications for nutrition counseling. *J Am Diet Assoc* 2003;103:231–234.

63. Physical Activity Guidelines for Americans 2008. Washington, DC: U.S. Department of Health and Human Services. Available at: www.hss.gov. Accessed: September 26, 2011.

64. Bouchard C. Childhood obesity: Are genetic differences involved? *Am J Clin Nutr* 2009;89:1494S–1501S.

65. Blackburn G, Wollner S, Heymsfield SB. Lifestyle interventions for the treatment of class III obesity: A primary target for nutrition medicine in the obesity epidemic. *Am J Clin Nutr* 2010;91:289–292.

66. Hill JO. Can a small-changes approach help address the obesity epidemic? A report of the joint task force of the American Society for Nutrition, Institute of Food Technologists, and International food Information Council. *Am J Clin Nutr* 2009;89:477–484.

2 Pathophysiology of Obesity

Theodore J. Angelopoulos, PhD, MPH

CONTENTS

INTRODUCTION

During the past 20 years, there has been a dramatic increase in obesity in developed countries. This increasing prevalence of obesity in developed countries has become a very important public health issue. The World Health Organization (WHO) estimates that there are more than 1.7 billion overweight adults in the world, with one-fifth of them meeting the definition of being clinically obese [1]. The prevalence of obesity was 32.2% among adult men and 35.5% among adult women in 2007–2008 [2]. Obesity is the most prevalent nutritional problem and plays a significant role in the pathogenesis of hypertension, diabetes mellitus (type 2 DM), heart disease, and some forms of cancer. It is associated with a moderate increase in all-cause mortality and contributes to morbidity and social disadvantage [3,4].

Adipose tissue is one of the largest organs in the body. Obesity generally is defined as an excess and abnormal accumulation of adipose tissue. Defining "excess," however, is not a simple task since adiposity is a continuous trait not marked by clear cut-offs into normal and abnormal. Typically, people classified as obese are 15%–20% or 20%–25% heavier than average for men and women, respectively. Body composition measurements are seminal in obesity from both research and clinical perspective. Examples of reliable methodologies in obtaining accurate measurements of total body fat are densitometry, bioelectrical impedance, dual x-ray absorptiometry, magnetic resonance imaging, and computed tomography. Although the methodology is advancing rapidly, one challenge, however, is that it is difficult to measure body fat directly. Consequently, obesity often is defined as excess body weight rather than as excess fat. In epidemiological studies, body mass index (BMI) calculated as weight in kilograms divided by height in meters squared is used to express weight adjusted for height.

Although the quantity of excess body fat is critical in the definition of obesity, its distribution within the body is clinically very important. For example, excess fat in the abdomen (central obesity) is associated with increased risk of developing heart disease, diabetes, breast cancer, and premature death [5,6]. The purpose of this chapter is to briefly review energy balance, examine the metabolic predictors of weight gain, discuss the role of adipokines, and explore the relative contributions of genetics and environment to the development of obesity.

ENERGY BALANCE

Obesity is caused by perturbations of the balance between food intake and energy expenditure, which is regulated by a complex physiological system that requires the integration of several peripheral signals and central coordination in the brain. Obesity is a multifactorial disease and involves the interaction of environmental and genetic factors resulting in a disorder of energy balance. Of particular importance, energy balance is usually tightly regulated. For example, even in societies where obesity is very prevalent, the average weight gain is only about 2.2 lb per year—reflecting an energy excess of about 20 kcal per day or less than 1% of daily energy expenditure [7].

Humans have a very complex and sophisticated system for regulating energy balance and fat stored in adipocytes. For example, changes in energy balance sufficient to alter body fat stores trigger a compensatory change in energy intake and energy expenditure that eventually returns fat stores to their preset level [8]. Obesity, as mentioned earlier, develops when energy intake exceeds energy output, leading to accumulation of adipose tissue. Energy balance is maintained through the control of appetite and metabolism. Appetite regulation is a very complex process affected by the integration of peripheral and central signals. In the gastrointestinal tract, orexin, ghrelin, and decreasing concentrations of macronutrients (i.e., glucose, fatty acids, and amino acids) stimulate hunger [9]. Following a meal, gastric and duodenal distension produce the feeling of satiety, aided by the release of gastrointestinal peptides such as cholecystokinin (CCK), glucagon-like peptide 1 (GLP-1), and peptide YY 3-36 [9]. Food intake is under short- and long-term control. In the short term, hunger develops in response to decreased circulating levels of glucose, fatty acids, and amino acids. Long-term signals depend on the magnitude of energy stores and include the adipose tissue hormone leptin.

The discovery of the obese (ob) gene and its product greatly enhanced our understanding of the physiological systems regulating energy balance [10]. The ob gene that is located on chromosome 7 encodes for a hormone called leptin (from the Greek leptos, meaning thin), which is secreted by adipocytes in proportion to the level of body adipose mass. Leptin plays a role in regulating energy intake and energy expenditure including appetite and metabolism [11]. Specifically, it inhibits pathways that stimulate food intake by inhibiting orexins such as melanin-concentrating hormone (MCH) in the paraventricular nucleus, neuropeptide Y (NPY), and agouti-related protein (AgRP) in the arcuate [9]. Leptin acts on receptors in the hypothalamus, inhibiting appetite by counteracting the effects of NPY. NPY is a potent feeding stimulant secreted by cells in the gut and in the hypothalamus. In the hypothalamus, NPY affects energy balance by stimulating appetite and increasing energy expenditure [12]. Further, leptin promotes the synthesis of melanocyte-stimulating hormone (MSH), an appetite suppressant. The absence of leptin (or its receptor) leads to uncontrolled food intake and the resulting obesity.

Leptin stimulates pathways that promote anorexia and weight loss, by stimulating anorexigenic signals, such as alpha MSH, which affects the melanocortin-4 receptors (MC4Rs), corticotrophin-releasing factor in the paraventricular nucleus, proopiomelanocortin precursor polypeptide (POMC), and cocaine- and amphetamine-regulated transcript (CART) in the arcuate nucleus [9]. Administration of recombinant leptin to these animals reverses these changes and induces weight loss.

Friedman proposed that reduction in fat depots causes a concomitant decrease in leptin production. Low leptin levels stimulate NPY in the hypothalamus, which triggers a series of events that leads to increased energy intake resulting in a positive energy balance. In contrast, an increase in fat depots causes an increase in leptin levels, which induces MSH to interact with its receptor. This interaction leads to decreased food intake, thus resulting in negative energy balance [13]. The precise areas within the brain and hypothalamus where these mediators interact to regulate eating behavior are not completely understood.

The three main components of energy expenditure are the resting metabolic rate (RMR), exercise-induced thermogenesis (physical activity), and food-induced thermogenesis. Thermogenesis refers to the physiological generation of heat and therefore the loss of energy. The RMR reflects the energy expended at rest. Metabolic rate contributes 60%–75% of total energy expenditure and depends on lean body mass, energy intake, physical fitness, and other factors such as age, height, stress, and environmental temperature [14,15]. Dietary thermogenesis is the energy required to digest and store food and is greatest for protein-rich foods, midway for carbohydrates, and lowest for fat [16]. Physical activity is influenced by behavioral and environmental factors.

The adrenergic system plays a major role in regulating energy expenditure. Beta-3 adrenoceptors are found in brown adipose tissue (BAT) and white adipose tissue (WAT) and appear to induce lipolysis and thermogenesis when activated by catecholamines [17].

METABOLIC PREDICTORS OF WEIGHT GAIN

Obesity develops when there is a mismatch between caloric intake and caloric output. In other words, the energy density of food consumed is disproportionate to the energy expended. Scientists have developed several techniques for the measurement of energy expenditure in order to better understand human bioenergetics. The metabolic chamber is considered the most accurate method of determining energy expenditure. Briefly, the metabolic chamber is a small room a subject can live in for a 24 h period, while metabolic rate is measured during meals, sleep, and light activities. It involves continuous measurements of heat output (direct calorimetry) or exhaled gas exchange (indirect calorimetry) in subjects confined to metabolic chambers. Researchers measure the heat released (direct calorimetry) from a person's body to determine how much energy each activity has burned for that person. In indirect calorimetry, researchers measure oxygen consumption, carbon dioxide production, and nitrogen excretion to calculate energy expenditure.

The doubly labeled water is another method of determining energy expenditure. It is a form of indirect calorimetry based on the elimination of deuterium and oxygen from urine. This method of determining energy expenditure is useful because it allows researchers to measure total carbon dioxide production over a long period of time (5–20 days) and requires only periodic sampling of urine. As such, it allows subjects to continue their normal routines. The doubly labeled water technique measures the turnover of hydrogen and oxygen into water and carbon dioxide, thus calculating energy expenditure. Researchers have also developed methods to measure energy expenditure in free-living situations. Such methods include monitoring heart rate and maintaining a daily activity log. Using a person's activity log, researchers can compute energy expenditure during various activities.

The major components of total energy expenditure are (1) RMR (amount of daily energy expended by humans and animals at rest), (2) thermic effect of food (the increment in energy above RMR due to metabolic cost of processing food), and (3) energy expanded during physical activity [18]. Metabolic factors such as RMR and levels of spontaneous activities have been shown to be good predictors of weight gain [19].

Early delicate studies on humans have established our understanding regarding the impact of metabolic factors on the development of obesity [20,21]. For example, Ravussin et al. [20] examined the contribution of energy expenditure to the development of obesity in Pima Indians and concluded that people with low energy expenditure were four times more likely to gain weight follow-up than those with high energy expenditure. They further observed that low rate of energy expenditure may contribute to aggregation of obesity in families, thus suggesting that energy expenditure may have a familial determinant. Although the study mentioned earlier provides strong evidence regarding the relationship of RMR to weight gain and the development of obesity, other studies failed to demonstrate similar observations [22].

Our understanding of the metabolic predictors of weight gain has improved as a result of subsequent well-controlled human studies and advances in biotechnology.

TABLE 2.1
Metabolic Predictors of Weight
Gain in Adults

RMR
Physical inactivity
Excess energy intake
Low fat oxidation
Insulin sensitivity
Low sympathetic nervous activity
Low plasma leptin
T3
Fasting insulin

These studies demonstrated that the insulin sensitivity, low fat oxidation, low sympathetic nervous system activity, low plasma leptin, fasting insulin, T3, and fasting serum insulin were significant predictors of weight gain [23,24]. Metabolic predictors of weight gain are depicted on Table 2.1.

FAT CELL AND ADIPOKINES

Adipose tissue plays an active role in energy homeostasis and various physiological processes, has complex interactions with the brain and peripheral organs, and has been recognized as a major endocrine organ [25–27]. Two types of adipose tissue exist: WAT and BAT. WAT is the predominant type of adipose tissue [1], and its depots are found in the subcutaneous region and around viscera where fat is stored in the form of triglycerides. As mentioned earlier, adipose tissue constitutes the largest endocrine organ that constantly communicates with other tissues by the synthesis and release of secretagogues, such as leptin, adiponectin, and visfatin, which along with insulin play an important role in regulating body-fat mass [28,29].

The pathophysiological basis of obesity is rooted to a great extent in the enlargement of fat cells. Large fat cells produce most of the pathogenic changes responsible for the complications associated with obesity. Specifically, in the obese state, the increase in WAT brings about histological and biochemical changes characteristic of inflammation [30], which produce inflammatory adipokines such as tumor necrosis factor (TNF), interleukin-6 (IL-6), and interleukin-1 (IL-1) [30,31]. These contribute to vascular dysfunction, which, along with free fatty acids, provide the pathophysiological basis for comorbid conditions associated with obesity such as insulin resistance and type 2 DM [32]. Further, C-reactive protein is increased in obesity as are intracellular adhesion molecule 1 and platelet-endothelial cell adhesion molecule-1, which induce adhesion and migration of monocytes in WAT endothelium. These conditions eventually may contribute to cardiovascular disease and atherosclerosis [33–35].

The role of inflammatory adipokines is depicted in Figure 2.1

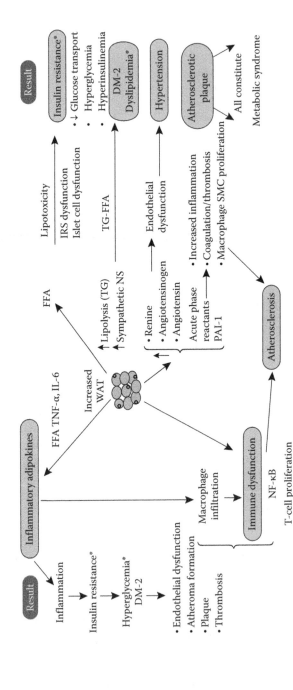

FIGURE 2.1 Role of lipotoxicity and inflammation on obesity. WAT releases pre-fatty acids and adipokines, which are lipotoxic and inflammatory and result in diverse effects, outlined in the left-hand columns. Their correlation to the metabolic syndrome is shown on the right-hand column, whereas all the effects culminate in atherosclerosis on the bottom of the figure. *Perturbed glucose and lipid metabolism. DM-2, diabetes mellitus-2; FFA, free fatty acids; IL, interleukin; IRS, insulin receptor substrate; NF-κB, nuclear factor kappa beta; NS, nervous system; PAI-1, plasminogen activator inhibitor-1; SMC, smooth muscle cell; TG, triglyceride; TNF, tumor necrosis factor.

CAUSES OF OBESITY

GENETICS

Obesity is caused by "a mismatch" of the balance between food intake and energy expenditure, a process that is regulated by complex physiological systems that require the integration of several signals of central and peripheral origin. As such, obesity is determined by an interaction of genetic and environmental factors. One of the earliest theories connecting genetics and obesity was proposed by James V. Neel in 1962 in his thrifty gene hypothesis [36].

The etiology of obesity has been evaluated extensively. Although it varies from study to study, 30% to ~50% of the variance in BMI can be attributed to genetics [37]. Such evidence for a genetic basis for obesity comes from a variety of studies including studies of resemblance and differences among family members, twins, and adoptees. These investigations suggest that a sizable portion of weight variation in adults is heritable [37–41].

The contribution of genes to human adiposity can be either single gene (one gene; monogenic obesity) or multiple genes (several genes; polygenic obesity). The development of DNA technology offered geneticists the opportunity to evaluate the genetic contribution to human body weight. The most frequent methodologies on the genetics of human obesity are genetic association studies and genome-wide scans. Genetic association studies are performed to determine whether a genetic variant is associated with a disease or trait. Genetic association can be between a phenotype (i.e., adiposity) and a genetic polymorphism, such as a single nucleotide polymorphism (SNP), or between two genetic polymorphisms. Association between genetic polymorphisms occurs when there is nonrandom association of their alleles as a result of their proximity on the same chromosome. Genome-wide association study is an approach that involves rapidly scanning markers across the complete sets of DNA, or genomes, of many people to find genetic variations associated with a particular disease. Once new genetic associations are identified, researchers can use the information to develop better strategies to detect, treat, and prevent the disease. Such studies are particularly useful in finding genetic variations that contribute to common, complex diseases, such as cancer, diabetes, and heart disease.

Monogenic Obesity

Direct evidence for monogenic obesity exists. Such evidence comes from several cases of extreme obesity due to mutations (changes in the genetic material) of single genes. Single-gene defects causing obesity are rare in humans. Examples include rare mutations in the gene encoding leptin or its receptor. Affected individuals suffer uncontrollable hunger and develop severe obesity at a young age. The first monogenic case to be reported was a leptin deficiency in two morbidly obese cousins [42]. Other syndromes have also been described that regulate signals downstream from leptin, in the POMC gene and the MC4R [43,44]. Several mutations in different genes have been linked to obesity. Monogenic obesity is rare and characterized by extreme phenotype and physiological perturbance in energy regulation [45,46].

Polygenic Obesity

Progress in identifying the multiple genes associated with the most common form of obesity is accelerating. In polygenic obesity, genetic factors exert their influences over a wide range of body mass. Further, in polygenic obesity, an individual's genetic background is susceptible to an environment that promotes positive energy balance. Genetic association studies and studies using genome-wide scans have focused on hundreds of groups of genes related to obesity. These genes have been linked to regulatory functions related to fat stores in adipose tissue, energy intake, and energy expenditure. Approximately 500 variants of 130 genes have been associated with obesity [47–50]. Recently, several independent population-based studies report that the FTO gene (fat mass and obesity-associated gene) might be responsible for up to 22% of all cases of common obesity in the general population. Several studies have been conducted regarding the role of genetics on adiposity and obesity. The FTO gene plays a pivotal role in energy balance. Of particular importance, the FTO gene is the first obesity-susceptibility gene identified by genome-wide association scans. Genetic variation in the FTO locus confers effect on BMI and adiposity [51]. Interestingly, this gene also shows a strong association with diabetes. The mechanism by which this gene operates is currently under intense scientific investigation, and it appears that it may regulate the transcription of genes involved in metabolism [52].

The interaction between genetics and environment is also important. In a given population, some people are genetically predisposed to develop obesity, but that genotype may be expressed only under certain adverse environmental conditions, such as high-fat diets and sedentary lifestyles in the United States, as well as in other Western countries, greater numbers of people are being exposed to these adverse environmental conditions, and consequently, the percentage of people expressing the obesity genotype has increased.

ENVIRONMENT

As mentioned previously in this chapter, the interplay between genes and environmental factors is seminal to the regulation of energy balance and adiposity. Although the genetic contributions on adiposity have received considerable attention in recent years, and despite the fact that a sizable portion of weight variation in adults is heritable [37–41], the dramatic increase in the prevalence of obesity over the last three decades is most likely due to recent environmental changes and effects. As such, individuals who are genetically susceptible are at risk for developing obesity in an environment that promotes high-density intake (i.e., food) and low energy expenditure (i.e., physical activity). The impact of such environment is best illustrated by a study of two groups of Pima Indians [53] living in Mexico and Arizona. These groups were separated more than 700 years ago and now differ in terms of both diet and physical activity. Pima Indians living in Mexico eat a diet with less caloric density, and they also have greater energy expenditure from various physical activities when compared to Arizona Pima Indians. Pima Indians residing in Arizona have among the highest prevalence of obesity and much higher BMI than those living in Mexico. The recent rapid increase in mean population BMI and obesity can be caused only by such environmental influences that disturb the homeostatic mechanisms described previously in this chapter.

Caloric Density

Profound changes in diet have occurred over the last three to four decades in industrialized societies [54–56]. Such changes involve increased consumption of energy-dense foods and soft drinks that are high in fat and/or sugar [57,58]. Estimates of food consumption in epidemiological studies are greatly confounded by underreporting by obese subjects. Specifically, from the early 1970s to the late 1990s, the average calories available per person per day (the amount of food bought) increased in almost all parts of the world. Total calorie consumption has been found to be related to obesity [54,55].

The availability of nutritional guidelines has done very little to address the problems associated with energy-dense foods, overeating, and poor dietary choice. Unfortunately, people become increasingly reliant on foods of high-calorie content, big portions, and fast-food meals. As such, the association between fast-food consumption and obesity becomes more of a concern [59]. A report from the USDA indicated that in the United States, consumption of fast-food meals tripled and food energy intake from these meals quadrupled between 1977 and 1995 [60].

Physical Inactivity

A sedentary lifestyle plays a significant role in obesity [61,62]. More than 60% of U.S. adults do not engage in the recommended amount of activity. Approximately 25% of U.S. adults are not active at all [63]. The U.S. population has become an inactive one. Similar trends are observed worldwide. In children, there appear to be declines in levels of physical activity due to less walking and physical education [64–66]. Further, in children, there is an association between television viewing time and the risk of obesity [67]. The Dietary Guidelines for Americans 2010 [68] concluded that there was "strong, consistent evidence" that physically active people are at reduced risk for becoming overweight or obese. Promoting regular activity and creating an environment that supports this behavior may reduce the obesity epidemic. Policy makers must strive to create and promote opportunities for regular physical activity in schools and communities.

SUMMARY

Body mass is regulated by metabolic factors, diet, and physical activity, all of which influenced by genetic traits. Despite scientific improvements in our understanding on the causes of obesity, the prevalence of obesity in industrialized societies has increased over the last 30 years. In contrast to monogenic obesity that is rare and involves mutation on a single gene, predisposition to more common forms of obesity is probably influenced by numerous susceptibility genes, accounting for variations in physiological system regulating energy balance. The worldwide changes in obesity prevalence during the last 30–40 years cannot be explained by changes in the gene pool. The contribution of the environment (i.e., energy density of food and physical attention) has been evaluated extensively by public health scientists. It is important to recognize society's difficulties in sustaining energy-restricted diets and adequate levels of physical activity and the relation of these behavioral attitudes to the obesity epidemic.

REFERENCES

1. www.who.int
2. Flegal KM, Carroll MD, Ogden CL, Curtin LR. Prevalence and trends in obesity among US adults, 1999–2008. *JAMA*. 2010;303(3):235–241.
3. Cohen DA, Finch BK, Bower A, Sastry N. Collective efficacy and obesity: The potential influence of social factors on health. *Soc Sci Med*. 2006;62(3):769–778.
4. Gray L, Hart CL, Smith GD, Batty GD. What is the predictive value of established risk factors for total and cardiovascular disease mortality when measured before middle age? Pooled analyses of two prospective cohort studies from Scotland. *Eur J Cardiovasc Prev Rehabil*. 2010;17(1):106–112.
5. Vague J. The degree of masculine differentiation of obesities: A factor determining predisposition to diabetes, atherosclerosis, gout and uric acid calculous disease. *Am J Clin Nutr*. 1956;4:20–34.
6. Despres J-P, Allard C, Tremblay A, Talbot J, Bouchard C. Evidence for a regional component of body fatness in the association with serum lipids in men and women. *Metabolism*. 1985;34:967–973.
7. Schwartz MW, Woods SC, Porte D Jr et al. Is the energy homeostasis system inherently biased toward weight gain? *Diabetes*. 2003;52:232–238.
8. Kennedy GC. The role of depot fat in the hypothalamus control of food intake in the rat. *Proc R Soc Lond (Biol)*. 1953;140:579–592.
9. Kumar P, Clarke M. *Clinical Medicine*, 7th edn. W.B. Saunders, Philadelphia, PA, online, available at http://www.kumarandclark.com/content Accessed: June, 2009.
10. Zhang Y, Proenca R, Maffel M, Barone M, Leopold L, Friedman JM. Positional cloning of the mouse obese gene and its human homologue. *Nature*. 1994;372:425–432.
11. Green ED, Maffei M, Braden VV, Proenca R, DeSilva U, Zhang Y, Chua SC Jr, Leibel RL, Weissenbach J, Friedman JM. The human obese (OB) gene: RNA expression pattern and mapping on the physical, cytogenetic, and genetic maps of chromosome 7. *Genome Res*. 1995;5(1):5–12.
12. Tomaszuk A, Simpson C, Williams G, Neuropeptide Y. The hypothalamus and the regulation of energy homeostasis. *Hormone Res*. 1996;46:53–58.
13. Friedman JM. The alphabet of weight control. *Nature*. 1996;385:119–120.
14. Olefsky JM. Obesity. In: Isselbacher KJ, Braunwald E, Wilson JD, Martin JB, Fauci AS, Kasper DL, eds. *Harrison's Principles of Internal Medicine*, 13th edn. New York: McGraw-Hill; 1994, pp. 446–452.
15. Zurlo F, Larson K, Bogardus C, Ravussin E. Skeletal muscle metabolism is a major determinant of resting energy expenditure. *J Clin Invest*. 1990;86:1423–1427.
16. Wilding J. Pathophysiology and aetiology of obesity. *Medicine*. 2003;31:4.
17. Insel PA. Adrenergic receptors—Evolving concepts and clinical implications. *N Engl J Med*. 1996;334:580–585.
18. Swinburn BA, Ravussin E. Energy and macronutrient metabolism. *Baillière's Clin Endocrinol Metab*. 1994;8:527–576.
19. Pi-Sunyer FX. The obesity epidemic: Pathophysiology and consequences of obesity. *Obes Res*. 2002;10:97S–104S.
20. Ravussin E, Lillioja S, Knowler WC, Christin L, Freymond D, Abbott WG, Boyce V, Howard BV, Bogardus C. Reduced rate of energy expenditure as a risk factor for body-weight gain. *N Engl J Med*. 1988;318:467–472.
21. Zurlo F, Lillioja S, Esposito-Del Puente A et al. Low ratio of fat to carbohydrate oxidation as predictor of weight gain: Study of 24-h RQ. *Am J Physiol*. 1990;259:E560–E567.
22. Weinsier RL, Nagy TR, Hunter GR, Darnell BE, Hensrud DD, Weiss HL. Do adaptive changes in metabolic rate favor weight regain in weight-reduced individuals? An examination of the set-point theory. *Am J Clin Nutr*. 2000;72:1088–1094.

23. Ravussin E, Gautier J-F. Metabolic predictors of weight gain. *Int J Obes Relat Metab Disord*. 1999;23:37–41.
24. Butte NF, Gai G, Cole SA, Wilson TA, Fisher JO, Zakeri IF, Ellis KJ, Comuzzie AG. Metabolic and behavioral predictors of weight gain in Hispanic children: The Viva la Familia Study. *Am J Clin Nutr*. 2007;85:1478–1485.
25. Flier JS. Obesity wars: Molecular progress confronts an expanding epidemic. *Cell*. 2004;23(116):337–350.
26. Kershaw EE, Flier JS. Adipose tissue as an endocrine organ. *J Clin Endocrinol Metab*. 2004;89(6):2548–2556.
27. Miner JL. The adipocyte as an endocrine cell. *J Anim Sci*. 2004;82:935–941.
28. Niswender KD, Baskin DG, Schwartz MW. Insulin and its evolving partnership with leptin in the hypothalamic control of energy homeostasis. *Trends Endocrinol Metab*. 2004;15:362–369.
29. Matsuzawa Y, Funahashi T, Kihara S, Shimomura I. Adiponectin and metabolic syndrome. *Arterioscler Thromb Vasc Biol*. 2004;24:29–33.
30. Weisberg SP, McCann D, Desai M, Rosenbaum M, Leibel RL, Ferrante AW Jr. Obesity is associated with macrophage accumulation in adipose tissue. *J Clin Invest*. 2003;112:1796–1808.
31. Xu H, Barnes GT, Yang Q et al. Chronic inflammation in fat plays a crucial role in the development of obesity-related insulin resistance. *J Clin Invest*. 2003;112:1821–1830.
32. McKeigue PM, Shah B, Marmot MG. Relation of central obesity and insulin resistance with high diabetes prevalence and cardiovascular risk in South Asians. *Lancet*. 1991;337:382–386.
33. Shirai K. Obesity as the core of the metabolic syndrome and the management of coronary heart disease. *Curr Med Res Opin*. 2004;20:295–304.
34. Rajala MW, Scherer PE. Minireview: The adipocyte—At the crossroads of energy homeostasis, inflammation, and atherosclerosis. *Endocrinology*. 2003;144:3765–3773.
35. Matsuzawa Y. White adipose tissue and cardiovascular disease. *Best Pract Res Clin Endocrinol Metab*. 2005;19:637–647.
36. Neel JV. Diabetes mellitus: A "thrifty" genotype rendered detrimental by "progress?" *Am J Hum Genet*. 1962;14:353–362.
37. Rice T, Perusse L, Bouchard C, Rao DC. Familial aggregation of body mass index and subcutaneous fat measures in the longitudinal Quebec family study. *Genet Epidemiol*. 1999;16(3):316–334.
38. Maes HH, Neale MC, Evans LJ. Genetic and environmental factors I relative body weight and human adiposity. *Behav Genet*. 1997;27:325–351.
39. Stunkard AJ, Sorensen TI, Hanis C et al. An adoption study of human obesity. *N Engl J Med*. 1986;314:193–198.
40. Stunkard AJ, Berkowitz RI, Stallings VA, Carter JR. Weights of parents and infants: Is there a relationship? *Int J Obes Relat Metab Disord*. 1999;23:159–162.
41. Bouchard C, Tremblay A, Després JP et al. The response to long-term overfeeding in identical twins. *N Engl J Med*. 1990;322:1477–1482.
42. Montague CT, Farooqi IS, Whitehead JP et al. Congenital leptin deficiency is associated with severe early-onset obesity in humans. *Nature*. 1997;387:903–908.
43. Clement K. Genetics of human obesity. *Proc Nutr Soc*. 2005;64:133–142.
44. Harrold JA, Williams G. Melanocorti-4 receptors, beta-MSH and leptin: Key elements in the satiety pathway. *Peptides* 2006;27:365–371.
45. Farooqi IS, O'Rahilly S. Monogenic obesity in humans. *Ann Rev Med*. 2005;56:443–458.
46. Farooqi IS, O'Rahilly S. Recent advances in the genetics of severe childhood obesity. *Arch Dis Child*. 2000;83:31–34.
47. Hunter DJ. Gene-environment interactions in human diseases. *Nat Rev Genet*. 2005;6:287–298.

48. Rankinen T, Zuberi A, Chagnon YC et al. The human obesity gene map: The 2005 update. *Obesity* (Silver Spring). 2006;14:529–644.
49. Bell CG, Walley AJ, Froguel P. The genetics of human obesity. *Nat Rev Genet.* 2005;6:221–223.
50. Mutch DM, Clement K. Unraveling the genetics of human obesity. *PLoS Genet.* 2006;2(12):1956–1962.
51. Loos RJ. Recent progress in the genetics of common obesity. *Br J Clin Pharmacol.* 2009;68:811–829.
52. Gerken T, Girard CA, Tung YC et al. The Obesity associated FTO gene encodes a 2-oxo-glutarate-dependent nucleic acid demethylase. *Science.* 2007;318:1469–1472.
53. Ravussin E, Valencia ME, Esparza J, Bennett PH, Schulz LO. Effects of a traditional lifestyle on obesity in Pima Indians. *Diabetes Care.* 1994;17:1067–1074.
54. Flegal KM, Carroll MD, Ogden CL, Johnson CL. Prevalence and trends in obesity among US adults, 1999–2000. *JAMA.* 2002;288(14):1723–1727.
55. Caballero B. The global epidemic of obesity: An overview. *Epidemiol Rev.* 2007;29:1–5.
56. Mozaffarian D, Hao T, Rimm EB, Willett WC, Hu FB. Changes in diet and lifestyle and long-term weight gain in women and men. *N Engl J Med.* 2011;364(25):2392–2404.
57. Malik VS, Schulze MB, Hu FB. Intake of sugar-sweetened beverages and weight gain: A systematic review. *Am J Clin Nutr.* 2006;84(2):274–288.
58. Olsen NJ, Heitmann BL. Intake of calorically sweetened beverages and obesity. *Obes Rev.* 2009;10(1):68–75.
59. Rosenheck R. Fast food consumption and increased caloric intake: A systematic review of a trajectory towards weight gain and obesity risk. *Obes Rev.* 2008;9(6):535–547.
60. Lin BH, Guthrie J, Frazao E. Nutrient contribution of food away from home. In: Frazão E, ed. *Agriculture Information Bulletin No. 750: America's Eating Habits: Changes and Consequences.* Washington, DC: U.S. Department of Agriculture, Economic Research Service, 1999, pp. 213–239.
61. Hu FB. Sedentary lifestyle and risk of obesity in type 2 diabetes. *Lipids.* 2003;38(2):103–108.
62. Jacobs RD. Fast food and sedentary lifestyle: A combination that leads to obesity. *Am J Clin Nutr.* 2006;83(2):189–190.
63. www.cdc.gov
64. Salmon J, Timperio A. Prevalence, trends and environmental influences on child and youth physical activity. *Med Sport Sci.* 2007;50:183–199.
65. Borodulin K, Laatikainen T, Juolevi A, Jousilahti P. Thirty-year trends of physical activity in relation to age, calendar time and birth cohort in Finnish adults. *Eur J Public Health.* 2008;18(3):339–344.
66. Brownson RC, Boehmer TK, Luke DA. Declining rates of physical activity in the United States: What are the contributors? *Annu Rev Public Health.* 2005;26:421–443.
67. Gortmaker SL, Must A, Sobol AM, Peterson K, Colditz GA, Dietz WH. Television viewing as a cause of increasing obesity among children in the United States, 1986–1990. *Arch Pediatr Adolesc Med.* 1996;150(4):356–362.
68. U.S. Department of Agriculture and U.S. Department of Health and Human Services. *Dietary Guidelines for Americans, 2010*, 7th edn. Washington, DC: U.S. Government Printing Office; December 2010.

3 Epidemiology of Obesity

Alan C. Utter, PhD, MPH, FACSM,
Richard R. Suminski, PhD, MPH, FACSM,
and Theodore J. Angelopoulos, PhD, MPH

CONTENTS

INTRODUCTION

Obesity may be viewed as the most daunting health condition of the present time. Many experts believe that the escalating rates of obesity in the United States will seriously impact the nation's health and place a huge burden on our health-care system. As of the year 2008, the World Health Organization (WHO) provided evidence suggesting that 1.5 billion individuals over the age of 20 were considered obese [1].

Obesity is not simply a cosmetic problem. There is a general agreement that obesity is a serious, chronic health problem. It is also a strong risk factor for type 2 diabetes mellitus (T2DM) and cardiovascular disease (CVD). Further, it is also associated with certain cancers (i.e., colorectal), osteoarthritis, liver disease, sleep apnea, depression, and other medical conditions that affect mortality, morbidity, and quality of life [2,3]. Although the mechanisms and causes of obesity are poorly understood, experts agree that obesity is largely the result of a chronic imbalance between caloric intake and caloric expenditure. This imbalance is likely the outcome of a complex interaction between genetic and environmental factors. Obesity also shortens life expectancy. For example, it has been estimated that the very severely obese (define body mass index [BMI] $\geq$ 40 kg/m^2) have an average life expectancy 5–20 years less than those who are not overweight or obese [4]. In addition to the increased risk of premature death associated with excess body weight, the obesity-related health-care costs were approximately $147 billion in the United States for the year 2008 [5].

Although obesity was once considered a problem only of high-income industrialized societies, obesity rates are rising worldwide. The WHO formally recognized obesity as a global epidemic [6]. The main objectives of this chapter are to provide some useful and practical information on the definition and assessment of obesity, present epidemiological trends, and discuss health complications associated with the obese state that underscore the impact of obesity on public health. These main topics are followed by a discussion regarding the impact of obesity on mortality and the importance of continuous efforts to develop preventive strategies.

The human body is primarily comprised of three structural components: muscle, bone, and fat. Excess adipose (fat) tissue is the principal characteristic of obesity. There are, however, different types of fat that are stored in various depots in the body with different clinical significance. For example, excess visceral fat (fat surrounding organs in the abdomen) appears to be a better predictor of obesity-related health consequences than the amount of total body or subcutaneous fat.

Assessing body fat is a tedious task making this approach impractical for use in large populations or epidemiological studies. As such, the American Heart Association and other organizations have adopted BMI as a practical clinical indicator of adiposity [7]. BMI, calculated as weight (kg) divided by height (m) squared (kg/m^2), correlates well with total body fat and is related to cardiovascular and all-cause mortality [8–11]. A set of cut points at five BMI intervals to classify overweight and obesity have been adapted by the National Heart, Lung, and Blood Institute and WHO [7]. BMI is a widely used index despite its limitations. For instance, BMI does not differentiate between weight from fat and weight from lean body compartments (i.e., muscle and bone) nor does it take into account regional adiposity (i.e., the distribution of body fat).

Overweight and obesity are classified for ranges of weight corresponding to BMI intervals that are greater than what is generally considered healthy for a given height. These BMI intervals have been shown to increase the likelihood of diseases (i.e., diabetes and cardiovascular) and other health problems.

DEFINITIONS FOR ADULTS AND CHILDREN

For most adults, BMI correlates well with the amount of adipose tissue; thus, it is considered a good indicator of adiposity for epidemiological studies. BMI is also used to classify children (ages 2–19) as overweight or obese based on growth charts that provide a means for determining age and gender specific BMI percentiles. Cut points of BMI intervals and percentiles use to classify adults and children as overweight or obese are depicted as follows [12]:

Adults		Children	
Overweight	25–29.9	Overweight	$85 \geq BMI \leq 95$
Obese	>30	Obese	$BMI \geq 95^{th}$ percentile

EPIDEMIOLOGICAL TRENDS

Generally, systematic data on obesity cannot be obtained from medical records or vital statistics and because of logistical difficulties, is based almost exclusively on BMI derived from measured height and weight. In the United States, the National Center for Health Statistics of the Center for Disease Control and Prevention conducts standardized physical examinations on large, representative samples of children, adolescents, and adults through the National Health and Nutrition Examination Survey (NHANES) program. Currently, NHANES includes oversampling of adolescents, Mexican Americans, African Americans, and other groups to improve estimates for these groups. The following description of obesity rates and trends in the United States is based on the NHANES data.

Rates of overweight and obesity have risen dramatically over the last 30 years in the United States (see Figure 3.1). During this time period, the prevalence of obesity increased 18% in adults (from 15% to 33%), while the prevalence of overweight in children tripled (6%–19%) [13,14]. The most recent estimates from 2010 indicate that 17% (or 12.5 million) of children and adolescents and 33.8% of adults are obese [15]. In some segments of the population, the rates of obesity are substantially higher, a possible result of interactions between culture, genetics, and environmental factors [16]. A most alarming trend is the rise in extreme obesity (grade III; BMI $\geq$ 40kg/m^2). Over a 7–8 year span, the percentage of adults 20 years of age or older with grade III obesity increased from 4.7% to 5.7%, which equates to about 2 million people in the United States [13].

Demographic characteristics are associated with overweight and obesity. Age-adjusted prevalence rates of obesity are generally higher in women than in men, older versus younger cohorts, and racial/ethnic groups compared with whites [13,14]. Approximately 32% of men (18.2% of male children and adolescents) and

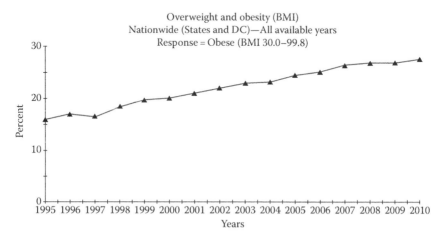

FIGURE 3.1 Overweight and obesity (BMI) nationwide (States and DC). (From Centers for Disease Control and Prevention (CDC), Overweight and obesity: US obesity trends, U.S. Department of Health and Human Services, Atlanta, GA, Centers for Disease Control and Prevention, 2010, available at: http://www.cdc.gov/obesity/data/trends.html, Accessed: October 31, 2011.)

35.5% of women (16.0% of female children and adolescents) were obese according to NHANES 2007–2008 with the odds of being obese higher in adult women than men but unrelated to gender in children and adolescents [14]. Non-Hispanic blacks and Mexican Americans display higher rates of obesity than whites. The most extreme example is found for women, where non-Hispanic adult, black women have a rate of obesity exceeding adult, white women by 24% (53.9% vs. 30.2%) [13]. Finally, age brings about increases in obesity especially for non-Hispanic white men and Hispanic females [14]. For example, the prevalence of obesity is 26.3% between 20 and 39 years of age in non-Hispanic white men but increases to 38.4% after age 60.

OBESITY AND DIABETES

An estimated 26 million Americans have diabetes, and over 79 million adults display evidence of "prediabetes" [17]. Obesity definitely plays a role in this phenomenon. A BMI $\geq 35\,kg/m^2$ is associated with a 42.1 times greater risk of T2DM in men and a 93.2 times greater risk in women compared to normal BMI controls, and the risk of developing T2DM is elevated the longer one is obese [18–20]. A meta-analysis on 32 articles published between 1966 and 2004 found the pooled relative risks for incident of T2DM to be 1.87, 1.87, and 1.88 per standard deviation of BMI, waist circumference, and waist/hip ratio, respectively [21]. A study on 84,000 female nurses conducted over a 16 year span showed that being overweight or obese was the single most important predictor of T2DM [22]. Another recent meta-analysis indicated that the pooled relative risk for developing T2DM increased across categories of BMI (normal to overweight to obese) and varied by gender [23]. The relative risks in this study were 2.4 and 6.7 for overweight and obese men and 3.9 and 12.4 for overweight and obese women. The association between waist circumference and T2DM is similar but weaker in comparison with BMI.

In the SEARCH for Diabetes in Youth study, it was estimated that the number of adolescents per year diagnosed with T2DM is approximately 3700 and increasing [23,24]. Not surprisingly, the relationships between obesity and both type 1 diabetes insipidus (T1DI) and T2DM are very strong among children and adolescents especially within minority populations [17,25,26]. For example, a dose–response relationship was supported evidence of a continuous association between childhood BMI and subsequent type T1DI with a pooled odds ratio of 1.25 per one standard deviation higher BMI [26]. Fasting insulin, insulin, and the insulin-to-glucose ratio are significantly higher in obese versus control 8–11 year olds, and impaired insulin sensitivity is more apparent as the duration of obesity increases [27–29]. Youth inflicted with T2DM compared with T1DI have a higher risk of retinopathy and nephropathy and display early signs of CVD [30–32].

The risk of developing T2DM increases significantly with increasing weight; however, weight loss has the potential to improve long-term risk [33,34]. Colditz et al. [33] observed a 2.3 average higher relative risk of T2DM for women gaining between 5 and 10.9 kg, while women who lost 5 kg experienced a 50% reduction in the risk of T2DM. In a 20 year prospective study of 7176 men, the relative risk of T2DM was 0.62 among men losing weight during that period compared with 1.76 among men who had a 10% gain in body weight [34]. In the Look AHEAD (Action for Health in Diabetes) study, an intensive 1 year lifestyle intervention resulted in significant weight loss (8.6% of body weight), which was associated with improved diabetes control and reductions in CVD risk factors and medication use [35].

OBESITY AND OTHER HEALTH COMPLICATIONS

The scientific literature abounds with evidence linking obesity with numerous health outcomes in addition to diabetes. Obesity is associated with the incidence of all cancers except esophageal and prostate cancer; CVDs including hypertension, congestive heart failure, coronary artery disease, stroke, and pulmonary embolism; asthma, chronic back pain, osteoarthritis, gallbladder disease; and all-cause mortality [23,36]. Two common findings are that the risk of disease is linearly and positively associated with BMI indicating a dose–response relationship and that weight loss results in disease risk reduction [23]. Furthermore, very few studies on the comorbidities related to obesity and overweight were conducted on racial/ethnic minorities. The proportion of racial/ethnic minorities examined in studies reporting this demographic ranged from 5% to 19% [23].

A number of long-term, large-scale studies have examined the influence of obesity on CVD risk. All CVDs examined in a recent meta-analysis by Guh et al. [23] were significantly associated with obesity. The relative risks for disease among obese men and women were 2.1 for hypertension, 1.5 for stroke, 2.4 for coronary artery disease, 1.8 for congestive heart failure, and 3.5 for pulmonary embolism [23]. Data from 5209 participants in the Framingham Heart study amassed over a 44 year period found the age-adjusted relative risks of CVD were 1.46 in men and 1.64 in women [37]. In a study on 7176 men followed for 20 years, the rate of major CVD was found to be 2.5% in obese subjects versus 1.4% among normal weight subjects [34]. Women with a BMI $\geq$ 35 kg/m^2 display odds ratios of 2.7 for coronary artery disease and 5.4 for hypertension [38]. In the Nord-Trondelag Health study, the risk for hypertension was increased $\geq$1.4-fold among men (n = 13,800) and women (n = 15,900) whose BMI increased from baseline compared with those who maintained a stable BMI [39]. A combination of cardiovascular risk factors known as the metabolic syndrome (MetS) is strongly associated with obesity especially abdominal obesity [40,41]. Weight reduction by itself or occurring in combination with lifestyle changes is associated with a significant drop in the prevalence of MetS [42,43]. Even a moderate 8 kg reduction in weight was shown to cause a significant reduction in the prevalence of MetS from 35% to 27% [43].

The evidence from several large-scale, prospective studies clearly indicates a significant association between obesity and cancer [23]. In a 16-year longitudinal study of nearly 1 million subjects, all-cause mortality from all cancers was 52% higher in men and 62% higher in women with a BMI > 40 kg/m^2 compared to subjects with a normal BMI [44]. Reeves et al. [45] found that increasing BMI in a sample of over 1.2 million women, aged 50–64 years, was associated with significantly higher incidence rates of 10 out of 17 of the most common types of cancer. In the meta-analysis conducted by Guh et al. [23], obesity was found to be associated with breast, endometrial, ovarian, colorectal, kidney, and pancreatic cancer. Relative risk estimates ranged from 1.13 for breast cancer to 3.22 for endometrial cancer. At present, the evidence suggests that obesity prevention may be more advantageous than weight loss in reducing the incidence of obesity-related cancer [46].

Obesity is significantly associated with several other disease risk factors and diseases in both men and women. Prepregnancy obesity and term obesity result in several maternal and fetal problems including maternal gestational diabetes, neonatal death, and fetal abnormalities (e.g., spina bifida) [47–49]. A 5 year, prospective study on a cohort of 2298 adults showed that the obese were at increased risk of becoming depressed (odds ratio = 2.11) [50]. Petry et al. [51] found significantly greater odds for a psychiatric disorder (odds ratio = 1.21) and a lifetime prevalence of major depressive disorder (odds ratio = 1.51) in obese compared with normal weight subjects. The prevalence of major depressive disorders is linearly related with BMI ranging from 6.5% for individuals having a BMI < 25%–25.9% for those with a BMI > 40 kg/m^2 [52]. Women with a diagnosis of knee osteoarthritis have an average BMI that is 24% higher than women without such an ailment [53]. Lementowski and Zelicof [54] demonstrated that for every two unit increase in BMI, the risk of osteoarthritis rises by 36%, and transitioning from obese to overweight may prevent 19% of new cases of severe knee pain. A randomized, clinical trial evaluating rapid weight loss found that a 10% weight reduction improved physical function by 28% in women with osteoarthritis [55]. In a study of 1.3 million women, 25% of hospital days for gallbladder disease (which has a considerable impact on health-care costs) were attributed to obesity [56]. A prospective study of nearly 30,000 men demonstrated that those with a BMI ≥ 28.5 kg/m^2 had a 2.49-fold greater risk of gallstones compared with men having a normal BMI [57]. The pooled relative risks of gallbladder disease are 1.43 and 2.32 for obese men and women, respectively [23]. Obesity is the most important risk factor for the development of obstructive sleep apnea, where 60%–90% of adults are overweight and the relative risk in obese patients (BMI > 29 kg/m^2) is ≥10 [58]. Finally, in an analysis of the NHANES database, overall years of life lost were 1–9 for those with low BMI (<17–19 kg/m^2) compared with 9–13 for those with a high BMI (≥35 kg/m^2) [4]. Importantly, patients undergoing gastric bypass surgery for morbid obesity have demonstrated as much as a 40% reduction in all-cause mortality with substantial weight loss [59]. Bariatric surgery also has been shown to improve hyperlipidemia in 70% of patients and hypertension in 62% of patients [60].

Obesity is significantly related to a number of comorbidities in children and adolescents. Goodman et al. [61] found that each component of the MetS worsens with increasing obesity in adolescents. Studies also demonstrate a significant association between obesity and hypertension, especially systolic hypertension, left ventricular hypertrophy, carotid intima media thickness and carotid elasticity, blood lipids, and sleep apnea [62–67]. Obese children and adolescents are more prone to psychosocial abnormalities such as depression, anxiety disorders, loneliness, poor self-perception, and suicidal tendencies [68–71]. In addition, obesity during childhood and adolescence is a determinant of a number of cardiovascular risk factors in adulthood [64–66,68].

PUBLIC HEALTH IMPLICATIONS

The National Institute of Health first officially recognized the health problems associated with obesity in 1985 [72]. The Center for Disease Control and Prevention's recent data indicates that obesity in the United States continues to be major public health problem [73,74]. Obesity is now considered one of the most important medical and public health issues of modern time and outranks both smoking and drinking in its deleterious effects on human health and health costs [75]. Sturm [75] reported that obesity was associated with a 36% increase in inpatient and outpatient spending compared with a 21% increase in spending for smoking and excessive drinking. Within the United States, there is currently no state that has achieved the Healthy People 2010 objective of reducing the proportion of adults who are obese to 15%. The 15% goal was carried over and is presently a Healthy People 2020 objective [76].

The National Institute of Health and several others have summarized the large number of health problems associated with obesity to include an increased psychological burden, blood pressure, levels of cholesterol and other lipids in the blood, risk of gallstones, osteoarthritis, early death, and heart disease [77]. As of the year 2000, the direct health-care costs for providing care for these obesity-related conditions in the United States was $117 billion [78], and $61 billion was spent in direct medical costs: the remainder was associated with indirect costs, such as lost work time, disability, and loss of income due to premature death [79]. During the period from 1998 to 2006, annual medical costs associated with obesity increased from 6.5% to 9.2% [73,74]. Overall, this computes to individuals who are obese spending $1429 annually, in 2006 dollars, for medical care, or 42% more than individuals of average weight [79].

In addition to the economic costs associated with obesity, the personal costs are equally as challenging. Given the strong pressures from society to be thin, obese individuals often suffer feelings of guilt, depression, anxiety, and low self-esteem [77]. From a psychological and suffering perspective, this may be the greatest burden of obesity, especially among children. Discrimination and prejudices against obese people are common in society at large and in the workplace [80]. Some of the social and economic consequences of being obese include reduced income and higher rates of poverty, decreased likelihood of getting married, and poorer academic performance and progress [81]. While legal ramifications and societal norms limit inappropriate responses and unfair treatment to individuals based on gender, race, religion, or sexual orientation, safeguards from a body weight bias do not exist. Future research, effective interventions, and potential legislation are needed to address both discrimination and prejudices that surround obese individuals.

There have been several studies that have investigated the economic impact of obesity in the workplace. Finkelstein et al. [82] studied per capita and aggregate medical expenditures and the value of lost productivity, including absenteeism and presenteeism (defined as lower work output), because of overweight and grade I, II, and III obesity among 33,015 U.S. male and female employees. Results indicated that the annual cost attributable to obesity among full-time employees is $73.1 billion. Individuals with a BMI > 35 represent 37% of the obese population but are responsible for 61% of excess costs. The authors concluded that successful efforts to reduce the prevalence of obesity, especially among those with a BMI > 35, could result in significant savings to employers [82]. When examining the total costs, obesity attributable, business expenditures on paid sick leave, life insurance, and disability insurance amounted to $2.4 billion, $1.8 billion, and $800 million, respectively [83]. Aside from the staggering health-care costs attributable to obesity, one must also ask the question: "Who pays for the health-care costs for the obese?" Thompson et al. [84] estimated that of the $12.7 billion obesity-related costs to U.S. businesses, $7.7 billion was paid out for health insurance expenditures.

One of the most significant public health concerns secondary to obesity is increased risk of early death. Numerous investigations have demonstrated that as body weight increases so does mortality from cancer, heart disease, and diabetes [4,44,85,86]. Minimal mortality has been associated with a body weight 10%–20% below the average for Americans, after the adjustment for smoking status [8]. If the American population lost its excess body mass, mortality would be reduced by 15% corresponding to 3 years of added life expectancy [77].

MORTALITY PREVENTION

As demonstrated, being overweight or obese can lead to a significant financial strain on our health-care system and workplace costs, in addition to increasing psychological burden and early mortality. Although there is still considerable debate as to the exact underlying causes of obesity, most experts will agree that the imbalance of increased caloric intake and decreased caloric expenditure is at its origin. Obesity is a complex chronic condition that is multicausal in nature with lifestyle, genetics, socioeconomic, cultural, and psychological factors all playing a role. Obesity is often treated and viewed as an acute condition, but the general consensus is that obesity should be viewed as a chronic condition much like heart disease and type 2 diabetes [87]. The treatment of obesity should include programmatic efforts not only at the individual level but also from a public health perspective at the community and national level.

Reversing the U.S. obesity epidemic will require a comprehensive and coordinated approach that implements policy and environmental change to transform communities into geographical locations that support and promote healthy lifestyle choices for all U.S. residents. An expert panel initiated by the CDC recently identified 24 recommended strategies for obesity prevention and a suggested measurement for each strategy that communities can use to assess performance and track progress over time [88]. A list of the recommended strategies from this report is outlined as follows:

Communities should engage in the following to prevent obesity and associated mortality:

- Increase availability of healthier food and beverage choices in public service venues.
- Improve availability of affordable healthier food and beverage choices in public service venues.
- Improve geographic availability of supermarkets in underserved areas.
- Provide incentives to food retailers to locate in and/or offer healthier food and beverage choices in underserved areas.
- Improve availability of mechanisms for purchasing foods from farms.
- Incentives for the production, distribution, and procurement of foods from local farms.
- Restrict availability of less healthy foods and beverages in public service venues.
- Institute smaller portion size options in public service venues.
- Limit advertisements of less healthy foods and beverages.
- Discourage consumption of sugar-sweetened beverages.
- Increase support for breastfeeding.
- Require physical education in schools.
- Increase the amount of physical activity in PE programs in schools.
- Increase opportunities for extracurricular physical activity.
- Reduce screen time in public service venues.
- Improve access to outdoor recreational facilities.
- Enhance infrastructure supporting bicycling.
- Enhance infrastructure supporting walking.
- Support locating schools within easy walking distance of residential areas.
- Improve access to public transportation.
- Zone for mixed-use development.
- Enhance personal safety in areas where persons are or could be physically active.
- Enhance traffic safety in areas where persons are or could be physically active.
- Communities should participate in community coalitions or partnerships to address obesity.

The goal of this report is to disseminate the recommended community strategies and suggested measurements for use by local governments and communities throughout the United States. To help accomplish this, an implementation and measurement guide will be published and made available through the CDC website (available at http://www.cdc.gov/nccdphp/dnpao/publications/index.html). The dissemination of these recommended obesity prevention strategies and proposed measurements is designed to inspire communities to consider implementing new policy and environmental change initiatives aimed at reversing the current obesity epidemic [88]. The recommended strategies and suggested measurements outlined in this report are presently being pilot tested in the Minnesota and Massachusetts state surveillance systems [88]. In addition to these community strategies, national policies to improve food-label information or providing financial and economic support for local community efforts are a few examples of what can be done to enhance the environmental support for individuals who are struggling to maintain on ideal body weight for overall health.

As discussed, obesity is a complex condition that will require a significant call for action, at all levels, for both adults and children in order to prevent early mortality. From a U.S. government perspective, our government can promote change. A recent example is First Lady Michelle Obama's "Let's Move" program (http://www.letsmove.gov/). The goal of this program is to eliminate childhood obesity within an entire generation. The campaign's main points are as follows:

- Empowering parents and caregivers
- Providing healthy food in schools
- Improving access to healthy, affordable foods
- Increasing physical activity

Strategies and actions at the state/community level are outlined earlier but are all focused on community initiatives to create environments that promote good nutrition and physical activity. Finally, as health-care providers and medical clinicians, we can counsel our patients to

- Eat more fruits and vegetables and fewer foods high in fat and sugar. See http://www.choosemyplate.gov/
- Drink more water instead of sugary drinks
- Limit TV watching in kids to less than 2 h a day and do not put one in their room at all
- Support breastfeeding
- Promote policies and programs at school, at work, and in the community that make the healthy choice the easy choice
- Try going for a 10 min brisk walk, three times a day, 5 days a week

REFERENCES

1. Kopelman PG, Caterson ID, Stock MJ, Dietz WH. *Clinical Obesity in Adults and Children*. Hoboken, NJ: Blackwell Publishing, p. 493, 2005.
2. Bray GA. Medical consequences of obesity. *J Clin Endocrinol Metab* 2004; 89(6):3583–3589.
3. Wyatt S, Winters K, Dubbert P. Overweight and obesity: Prevalence, consequences and causes of a growing public health problem. *Am J Med Sci* 2006; 331(4):166–174.
4. Fontaine KR, Redden DT, Wang C, Westfall AO, Allison DB. Years of life lost due to obesity. *JAMA* 2003; 289(2):187–193.
5. Levine JA, Koepp GA. Federal health-care reform: Opportunities for obesity prevention. *Obesity* 2011; 19:897–899.
6. Caballero B. The global epidemic of obesity: An overview. *Epidemiol Rev* 2007; 29:1–5.
7. Eckel RH, Krauss RM. American Heart Association call to action: Obesity as a major risk factor for coronary heart disease. AHA Nutrition Committee. *Circulation* 1998; 97(21):2099–2100.
8. Lee IM, Manson JE, Hennekens, CH, Paffenbarger RS, Jr. Body weight and mortality. A 27-year follow-up of middle-aged men. *JAMA* 1993; 270(23):2823–2828.

9. Manson JE, Willett WC, Stampfer MJ et al. Body weight and mortality among women. *N Engl J Med* 1995; 333(11):677–685.

10. Stevens J, Cai J, Pamuk ER, Williamson DF, Thun MJ, Wood JL. The effect of age on the association between body-mass index and mortality. *N Engl J Med* 1998; 338(1):1–7.

11. WHO. Obesity: Preventing and managing the global epidemic. Geneva, Switzerland: WHO WHO/NUT/NCD/98.1. 1998.

12. Barlow SE and the Expert Committee. Expert committee recommendations regarding the prevention, assessment, and treatment of child and adolescent overweight and obesity: Summary report. *Pediatrics* 2007; 120(Suppl):S164–S192.

13. Ogden CL, Carroll MD, Curtin LR, McDowell MA, Tabak CJ, Flegal KM. Prevalence of overweight and obesity in the United States, 1999–2004. *JAMA* 2006; 295:1549–1555.

14. Flegal KM, Carroll MD, Ogden CL, Curtin LR. Prevalence and trends in obesity among US adults, 1999–2008. *JAMA* 2010; 303:235–241.

15. Centers for Disease Control and Prevention (CDC). 2010. Overweight and obesity: US obesity trends. Atlanta, GA: U.S. Department of Health and Human Services, Centers for Disease Control and Prevention. Available at: http://www.cdc.gov/obesity/data/trends.html Accessed: October 31, 2011.

16. Suminski RR, Poston WS, Jackson AS, Foreyt JP. Early identification of Mexican American children who are at risk for becoming obese. *Int J Obes* 1999; 23:823–829.

17. Centers for Disease Control and Prevention (CDC). 2011. National diabetes fact sheet: National estimates and general information on diabetes and prediabetes in the United States, 2011. Atlanta, GA: U.S. Department of Health and Human Services, Centers for Disease Control and Prevention.

18. Carey VJ, Walters EE, Colditz GA, Solomon CG, Willet WC, Rosner BA, Speizer FE, Manson JE. Body fat distribution and risk of non-insulin dependent diabetes mellitus in women: The Nurses' Health Study. *Am J Epidemiol* 1997; 145(7):614–619.

19. Chan JM, Rimm EB, Colditz GA, Stampfer MJ, Willett WC. Obesity, fat distribution, and weight gain as risk factors for clinical diabetes in men. *Diabetes Care* 1994; 17(9):961–969.

20. Mokdad AH, Ford ES, Bowman BA, Dietz WH, Vinicor F, Bales VS, Marks JS. Prevalence of obesity, diabetes, and obesity-related health risk factors, 2001. *JAMA* 2003; 289:76–79.

21. Vazquez G, Duval S, Jacobs DR Jr, Siventoinen K. Comparison of body mass index, waist circumference, and waist/hip ratio in predicting incident diabetes: A meta-analysis. *Epidemiol Rev* 2007; 29:115–128.

22. Maggio CA, Pi-Sunyer FX. Obesity and type 2 diabetes. *Endocrinol Metab Clin N Am* 2003; 32:805–822.

23. Guh DP, Zhang W, Bansback N, Amarsi Z, Birmingham CL, Anis AH. The incidence of comorbidities related to obesity and overweight: A systematic review and meta-analysis. *Am J Med* 2009; 122:248–256.

24. Writing Group for the SEARCH for Diabetes in Youth Study Group, Dabelea D, Bell RA et al. Incidence of diabetes in youth in the United States. *JAMA* 2007; 297:2716–2724.

25. Nadeau K, Dabelea D. Epidemiology of type 2 diabetes in children and adolescents. *Endocr Res* 2008; 33:35–58.

26. Verbeeten KC, Elks CE, Daneman D, Ong KK. Association between childhood obesity and subsequent Type 1 diabetes: A systematic review and meta-analysis. *Diabet Med* 2011 January; 28(1):10–18.

27. Gutin B, Islam S, Manos T, Cucuzzo N, Smith C, Stachura ME. Relation of percentage body fat and maximal aerobic capacity to risk factors for atherosclerosis and diabetes in black and white seven- to eleven-year-old children. *J Pediatr* 1994; 125:847–852.

28. Legido A, Sarria A, Bueno M, Garagorri J, Fleta J, Ramos F, Abos MD, Perez-Gonzalez J. Relationship of body fat distribution to metabolic complications in obese prepubertal boys: Gender related differences. *Acta Paediatr Scand* 1989; 78:440–446.
29. Le Stunff C, Gougneres P. Early changes in postprandial insulin secretion, not in insulin sensitivity, characterize juvenile obesity. *Diabetes* 1994; 43:696–702.
30. Yokoyama H, Okudaira M, Otani T et al. Higher incidence of diabetic nephropathy in type 2 than in type 1 diabetes in early onset diabetes in Japan. *Kidney Int* 2000; 58:302–311.
31. Yoshida Y, Hagura R, Hara Y, Sugasawa G, Akanuma Y. Risk factors for the development of diabetic retinopathy in Japanese type 2 diabetic patients. *Diabetes Res Clin Pract* 2001; 51:195–203.
32. Gungor N, Thompson T, Sutton-Tyrrell K, Janosky J, Arslanian S. Early signs of cardiovascular disease in youth with obesity and type 2 diabetes. *Diabetes Care* 2005; 28:1219–1221.
33. Colditz GA, Willett WC, Rotnitzky A, Manson JE. Weight gain as a risk factor for clinical diabetes mellitus in women. *Ann Intern Med* 1995; 122:481–486.
34. Wannamethee SG, Shaper AG, Walker M. Overweight and obesity and weight change in middle aged men: Impact on cardiovascular disease and diabetes. *J Epidemiol Community Health* 2005; 59:134–139.
35. Look AHEAD Research Group, Pi-Sunyer X, Blackburn G et al. Reduction in weight and cardiovascular disease risk factors in individuals with type 2 diabetes: One-year results of the look AHEAD trial. *Diabetes Care* 2007; 30:1374–1383.
36. Lenz M, Richter T, Muhlhauser I. The morbidity and mortality associated with overweight and obesity in adulthood. *Dtsch Arztebl Int* 2009 October; 106(40):641–648.
37. Wilson PW, D'Agostino RB, Sullivan L, Parise H, Kannel WB. Overweight and obesity as determinants of cardiovascular risk: The Framingham experience. *Arch Intern Med* 2002; 162:1867–1872.
38. Patterson RE, Frank LL, Kristal AR, White E. A comprehensive examination of health conditions associated with obesity in older adults. *Am J Prev Med* 2004; 27:385–390.
39. Droyvold WB, Midthjell K, Nilsen TI, Holmen J. Change in body mass index and its impact on blood pressure: A prospective population study. *Int J Obes* 2005; 29:650–655.
40. Gao W, DECODE Study Group. Does the constellation of risk factors with and without abdominal adiposity associate with different cardiovascular mortality risk? *Int J Obes* 2008; 32:757–762.
41. Chen K, Lindsey JB, Khera A et al. Independent associations between metabolic syndrome, diabetes mellitus and atherosclerosis: Observations from the Dallas Heart Study. *Diab Vasc Dis Res* 2008; 5:96–101.
42. Ilanne-Parikka P, Eriksson JG, Lindstrom J et al. Finnish Diabetes Prevention Study Group. Effect of lifestyle intervention on the occurrence of metabolic syndrome and its components in the Finnish Diabetes Prevention Study. *Diabetes Care* 2008; 31:805–807.
43. Phelan S, Wadden TA, Berkowitz RI et al. Impact of weight loss on the metabolic syndrome. *Int J Obes* 2007; 31:1442–1448.
44. Calle EE, Rodriquez C, Walker-Thurmond K, Thun MJ. Overweight, obesity, and mortality from cancer in a prospectively studied cohort of U.S. adults. *N Engl J Med* 2003; 348:1625–1638.
45. Reeves GK, Pirie K, Beral V, Green J, Spencer E, Bull D, Million Women Study Collaboration. Cancer incidence and mortality in relation to body mass index in the Million Women Study: Cohort study. *BMJ* 2007; 335:1134.
46. Ostlund MP, Lu Y, Lagergren J. Risk of obesity-related cancer after obesity surgery in a population-based cohort study. *Ann Surg* 2010 December; 252(6):972–976.
47. Chu SY, Callaghan WM, Kim SY et al. Maternal obesity and risk of gestational diabetes mellitus. *Diabetes Care* 2007; 30:2070–2076.

48. Kristensen J, Vestergaard M, Wisborg K, Kesmodel U, Secher NJ. Pre-pregnancy weight and the risk of stillbirth and neonatal death. *BJOG* 2005; 112:403–408.
49. Weintraub AY, Levy A, Levi I, Mazor M, Wiznitzer A, Sheiner E. Effect of bariatric surgery on pregnancy outcome. *Int J Gynaecol Obstet* 2008; 103:246–251.
50. Istvan J, Zavela K, Weidner G. Body weight and psychological distress in NHANES I. *Int J Obes Relat Metab Disord* 1992; 16:999–1003.
51. Petry NM, Barry D, Pietrzak RH, Wagner JA. Overweight and obesity are associated with psychiatric disorders: Results from the National Epidemiologic Survey on Alcohol and Related Conditions. *Psychosom Med* 2008; 70:288–297.
52. Simon GE, Ludman EJ, Linde JA et al. Association between obesity and depression in middle-aged women. *Gen Hosp Psychiatry* 2008; 30:32–39.
53. Sowers MF, Yosesf M, Jamadar D, Jacobson J, Karvonen-Gutierrez C, Jaffe M. BMI vs. body composition and radiographically defined osteoarthritis of the knee in women: A 4-year follow-up study. *Osteoarthr Cartil* 2008; 16:67–72.
54. Lementowski PW, Zelicof SB. Obesity and osteoarthritis. *Am J Orthop* 2008 March; 37(3):148–151.
55. Christensen R, Astrup A, Bliddal H. Weight loss: The treatment of choice for knee osteoarthritis? A randomized trial. *Osteoarthr Cartil* 2005; 13:20–27.
56. Liu B, Balkwill A, Spencer E, Beral V, Million Women Study Collaborators. Relationship between body mass index and length of hospital stay for gallbladder disease. *J Public Health* 2008; 30:161–166.
57. Tsai CJ, Leitzmann MF, Willett WC, Giovannucci EL. Prospective study of abdominal adiposity and gallstone disease in US men. *Am J Clin Nutr* 2004; 80:38–44.
58. Resta O, Foschino-Barbaro MP, Legari G et al. Sleep-related breathing disorders, loud snoring and excessive daytime sleepiness in obese subjects. *Int J Obes Relat Metab Disord* 2001; 25:669–675.
59. Adams TD, Gress RE, Smith SC et al. Long-term mortality after gastric bypass surgery. *N Engl J Med* 2007; 357:753–761.
60. Buchwald H, Avidor Y, Braunwald E et al. Bariatric surgery: A systematic review and meta-analysis. *JAMA* 2004; 292:1724–1737.
61. Goodman E, Dolan LM, Morrison JA, Daniels SR. Factor analysis of clustered cardio-vascular risks in adolescence: Obesity is the predominant correlate of risk among youth. *Circulation* 2005; 111:1970–1977.
62. Sorof JM, Lai D, Turner J, Poffenbarger T, Portman RJ. Overweight, ethnicity, and the prevalence of hypertension in school-aged children. *Pediatrics* 2004; 113:475–482.
63. Sivanandam S, Sinaiko AR, Jacobs DR Jr, Steffen L, Moran A, Steinberger J. Relation of increase in adiposity to increase in left ventricular mass from childhood to young adulthood. *Am J Cardiol* 2006; 98:411–415.
64. Raitakari OT, Juonala M, Viikari JS. Obesity in childhood and vascular changes in adult-hood: Insights into the Cardiovascular Risk in Young Finns Study. *Int J Obes* 2005; 29(Suppl 2):S101–S104.
65. Berenson GS, Srinivasan SR, Bao W, Newman WP 3rd, Tracy RE, Wattigney WA. Association between multiple cardiovascular risk factors and atherosclero-sis in children and young adults: The Bogalusa Heart Study. *N Engl J Med* 1998; 338:1650–1656.
66. Lauer RM, Lee J, Clarke WR. Factors affecting the relationship between childhood and adult cholesterol levels: The Muscatine Study. *Pediatrics* 1988; 82:309–318.
67. Gozal D, Capdevila OS, Kheirandish-Gozal L. Metabolic alterations and systemic inflammation in obstructive sleep apnea among nonobese and obese prepubertal chil-dren. *Am J Respir Crit Care Med* 2008; 177:1142–1149.
68. Herva A, Laitinen J, Miettunen J et al. Obesity and depression: Results from the longi-tudinal Northern Finland 1966 Birth Cohort Study. *Int J Obes* 2006; 30:520–527.

69. Anderson SE, Cohen P, Naumova EN, Jacques PF, Must A. Adolescent obesity and risk for subsequent major depressive disorder and anxiety disorder: Prospective evidence. *Psychosom Med* 2007; 69:740–747.

70. Hayden-Wade HA, Stein RI, Ghaderi A et al. Prevalence, characteristics, and correlates of teasing experiences among overweight children vs. non-overweight peers. *Obes Res* 2005; 13:1381–1392.

71. Ackard DM, Neumark-Sztainer D, Story M, Perry C. Overeating among adolescents: Prevalence and associations with weight-related characteristics and psychological health. *Pediatrics* 2003; 111:67–74.

72. Must A, Spadano J, Coakley EH, Field AE, Colditz G, Dietz WH. The disease burden associated with overweight and obesity. *JAMA* 1999 October; 282(16):1523–1529.

73. Centers for Disease Control and Prevention (CDC). 2009. Study estimates medical cost of obesity may be as high as $147 billion annually. Available at: http://www.cdc.gov/media/pressrel/2009/r090727.htm Accessed: October 31, 2011.

74. Centers for Disease Control and Prevention (CDC). 2009. Behavioral risk factor surveillance system. Available at: http://www.cdc.gov/brfss/. Accessed: October 31, 2011.

75. Sturm R. The effects of obesity, smoking and drinking on medical problems and costs. *Health Aff (Millwood)* 2002; 21(2):245–253.

76. U.S. Department of Health and Human Services (DHHS Healthy People. http://www.healthypeople.gov/Data/, Accessed: October 31, 2011). 2009.

77. Nieman DC. *Exercise Testing and Prescription: A Health Related Approach*, 7th edn. New York: McGraw Hill Companies, Inc., pp. 444–447, 2011.

78. U.S. Department of Health and Human Service (DHHS). Office of the U.S. Surgeon General. 2000. *The Surgeon General's Call to Action to Prevent and Decrease Overweight and Obesity, 2001*. Rockville, MD: U.S. Government Printing Office.

79. Ward-Smith P. Obesity—America's health crisis. *Urol Nurs* 2010 July–August; 30(4):242–245.

80. Stunkard AJ, Wadden TA. Psychological aspects of severe obesity. *Am J Clin Nutr* 1992 February; 55(2 Suppl):524S–532S.

81. Gortmaker SL, Must A, Perrin JM, Sobol AM, Dietz WH. Social and economic consequences of overweight in adolescence and young adulthood. *N Engl J Med* 1993 September; 329(14):1008–1012.

82. Finkelstein EA, DiBonaventura M, Burgess SM, Hale BC. The costs of obesity in the workplace. *J Occup Environ Med* 2010 October; 52(10):971–976.

83. Russell GV, Pierce CW, Nunley L. Financial implications of obesity. *Orthop Clin N Am* 2011 January; 42(1):123–127.

84. Thompson D, Edelsberg J, Kinsey KL et al. Estimated costs of obesity to U.S. business. *Am J Health Promot* 1998; 13(2):120–127.

85. National Institutes of Health Consensus Development Conference Statement. Health implications of obesity. *Ann Intern Med* 1985; 103:981–1077.

86. Stevens J, Cai J, Juhaeri J, Thun MJ, Wood JL. Evaluation of WHO and NHANES II standards for overweight using mortality rates. *J Am Diet Assoc* 2000 July; 100(7):825–827.

87. Tsai AG, Wadden TA. Systematic review: An evaluation of major commercial weight loss programs in the United States. *Ann Intern Med* 2005 January; 142(1):56–66.

88. Kahn LK, Sobush K, Keener D et al. Recommended community strategies and measurements to prevent obesity in the United States. *MMWR* 2009; 58(RR-7):1–26.

4 Identification, Evaluation, and Treatment of Overweight and Obesity

George A. Bray, MD

CONTENTS

INTRODUCTION

Overweight is now recognized as a risk factor for overall mortality and cardiovascular disease, diabetes, gallbladder disease, cancer, and many other diseases.[1,2] In this context, it is important to evaluate and treat obesity and other risk factors to reduce the overall likelihood for developing these comorbid diseases and to reduce the social consequences of being obese.

This chapter addresses identification and evaluation of the overweight patient as a guide to selection of treatment.[3-5] Both clinical and laboratory information are needed for this evaluation. To make this evaluation effective, it must be done in the context of a sympathetic office practice concerned with the care and treatment of overweight patients. For additional insights into care of the obese patient in a primary care setting, the reader is referred elsewhere.[6]

IDENTIFICATION OF OBESITY

Obesity has a long tradition in clinical practice and has often been identified simply by observing the individual. As the implications of obesity on health have become clearer, definitions and methods of measurement have become more important in helping to define risk. Obesity refers to an increase in body fat, a measurement that is not easily done in clinical practice. Moreover, interpretation of body fatness depends on such factors as gender, age, ethnic group, and level of physical activity. "Overweight" is an increase in body weight relative to some standard and has become a surrogate for "obesity" both clinically and epidemiologically. This will be the focus of techniques described later. The importance of centrally located fat has also become evident. Central adiposity refers to conditions where fat is located more in the abdominal area than on the hips, thighs, or arms. Techniques for quantifying this are also described. Central adiposity is a key element of the metabolic syndrome, a collection of measurements that reflect resistance to the action of insulin, and which have central adiposity as a key component, along with elevated blood pressure, elevated plasma glucose, elevated triglycerides, and low levels of high-density lipoprotein (HDL) cholesterol.

EVALUATION OF THE OBESE/OVERWEIGHT PATIENT

INFORMATION FROM THE CLINICAL INTERVIEW

The clinician or therapist who sees an overweight patient needs to obtain certain basic information, which is relevant to assessing the patient's risk from obesity. This includes an understanding of the events that led to the development of obesity, what the patient has done to deal with the problem, and how successful or unsuccessful he or she was in these efforts. The family constellation is important for identifying attitudes about obesity and the possibility of finding rare genetic causes. Information about the amount of weight gain (>22 lb or >10 kg) since ages 18–20 and the rate of weight gain is important because this is related to the risk of developing complications from obesity.[7] The type and regularity of physical activity is also important since physical inactivity increases cardiovascular risk, particularly in overweight individuals.[8] Information about comorbid conditions such as diabetes, hypertension, heart disease, sleep apnea, and gall gladder disease also needs to be elicited. Since a number of drugs can cause significant weight gain (Table 4.1), a history of medication use for mental health problems, depression, convulsive disorders, diabetes, and the use of steroids for asthma should be elicited as well.[1,8] Information about whether the patient/client is "ready" to put in the effort needed to lose weight can help the

TABLE 4.1
Drugs That Produce Weight Gain and Alternatives

Category	Drugs That Cause Weight Gain	Possible Alternatives
Neuroleptics	Thioridazine, olanzapine, quetiapine, risperidone, and clozapine	Molindone, haloperidol, and ziprasidone
Antidepressants		
Tricyclics	Amitriptyline and nortriptyline	
Monoamine oxidase inhibitors	Imipramine	Protriptyline
Selective serotonin reuptake inhibitors	Mirtazapine	Bupropion and nefazodone
	Paroxetine	Fluoxetine and sertraline
Anticonvulsants	Valproate, carbamazepine, and gabapentin	Topiramate, lamotrigine, and zonisamide
Antidiabetic drugs	Insulin	Acarbose, miglitol, and sibutramine
	Sulfonylureas	
	Thiazolidinediones	Metformin and orlistat
Antiserotonin	Pizotifen	
Antihistamines	Cyproheptadine	Inhalers and decongestants
β-Adrenergic blockers	Propranolol	Angiotensin-converting enzyme inhibitors and calcium channel blockers
α-Adrenergic blockers	Terazosin	
Steroid hormones	Contraceptives	Barrier methods
	Glucocorticoids	Nonsteroidal anti-inflammatory agents
	Progestational steroids	

health-care professional decide with the patient whether this is the right time to proceed with treatment. Information about possible etiologies for obesity also needs to be obtained, for example, altered menstrual history in women, suggesting polycystic ovary syndrome, or purplish abdominal striae, suggesting Cushing's disease.

Information from Physical Evaluation

Step 1: Measure Body Mass Index

As part of any clinical encounter, the nurse or physician should measure several vital signs including height and weight to calculate body mass index (BMI), waist circumference, pulse, blood pressure, and, if indicated by the patient's complaints, temperature.[1,9] Accurate measurements of height with a wall-mounted stadiometer and weight with a regularly calibrated scale are used to calculate the BMI.[9,10] The body mass or Quetelet index is calculated as the body weight (kg) divided by the stature (height [m]) squared (wt/ht^2), or body weight (lb) × 703 divided by the height (stature) squared (wt [lb] × 703/[ht (in.)])^2. Table 4.2 lists BMI values for height in centimeters or inches and weight in kilograms or pounds. BMI correlates well with body fat and is relatively unaffected by height.

TABLE 4.2
Body Mass Index (Using Either Pounds and Inches or Kilograms and Centimeters)

BMI (kg/m²)

Inches	19	20	21	22	23	24	25	26	27	28	29	30	31	32	33	34	35	36	37	38	39	40	Centimeters
58	91	95	100	105	110	115	119	124	129	134	138	143	148	153	158	162	167	172	177	181	186	191	147
	41	*43*	*45*	*48*	*50*	*52*	*54*	*56*	*58*	*61*	*63*	*65*	*67*	*69*	*71*	*73*	*76*	*78*	*80*	*82*	*84*	*86*	
59	94	99	104	109	114	119	124	128	133	138	143	148	153	158	163	168	173	178	183	188	193	198	150
	43	*45*	*47*	*50*	*52*	*54*	*56*	*59*	*61*	*63*	*65*	*68*	*70*	*72*	*74*	*77*	*79*	*81*	*83*	*86*	*88*	*90*	
60	97	102	107	112	118	123	128	133	138	143	148	153	158	164	169	174	179	184	189	194	199	204	152
	44	*46*	*49*	*51*	*53*	*55*	*58*	*60*	*62*	*65*	*67*	*69*	*72*	*74*	*76*	*79*	*81*	*83*	*85*	*88*	*90*	*92*	
61	100	106	111	116	121	127	132	137	143	148	153	158	164	169	174	180	185	190	195	201	206	211	155
	46	*48*	*50*	*53*	*55*	*58*	*60*	*62*	*65*	*67*	*70*	*72*	*74*	*77*	*79*	*82*	*84*	*86*	*89*	*91*	*94*	*96*	
62	104	109	115	120	125	131	136	142	147	153	158	164	169	175	180	186	191	196	202	207	213	218	158
	47	*50*	*52*	*55*	*57*	*60*	*62*	*65*	*67*	*70*	*72*	*75*	*77*	*80*	*82*	*85*	*87*	*90*	*92*	*95*	*97*	*100*	
63	107	113	118	124	130	135	141	146	152	158	163	169	175	180	186	192	197	203	208	214	220	225	160
	49	*51*	*54*	*56*	*59*	*61*	*64*	*67*	*69*	*72*	*74*	*77*	*79*	*82*	*84*	*87*	*90*	*92*	*95*	*97*	*100*	*102*	
64	110	116	122	128	134	140	145	151	157	163	169	174	180	186	192	198	203	209	215	221	227	233	162
	50	*52*	*55*	*58*	*60*	*63*	*66*	*68*	*71*	*73*	*76*	*79*	*81*	*84*	*87*	*89*	*92*	*94*	*97*	*100*	*102*	*105*	
65	114	120	126	132	138	144	150	156	162	168	174	180	186	192	198	204	210	216	222	228	234	240	165
	52	*54*	*57*	*60*	*63*	*65*	*68*	*71*	*74*	*76*	*79*	*82*	*84*	*87*	*90*	*93*	*95*	*98*	*101*	*103*	*106*	*109*	
66	117	124	130	136	142	148	155	161	167	173	179	185	191	198	204	210	216	223	229	235	241	247	168
	54	*56*	*59*	*62*	*65*	*68*	*71*	*73*	*76*	*79*	*82*	*85*	*87*	*90*	*93*	*96*	*99*	*102*	*104*	*107*	*110*	*113*	
67	121	127	134	140	147	153	159	166	172	178	185	191	198	204	210	217	223	229	236	242	248	255	170
	55	*58*	*61*	*64*	*66*	*69*	*72*	*75*	*78*	*81*	*84*	*87*	*90*	*92*	*95*	*98*	*101*	*104*	*107*	*110*	*113*	*116*	

in	19	20	21	22	23	24	25	26	27	28	29	30	31	32	33	34	35	36	37	38	39	40	cm
68	*125*	*131*	*138*	*144*	*151*	*158*	*164*	*171*	*177*	*184*	*190*	*197*	*203*	*210*	*217*	*223*	*230*	*236*	*243*	*249*	*256*	*263*	**173**
	57	**60**	**63**	**66**	**69**	**72**	**75**	**78**	**81**	**84**	**87**	**90**	**93**	**96**	**99**	**102**	**105**	**108**	**111**	**114**	**117**	**120**	
69	*128*	*135*	*142*	*149*	*155*	*162*	*169*	*176*	*182*	*189*	*196*	*203*	*209*	*216*	*223*	*230*	*237*	*243*	*250*	*257*	*264*	*270*	**175**
	58	**61**	**64**	**67**	**70**	**74**	**77**	**80**	**83**	**86**	**89**	**92**	**95**	**98**	**101**	**104**	**107**	**110**	**113**	**116**	**119**	**123**	
70	*132*	*139*	*146*	*153*	*160*	*167*	*174*	*181*	*188*	*195*	*202*	*209*	*216*	*223*	*230*	*236*	*243*	*250*	*257*	*264*	*271*	*278*	**178**
	60	**63**	**67**	**70**	**73**	**76**	**79**	**82**	**86**	**89**	**92**	**95**	**98**	**101**	**105**	**108**	**111**	**114**	**117**	**120**	**124**	**127**	
71	*136*	*143*	*150*	*157*	*165*	*172*	*179*	*186*	*193*	*200*	*207*	*215*	*222*	*229*	*236*	*243*	*250*	*258*	*265*	*272*	*279*	*286*	**180**
	62	**65**	**68**	**71**	**75**	**78**	**81**	**84**	**87**	**91**	**94**	**97**	**100**	**104**	**107**	**110**	**113**	**117**	**120**	**123**	**126**	**130**	
72	*140*	*147*	*155*	*162*	*169*	*177*	*184*	*191*	*199*	*206*	*213*	*221*	*228*	*235*	*243*	*250*	*258*	*265*	*272*	*280*	*287*	*294*	**183**
	64	**67**	**70**	**74**	**77**	**80**	**84**	**87**	**90**	**94**	**97**	**100**	**104**	**107**	**111**	**114**	**117**	**121**	**124**	**127**	**131**	**134**	
73	*144*	*151*	*159*	*166*	*174*	*182*	*189*	*197*	*204*	*212*	*219*	*227*	*234*	*242*	*250*	*257*	*265*	*272*	*280*	*287*	*295*	*303*	**185**
	65	**68**	**72**	**75**	**79**	**82**	**86**	**89**	**92**	**96**	**99**	**103**	**106**	**110**	**113**	**116**	**120**	**123**	**127**	**130**	**133**	**137**	
74	*148*	*155*	*163*	*171*	*179*	*187*	*194*	*202*	*210*	*218*	*225*	*233*	*241*	*249*	*256*	*264*	*272*	*280*	*288*	*295*	*303*	*311*	**188**
	67	**71**	**74**	**78**	**81**	**85**	**88**	**92**	**95**	**99**	**102**	**106**	**110**	**113**	**117**	**120**	**124**	**127**	**131**	**134**	**138**	**141**	
75	*152*	*160*	*168*	*176*	*184*	*192*	*200*	*208*	*216*	*224*	*232*	*240*	*247*	*255*	*263*	*271*	*279*	*287*	*295*	*303*	*311*	*319*	**190**
	69	**72**	**76**	**79**	**83**	**87**	**90**	**94**	**97**	**101**	**105**	**108**	**112**	**116**	**119**	**123**	**126**	**130**	**134**	**137**	**141**	**144**	
76	*156*	*164*	*172*	*180*	*189*	*197*	*205*	*213*	*221*	*230*	*238*	*246*	*254*	*262*	*271*	*279*	*287*	*295*	*303*	*312*	*320*	*328*	**193**
	71	**74**	**78**	**82**	**86**	**89**	**93**	**97**	**101**	**104**	**108**	**112**	**115**	**119**	**123**	**127**	**130**	**134**	**138**	**142**	**145**	**149**	
BMI	**19**	**20**	**21**	**22**	**23**	**24**	**25**	**26**	**27**	**28**	**29**	**30**	**31**	**32**	**33**	**34**	**35**	**36**	**37**	**38**	**39**	**40**	**BMI**

Source: Bray, G.A., Classification and evaluation of the overweight patient in *Handbook of Obesity*, G.A. Bray, C. Bouchard, W.P.T. James eds., Marcel Dekker, Inc., New York, 1998, pp. 831–854.

Note: The BMI is shown as bold underlined numbers at the top and bottom. To determine your BMI, select your height in either inches or centimeters and move across the row until you find your weight in pounds or inches. Your BMI can be read at the top or bottom.
The italics are for pounds and inches; the bold is for kilograms and centimeters.

Step 2: Measure Waist Circumference

Waist circumference is the most practical clinical approach to assessing visceral fat. Waist circumference is measured with a flexible tape placed horizontally at the level of the superior iliac crest.[9,10] Measuring the change in waist circumference is a good tool for following the progress of weight loss. It is particularly valuable when patients become more physically active. Physical activity may slow loss of muscle mass and thus slow weight loss while fat continues to be mobilized. Changes in waist circumference can help in making this distinction. As with BMI, the relationship of central fat to risk factors for health varies among populations as well as within them.

Current classifications of obesity are based on BMI and waist circumference. The one recommended by the World Health Organization[5] and the National Heart, Lung, and Blood Institute (NHLBI)[4] is shown in Table 4.3.

BMI has a curvilinear relationship to risk. Several levels of risk can be identified using the BMI (Figure 4.1).[8] These cut points are derived from data collected on Caucasians. It is now clear that different ethnic groups have different percentages of body fat for the same BMI. Thus, the same BMI presumably carries a different risk in each of these populations. The percent body fat for the same BMI in Caucasians is somewhat different from that of African Americans, Asians, and Latinos.[12] For Japanese, a BMI of 23 or 24 kg/m² has the same percent fat as that of a BMI of 25 in Caucasians or 28–29 in African Americans. Based on these differences and the observations that the risk for diabetes and hypertension had doubled when the BMI was 25 kg/m², a task force from the Asia-Oceania section of the International Association for the Study of Obesity[13] has proposed an alternative table, where

TABLE 4.3
Classification of Overweight and Obesity as Recommended by the NHLBI Guidelines

Disease Risk[a] Relative to Normal Weight and Waist Circumference

	BMI (kg/m²)	Obesity Class	Waist Circumference	
			<102 cm (Men) <88 cm (Women)	>102 cm (Men) >88 cm (Women)
Underweight	<18.5		—	—
Normal[b]	18.5–24.9		—	—
Overweight	25.0–29.9		Increased	High
Obesity	30.0–34.9	1	High	Very high
	35.0–39.9	2	Very high	Very high
Extreme obesity	≥40.0	3	Extremely high	Extremely high

Source: NHLBI Obesity Education Initiative Expert Panel on the Identification, Evaluation, and Treatment of Overweight and Obesity in Adults, *Obes. Res.*, 6(Suppl 2), 51S, 1998.

BMI, body mass index.

[a] Disease risk for type 2 diabetes, hypertension, and cardiovascular disease.

[b] Increased waist can also be a marker for increased risk in normal weight individuals.

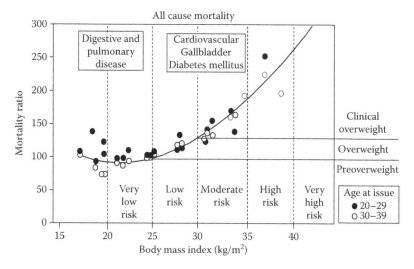

FIGURE 4.1   Curvilinear relationship between BMI and risk. (From Bray, G.A., *Obesity and the Metabolic Syndrome*, Humana Press, Inc., Totowa, NJ, 2007; Bray, G.A., Classification and evaluation of the overweight patient. In *Handbook of Obesity*, G.A. Bray, C. Bouchard, and W.P.T. James (eds)., Marcel Dekker, Inc., New York, 1998, pp. 831–854.)

obesity is defined as a BMI > 25 kg/m² and high-risk waist circumference at >90 cm for men and >80 cm for women (Table 4.4).

Data from Hispanics and African Americans suggest that increased body fat carries a greater risk of diabetes but has less impact on heart disease. After treatment begins, regular measurement of body weight is one important way to follow the progress of any treatment program.

TABLE 4.4

Classification of Obesity as Recommended by the Asia-Pacific Task Force

| | | Risk of Comorbidities | |
| | | Waist Circumference | |
Classification	BMI (kg/m²)	<90 cm (Men) <80 cm (Women)	≥90 cm (Men) ≥80 cm (Women)
Underweight	<18.5	Low (but increased risk of other clinical problems)	Average
Normal range	18.5–22.9	Average	Increased
Overweight	≥23		
At risk	23–24.9	Increased	Moderate
Obese I	25–25.9	Moderate	Severe
Obese II	≥30	Severe	Very severe

BMI, body mass index.

Other Aspects of the Physical Examination of Obesity

A number of physical features of an obese individual may help identify a specific cause for the individual's problem. Hypothalamic obesity is a rare syndrome resulting from brain injury that produces variable degrees of obesity and neurologic findings.[14] Cushing's syndrome with its striae, obesity, and hypertension represents the consequences of increased levels of adrenal steroids.[15] Polycystic ovarian disease is a common cause of obesity in younger women.[16] It is associated with mild excess of androgen and with marked insulin resistance. Among the various genetic diseases that produce obesity, the Prader–Willi is the most common. It includes hypotonia, mental retardation, and sexual immaturity and can usually be recognized clinically. The Bardet–Biedl syndrome with its polydactyly and retinal disease is distinctive. A child with obesity and red hair might suggest a defect in the processing of proopiomelanocortin.[17] Detection of acanthosis nigricans should suggest significant insulin resistance. This is a clinical finding of increased very dark pigmentation in the folds of the neck, along the exterior surface of the distal extremities, and over the knuckles. It may signify increased insulin resistance or malignancy, and these possibilities should be evaluated. Although 40 other genes have been associated with obesity, individually they only contribute a small amount.

INFORMATION FROM LABORATORY TESTS

The third part of the evaluation comes from laboratory tests. At the present time, laboratory tests often come in "batteries" that provide a larger number of tests than may be needed, but where unbundling these tests is more expensive than any benefits it gains. It is thus important to focus attention on the laboratory tests that are most relevant to decision making about the overweight patient.

Plasma glucose: Over 7% of the adult American population has diabetes, and in the face of an epidemic, measurement and, if needed, confirmation of a high glucose or a high 2 h value from a glucose tolerance test may be indicated.

Plasma lipids: A low level of HDL cholesterol and a high triglyceride level provide one combination of laboratory values that are included in the diagnosis of the metabolic syndrome and are thus important values to determine. LDL cholesterol is the pivotal lipoprotein in decisions about the prevention and treatment of coronary heart disease.[18] In the presence of diabetes, the target values for beginning treatment are lowered.

Thyroid-stimulating hormone: Thyroid-stimulating hormone (TSH) is important as an index of hypothyroidism, which can occur in up to 4% of older women and may be a factor in weight gain at this time in life.

Prostate-specific antigen: Prostate cancer is one of the male cancers associated with obesity. Although prostate-specific antigen (PSA) is a common screening test in men, the relationship of obesity to prostate cancer highlights its value when screening overweight men.

SPECIALIZED TESTS

Because diabetes, gallbladder disease, heart disease, sleep apnea, and cancer have a relationship to obesity,[2,8] these are important conditions to evaluate with specialized tests.

Sleep study: Sleep apnea is common in obesity.[8] If suspected, a sleep study can make the diagnosis. Continuous positive airway pressure (CPAP) can be used to treat this condition.

Ultrasound of the gallbladder: The high prevalence of gall stones in obese men and women would suggest the desirability of an ultrasound, especially if there are any abdominal complaints of indigestion.[2]

Electrocardiograms and echocardiography: An ECG is commonly done as part of a physical examination. Echocardiography and other specialized test may be indicated if the patient has symptoms of chest pain.

Mammography: Breast cancer is increased in obese women. The presence of obesity may suggest the need for mammography on an individualized basis.

METABOLIC SYNDROME

The metabolic syndrome is a complex of traits that are associated with the risk of diabetes and cardiovascular disease. Although it includes a variety of factors, diagnosis can be made when three of the following five measures are abnormal: adiposity, blood pressure, HDL cholesterol, triglycerides, or glucose[1,18] (Table 4.5). The syndrome is associated with abdominal obesity, measured in this definition by waist circumference. The recognition that different ethnic populations have different

TABLE 4.5
Clinical Features of the Metabolic Syndrome

Risk Factor	Defining Level
Abdominal obesity (waist circumference)	
Men	>102 cm (>40 in.)
Women	>88 cm (>35 in.)
HDL cholesterol	
Men	<40 mg/dL
Women	<50 mg/dL
Triglycerides	≥150 mg/dL
Fasting glucose	≥100 mg/dL
Blood pressure (systolic/diastolic)	≥130/≥85 mmHg

HDL, high-density lipoprotein.

relations of abdominal fat and its risks indicates that these definitions, like BMI, need ethnic sensitivity in their interpretation. Individuals of Asian descent (Chinese, Japanese, and South Indians) may have more abdominal fat for a given BMI and body fat than Caucasians.

GUIDELINES FOR TREATMENT

Once the workup for etiologic and complicating factors is complete, the risk associated with elevated BMI, fat distribution, weight gain, and level of physical activity can be evaluated. Several algorithms have been developed for this purpose, but the one we will use is from the NHLBI (Figure 4.2).[4]

The BMI (Table 4.2) provides the first assessment of risk. Individuals with a BMI below 25 kg/m^2 are at very low risk, but, nonetheless, nearly half of those in this category at ages 20–25 will become overweight by ages 60–69. Thus, a large group of preoverweight individuals are at risk for further weight gain. Health risk rises with a BMI above 25–30 kg/m^2. The presence of complicating factors further increases this risk.

Treatments for obesity can be risky. In many cases, treatment for obesity needs to be chronic, hence the emphasis on risk–benefit evaluation and safety. Each treatment listed in Table 4.6 has been associated with an unwanted therapeutic outcome. This must temper enthusiasm for new treatments unless the risk is very low. Because obesity is stigmatized, any treatment approved by the FDA will be used for cosmetic purposes by preoverweight people who suffer the stigma of obesity. Thus, drugs to treat obesity must have very high safety profiles.

IS THE PATIENT READY TO LOSE WEIGHT?

Before initiating any treatment, it is important to know that the patient is ready to make changes. A series of questions developed by Brownell[19] in *The Dieting Readiness Test* can be used to assess this.

When counseling patients who are ready to lose weight, accommodation of their individual needs, as well as ethnic factors, age, and other differences, is essential. The approach outlined earlier is not rigid and must be used to help guide clinical decision making, not to serve as an alternative to considering individual factors in developing a treatment plan. Because of increasing complications of obesity, more aggressive efforts at therapy should be directed at people in each of the successively higher risk classifications, as defined in the table by BMI. This is shown in Table 4.7.

DO PATIENT AND DOCTOR HAVE REALISTIC EXPECTATIONS?

The doctor and his or her assistant who find an elevated BMI should take a moment to make sure the patient knows his or her BMI and waist circumference and how to interpret them. If the patient knows his or her BMI, it suggests that the physician or assistant also knows the BMI. However, a clinical survey showed that only 42% of obese patients seen for a routine checkup were told they needed to lose weight.[20] We need to do better for our patients.

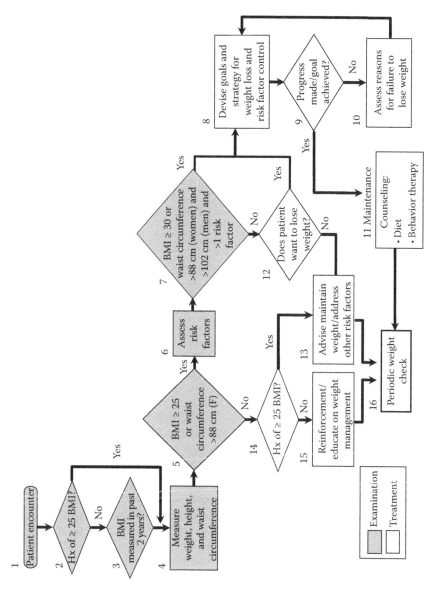

FIGURE 4.2   Treatment algorithm from the NHLBI. BMI, body mass index; Hx, history.

TABLE 4.6
Unintended Consequences from Treatments for Obesity

Year	Drug	Consequences
1892	Thyroid extract	Hyperthyroidism
1932	Dinitrophenol	Neuropathy/cataracts
1937	Amphetamine	Addiction
1968	Multicolored pills with diuretics and digitalis	Deaths from arrhythmias
1985	Gelatin-based very-low-calorie formula diets	Cardiovascular deaths
1997	Phentermine/fenfluramine combined therapy	Cardiac valvular regurgitation and pulmonary hypertension
1998	Phenylpropanolamine	Strokes
2003	Ma huang (ephedra alkaloids)	Heart attacks and stroke
2008	Rimonabant	Suicidality
2010	Sibutramine	Cardiovascular deaths

TABLE 4.7
Selection of Treatments Based on the BMI

Treatment	25–29.9	27–29.9	30–34.9	35–39.9	>40
Diet, exercise, and lifestyle	+	+	+	+	+
Pharmacotherapy		With comorbidities	+	+	+
Surgery				With comorbidities	+

The realities of treatment for obesity are often at odds with a patient's expectations. Patients were asked to give the weights they wanted to achieve in several categories, from their dream weight to a weight loss that would leave them disappointed.[21] When we compare the goals of these patients with reported outcomes, we find that many treatments will leave patients disappointed. Note that only the surgical intervention produced a "dream" weight loss. None of the other treatments produced weight loss that would allow patients to achieve their dream weight, which was on average 38% below baseline. Nearly half failed to achieve even a weight-loss outcome that would disappoint them (>15% weight loss). The desire to lose weight from a cosmetic standpoint almost always conflicts with the reality of weight loss. This mismatch between patient expectations and the realities of weight loss provides clinicians and their patients with an important challenge as they begin treatment. A weight-loss goal of 5%–15% can be achieved by most patients and will improve many of the risk factors associated with obesity. Larger weight losses are only consistently produced with surgery.

One complaint about treatments for obesity is that they frequently fail. By this, patients mean that weight loss stops well short of their desired level. An alternative interpretation may be better.[26] Overweight is not curable. However, it can be treated in many ways, but in all cases, weight loss reaches a "plateau." When treatment is stopped, weight is regained. This is similar to what happens in patients with hypertension who stop taking their antihypertensive drugs, or in patients with high cholesterol who stop taking their hypocholesterolemic drugs. In each case, blood pressure or cholesterol rises. Like overweight, these chronic diseases have not been cured, but rather palliated. When treatment is stopped, the risk factor recurs.

Patients who are ready to lose weight and have a reasonable expectation for their weight-loss goals are ready to begin. An ideal outcome is a return of body weight to normal range, with no weight gain thereafter.[1]

However, this is rarely achieved and is unrealistic for most patients. Rather, they need guidance in accepting a realistic goal. A satisfactory outcome is a maintenance of body weight over the ensuing years. A good outcome would be a loss of 5%–15% of initial body weight and regain no faster than the increase in body weight of the population.[22] Patients who achieve this should be applauded. An excellent outcome would be weight loss of more than 15% of body weight. An unsatisfactory outcome is a loss of less than 5% with regain above the population weight. If weight loss is <5%, therapy should be modified or discontinued.

QUALITY OF LIFE

Quality of life is important for all patients. This has effects in many areas. From the health-care perspective, a reduction in comorbidities is a significant improvement. Remission of type 2 diabetes or hypertension can reduce costs of treating these conditions, as well as delay or prevent the development of disease.[22,23] Weight loss can reduce the wear and tear on joints and slows the development of osteoarthritis. Sleep apnea usually resolves.[8]

Psychosocial improvement is of great importance to patients. Studies of patients who achieved long-term weight loss from surgical intervention show improved social and economic function of previously disabled overweight patients.[24] Loss of 5% or more of initial weight almost always translates into improved mobility, improvement in sleep disturbances, increased exercise tolerance, and heightened self-esteem. A focus on these, rather than cosmetic outcomes, is essential.

REALITIES OF OVERWEIGHT

Overweight is a chronic, stigmatized disease that is increasing in prevalence, with more than 60% of the American population now overweight (BMI > 25kg/m^2).[25] This represents more than 100 million people. The prevalence of obesity (BMI > 30kg/m^2) has risen more than 100% in the last 30 years and continues to increase. The social disapproval of obesity and the lengths people go to prevent or reverse it fuels a $100 billion/year set of industries. Nearly 65% of American women consider themselves overweight, and even more (66%–75%) want to weigh less. The figures for men are somewhat less. More than 50% of the women with a BMI < 21kg/m^2 (normal weight) want to weigh less. This individual perception of a "desirable" weight for them indicates the degree of both the stigmatization for those who are not "thin" and the drive to lose weight.[8]

The stigma of obesity is also evident in the general public disapproval of corpulence and in the disapproving moral attitudes of many health-care professionals. For example, mental health workers are more likely to assign negative psychological symptoms to the obese than to normal-weight people. Nursing, medical, and ancillary health-care personnel also carry these negative stereotypes. Sensitivity training for health professionals dealing with overweight patients is important in any office or clinic offering treatment for obesity.[6]

Overweight has many causes. The natural history of obesity indicates that it occurs gradually. Although overweight in childhood carries a serious adverse prognosis, particularly if the parents are overweight, nearly two-thirds of overweight adults developed their problem in adult life.

Results from most long-term clinical studies of treatment for overweight patients show a high prevalence of weight regain. In the Institute of Medicine report "Weighing the Options,"[26] for those who achieved weight loss, more than one-third of the weight typically was regained within 1 year, and nearly all within 5 years. Despite this gloomy report, many long-term successes have occurred. A study of secondary prevention in successful weight maintainers showed no differences between those who regained weight in reported level of energy expenditure from exercise. However, those who successfully maintained weight loss showed greater control of fat intake, which included avoiding fried foods and substituting low-fat foods for high-fat foods. Several other programs have also reported long-term weight loss or prevention, especially in children.[1]

Overweight, central or abdominal fat, weight gain after age 20, and a sedentary lifestyle all increase health risks and increase economic costs of obesity. Intentional weight loss by overweight individuals, on the other hand, reduces these risks. Although data are not yet available, researchers widely believe that long-term intentional weight loss lowers overall mortality, particularly from diabetes, gallbladder disease, hypertension, heart disease, and some types of cancer.[8]

GUIDELINES FOR TREATMENT BY AGE GROUP

After evaluating a patient and deciding that he or she is ready to lose weight, the potential treatments can be grouped by age and BMI.

AGES 1–10 YEARS

Table 4.8 shows the strategies available for overweight children. A variety of genetic factors can enhance obesity in this age group. This age group also contains a high percentage of preoverweight individuals. Identifying individuals at highest risk for becoming overweight in adult life allows us to focus on preventive strategies. Among these strategies is the need to develop patterns of physical activity and good eating habits, including a lower fat intake, lower energy-density diet, and smaller portion sizes. For growing children, medications should be used to treat the comorbidities directly. Drugs for weight loss are generally inappropriate until the patient reaches adult height, and surgical intervention should only be considered after consultation with medical and surgical experts.

TABLE 4.8
Therapeutic Strategies: Ages 1–10 Years

Predictors of Overweight	Therapeutic Strategies		
	Preoverweight at Risk	Preclinical Overweight	Clinical Overweight
Positive family history	Family counseling	Family behavior therapy	Treat comorbidities
Genetic defects	Reduce inactivity	Exercise	Exercise
(dysmorphic)		Low-fat/low-energy-	Low-fat/low-energy-
Prader–Willi		dense diet	dense diet
syndrome			
Bardet–Biedl; Cohen			
Hypothalamic injury			
Low metabolic rate			
Diabetic mother			

AGES 11–50 YEARS

Table 4.9 outlines the available strategies for overweight and obese adults. Since nearly two-thirds of preoverweight individuals move into the overweight and obese categories in this age range, this age is quantitatively the most important. Preventive strategies should be used for patients with predictors of weight gain. These should include advice on lifestyle changes, including increased physical activity, which would benefit almost all adults, and good dietary practices, including a diet lower in saturated fat.

For patients in the overweight category, behavioral strategies should be added to these lifestyle strategies. This is particularly important for overweight adolescents, because good 10-year data show that intervention for this group can reduce the degree of overweight in adult life. Data on the efficacy of behavioral programs carried out in controlled settings show that weight losses average of 7%–10% in trials

TABLE 4.9
Therapeutic Strategies: Appropriate for Individuals from Ages 11 to 50

Predictors of Overweight	Therapeutic Strategies		
	Preoverweight at Risk	Preclinical Overweight	Clinical Overweight
Positive family history	Reduce sedentary	Behavior therapy	Treat comorbidities
of diabetes or obesity	lifestyle	Low-fat/low-energy-	Drug treatment for
Endocrine disorders	Low-fat/low-energy-	dense diet	overweight
(polycystic ovary	dense diet	Reduce sedentary	Reduce sedentary
syndrome)	Portion control	lifestyle	lifestyle
Multiple pregnancies			Low-fat/low-energy-
Marriage			dense diet
Smoking cessation			Behavior therapy
Medication			Surgery

lasting more than 16 weeks. The limitation is the likelihood of regaining weight once the behavioral treatment ends, although a long-term behavioral therapy study did provide long-term weight loss.[1]

Medication should be seriously considered for clinically overweight individuals in this group. Two strategies can be used. The first is to use drugs to treat each comorbidity, that is, individually treating diabetes, hypertension, dyslipidemia, and sleep apnea. Alternatively, or in addition, patients with a BMI > $30 kg/m^2$ could be treated with antiobesity drugs. Current FDA-approved drugs include appetite suppressants that act on the central nervous system and orlistat, which blocks pancreatic lipase. The availability of these agents differs from country to country, and any physician planning to use them should be familiar with the local regulations. Most of the drugs on the market were reviewed and approved more than 20 years ago and are approved for short-term use only.[8] The basis for the short-term use is twofold. First, almost all the studies of these agents are short term. Second, the regulatory agencies are concerned about the potential for abuse and thus have restricted most of them to prescription use with limitations. The withdrawal of fenfluramine and dexfenfluramine from the market in 1997 following in the development of valvular heart disease, and rimonabant in 2008 for psychiatric side effects, further compounds the concern of health authorities about the safety of these drugs. Because of the regulatory limitations and the lack of longer-term data on safety and efficacy, the use of the drugs approved for short-term treatment must be carefully justified. They may be useful in initiating treatment and in helping a patient who is relapsing.

Only one drug, orlistat, is currently approved for long-term use. Orlistat (Xenical®), a drug that blocks intestinal lipase, is approved for long-term use in most countries. In clinical trials lasting up to 2 years, orlistat was associated with a mean weight loss of up to 10% at the end of 1 year in patients who were prescribed a 30% fat diet. As might be expected, because the drug blocks pancreatic lipase in the intestine, fecal fat loss is increased. Major side effects reported early were markedly reduced over time, implying that patients learned to use the drug effectively in relation to dietary intake of fat. The effective use of this medication requires that physicians and their staffs provide good dietary control counseling to patients.[8] Orlistat in a lower dose is also available without prescription in some countries.[27]

AGE OVER 51 YEARS

Table 4.10 shows the proposed treatments for this age group. By age 50, almost all of the people who will become overweight have done so. Thus, preventive strategies are no longer important, and the focus is on treatment for those who are overweight or obese. The basic treatments and treatment considerations are similar to those of the younger group. However, in this age group, the argument may be stronger for directly treating comorbidities and paying less attention to weight loss. For patients in this group who wish to lose weight, however, the considerations for patients between ages 11 and 50 still apply. Surgery should only be considered for individuals with class II or III obesity, or who are severely overweight.[28] This form of treatment requires skilled surgical intervention and should only be carried out at specialized centers.

TABLE 4.10

Therapeutic Strategies: Appropriate for Individuals over 51 Years of Age

Predictors of Overweight	Therapeutic Strategies		
	Preoverweight at Risk	Preclinical Overweight	Clinical Overweight
Menopause	Few individuals remain	Behavior therapy	Treat comorbidities
Declining growth hormone	in this subgroup	Low-fat/low-energy-dense diet	Drug treatment for overweight
Declining testosterone		Reduce sedentary lifestyle	Reduce sedentary lifestyle
Smoking cessation			Low-fat/low-energy-dense diet
Medication			Behavior therapy
			Surgery

CONCLUSIONS

This chapter has examined some of the guidelines for evaluation and treatment of obesity. They provide a reasonable basis for approaching the obese patient.

REFERENCES

1. Bray GA. *A Guide of Obesity and the Metabolic Syndrome*. Taylor & Francis, New York, 2011.
2. Klein S, Burke LE, Bray GA et al. American Heart Association Council on Nutrition, Physical Activity, and Metabolism. Clinical implications of obesity with specific focus on cardiovascular disease: A statement for professionals from the American Heart Association Council on Nutrition, Physical Activity, and Metabolism: Endorsed by the American College of Cardiology Foundation. *Circulation* 2004; 110:2952–2967.
3. National Institutes of Health, National Heart, Lung, and Blood Institute, North American Association for the Study of Obesity. *The Practical Guide. Identification, Evaluation, and Treatment of Overweight and Obesity in Adults*. National Institutes of Health, Bethesda, MD, October 2000, NIH Publication Number 00–4084.
4. NHLBI Obesity Education Initiative Expert Panel on the Identification, Evaluation, and Treatment of Overweight and Obesity in Adults. Clinical guidelines on the identification, evaluation, and treatment of overweight and obesity in adults—The evidence report. *Obes Res* 1998; 6(Suppl 2):51S–209S.
5. Obesity Preventing and managing the global epidemic. Report of a WHO consultation. World Health Organization Technical Report Series 894, pp. i–xii, 1–253.
6. Kushner RF, Aronne LJ. Obesity and the primary care physician. In: *Handbook of Obesity: Clinical Applications*, 3rd edn., Bray GA, Bouchard C, eds. Informa Healthcare, New York, 2008, pp. 117–129.
7. Willett WC, Manson JE, Stampfer MJ et al. Weight, weight change, and coronary heart disease in women: Risk within the 'normal' weight range. *JAMA* 1995; 273(6):461–465.
8. Bray GA. *Obesity and the Metabolic Syndrome*. Humana Press, Inc., Totowa, NJ, 2007.
9. U.S. Department of Health and Human Services. Body measurements. In: *Clinician's Handbook of Preventive Services: Put Prevention into Family Practice*. U.S. Government Printing Office, Washington, DC, 1994, pp. 141–146.

10. Roche A, Heymsfield SB, Lohman T. *Human Body Composition*. Human Kinetics, Champaign, IL, 1996.
11. Bray GA. Classification and evaluation of the overweight patient. In: *Handbook of Obesity*, Bray GA, Bouchard C, James WPT, eds. Marcel Dekker, Inc, New York, 1998, pp. 831–854.
12. Gallagher D, Heymsfield SB, Heo M et al. Healthy percentage body fat ranges: An approach for developing guidelines based on body mass index. *Am J Clin Nutr* 2000; 72(3):694–701.
13. Asian Task Force: Li G, Chen X, Jang Y et al. Obesity, coronary heart disease risk factors and diabetes in Chinese: An approach to the criteria of obesity in the Chinese population. *Obes Rev* 2002; 3:167–172.
14. Srinivasan S, Ogle GD, Garnett SP, Briody JN, Lee JW, Cowell CT. Features of the metabolic syndrome after childhood craniopharyngioma. *J Clin Endocrinol Metab* 2004; 89(1):81–86.
15. Arnaldi G, Angeli A, Atkinson AB et al. Diagnosis and complications of Cushing's syndrome: A consensus statement. *J Clin Endocrinol Metab* 2003 Dec; 88(12):5593–5602.
16. Welt CK, Gudmundsson JA, Arason G, Adams J, Palsdottir H, Gudlaugsdottir G, Ingadottir G, Crowley WF. Characterizing discrete subsets of polycystic ovary syndrome as defined by the Rotterdam criteria: The impact of weight on phenotype and metabolic features. *J Clin Endocrinol Metab* 2006 Dec; 91(12):4842–4848.
17. O'Rahilly S, Farooqi IS. Human obesity: A heritable neurobehavioral disorder that is highly sensitive to environmental conditions. *Diabetes* 2008 Nov; 57(11):2905–2910.
18. Expert Panel on Detection, Evaluation, and Treatment of High Blood Cholesterol in Adults. Executive summary of the Third Report of the National Cholesterol Education Program (NCEP) expert panel on detection, evaluation, and treatment of high blood cholesterol in adults (Adult Treatment Panel III). *JAMA* 2001; 285(19):2486–2497.
19. Brownell KD. Dieting readiness. *Weight Control Dig* 1990; 1:1–9.
20. Galuska DA, Will JC, Serdula MK et al. Are health care professionals advising obese patients to lose weight? *JAMA* 1999; 282(16):1576–1578.
21. Foster GD, Wadden TA, Vogt RA et al. What is a reasonable weight loss? Patients' expectations and evaluations of obesity treatment outcomes. *J Consult Clin Psychol* 1997; 65(1):79–85.
22. Knowler WC, Barrett-Connor E, Fowler SE, Hamman RF, Lachin JM, Walker EA, Nathan DM, Diabetes Prevention Program Research Group. Reduction in the incidence of type 2 diabetes with lifestyle intervention or metformin. *N Engl J Med* 2002 Feb 7; 346(6):393–403.
23. Herman WH, Hoerger TJ, Brandle M, Hicks K, Sorensen S, Zhang P, Hamman RF, Ackermann RT, Engelgau MM, Ratner RE, Diabetes Prevention Program Research Group. The cost-effectiveness of lifestyle modification or metformin in preventing type 2 diabetes in adults with impaired glucose tolerance. *Ann Intern Med* 2005 Mar 1; 142(5):323–332.
24. Sjostrom L. Surgical treatment of obesity. In: *Handbook of Obesity Clinical Applications*, 2nd edn., Bray GA, Bouchard C, eds. Marcel Dekker, Inc., New York, 2004, pp. 359–389.
25. Bray GA. Obesity is a chronic, relapsing neurochemical disease. *Int J Obes Relat Metab Disord* 2004; 28(1):34–38.
26. Institute of Medicine: Thomas P, ed. *Weighing the Options*. National Academy Press, Washington, DC, 1995.
27. Bray GA. Are non-prescription medications needed for weight control? *Obesity (Silver Spring)* 2008 Mar; 16(3):509–514. Erratum in: *Obesity (Silver Spring)* 2008 Jul; 16(7):1723.
28. Buchwald H, Estok R, Fahrbach K, Banel D, Jensen MD, Pories WJ, Bantle JP, Sledge I. Weight and type 2 diabetes after bariatric surgery: Systematic review and meta-analysis. *Am J Med* 2009 Mar; 122(3):248–256.

5 Nutritional Aspects of Obesity Management

Johanna Dwyer, DSc and Nikita Kapur, MS, RD

CONTENTS

INTRODUCTION

This chapter reviews the nutritional aspects of obesity treatment and management. It begins with a brief discussion of the reasons for concern about obesity. Obesity assessment methods and the goals of weight management are then reviewed. The process of designing and implementing appropriate dietary recommendations during the weight loss phase of obesity management is described including reducing diets, physical activity, dietary supplements, and drugs (which are sometimes useful). The changes in diet that must accompany bariatric surgery are also reviewed. This chapter concludes with a discussion of nutrition management during the maintenance phase of weight management.

REASONS FOR CONCERN ABOUT OBESITY

The rationale for treating obesity is that it is widely prevalent and is associated with the increased severity and incidence of several chronic diseases in addition to discontent about appearance.

MANY AMERICANS ARE OBESE

Obesity is defined as a body mass index (BMI) of ≥ 30 and overweight as a BMI between 25 and 29 [1]. Obesity prevalence increased from 1988–1994 to 2007–2008 among adults at all income and education levels in the United States, and almost two-thirds of adults in the United States who are currently overweight or obese [2]. According to the 2008 National Health Interview Survey (NHIS), 35% of all American adults were overweight and 27% were obese [3]. In the 2007–2008 National Health and Nutrition Examination Survey (NHANES), obesity prevalence was 32% among men and 36% among women [1]. Compared to the great increases in obesity prevalence evident over the previous 30 years, this upward trend appears to at last be slowing, especially in women and children, although the numbers are still very high [1]. These trends signify the need for continued attention to the obesity problem and development of better approaches to treating it. The 2010 Dietary Guidelines for Americans emphasize the importance of avoiding obesity by balancing calories in order to maintain a healthy body weight [4]. But for many Americans, the problem is not maintaining but achieving a healthy body weight. This chapter assists health professionals to counsel obese adults on managing their weight through conventional dietary therapy with low-calorie diets and increased physical activity, which is an appropriate treatment modality for most overweight and obese individuals. However, for some individuals such as those who are severely obese with BMIs > 40, other weight reduction methods such as very-low-calorie diets or bariatric surgery should be considered. Others, such as those who are pregnant, lactating, or suffering from an eating disorder, depression, or other serious comorbidities like advanced cancer, should not diet until their conditions have resolved.

Obesity Increases the Prevalence and Severity of Comorbidities*

The major medical reason for treating obesity is that it increases the risks and/or severity of many other health problems and decreases quality of life. Some of the health problems are orthopedic (such as osteoarthritis of the knees) and are worsened simply because of the sheer bulk of weight and fat tissue. Other health problems arise due to the metabolic changes that ensue with obesity. Table 5.1 highlights some of the conditions that are associated with or exacerbated by overweight and obesity [1]. For example, obesity tends to increase the prevalence of and health risks from high blood pressure and type 2 diabetes [1]. Some of the hormone-dependent cancers (such as breast, colon, and prostate cancers) also seem to be more prevalent among those who are very heavy. In addition to these ill effects, obesity also increases risks of morbidity and mortality associated with smoking [1].

ASSESS THE OBESE PATIENT'S CHARACTERISTICS†

The first step in approaching an overweight patient is to assess his or her weight, health status, dietary patterns, and attitudes toward weight loss.

---

* See also Chapters 11 through 15 for discussion of specific comorbidities associated with obesity.
† See also Chapter 4 for a detailed discussion of the clinical approach to the obese patient.

TABLE 5.1

Comorbidities and Examples of Conditions That Are Associated with Overweight and Obesity

Problem	Condition or Comorbidity
Metabolic	Type 2 diabetes
	Impaired glucose tolerance
	Insulin resistance
	Hyperlipidemia
	Dyslipidemia
	Metabolic syndrome
	Gout
	Liver disease
Cardiovascular and vascular	Hypertension
	Coronary heart disease
	Congestive heart failure
	Stroke
Reproductive	Infertility
	Poor pregnancy outcomes
	Sexual dysfunction
Structural	Osteoarthritis
	Falls
Psychiatric	Mood disorders
	Depression
	Anxiety
Cancer	Endometrial cancer
	Postmenopausal breast cancer
	Colorectal cancer
	Esophageal adenocarcinoma
Respiratory	Obstructive sleep apnea
	COPD (chronic obstructive pulmonary disease)

Source: Expert panel on the identification, evaluation, and treatment of over-weight in adults, *Am. J. Clin. Nutr.*, 68(4), 899, 1998.

Assess the Patient's Weight for Height (BMI) as an Estimate of Body Fatness

Weight should be measured, without clothing, on an electronic scale (which does not require constant adjustment), and height should be measured against a wall or by using a wall-mounted stadiometer. BMI should then be calculated using the following formulas [1]:

$$BMI = \frac{(weight\,lb \times 703)}{height\,in\,inches^2}$$

TABLE 5.2
Classification of Weight Status by BMI

Classification	BMI (kg/m²)
Underweight	<18.5
Normal weight	18.5–24.9
Overweight	25–29.9
Obesity class 1	30–34.9
Obesity class 2	35–39.9
Extreme obesity class 3	>40

Source: Expert panel on the identification, evaluation, and treatment of overweight in adults,
Am. J. Clin. Nutr., 68(4), 899, 1998.

or

$$BMI = \frac{weight\ kilograms}{height\ in\ meters}$$

$1\,kg = 2.2\,lb$
$1\,m = 39.37\,in.$

Measuring body fat directly in clinical practice is difficult. Instead, BMI is calculated from weight and height and used as a proxy for body fatness. It is good enough for most clinical purposes.

Table 5.2 presents the classification of adult BMI values used by the National Institutes of Health (NIH) [1].

USE WAIST CIRCUMFERENCE MEASUREMENTS TO FURTHER QUANTIFY RISKS RELATED TO BODY FAT DISTRIBUTION

Waist circumference is measured at the level of the umbilicus ("belly button") using a nonstretchable plastic tape. A waist circumference greater than 35 in. in women and greater than 40 in. in men indicates an increased risk of developing certain diseases associated with overweight and obesity [1]. The amount and distribution of fat on the body also alter health risk [1]. Central obesity (in the torso and abdomen) poses a greater risk than peripheral obesity (in the hips and extremities). Excessive mesenteric fat around the vital organs in the abdomen is now recognized as an independent risk factor for morbidity associated with central obesity [1]. Waist circumference is directly related to it and is therefore a proxy for the extent of abdominal obesity [1]. A more recent innovation used in the United Kingdom is the waist-to-height ratio [5]. It is also a proxy for central obesity such that a waist-to-height ratio above 0.5 denotes increased risk, providing patients the message to "keep your waist circumference to less than half your height" [5]. The waist-to-height ratio, which is claimed to be a better predictor of metabolic risk factors as compared to BMI, is an effective screening tool for cardiovascular disease risk factors [5]. It is helpful to periodically monitor the patient's weight change, BMI and waist circumference, or waist-to-height ratio to provide both the patient and the counselor with some benchmarks on progress.

ASSESS RELATED HEALTH RISKS

Obesity and overweight are associated with the development of a number of diseases and conditions [6]. Table 5.3 shows that risk of weight-related conditions increases with both greater BMI and waist circumference [1]. Risks include type 2 diabetes, hypertension, dyslipidemia, coronary heart disease, cardiovascular disease, congestive heart failure, stroke, gallstones, cancer, osteoarthritis, hormone-dependent cancers, sleep apnea, and certain reproductive problems [6]. Clinicians need to be aware of these problems in order to take steps to reduce complications, reverse the burden of illness, and ultimately improve the patient's quality of life.

In addition to the clinical tools discussed earlier, there are several other measures that may be useful for research or other purposes. These are listed in Appendix A.

EVALUATE THE PATIENT'S MOTIVATIONS AND ATTITUDES TOWARD WEIGHT CONTROL

Patients vary in their motivations, willingness, and readiness to lose weight. Since weight loss and maintenance both require behavioral change, patients must be motivated and ready before they attempt to lose weight. Although the clinician's primary interest in weight loss is to reduce medical problems, most patients are motivated chiefly by cosmetic considerations, with health often playing a minor role.

TABLE 5.3
Health Risks Associated with Obesity

	Disease Risk in Relation to BMI and Waist Circumference	
Classification of Weight by BMI	Waist Circumference Women < 35 in. Men < 40 in.	Waist Circumference Women > 35 in. Men > 40 in.
Underweight (BMI < 18.5)		
Normal (BMI 18.5–24.9)		
Overweight (BMI 25–29.9)	Increased	High
Obese class 1 (BMI 30–34.9)	High	Very high
Obese class 2 (BMI 35–39.9)	Very high	Very high
Extreme obesity class 3 (BMI > 40)	Extremely high	Extremely high

Source: Expert panel on the identification, evaluation, and treatment of overweight in adults, *Am. J. Clin. Nutr.*, 68(4), 899, 1998.

TABLE 5.4
Prochaska's Transtheoretical Model of Behavior Change Applied to Obesity Readiness

Stage	Characteristics	Patient Verbal Cues
Precontemplation	Unaware of problem, no interest in behavior change	"I'm not really interested in weight loss. It's not a problem."
Contemplation	Aware of problem, beginning to think of changing	"I need to lose weight but with all that's going on in my life right now, I'm not sure if I can."
Preparation	Realizes benefits of making changes and thinking about how to make those changes	"I have to lose weight, and I'm planning to do that."
Action	Actively taking steps toward achieving the behavioral goal, but only for a brief period (less than 6 months)	"I'm doing my best. This is harder than I thought."

Sources: Kushner, R.F. and Kushner, N., *Counseling Overweight Adults: The Lifestyle Patterns Approach and Toolkit*, American Dietetic Association, Chicago, IL, 2008; American Psychiatric Association (ed.), *Diagnostic and Statistical Manual of Mental Disorders*, 4th edn., American Psychiatric Press, Washington, DC, 1994.

Table 5.4 describes the various stages of behavior change in obesity as Kushner described it using Prochaska's transtheoretical model of behavior change [7,8].

A patient's readiness for weight loss is best determined by first discussing their motivations and understanding of the requirements, risks, and benefits of treatment [1]. A history of previous weight loss attempts and reasons for failure may also provide clues for shaping more successful strategies in the future.

EVALUATE THE PATIENT'S HEALTH-RELATED QUALITY OF LIFE

Health-related quality of life (HRQOL) tools document an individual's subjective opinion of his or her health that can include, but is not limited to, general health, physical, cognitive, social, and emotional functioning [9]. HRQOL provides a comprehensive description of the impact of a complex condition like obesity on the patient. The Short Form 8 (SF8) is an eight-item questionnaire that takes only a few minutes for the patient to complete, and is worth considering to assess the broader psychosocial impacts of obesity [9]. Findings from HRQOL are helpful for designing treatments that address factors that are particularly important to the individual's health and quality of life [9].

ASSESS EATING PATTERNS AND HABITS

The patient's current dietary intake is the foundation upon which a customized and appealing moderate-to-low-calorie diet is developed. Although inexact for energy intake, much useful information on eating patterns can be obtained by administering a food frequency questionnaire, diet history, a food record, or a 24 h dietary recall [9].

Food frequency questionnaires are self-administered questionnaires that ask individuals to report their usual consumption of certain foods over a specific time period, usually a year [9]. The questionnaires provide an idea of an individual's food pattern that is useful for customizing dietary therapy, but, as mentioned, only a very imprecise estimate of energy intake. The diet history is another retrospective method for assessing intake [9]. The counselors, usually a registered dietitian (RD), question the patient about the type and amount of food that was eaten. The diet history's main disadvantage is that it requires a trained interviewer to ask the questions and, thus, takes 45 min or more to complete [9]. Food records are obtained by asking patients to record the type and amount of food they eat for several days [9]. Food intake is typically underreported, and also, several days are needed to appropriately capture an individual's usual intake pattern. The very act of keeping a food record may help the patient to identify how intake contributes to dietary excess and what to cut down on to reduce energy intake. Twenty-four hour dietary recalls are usually administered to the patient by a counselor, and these too provide only a snapshot about intake [9]. Although none of the various dietary assessment tools provide precise estimates of energy intake, they do provide the counselor with a sense of what the patient is generally eating.

Obtain a Rough Estimate of Current Energy Intake

There is no single accurate method for assessing energy intake, but there are several methods that provide a rough estimate of the patient's caloric intake. There are several reasons why it is so difficult to obtain good estimates of energy intake. Generally, energy intake cycles over a period of time and therefore many days or weeks of collection are needed to accurately estimate usual energy intake. Moreover, the obese are sensitive about their food intake and may inadvertently or deliberately underreport their intakes. Also, individuals tend to forget what they eat (particularly snacks, which are likely to be high in energy), and so underreporting is common with all methods particularly with retrospective methods based on recall. With prospective methods such as a food diary, individuals are also more inclined to change their intakes, usually decreasing them, to simplify record keeping and to be more in line with norms.

The USDA My Pyramid tracker provides one simple way for patients to record and assess their food intake and physical activity pattern [10]. It provides an easy-to-use online tool for patients to track their current energy intake and physical activity and can be accessed at http://www.mypyramidtracker.gov/ [10]. One way to estimate current and projected daily energy needs on a weight reduction diet is to estimate resting metabolic rate (RMR) from height and weight. The Mifflin–St. Jeor equation is one of the most accurate ways to determine the RMR for overweight and obese individuals [11].

RMR for males > 19 years old:

(10 × weight in kilograms + (6.25 × height in centimeters) − (5 × age in years) + 5)

RMR for women > 19 years old:

(10 × weight in kilograms)(6.25 × height in centimeters) − (5 × age in years) − 161

TABLE 5.5

Activity Factors for Different Physical Activity Levels

	Sedentary	Low Active	Active	Very Active
	Light physical activity for daily activities	Walking about 1.5–3 miles/day at 3–4 miles/h in addition to activities of daily living	60 min of moderate-intensity physical activity, walking 3 miles/day at about 3–4 miles/h	60 min of moderate to vigorous physical activity or walking more than 7.5 miles/day at 3–4 miles/h
Males	1.0	1.11	1.25	1.48
Females	1.0	1.12	1.27	1.45

Source: Dwyer, J. and Melanson, K.J., Dietary treatment of obesity, in *Endotext*, 2nd edn., 2007. Caro, J. (ed.), http://www.endotext.com/obesity/index.htm.

The RMR is multiplied by an appropriate physical activity factor to determine the total energy needs of the patient for weight maintenance [12]. Activity factors are estimated based on various physical activity levels such as sedentary, low active, active, and very active [13]. Table 5.5 outlines the different activity factors that should be used to determine adequate energy needs for weight maintenance based on the level of physical activity [13]. A 500 cal deficit from the baseline energy needs is typically used to achieve weight loss of 1 lb a week [6].

OBTAIN OTHER RELEVANT DIET-RELATED INFORMATION

Information about food allergies, food preferences, use of dietary supplements (especially nutrient containing dietary supplements), and any special dietary constraints due to ethnic, cultural, or religious considerations should also be obtained as it is useful for prescribing and planning the weight reduction diets.

SCREEN PROPENSITY TO EATING DISORDERS IF THE PATIENT IS LIKELY TO BE AT RISK

Table 5.6 defines the criteria for anorexia nervosa, Table 5.7 provides similar information on bulimia nervosa, and Table 5.8 outlines eating disorders not otherwise specified (EDNOS) from the *Diagnostic and Statistical Manual of Mental Disorders*, fourth edition, text revision (DSM IV-TR1) [8]. These are serious conditions and those who are affected should not be on weight loss diets at all or, at the very minimum, not until their condition resolves. If such individuals do undertake weight loss later on, it should be carefully monitored both medically and psychiatrically to avoid relapse.

Eating-related pathology also needs to be assessed and ruled out. Short, easily administered screening instruments for eating disorders and restrained eating

TABLE 5.6
DSM IV-TR Criteria for Anorexia Nervosa

- Refusal to maintain body weight at or above a minimally normal weight for age and height: Weight loss leading to maintenance of body weight <85% of that expected or failure to make expected weight gain during period of growth, leading to body weight less than 85% of that expected
- Intense fear of gaining weight or becoming fat, even though under-weight
- Disturbance in the way one's body weight or shape is experienced, undue influence of body weight or shape on self evaluation, or denial of the seriousness of the current low body weight
- Amenorrhea (at least three consecutive cycles) in postmenarchal girls and women: Amenorrhea is defined as periods occurring only following hormone (e.g., estrogen) administration

Source: American Psychiatric Association (ed.), *Diagnostic and Statistical Manual of Mental Disorders*, 4th edn., American Psychiatric Press, Washington, DC, 1994.

TABLE 5.7
DSM IV-TR Criteria for Bulimia Nervosa

1. Recurrent episodes of binge eating characterized by both:
    a. Eating, in a discrete period of time (e.g., within any 2 h period), an amount of food that is definitely larger than most people would eat during a similar period of time and under similar circumstances
    b. A sense of lack of control over eating during the episode, defined by a feeling that one cannot stop eating or control what or how much one is eating
2. Recurrent inappropriate compensatory behavior to prevent weight gain
3. Self-induced vomiting
4. Misuse of laxatives, diuretics, enemas, or other medications
5. Fasting
6. Excessive exercise
7. The binge eating and inappropriate compensatory behavior both occur, on average, at least twice a week for 3 months
8. Self-evaluation is unduly influenced by body shape and weight

Source: American Psychiatric Association (ed.), *Diagnostic and Statistical Manual of Mental Disorders*, 4th edn., American Psychiatric Press, Washington, DC, 1994.

behaviors are available [9]. The most accurate screening tool for assessing eating disorder psychopathology is the Eating Disorder Examination Questionnaire (EDE-Q), which takes 30 min, making it far too long to use clinically in most instances [9]. A better alternative for clinical screening purposes when an eating disorder is suspected is the SCOFF (sickness, control, one stone, fatness, and food) questionnaire; it has five items and takes only a few minutes [14]. The five questions comprise of items measuring sickness, control, weight loss (one stone = 14 lb), and the individual's perception about their fatness and food [14]. If the screen or

TABLE 5.8
DSM IV-TR Criteria for Eating Disorder Not Otherwise Specified

- Eating disorder not otherwise specified includes disorders of eating that do not meet the criteria for any specific eating disorder
- For female patients, all of the criteria for anorexia nervosa are met except that the patient has regular menses
- All of the criteria for anorexia nervosa are met except that, despite significant weight loss, the patient's current weight is in the normal range
- All of the criteria for bulimia nervosa are met except that the binge eating and inappropriate compensatory mechanisms occur less than twice a week or for less than 3 months
- The patient has normal body weight and regularly uses inappropriate compensatory behavior after eating small amounts of food (e.g., self-induced vomiting after consuming two cookies)
- Repeatedly chewing and spitting out, but not swallowing, large amounts of food
- Binge-eating disorder is recurrent episodes of binge eating in the absence of regular inappropriate compensatory behavior characteristic of bulimia nervosa

Source: American Psychiatric Association (ed.), *Diagnostic and Statistical Manual of Mental Disorders*, 4th edn., American Psychiatric Press, Washington, DC, 1994.

the medical history suggests an eating disorder, the patient should be referred for further evaluation and appropriate treatment before beginning dietary treatment. Patients with anorexia nervosa and bulimia nervosa that are already clinically evident should not embark upon reducing diets.

ESTIMATE CURRENT ENERGY INTAKE AND DEFICIT NEEDED TO LOSE WEIGHT

A caloric deficit of 500–1000 kcal/day less than the patient's current intake over time will help achieve a weight loss of 1–2 lb/week [1]. The actual level of energy intake necessary to achieve weight loss on a reducing diet will vary depending on the calories needed to achieve and maintain the desired weight goal [1]. For example, a sedentary woman who weighs 180 lb with a 10 lb weight loss goal will have very different energy needs than a physically active man who weighs 180 lb with a similar weight loss target of 10 lb. This is because the woman has a lower RMR (due to less actively metabolizing lean tissue than a male) and also less energy from physical activity, therefore resulting in less overall energy needs.

DETERMINE MEDICAL/HEALTH OBJECTIVES FOR WEIGHT MANAGEMENT

DISCUSS WHETHER DIETARY TREATMENT IS THE APPROPRIATE OPTION AND WHAT OPTIONS MAKE MORE SENSE TO THE PATIENT IF IT IS NOT

All individuals with a BMI of 25–30 with comorbidities and all patients with a BMI over 30 are likely to require some sort of dietary modification in order to lose weight. However, dietary treatment is not an appropriate option for everyone who needs to lose weight [1]. For example, for the very obese with a BMI > 35, other measures may be more effective; a moderately hypocaloric diet would take many months or even years to achieve the healthier weight objective. Such extremely obese patients should be referred to a multidisciplinary obesity consulting team that can develop an appropriate treatment plan (such as a very-low-calorie diet or bariatric surgery) for achieving sustainable weight loss.

SET REALISTIC GOALS AND DEFINE SUCCESSFUL OUTCOMES WITH THE PATIENT

The goal of the counselor and the patient should be to achieve an acceptable weight target for optimal health. Goals and weight reduction targets vary and depend on several factors, including existing comorbidities. In general, the recommended weight loss target is between 1/2 and 2 lb of body weight per week over 6 months, which equals roughly a 5%–10% reduction in body weight [1]. After the first 6 months of weight loss therapy, the focus should shift toward weight maintenance through a combination of diet therapy and physical activity [1].

IMPLEMENT THE WEIGHT LOSS PHASE WITH AN APPROPRIATE REDUCING DIET

CONSIDER ENERGY LEVELS OF THE DIET

The lower the caloric level, the greater the metabolic effects such as decreased RMR, increased breakdown of lean tissue, mild ketosis, and, in turn, increased risk of dehydration and electrolyte imbalances [15–17]. These and other weight loss diets are discussed in greater length elsewhere [13]. The energy levels used to achieve weight reduction include very-low-calorie diets (<800 kcal), low-calorie diets (<1000 kcal), and moderately low-calorie diets (1200 kcal) [15,16]. Fasting is not recommended. Very-low-calorie diets are recommended only for patients who have failed on more moderate regimens and for those who must lose weight immediately for medical reasons [15]. These diets involve considerable metabolic perturbation and therefore need a considerable amount of medical supervision to avoid complications.

ENSURE THAT THE DIETARY COMPOSITION OF THE REDUCING DIET IS APPROPRIATE

The composition of the diet should be considered because it has a direct effect on weight loss and nutritional status. Recommendations for nutritionally balanced hypocaloric diets (also called "balanced deficit diets") include diets containing 35%–50% of energy as carbohydrate, 25%–35% of energy as fat, and 25%–30% as protein [18]. Carbohydrate-restricted diets with <35% of total calories from carbohydrates are associated with a slightly greater short-term weight loss for the first 6 months, compared to traditional hypocaloric or reducing diets, but with other disadvantages and no clear advantages over the long term [18]. The main concern with diets that have unbalanced macronutrient composition is nutrient inadequacy; vitamin and mineral supplementation may be required since the usual food sources of nutrients may not be included [16]. Current evidence on reducing diets for weight loss recommends balanced deficit hypocaloric diets with moderate amounts of fat, carbohydrate, and protein [18].

Referral to an RD is one way of implementing an individualized weight loss regimen and any other medical nutrition therapeutic measures that may be necessary for patients who are also afflicted with other medical problems requiring medical nutrition therapy. RDs have the skills and expertise to work collaboratively with other members of the medical team in order to translate scientific knowledge into practical applications that promote a healthy lifestyle [11]. They are experts in implementing specialized diets for specific populations including but not limited to celiac disease, type 2 diabetes, cardiovascular disease and diets for hypertension, renal disease, and for various inborn errors of metabolism. However, dietitian visits may be more expensive than some commercial weight loss programs, so it is important to determine if the patient's medical insurance covers the diet therapy.

REVIEW AND RECOMMEND REDUCING DIET OPTIONS

Table 5.9 provides a description of different reducing diet options, the ideal candidates for them, and the safety and effectiveness of each option [15–17].

SCREEN WEIGHT LOSS BOOKS FOR APPROPRIATENESS

Some individuals prefer to follow weight loss regimens discussed in the hundreds of books that are now available in the market on this topic. Table 5.10 highlights examples of weight loss books currently available [19–21]. Only a few of them can be recommended; many more have little sound advice to offer to patients. While a good book may be helpful to patients, it is rarely enough by itself to achieve success in weight loss as most individuals require medical and nutrition advice along with social support.

The Internet is another tool that may be a useful adjunct to the patient's reducing diet. Table 5.11 features a list of recommended web-based weight loss programs that provide dieters with online tools and resources that may be helpful in achieving weight loss goals [22,23]. These resources primarily provide tools for tracking progress and offer online support to the dieter. Although they can be helpful, they do not serve as a substitute for group support and face-to-face interaction with a counselor.

REVIEW THE PROS AND CONS OF COMMERCIAL WEIGHT LOSS PROGRAMS

There are many commercial weight loss programs available to dieters today. They can be helpful particularly if they are combined with some attention from the healthcare provider to initially assess the advisability of the therapy and to encourage the patient as progress is made. Table 5.12 includes a list of the most popular commercial weight loss programs, including a brief description of both medically supervised and self-help-type programs [24,25].

TABLE 5.9

Characteristics of Various Weight Loss Schemes and Appropriate Candidates for Therapy

What It Is	Ideal Candidates for Therapy	Safety	Effectiveness	Formulations	Use: Pros and Cons
Total Fasting Rapid weight loss consists of lean body mass and water weight and is thus undesirable	None	Ketosis, lethargy, weakness, menstrual irregularity, hair loss, and insufficient vitamin and mineral intake	NA	NA	Contraindicated; causes excessive breakdown of lean tissue, diuresis, and ketosis; decreases RMR and physical activity resulting in lower energy output and impeding rate of weight loss
Very-Low-Calorie Diets <800cal/day 50–80 g of protein Typically consists of commercially prepared meal replacement liquid formulas for quick weight loss	Patients with BMIs > 30 Patients with high medical risks from obesity-related coexisting conditions (obstructive sleep apnea, poorly controlled type 2 diabetes, impaired mobility, and hypertriglyceridemia)	Physiological effects: mild ketosis, increased risk of dehydration, and electrolyte imbalances Minor side effects: fatigue, dizziness, muscle cramps, gastrointestinal distress, cold intolerance, and increased risk of cholelithiasis	Produces greater initial weight loss than low-calorie diets although mostly through shifts in water balance Little difference in outcomes between commercial and properly formulated homemade VLCDs	*Commercial preparations:* HMR™ (Health Management Resources) Medifast Optifast™ (Novartis Nutrition) Slimfast	May be safe and effective for weight loss under appropriate medical supervision Requires careful evaluation of health risks and constant physician monitoring

	Medical contraindications include recent myocardial infarction, cardiac conduction disorders, history of cardiovascular disease, renal or hepatic disease, cancer, type 1 diabetes, and pregnancy	Multivitamin and multimineral supplement if incomplete formula	Weight regain is common over long term, although combining a VLCD with behavior therapy, physical activity, and active physician follow-up may help to prevent some of the weight regain and aid in greater weight loss	*Homemade preparations:* sometimes referred to as "protein-sparing fasts," or "protein-sparing modified fasts" (PSMF)	
Low-Calorie Diets 800–1000 kcal	Behavioral contraindications include bulimia nervosa, major depression, bipolar disorder, substance abuse, and acute psychiatric illness	Fatigue, nausea, diarrhea, and constipation	May help reduce body weight by an average of 8% and decrease abdominal fat over 6 months No improvement in cardiovascular and respiratory fitness	Prepackaged meals including Weight Watchers® meals, Jenny Craig®, Nutrisystem, and frozen entrees including Healthy Choice, Lean Cuisine, and Smart ones	Slow weight loss

(continued)

TABLE 5.9 (continued)

Characteristics of Various Weight Loss Schemes and Appropriate Candidates for Therapy

What It Is	Ideal Candidates for Therapy	Safety	Effectiveness	Formulations	Use: Pros and Cons
Moderately Low Calorie Diets 1000–1200 kcal "Balanced deficit" diets because they maintain a reasonable balance among macronutrients based on recommended levels	For slow progressive weight loss of 1–2 lb a week	Minimal metabolic effects and greater exercise tolerance		Some examples of balanced deficit diets are the Weight Watchers Diet, Jenny Craig, diets based on the food pyramid, the DASH diet, the Shape Up and Drop 10 diet of Shape Up! America	Slow and gradual weight loss

Sources: Tsai, A.G. and Wadden, T.A., *Obesity (Silver Spring, Md.)*, 14(8), 1283, 2006; National Heart, Lung and Blood Institute (NHLBI) Obesity Education Initiative Expert Panel, *Clinical Guidelines on the Identification, Evaluation, and Treatment of Overweight and Obesity in Adults*, National Institute of Health, Bethesda, MD, 1998; Wadden, T.A. and Stunkard, A.J., *Handbook of Obesity Treatment*, Guilford Press, New York, 2002.

TABLE 5.10
Examples of Some Popular Weight Loss Books

Weight Loss Books	Brief Description	Comments
Recommended Books		
The Complete Food Counter Annette B. Natow and Jo-Ann Heslin New York: Pocket Books, 2009	Calorie counting resource that provides nutrition information on over 17,000 foods and provides information on the adequate use of various nutrients	Helpful for providing nutrition information of various foods
Eat Out, Eat Right: The Guide to Healthier Restaurant Eating, 3rd edn Hope Warshaw Chicago, IL: Surrey Books, 2008	A guide for healthy restaurant eating that includes tips and skills useful in making healthier choices while eating out	
The Supermarket Diet Janis Jibrin MS, RD New York: Hearst, 2007	Written by a dietitian to promote portion control and label reading. The book also includes shopping lists, meal plans, recipes, and snacks	
Thin for Life: 10 Keys to Success From People Who Have Lost Weight and Kept It Off Anne M. Fletcher New York: Houghton Mifflin, 2003	Resource for weight management based on people's success stories and findings from the National Weight Control Registry	
No-Fad Diet: A Personal Plan for Healthy Weight Loss American Heart Association New York: Clarkson Potter, 2005	Weight loss planning tool that encourages three key behaviors: think smart, eat well, and move more	

(continued)

TABLE 5.10 (continued)
Examples of Some Popular Weight Loss Books

Weight Loss Books	Brief Description	Comments
Books Not Recommended		
Atkins For Life Dr. Robert C. Atkins™, MD St. Martin's Giffin, 2004	Designed for individuals who have lost weight on the original Atkins Diet. It recommends a lower-carbohydrate plan for continued weight loss	Fails to meet the RDA/AI for calcium, magnesium, potassium, and iron, and thus a daily multivitamin is recommended
Body for Life Bill Phillips, Michael D'Orso William Morrow, 1999	Six meals per day for 6 weeks including whole grains, vegetables, lean meats, vegetables, healthy fats, and fish along with regular exercise	A flexible and adaptable diet approach that is primarily focused on exercise
5-Factor Diet Harley Pasternak Ballantine Books, 2009	5 week plan, 5 meals per day, 5 min preparation time per meal, recipes with only 5 ingredients, 5 cheat days in 5 weeks, and 25 min workouts 5 days a week for 5 weeks	
The Cheaters Diet Paul Rivas, MD HCI, 2005	Based on the plate method: 1/2 plate vegetables, 1/4 whole grains, 1/4 lean protein. Allow cheating on the weekends for boosting metabolism and weight loss	
Eat This Not That David Zinczenko with Matt Goulding Rodale Books, 2009	Targets male readers with an attempt to provide healthier alternatives to calorie-laden fast-food choices	
Abs Diet David Zinczenko, Editor-in-Chief of *Men's Health* Rodale Books, 2005	Abs Diet Acronym (Almonds, beans, spinach, dairy, instant oatmeal, turkey, peanut butter, olive oil, whole grains, extra protein, and raspberries)	More appropriate for weight maintenance than for weight loss

Flat Belly Diet Liz Vaccariello and Cynthia Sass Rodale Books, 2009	Recommends a 1600 kcal diet that includes a monounsaturated fatty acid at every meal. In conjunction, also suggests frequent eating and regular exercise	
French Women Don't Get Fat Mireille Guiliano Vintage, 2007	Low-calorie diet that incorporates lifestyle changes	Emphasis on lifestyle changes without a recommended diet plan
Change Your Genetic Destiny (The Genotype Diet) Dr. Peter J. D'Adamo and Catherine Whitney Broadway, 2009	Diet based on an individual's genetic makeup and is based on the six genotypes: the Hunter, the Gatherer, the Teacher, the Explorer, the Warrior, and the Nomad	Diet based on unsubstantiated research
The Perricone Prescription Dr. Nicholas Perricone Harper Paperbacks, 2004	Recommends anti-inflammatory foods such as salmon	
Joy's LIFE Diet: Four Steps to Thin Forever Joy Bauer New York: HarperCollins, 2009	Provides four steps for successful weight loss: "release" old habits, "relearn" how to eat healthfully, "reshape" an eating plan, and "reveal" weight loss success	
Sensa Weight-Loss Program (The Sprinkle Diet) Dr. Alan Hirsch, MD, FACP Hilton Publishing, 2009	Flavored sprinkles that reduces appetite and increases satiety	
The Serotonin Power Diet Judith J. Wurtman, PhD Nina T. Frusztajer, MD Rodale Books, 2006	Recommends carbohydrate-rich snack eating, which helps produce serotonin to decrease stress and reduce weight	

(continued)

TABLE 5.10 (continued)
Examples of Some Popular Weight Loss Books

Weight Loss Books	Brief Description	Comments
South Beach Diet Dr. Arthur Agatston Rodale, Inc., 2003	Low-carbohydrate diet	Does not provide any specific recommendations for fluid intake
The Spectrum Diet Dr. Dean Ornish, MD Ballantine Books, 2008	Uses Ornish's food spectrum (Group 1 being the healthiest, Group 5, the least healthy) to make changes based on desired health outcomes (e.g., weight loss, weight maintenance, and reduced risk of cancer)	
The Volumetrics Weight-Control Plan Barbara Rolls New York: Harper Collins Publishers, 2000	Based on the concept of satiety by filling up on high-volume foods with low energy density	The long-term effects are not demonstrated, and longer-term studies in obese individuals need to be conducted to determine the effect of dietary energy density and food intake regulation
YOU: On a Diet (Revised Edition) Dr. Mehmet Oz and Dr. Michael Roizen New York: Free Press, 2009	Based on achieving weight loss through waist measurement and its relationship to health	
Eat More Weigh Less Dean Ornish New York: Harper Collins, 1993	Vegetarian, plant-based diet that emphasizes low-fat, highly complex carbohydrates and fiber	Emphasis on achieving satiety from whole grains, fruits, vegetables, and water
Mindless Eating, Brian Wansink New York: Bantam Dell, 2006	Describes mindless eating behaviors and ways to identifying and preventing such behaviors	

Sources: Stevens, A., E. Dionne, and J. Dwyer; Popular and fad diet programs: Nutritional adequacy, safety and efficacy, in *Self-Help Approaches for Obesity and Eating Disorders*, J. Latner and T. Wilson (eds)., The Guilford Press, New York, pp. 21–52; Melanson, K. and Dwyer, J., Popular diets for treatment of overweight and obesity, T.A. Wadden and A.J. Stunkard (eds), in *Handbook of Obesity Treatment*, Guilford Press, New York, 2002, pp. 249–275; Food and Nutrition Information Center, National Agricultural Library, USDA, Weight management and obesity resource list, available from http://www.nal.usda.gov/fnic/pubs/bibs/topics/weight/consumer.pdf, Accessed, February 24, 2011, 2009.

TABLE 5.11
Examples of Web-Based Weight Loss Programs

Type of Website	Brief Description
The Diet Solution	www.thedietsolutionprogram.com
	Based on the metabolic typing principle that helps identify the type of diet, carbohydrate, protein, or mixed through a diet type analysis
Cyberdiet.com	www.cyberdiet.com
	The program provides resources on fitness, nutrition, behavioral motivation, recipes, and emotional health. Counseling is provided by accredited health professionals to individualize diet program
WebMD Nutrition Resources	http://www.webmd.com/diet/default.htm
	Website for patients that provides various useful tools including a calorie counter, BMI calculator, nutrient and food database, helpful articles, and videos to help live healthfully
Ediets.com	www.ediets.com
	A meal delivery system that provides weight loss resources including food lists, healthy recipes, fitness information, and an opportunity for social networking in the community
Weight Watchers® Online	www.weightwatchers.com
	Customized online weight loss program used to help personalize diet plan. Based on a daily point system that allows a certain calorie range per day and encourages eating all foods including fruits, vegetables, whole grains, and lean proteins within that set range
Lifepractice.com	www.lifepractice.com
	The Life Practice program centers its recommendations around adequate exercise, nutrition, sleep habits, and stress management
Fitday.com	http://fitday.com
	Weight loss website that helps track weight loss, food intake, and exercise in the form of an online journal
Caloriescount.com	www.caloriescount.com
	Weight loss website that provides calorie counts for over 20,000 foods and acts like an online journal to help track weight loss goals by keeping a record of exercise and caloric intake. Also offers online diet meal plans and additional weight loss tools
Spark People®	www.sparkpeople.com
	Weight loss tracking website that offers a large online social network by providing support groups and resources for maintaining weight loss approaches. Provides a wide variety of free nutrition information, health and fitness tools, and resources
Diet.com	www.diet.com
	Health website that provides tools and resources for weight loss, exercise, and general wellness

Sources: Augustin, J., *Nutr. Clin. Care*, 4, 272, 2001; Fitday, Free internet tools for tracking weight, diet, exercise, and more, available from http://www.fitday.com/, Accessed February 24, 2011, 2009.

TABLE 5.12
Commercial Weight Loss Programs

Type of Program	Description	Comments
Weight Watchers™ Points Plus System	Based on a point counting system that provides a framework for creating a caloric deficit by calculating points from various macronutrients. The current Points Plus program offers unlimited quantities of fruits and vegetables. This model encourages slow healthy weight loss with adequate exercise, behavior modification, and support	The point-based plan allots points to foods based on calories, fat, and fiber. Dieters receive a daily point allotment based on current weight with an emphasis toward meal planning integrated with exercise, behavior modification, and social support
Nutrisystem™ Diet Plan	Diet plan that provides ready-to-eat, portion-controlled, balanced meals through an Internet-based diet program. Focuses on providing meals low in sodium, saturated fat, and trans fats and high in whole grains, fiber, and healthy proteins	Preportioned foods are conveniently provided. The program also provides social support and online tools and tips for dieters. However, it does not mirror realistic eating patterns to achieve lifestyle changes and can be expensive
Take Off Pounds Sensibly (TOPS)	Weight loss program based on a regular diet with standard foods combined with healthy eating, regular exercise, and support for overall wellness	Nonprofit program that emphasizes slow and gradual weight loss
Jenny Craig®	Diet program that offers both preportioned and grocery store foods along with regular counseling and information on nutrition and lifestyle management	Primary focus on weight management with behavior modifications and healthy lifestyle changes
Overeaters Anonymous (OA)	Weight loss program based on a social support network where compulsive eating is addressed using the 12-step program outlined by the OA principles and traditions	Does not focus on a "diet" and instead focuses on providing support and professional advice for managing emotional eating
Medifast™ Diet Plan	Medical weight loss program that provides meal replacement products from an assortment of portion-controlled, low-calorie, high-protein food products	Balanced, diet meal replacement program that provides a structured environment for weight loss and weight maintenance. The program does not provide support groups, is expensive, and is available only in the United States
Health Management Resources (HMR)	Medically supervised weight management programs with a prime focus on lifestyle change. Modified form of a VLCD diet combined with individualized diet plans and counseling. HMR products mostly contain of preprepared meals including shakes, puddings, bars, soups, and entrees	A very expensive clinically focused weight loss program that provides a convenient portion-controlled meal replacement food products. HMR foods tend to be very high in soy and very low in calories, and dieters on this program should be under medical supervision

Sources: Anderson, J., Young L., and Roach J., Weight Loss Products and Programs, 2008, http://www. ext.colostate.edu/pubs/foodnut/09363.html (Accessed February 24, 2011); Tsai, A.G. and Wadden, T.A., *Ann. Intern. Med.*, 142(1), 56, 2005.

SHOW THE PATIENT HOW FOOD LABELS FOR CALORIE
AND NUTRITION INFORMATION CAN BE USEFUL

SHOW THE PATIENT HOW FOOD LABELS FOR CALORIE AND NUTRITION INFORMATION CAN BE USEFUL

The Nutrition Facts label found on all processed and many other foods provides calories-per-serving information [26]. This label is useful as an information source for those on reducing diets as long as they are aware of the standard size that the calorie statement refers to; often, the serving specified is very much smaller than what people usually eat. A variety of different nutrition labeling schemes exist on the front of food packages, and some of them prominently display calories, which can also be helpful to dieters. The Food and Drug Administration (FDA) assessment of the effectiveness of various front of pack (FOP) labeling approaches for calories and other nutrients currently suggests that calories should be prominently displayed to provide consumers with a tool to notice, understand, and use in order to make more nutritious choices for themselves and their families [26].

MAKE PATIENT AWARE OF THE LIMITATIONS OF POPULAR THEORIES AND FAD DIETS

Popular theories and fad diets abound in the field of weight control are aided and abetted by diet books, talk shows, and Internet sales of various "cures" for obesity. Some of the unproven current theories are described in the following.

FOOD ADDICTION THEORY AS A PURPORTED CAUSE OF OBESITY

A small number of individuals who are obese clearly suffer from food addiction and should be referred for psychological counseling in order to be treated. However, some argue that many obese people suffer from food addiction and that the cause of their problems can be attributed to this very reason. David Kessler has popularized this theory in his book and numerous television appearances [27]. Unfortunately, there is little evidence to support the contention that food addiction is the major cause of obesity and that most or all obese patients are "addicted" to food. The food addiction hypothesis relies primarily on the similarities between food and drug cravings and the observation that the same neurobiological pathways implicated in drug abuse are also involved in the modulation of food consumption and the regulation of food intake. Both behaviors involve a complex set of peripheral and central signaling networks, including homeostatic and hedonic neural pathways [28,29]. The homeostatic pathway increases the motivation to eat during periods of decreased energy levels and stores. The hedonic pathway regulates food intake based on a reward system by increasing the desire to eat even during periods of relative energy abundance [29]. The interactions of these homeostatic and hedonic neural pathways play a major role in the control of food intake and food cravings, and certain changes in diet, such as ceasing a high-fat diet, lead to neurochemical responses that are similar to those induced by withdrawal from a drug [29]. Proponents of the food addiction theory believe that depression can also modify endogenous signals involved in food intake regulation, just as it does in drug withdrawal [29]. They claim that binging on sugar in rats induces behavioral and neuronal changes including dopaminergic, cholinergic, and opioid effects, similar to those induced by drugs of abuse [30]. However, external stimuli, such as environmental or social cues, can modulate food-seeking behaviors and food intake in important ways via classical conditioning in experimental animals [28]. Although animal models are useful for generating hypotheses on the basic mechanisms common to the consumption of food and drugs, humans are also influenced by their cultural and social environments. This adds a complexity not observed and studied in such animal models. Therefore, although it is true that food acts on some of the same neuronal systems as do drugs of abuse in both rats and human beings, the use of rat behavior to predict human behavior is fraught with difficulties.

More research is needed on the effects of highly palatable foods and compulsive food intake in both lean and obese individuals, and on their role in the development of obesity. For the small number of individuals who truly appear to be addicted to food, psychological counseling is in order.

LOW-GLYCEMIC-INDEX DIETS TO TREAT OBESITY

The glycemic index (GI) was originally developed for the therapy of diabetes [31]. It is now used in classifying carbohydrate-containing foods according to the postprandial blood glucose responses that ensue when food portions containing standardized amounts of carbohydrates are eaten [31,32]. Some observational studies suggest that foods that have a low GI are associated with a reduced risk of obesity-related conditions such as type 2 diabetes and cardiovascular disease [32]. Other short-term clinical studies suggest an association between diets of low-GI foods and weight loss due to their supposed effects on satiety, appetite control, and metabolism [33]. However, no long-term studies have demonstrated that low-GI diets promote greater weight loss [33]. At present, the concept appears to be of limited use in weight loss. Before low-GI diets can be adopted as a bona fide weight loss intervention, longer-term randomized controlled clinical trials of efficacy need to be conducted [33]. Until then, the use of low-GI diets should be limited to those that are hypocaloric and seem to help the patient.

THEORY OF VITAMIN D AS CAUSE OR TREATMENT OF OBESITY

There is a strong association between obesity over a BMI of 30 and lower levels of serum 25-hydroxy vitamin D levels in blood [34], probably because, compared to leaner individuals, more vitamin D is sequestered in fat tissue [34]. Whether this is clinically relevant as a cause of obesity is questionable, however. There is no evidence that treatment with vitamin D reverses obesity, and at present, there is no reason to prescribe vitamin D above RDA levels to obese people [34].

THEORY THAT DIETARY SUPPLEMENTS ARE AVAILABLE TO ACHIEVE WEIGHT LOSS

A dietary supplement is a product intended to supplement the diet that contains dietary ingredients such as vitamins, minerals, herbs, or botanicals [35,36]. According to a recent national survey, 34% of adults reported using a dietary supplement for weight loss [37]. The 2007 NHIS found that 18% of U.S. adults had used some sort of a non-vitamin, nonmineral dietary supplement for weight loss [38]. About one-third of U.S. adults use a multivitamin and mineral supplement regularly [35,39]. Dietary supplements are used on weight reduction diets for two reasons [40]. The first is a legitimate one, involving the supplementation of nutrients such as calcium and trace elements that tend to be low on calorie-restricted diets [40]. When reducing diets such as very-low- or low-calorie diets fail to provide the required RDA/AI of a nutrient, dietary supplements in RDA/AI amounts can help prevent deficiency by providing adequate amounts of the nutrients that are lacking [40]. A second and unjustified reason consumers have for using dietary supplements is their belief that they actually cause weight loss [40]. The evidence for the claim that dietary supplements enhance or stimulate weight loss is poor and inconclusive, and the use of some of these products advertised as weight loss supplements is fraught with safety concerns [40]. *Ephedra* (ma huang), first isolated from an herb used in traditional Chinese medicine, is an example of a potentially dangerous herbal product that was so widely marketed as a weight loss supplement in the 1990s that by the late 1990s, their sales had reached $6.8 billion [41]. *Ephedra* has anorectic, lipolytic, and thermogenic effects and did increase weight loss slightly over placebos, but not without other risks [36]. Due to its adverse side effects, which included high blood pressure, myocardial infarctions, cerebrovascular accidents, seizures, and death, the Food and Drug Administration (FDA) banned the use of *Ephedra* in 2004 and prohibited its sale in supplements [41]. Bitter orange, or *Citrus aurantium*, has a similar compound in it, and it may also have adverse effects. There are currently no dietary supplements in the market that are effective for weight loss and that do not also carry risks of adverse events [40]. Many supplements contain caffeine in relatively high doses, and these are often combined with other stimulants such as ma huang, bitter orange, yohimbe, and guarana [42]. The amounts of caffeine in some of them are high enough to cause diuresis and caffeinism in some individuals, in addition to adverse effects from other botanicals that are also often present [42]. Caffeine can temporarily increase RMR slightly, but the effects are not large, specific, nor necessarily chronic, and, at very high doses, caffeine may also decrease appetite. Green tea and green tea extracts at doses of 100–300 mg may also temporarily increase thermogenesis. In combination with a low-calorie diet, there may be slightly increased weight loss, but these effects may not be evident in individuals who drink large amounts of coffee, perhaps because their metabolism disposes of the caffeine more effectively [43,44]. Data on efficacy are lacking for other products that purport to produce weight loss, including conjugated linolenic acid (CLA), L-carnitine, hydroxycitrate (isolated from the rind of *Garcinia camboglia*), pyruvate, and chromium picolinate [45,46]. Recently, weight loss supplements have been illegally spiked with active and undeclared prescription drugs, including diuretics. The U.S. FDA website (http://www.cfsan.fda.gov) is helpful for obtaining the most up-to-date information on product warnings and problems associated with dietary supplements [41].

The National Institutes of Health's Office of Dietary Supplements (ODS) (http://ods.od.nih.gov/) and the National Center for Complementary and Alternative Medicine (NCCAM) (http://nccam.nih.gov/) provide objective fact sheets and other information for consumers and health professionals on dietary supplements that may be useful to patients.

INCLUDE PHYSICAL ACTIVITY IN WEIGHT MANAGEMENT*

PHYSICAL ACTIVITY GUIDELINES FOR AMERICANS

It is essential to draw attention to physical activity in weight management. Table 5.13 outlines the 2008 Physical Activity Guidelines for Americans [47]. Weight control and weight loss require more physical activity than weight maintenance, and therefore the recommendation for weight loss is 45–75 min of moderate-intensity activity or 22 min of vigorous activity per day [47,48]. Moderate-intensity activities include walking, gardening, and aerobics, whereas examples of vigorous activity include jogging, bicycling, rock climbing, and swimming. Recommendations for weight maintenance include 60 min of moderate activity or 30 min of vigorous activity per day [48]. The benefits of regular physical activity extend beyond weight control to general wellness, improved sleep and mood in addition to decreased risk of health problems including type 2 diabetes, blood pressure, heart disease, high serum cholesterol, and osteoporosis [48].

PHYSICAL ACTIVITY GUIDELINES DURING THE WEIGHT LOSS PHASE OF DIETING

The amount and type of physical activity required for achieving a healthy weight varies from person to person [48]. Each week, at least 5 h of moderate-intensity physical activity or 150 min of vigorous-intensity physical activity is required for optimal weight control [48]. However, physical activity alone leads to little weight loss unless appropriate adjustments are also made in the type and amount of foods being eaten through a hypocaloric diet [49]. According to the 2010 Dietary Guidelines for Americans, both physical activity and a caloric deficit are necessary to maintain weight and prevent weight regain [4] since the lighter body takes less energy to move around, and the lower lean body mass contributes to a lower RMR. There is an association between regular physical activity, weight maintenance, and long-term body weight control, especially for obese individuals who have reduced their weights [50]. Data from the National Weight Control Registry, a registry of more than 3000 individuals who have successfully maintained at least a 30 lb weight loss for a minimum of 1 year, show that 90% of the individuals exercise 1 h/day on average for long-term weight maintenance [11].

CONSIDER WEIGHT LOSS DRUGS AS AN ADJUNCT TO DIET THERAPY†

Prescription weight loss medications are sometimes useful adjuncts to the dietary therapy of obesity for patients who are very heavy but also at an increased medical risk secondary to their weight (e.g., individuals with a BMI of 30 and above or a BMI of 27 and with obesity-related comorbidities [51]).

---

* See also Chapter 6 for a detailed discussion of the role of exercise in the management of the obese patient.
† See also Chapter 9 for a detailed discussion of pharmacologic options for management of the obese patient.

TABLE 5.13
2008 Physical Activity Guidelines for Americans

Population/Focus Area	Key Guidelines
Children and adolescents (6–17 years old)	Children and adolescents should do 60 min (1 h) or more of physical activity daily
	• *Aerobic*: Most of the 60 or more minutes a day should be either moderate- or vigorous-intensity aerobic physical activity, and should include vigorous-intensity physical activity at least 3 days a week
	• *Muscle-strengthening*: As part of their 60 or more minutes of daily physical activity, children and adolescents should include muscle-strengthening physical activity on at least 3 days of the week
	• *Bone-strengthening*: As part of their 60 or more minutes of daily physical activity, children and adolescents should include bone-strengthening physical activity on at least 3 days of the week
	It is important to encourage young people to participate in physical activities that are appropriate for their age, that are enjoyable, and that offer variety
Adult (18–64 years old)	• All adults should avoid inactivity. Some physical activity is better than none, and adults who participate in any amount of physical activity gain some health benefits
	• For substantial health benefits, adults should do at least 150 min (2 h and 30 min) a week of moderate-intensity, or 75 min (1 h and 15 min) a week of vigorous-intensity aerobic physical activity, or an equivalent combination of moderate- and vigorous-intensity aerobic activity. Aerobic activity should be performed in episodes of at least 10 min, and preferably, it should be spread throughout the week
	• For additional and more extensive health benefits, adults should increase their aerobic physical activity to 300 min (5 h) a week of moderate-intensity, or 150 min a week of vigorous-intensity aerobic physical activity, or an equivalent combination of moderate- and vigorous-intensity activity. Additional health benefits are gained by engaging in physical activity beyond this amount
	• Adults should also do muscle-strengthening activities that are moderate or high intensity and involve all major muscle groups on 2 or more days a week for additional benefits

(continued)

TABLE 5.13 (continued)
2008 Physical Activity Guidelines for Americans

Population/Focus Area	Key Guidelines
Older adults (65 years and older)	The key guidelines for adults also apply to older adults. In addition, the following Guidelines are for older adults:
	• When older adults cannot do 150 min of moderate-intensity aerobic activity a week because of chronic conditions, they should be as physically active as their abilities and conditions allow
	• Older adults should do exercises that maintain or improve balance if they are at risk of falling
	• Older adults should determine their level of effort for physical activity relative to their level of fitness
	• Older adults with chronic conditions should understand whether and how their conditions affect their ability to do regular physical activity safely
Adults with disabilities	• Adults with disabilities, who are able to, should get at least 150 min a week of moderate-intensity, or 75 min a week of vigorous-intensity aerobic activity, or an equivalent combination of moderate- and vigorous-intensity aerobic activity. Aerobic activity should be performed in episodes of at least 10 min, and preferably, it should be spread throughout the week
	• Adults with disabilities, who are able to, should also do muscle-strengthening activities of moderate or high intensity that involve all major muscle groups on 2 or more days a week, as these activities provide additional health benefits
	• When adults with disabilities are not able to meet the Guidelines, they should engage in regular physical activity according to their abilities and should avoid inactivity
	• Adults with disabilities should consult their health-care provider about the amounts and types of physical activity that are appropriate for their abilities

Source: U.S. Department of Health and Human Services, U.S. Department of Agriculture, *Physical Activity Guidelines for Americans.* 2008, U.S. Government Printing Office, Washington, DC, 2008.

TABLE 5.14

Prescription Medications Available for Weight Loss in the United States

Generic Name	FDA Approval for Weight Loss	Drug Type	Common Side Effects
Phentermine (Obenix™)	Yes; short term (up to 12 weeks) for adults	Appetite suppressant	Increased blood pressure and heart rate, sleeplessness, and nervousness
Diethylpropion (Tenuate™)	Yes; short term (up to 12 weeks) for adults	Appetite suppressant	Dizziness, headache, sleeplessness, and nervousness
Phendimetrazine (Adipost™)	Yes; short term (up to 12 weeks) for adults	Appetite suppressant	Sleeplessness and nervousness
Orlistat (prescription: Xenical™)	Yes; long term (up to 1 year) for adults and children age 12 and older	Lipase inhibitor	Gastrointestinal issues (cramping, diarrhea, and oily spotting)
Bupropion (Wellbutrin™)	No	Depression treatment	Dry mouth and insomnia
Topiramate (Topamax™)	No	Seizure treatment	Numbness of skin and change in taste
Zonisamide (Zonegran™)	No	Seizure treatment	Drowsiness, dry mouth, dizziness, headache, and nausea
Metformin (Glucophage™)	No	Diabetes treatment	Weakness, dizziness, metallic taste, and nausea

Source: Weight control information network, U.S. Department of Health and Human Services, National Institutes of Health [database online]. 2010. http://win.niddk.nih.gov/publications/prescription.htm (Accessed: February 26, 2011).

Table 5.14 provides an overview of prescription medications available in the United States for weight loss [51]. The mechanisms of their actions vary, as do their side effects.

APPETITE SUPPRESSANTS

Appetite suppressants, also called anorectic agents, promote weight loss by decreasing appetite or increasing satiety [51]. Until recently, sibutramine (Meridia™), a centrally acting appetite suppressant, was the only FDA-approved appetite suppressant that was available for long-term use (up to 2 years) [51]. However, it was withdrawn from the market in October 2010 because of increased cardiovascular disease risks associated with its use, including stroke and heart attacks [51].

Currently, the most commonly prescribed appetite suppressant in the United States is phentermine, which also carries only limited efficacy and its share of unpleasant side effects [51]. Concerns and issues with other anorectic weight loss drugs include drug abuse and dependence or development of tolerance [51]. Thus, when prescribing medications for weight loss, clinicians should review and evaluate with patients the potential side effects associated with the drug as well as its efficacy.

AGENTS CAUSING MALABSORPTION

The only drug that is currently approved by the FDA for long-term use in weight reduction is orlistat. The trade name of orlistat is Xenical™, available by prescription or over the counter in half strength, marketed as Alli™ [51]. Orlistat is a lipase inhibitor that inhibits fat absorption by blocking the enzyme lipase, involved in fat absorption [51]. A low-fat hypocaloric diet is vital if orlistat is to be effective, as it helps the individual to achieve the needed caloric deficit while minimizing the adverse side effects of the drug by decreasing the degree of malabsorption [51]. The major side effects of orlistat include cramping, intestinal discomfort, flatulence, diarrhea, and anal leakage [51]. Furthermore, patients suffering from kidney disease and pancreatitis should avoid using orlistat without medical supervision [51]. Since orlistat decreases fat-soluble vitamin absorption, a multivitamin supplement containing fat-soluble vitamins is recommended to ensure adequate nutritional status [51].

CONSIDER THE SAFETY OF WEIGHT LOSS MEDICATIONS

Medications and drugs are usually associated with potential risks and side effects, which should be taken into account when their use in the treatment of obesity is being considered. In the 1990s, the indiscriminate use of untested combinations of weight loss drugs such as phentermine–fenfluramine ("phen/fen") combinations and dexfenfluramine for long-term weight management led to some serious and even fatal side effects, including the development of cardiac valvular disease and serious abnormalities in mitral, aortic, and tricuspid heart valves in addition to pulmonary hypertension [52]. Based on these adverse effects and associated safety concerns, fenfluramine and dexfenfluramine were subsequently banned from the U.S. market [52].

BARIATRIC SURGERY AS AN OPTION FOR SEVERE OBESITY*

Bariatric surgery for obesity has increased dramatically: from 10,000 cases in 1996 to approximately 70,000 cases in 2002, to 170,000 cases in 2005, and to the most recent estimate of 220,000 cases in 2008 in the United States [53,54].

Table 5.15 describes the NIH's guidelines and eligibility criteria for surgical therapy for weight loss [55]. The criteria for weight loss surgery are a BMI $\geq 40\,\text{kg/m}^2$ or a BMI $\geq 35\,\text{kg/m}^2$ in association with obesity-related comorbidities such as cardiovascular disease, type 2 diabetes, and sleep apnea [1].

Table 5.16 outlines the different types of bariatric surgical procedures and the risks and potential nutritional complications associated with those procedures. It also summarizes key nutritional implications for clinicians involved in the care and management of patients undergoing them [54–57].

BENEFITS ASSOCIATED WITH WEIGHT LOSS SURGERY

Several studies of postoperative outcomes for severely obese individuals show beneficial effects of surgery on the resolution of comorbidities, mortality, survival

---

* See also Chapter 10 for a detailed discussion of surgical treatment of obesity.

TABLE 5.15

Candidates for Weight Loss Surgery

Eligibility Criteria for Bariatric Surgery

- BMI > 35 and who also have two or more comorbidities (high cholesterol, sleep apnea, diabetes, heart disease, and hypertension)
- BMI ≥ 40 without comorbidities
- Between 18 and 65 years of age
- Previously exhausted nonsurgical weight loss methods

Sources: Expert panel on the identification, evaluation, and treatment of overweight in adults, *Am. J. Clin. Nutr.*, 68(4), 899, 1998; Flegal, K.M. et al., *JAMA*, 303(3), 235, 2010; American Society for Metabolic and Bariatric Surgery, *Fact Sheet: Metabolic & Bariatric Surgery*, 2009. www.asbs.org/Newsite07/media/asbs_presskit.html (Accessed: March 9, 2011).

rates, and quality of life, but only if weight loss can be maintained for several years [58,59]. Weight regain after surgery is common [60]. Various long-term studies indicate weight regain postsurgery is between 7% and 50% [60]. Over a period of 10 years, 20%–25% of the lost weight is usually regained even among those who successfully lost significant amount of weight [60,61]. The prospective, controlled SOS study involving 4047 obese subjects showed that mean weight loss was maximum after 1–2 years and had stabilized after 10 years [62]. Patients who have lost weight after bariatric surgery and who have maintained it for at least 8 years tend to have improved outcomes with obesity-related comorbidities such as type 2 diabetes, blood pressure, and dyslipidemia [63]. The immediate effect of bariatric surgery on type 2 diabetes is dramatic with resolution of type 2 diabetes in 83% of some patients who underwent gastric bypass surgery [64]. Weight loss surgery also has positive effects on hypertension [65] and on lipid markers and dyslipidemia [66]. However, none of these positive effects remain if the weight is regained [61].

RISKS AND COMPLICATIONS ASSOCIATED WITH BARIATRIC SURGERY

Bariatric surgery is associated with several risks and complications, making postoperative care critical to obtain optimal health effects in order to avoid unnecessary adverse events. These can be minimized by referring patients to a specialist in the field and not to general surgeons. Many of the other postoperative risks involve secondary malnutrition and these are more immediate [60]. Protein calorie malnutrition is a severe complication of the malabsorptive bariatric surgical procedures such as Roux-en-Y gastric bypass, gastric sleeve, and biliopancreatic diversion, typically occurring 2–6 months postsurgery [60]. Malabsorptive surgical procedures increase the risk for various vitamin and mineral deficiencies especially within the first year of surgery [60]. Supplementation with a multivitamin, multimineral, calcium, vitamin D, iron, and vitamin B12 is critical to prevent any of these micronutrient nutritional deficiencies [60].

TABLE 5.16

Types of Surgical Procedures: Safety and Nutritional Implications

Type of Procedure and Description	Safety and Associated Risks	Nutritional Implications	Implications for Clinicians
Gastric Bypass—Roux-en-Y Procedure: The upper part of the stomach is stapled resulting in two different sections: the top part of the stomach called the pouch attached to the esophagus and the remaining part of the stomach without any food being passed through it. The food enters into the pouch through the esophagus and directly enters into the intestine "bypassing" the remaining part of the stomach. Due to the reduced size and capacity of the stomach, patients have a reduced appetite and thus eat less food and get full faster, which in turn aids in weight loss	Stomach ulcers, lactose intolerance, dehydration, constipation/bowel obstruction, surgical complications including bleeding, anastomotic leak, pulmonary embolism, deep vein thrombosis, staple line failure, and mortality	Vitamin and mineral malabsorption (calcium, iron, vitamins A, D, E, K, C, B6, and B12) Dumping syndrome	Patients need informed dietary advice postsurgery Vitamins, mineral, and dietary supplements may be required
Adjustable Gastric Band: The adjustable gastric band operation is a type of restrictive surgical weight loss procedure where an adjustable saline-filled silicone band is placed near the upper part of the stomach creating a small pouch. This procedure is minimally invasive, adjustable, and reversible. This smaller pouch reduces the functional capacity of the stomach and makes the patient feel full faster and longer and thus results in weight loss	Surgical complication including infection, slippage, malposition of the band, gastritis, and internal bleeding	Nutritional complication: nausea, vomiting, gastroesophageal reflux, stomach obstruction, constipation, diarrhea, difficulty swallowing, gallstones Nutritional deficiencies including iron, B12, and calcium	Patients need informed dietary advice postsurgery Vitamins, mineral, and dietary supplements may be required

Procedure	Postoperative complications	Nutritional deficiencies	Supplementation
Biliopancreatic Diversion with Duodenal Switch (BPD/DS): A malabsorptive procedure that includes removal of a large portion of the stomach to promote smaller meal sizes, rerouting of food away from much of the small intestine to partially prevent absorption of food, and rerouting of bile and other digestive juices that impair digestion	Postoperative complications	Severe malabsorption—Fe, Ca, Mg, Zn, vitamins C and B-complex Protein malabsorption, fat malabsorption, and subsequent fat soluble vitamin deficiency including vitamins A, D, E, K	Vitamin and mineral supplementation required. Malabsorption may be severe
Vertical Sleeve Gastrectomy (VSG): A large portion of the stomach is removed to form a more tubular "gastric sleeve." The smaller stomach sleeve remains connected to a very short segment of the duodenum, which is then directly connected to a lower part of the small intestine. This small portion of the duodenum performs absorption although the food eaten bypasses majority of the duodenum	Stomach leak: leaking of the sleeve, blood clots and wound infection, and weight regain	Nutritional def including iron, B12, and calcium, Mg, Zn, and vitamins C and B-complex	

Sources: American Society for Metabolic and Bariatric Surgery, *Fact Sheet: Metabolic & Bariatric Surgery*, 2009. www.asbs.org/Newsite07/media/asbs_presskit.html (Accessed: March 9, 2011). NIH conference, Gastrointestinal surgery for severe obesity, Consensus development conference panel, *Ann. Intern. Med.*, 115(12), 956, 1991; Leff, D.R. and Heath, D., *BMJ (Clin. Res. Ed.)* 339, b3402, 2009; Colquitt, J.L. et al., Surgery for obesity. *Cochrane Database Syst. Rev. Issue 2*, CD003641, doi:10.1002/14651858.CD003641.pub3, 2009.

TABLE 5.17

Post–Gastric Bypass Surgery Diet Used at Tufts Medical Center, Boston, MA

Stage 1	One ounce of water per hour, typically in the hospital on the day of surgery
Stage 2	Noncaloric clear liquids, usually in the hospital the day after surgery (e.g., sugar-free Jell-O, flat diet soda, and diet juice)
Stage 3	Three to four small meals per day, each consisting of a high-protein, no added sugar shake, such as Isopure or Sugar-Free Carnation® Instant Breakfast™
	Water or noncaloric, noncarbonated clear liquids between meals
	Goals of this stage are to drink 64 oz fluid/day, 50–60 g of protein a day for women and 60–70 g of protein per day for men
	This stage lasts 2–3 weeks
Stage 4	Small portions of moist, ground/pureed foods
	Begin supplementing with a multivitamin plus minerals, vitamin D with calcium (specifically calcium and sublingual vitamin B12)
	Aim for 60–70 g of protein per day
	This stage lasts 4–5 weeks
Stage 5	Small portions of low-fat (<3–5 g/serving) or low-sugar (<14 g/serving) solid foods
	At least 64 oz of fluid/day
	Aim for 60–80 g of protein
	Continue to take supplements
	Follow this 6–8 weeks after surgery and follow up with an RD

Source: Kolasa, K.M. et al., *N. C. Med. J.*, 67(4), 283, 2006.

Surgical complications of bariatric surgery include bleeding, staple line failures, intestinal obstructions, anastomotic leaks, and internal hernias [59]. Postoperative follow-up and clinical management of the surgical patient is crucial in preventing and treating nutritional and surgical complications associated with such bariatric procedures [59]. Referral to an RD along with close monitoring and regular follow-up, coupled with long-term management of surgical patients by a multidisciplinary medical team, is the best way to reduce risks from a host of postoperative complications and to avoid weight regain, which is a common risk [59].

Table 5.17 outlines a post–gastric bypass surgery diet used by the bariatric group at the Tufts Medical Center [67]. It explains the various diet stages recommended for patients undergoing gastric bypass at the Tufts Weight and Wellness Center.

PLAN AND IMPLEMENT THE WEIGHT MAINTENANCE PHASE FOLLOWING WEIGHT LOSS

Successful weight loss should be followed by a well-designed weight loss maintenance regimen. Prevention of weight regain and maintenance of weight loss can be achieved by a combination of a diet that is modestly reduced in calories, regular physical activity, and behavior modification [13]. According to the National Weight

Control Registry, dieters have successfully maintained their weight loss report following a reduced-calorie, low-fat diet, in addition to increased levels of regular physical activity [15].

CONSIDER ENERGY INTAKE AND NUTRIENT NEEDS IN WEIGHT MAINTENANCE

The main goal of weight maintenance is to prevent weight gain and to maintain a lower body weight and health over long term [13]. The diet needs to be lower in calories than it was prior to weight loss during maintenance since energy needs are reduced because of less lean body mass (thus lower RMR) and the lesser energy cost of moving the lighter body. The diet should include RDA/AI levels of nutrients and be balanced in energy-providing nutrients. Weight maintenance strategies should also include adequate amounts of physical activity and psychological and social support [16].

INCLUDE PHYSICAL ACTIVITY IN WEIGHT MAINTENANCE

Regular amounts of physical activity continue to remain important once an individual has lost weight. Recommendations for weight maintenance include 60 min of moderate-intensity activity or 30 min of vigorous-intensity activity per day [48]. Physical activity is one of the best predictors of long-term weight maintenance and plays a vital role in promoting general wellness and preventing risk for chronic disease [15].

INCLUDE BEHAVIOR MODIFICATION AND SUPPORT TO MAINTAIN WEIGHT LOSS*

Long-term weight reduction and maintenance are aided by self-monitoring of diet, activity, stress management, approaches to problem solving, and stimulus control [13]. A strong social support network of family and friends in addition to self-management helps provide the motivation to continue and achieve weight maintenance goals [21].

PUT PUBLIC HEALTH AND POLICY RECOMMENDATIONS IN PLACE FOR FUTURE PROGRESS†

Table 5.18 outlines some relevant public health and policy recommendations on overweight and obesity for Americans. Current recommendations include the president's White House Task Force on Childhood Obesity, the Dietary Guidelines for Americans 2010, the U.S. Department of Health and Human Services Healthy People 2020, and the U.S. Preventive Services Task Force Report [68–70]. Taken together, these documents chart the way forward in the battle to control weight. Now they must be implemented.

---

* See also Chapter 7 for a detailed discussion of behavioral issues in obesity management.
† See also Chapter 11 for a detailed discussion of public policy issues related to obesity.

TABLE 5.18

Recent Public Health and Public Policy Recommendations on Overweight and Obesity

Recommendation	Specific Objectives	Implications for Clinicians
President's Task Force on Childhood Obesity	Empower parents and caregivers Provide healthy foods in schools Improve access to healthy, affordable foods Increase physical activity	Implement strategies that will strengthen prenatal care and promote breastfeeding Initiatives that will strengthen the role of health-care providers Provide adequate resources for patients to make healthful choices Efforts to encourage physical activity in schools and in activities outside of the school
"Let's Move" Campaign For Children	Empower parents to make healthier family choices Provide healthier foods in schools Increase access to healthy and affordable food Increase physical activity	Calls for a multidisciplinary approach to treating obesity by encouraging collaboration among child care professionals, clinicians, politicians, and government and community leaders to promote the health and wellness of families and communities Integrate exercise into every patient–client interaction The National Initiative for Children's Healthcare Quality (NICHQ) and the "Healthy Care for Healthy Kids: a Collaborative to Prevent, Identify and Manage Childhood Overweight," have developed a toolkit to assist clinicians and primary care practice teams in providing and delivering coordinated, integrated and multidisciplinary services to prevent overweight and improve care for children who are already overweight or at risk The American Academy of Pediatrics (AAP) has partnered with the White House on the First Lady's Let's Move campaign. As part of the program, the AAP is asking every pediatrician to calculate BMI for every child over the age of 2 at every well-child visit
Healthy People 2020	Goals include Attain high-quality, longer lives free of preventable disease, disability, injury, and premature death Achieve health equity, eliminate disparities, and improve the health of all groups	Increase the proportion of physician offices visits that include counseling or education related to nutrition or weight Increase the proportion of primary care physicians who regularly measure the BMI of their patients

Create social and physical environments that promote good health for all

Promote quality of life, healthy development, and healthy behaviors across all life stages

Increase the proportion of physician office visits for chronic health diseases or conditions that include counseling or education related to exercise

USDA Dietary Guidelines 2010

Maintain caloric balance over time to achieve and sustain a healthy weight

- Control total calorie intake to manage body weight
- Increase physical activity and reduce time spent in sedentary behaviors
- Consume nutrient-dense foods and beverages
- Reduce daily sodium intake to less than 2300 (mg)
- Consume less than 10% of calories from saturated fatty acids by replacing them with monounsaturated and polyunsaturated fatty acids
- Consume less than 300 mg/day of dietary cholesterol
- Keep trans-fatty acid consumption as low as possible by limiting foods that contain synthetic sources of trans fats, such as partially hydrogenated oils, and by limiting other solid fats
- Reduce the intake of calories from solid fats and added sugars
- Limit consumption of foods that contain refined grains, especially refined grain foods that contain solid fats, added sugars, and sodium
- Increase vegetable and fruit intake
- Consume at least half of all grains as whole grains
- Increase intake of fat-free or low-fat milk and milk products, such as milk, yogurt, cheese, or fortified soy beverages
- Choose a variety of protein foods, which include seafood, lean meat and poultry, eggs, beans and peas, soy products, and unsalted nuts and seeds
- Increase the amount and variety of seafood consumed by choosing seafood in place of some meat and poultry

(continued)

TABLE 5.18 (continued)

Recent Public Health and Public Policy Recommendations on Overweight and Obesity

Recommendation	Specific Objectives	Implications for Clinicians
US Preventive Service Task Force (USPSTF)	Reviews preventive clinical health-care services like screening, and counseling and accordingly provides recommendations for primary care physicians	The USPSTF recommends that clinicians screen all adult patients for obesity and offer intensive counseling and behavioral interventions to promote sustained weight loss for obese adults
		The USPSTF recommends that clinicians screen children aged 6 years and older for obesity and offer them or refer them to comprehensive, intensive behavioral interventions to promote improvement in weight status

Sources: White House Task Force on Childhood Obesity, *Solving the Problem of Childhood Obesity Within a Generation*, White House Task Force on Childhood Obesity, Office of the U.S. President, Washington, DC, 2010; U.S. Department of Health and Human Services, *Healthy People 2020*, Office of Disease Prevention and Health Promotion, Washington, DC, 2010; U.S. Department of Health and Human Services, *U.S. Preventive Services Task Force (USPSTF)*, Agency for Healthcare Research and Quality, Rockville, MD, 2010.

CONCLUSION

Overweight and obesity are major health problems in the United States. The dietary management of obesity involves the medical, nutritional, psychological, and social assessment of the individual; identification of health and medical objectives; and the selection and implementation of the appropriate dietary therapy for the patient. The nutritional treatment of obesity is only a part of a comprehensive program of weight control that incorporates physical activity, psychological and social support, and medical assistance for related health problems in order to focus on establishing and achieving weight loss and long-term weight maintenance.

APPENDIX A

RESEARCH TOOLS FOR ASSESSING BODY FATNESS

SKINFOLDS

Skinfold thickness is used in research settings as another rough measure of body fatness. It is used to measure subcutaneous fat at specific sites, including the subscapular, suprailiac, triceps, pectoral (chest), midaxillary, abdominal, thigh, and other sites including biceps and calf [9]. A metal skinfold caliper is used to measure the fat fold; it provides a very rough estimate of body fatness [9]. In most cases, this is insufficiently precise to calculate percent body fat, but it does provide a relatively inexpensive method that is appropriate for large-scale studies [9]. However, it requires trained technicians and health professionals to ensure accuracy and reliability of the measurements [9].

BIOELECTRICAL IMPEDANCE

Bioelectrical impedance (BIA) is commonly used to assess body composition [9]. The resistance or impedance to a small electrical current through the body's water is measured to estimate total body water, which is then used to assess total body fat-free mass [9]. The difference between body weight and fat-free mass provides the total body fat. It is low cost and easy to use, but does not give accurate measurements for the amount of the fat as it is hydration dependent and is not accurate in patients with disturbances in body fluids [9].

DUAL-ENERGY X-RAY ABSORPTIOMETRY

Dual-energy x-ray absorptiometry (DEXA) is considered the gold standard for measuring body composition. This technique scans the whole body to provide estimates of the three main body compartments (bone mineral, fat-free mass, and fat mass) [9]. It is a highly accurate and reliable method used for estimating body composition. However, it is an expensive method, and the machine cannot accommodate very large individuals, given its weight and height limit. Moreover, trained technicians are required, and it cannot be used in field studies.

ACKNOWLEDGMENTS

This work was supported in part with resources from the U.S. Department of Agriculture, Agricultural Research Service, under agreement No. 58-1950-7-707.*

REFERENCES

1. Expert panel on the identification, evaluation, and treatment of overweight in adults. Oct 1998. Clinical guidelines on the identification, evaluation, and treatment of overweight and obesity in adults: Executive summary. *The American Journal of Clinical Nutrition* 68(4): 899–917.
2. Flegal, K. M., M. D. Carroll, C. L. Ogden, and L. R. Curtin. Jan 20, 2010. Prevalence and trends in obesity among US adults, 1999–2008. *JAMA* 303(3): 235–241.
3. Pleis, J. R., J. W. Lucas, and B. W. Ward. Dec 2009. Summary health statistics for U.S. adults: National health interview survey, 2008. *Vital and Health Statistics. Series 10, Data from the National Health Survey* 242: 1–157.
4. U.S. Department of Agriculture and U.S. Department of Health and Human Services. Dec 2010. *Dietary Guidelines for Americans, 2010.* 7th edn., Washington, DC: U.S. Government Printing Office.
5. Mokha, J. S., S. R. Srinivasan, P. Dasmahapatra, C. Fernandez, W. Chen, J. Xu, and G. S. Berenson. 2010. Utility of waist-to-height ratio in assessing the status of central obesity and related cardio-metabolic risk profile among normal weight and overweight/obese children: The Bogalusa heart study. *BMC Pediatrics* 10: 73. doi:10.1186/1471-2431-10-73
6. Khan Afridi, A., M. Safdar, M. M. A. K. Khattak, and A. Khan. 2003. Health risks of overweight and obesity—An overview. *Pakistan Journal of Nutrition* 2(6): 350–360.
7. Kushner, R. F. and N. Kushner. 2008. *Counseling Overweight Adults: The Lifestyle Patterns Approach and Toolkit.* Chicago, IL: American Dietetic Association.
8. American Psychiatric Association, ed. 1994. *Diagnostic and Statistical Manual of Mental Disorders.* 4th edn., Washington, DC: American Psychiatric Press.
9. Allison, D. B. and M. L. Baskin. 2009. *Handbook of Assessment Methods for Eating Behaviors and Weight-Related Problems: Measures, Theory, and Research.* Thousand Oaks, CA: Sage Publications, Inc.
10. USDA Center for Nutrition Policy and Promotion. My pyramid tracker. In United States Department of Agriculture [database online]. 2011. http://www.mypyramidtracker.gov/ (Accessed: April 12, 2011).
11. Seagle, H. M., G. W. Strain, A. Makris, and R. S. Reeves. 2009. Position of the American dietetic association: Weight management. *Journal of the American Dietetic Association* 109(2): 330–346.
12. Lin, P. H., M. A. Proschan, G. A. Bray, C. P. Fernandez, K. Hoben, and M. Most-Windhauser, DASH Collaborative Research Group. (2003). Estimation of energy requirements in a controlled feeding trial. *The American Journal of Clinical Nutrition* 77(3): 639–645.
13. Dwyer, J. and K. J. Melanson. 2002. Dietary treatment of obesity. In *Endotext*, 2nd edn. Caro, J., ed., 2007. Available from http://www.endotext.com/obesity/index.htm
14. Mond, J. M., T. C. Myers, R. D. Crosby, P. J. Hay, B. Rodgers, J. F. Morgan, J. H. Lacey, and J. E. Mitchell. May 2008. Screening for eating disorders in primary care: EDE-Q versus SCOFF. *Behavior Research and Therapy* 46(5): 612–622.
15. Tsai, A. G. and T. A. Wadden. Aug 2006. The evolution of very-low-calorie diets: An update and meta-analysis. *Obesity (Silver Spring, Md.)* 14(8): 1283–1293.

---

* Any opinions, findings, conclusions, or recommendations expressed here are those of the authors and do not necessarily reflect the view of the U.S. Department of Agriculture.

16. National Heart, Lung and Blood Institute (NHLBI) Obesity Education Initiative Expert Panel. 1998. *Clinical Guidelines on the Identification, Evaluation, and Treatment of Overweight and Obesity in Adults.* Bethesda, MD: National Institute of Health.
17. Wadden, T. A. and A. J. Stunkard. 2002. *Handbook of Obesity Treatment.* New York: The Guilford Press.
18. Schoeller, D. A. and A. C. Buchholz. 2005. Energetics of obesity and weight control: Does diet composition matter? *Journal of the American Dietetic Association* 105(5 Suppl 1): S24–S28. doi:10.1016/j.jada.2005.02.025
19. Stevens, A., E. Dionne, and J. Dwyer. 2007. Popular and fad diet programs: Nutritional adequacy, safety and efficacy. In *Self-Help Approaches for Obesity and Eating Disorders,* J. Latner and T. Wilson (eds)., New York: The Guilford Press, pp. 21–52.
20. Melanson, K. and J. Dwyer. 2002. Popular diets for treatment of overweight and obesity. T. A. Wadden and A. J. Stunkard (eds)., In *Handbook of Obesity Treatment.* New York: The Guilford Press, pp. 249–275.
21. Food and Nutrition Information Center, National Agricultural Library, USDA. 2009. Weight management and obesity resource list. http://www.nal.usda.gov/fnic/pubs/bibs/topics/weight/consumer.pdf (Accessed: February 24, 2011).
22. Augustin, J. 2001. Web based resources for weight loss. *Nutrition in Clinical Care* 4: 272–274.
23. Fitday. Free internet tools for tracking weight, diet, exercise, and more. 2009. http://www.fitday.com/ (Accessed: February 24, 2011).
24. Anderson, J., L. Young, and J. Roach. 2008. Weight Loss Products and Programs. http://www.ext.colostate.edu/pubs/footnut/09363.html (Accessed: February 24, 2011).
25. Tsai, A. G. and T. A. Wadden. Jan 4, 2005. Systematic review: An evaluation of major commercial weight loss programs in the United States. *Annals of Internal Medicine* 142(1): 56–66.
26. Institute of Medicine (U.S.), E. Wartella, A. H. Lichtenstein, and C. S. Boon. 2010. Front-of-package nutrition rating systems and symbols: Phase I Report. Washington, DC: National Academies Press.
27. Freudenberg, N. 2010. The biology and politics of obesity. *The Lancet* 375(9712): 365–366.
28. Pelchat, M. L. Mar 2009. Food addiction in humans. *The Journal of Nutrition* 139(3): 620–622.
29. Lutter, M. and E. J. Nestler. Mar 2009. Homeostatic and hedonic signals interact in the regulation of food intake. *The Journal of Nutrition* 139(3): 629–632.
30. Avena, N. M., P. Rada, and B. G. Hoebel. 2008. Evidence for sugar addiction: Behavioral and neurochemical effects of intermittent, excessive sugar intake. *Neuroscience and Biobehavioral Reviews* 32(1): 20–39.
31. Jenkins, D. J., T. M. Wolever, R. H. Taylor, H. Barker, H. Fielden, J. M. Baldwin, A. C. Bowling, H. C. Newman, A. L. Jenkins, and D. V. Goff. Mar 1981. Glycemic index of foods: A physiological basis for carbohydrate exchange. *The American Journal of Clinical Nutrition* 34(3): 362–366.
32. Barclay, A. W., P. Petocz, J. McMillan-Price, V. M. Flood, T. Prvan, P. Mitchell, and J. C. Brand-Miller. Mar 2008. Glycemic index, glycemic load, and chronic disease risk—A meta-analysis of observational studies. *The American Journal of Clinical Nutrition* 87(3): 627–637.
33. Esfahani, A., J. M. Wong, A. Mirrahimi, C. R. Villa, and C. W. Kendall. Jan 2011. The application of the glycemic index and glycemic load in weight loss: A review of the clinical evidence. *International Union of Biochemistry & Molecular Biology (IUBMB)* 63(1): 7–13.
34. Institute of Medicine, Food and Nutrition Board. 2010. *Dietary Reference Intakes for Calcium and Vitamin D.* Washington, DC: National Academy Press.

35. U.S. Food and Drug Administration. Dietary Supplement Health and Education act of 1994. http://www.fda.gov/RegulatoryInformation/Legislation/FederalFoodDrugandCosmeticActFDCAct/SignificantAmendmentstotheFDCAct/ucm148003.htm (Accessed: February 26, 2011).

36. National Center for Complementary and Alternative Medicine, National Institutes of Health. 2009. Using dietary supplements wisely. http://nccam.nih.gov/health/supplements/wiseuse.htm (Accessed: February 26, 2011).

37. Pillitteri, J. L., S. Shiffman, J. M. Rohay, A. M. Harkins, S. L. Burton, and T. A. Wadden. Apr 2008. Use of dietary supplements for weight loss in the United States: Results of a national survey. *Obesity (Silver Spring, Md.)* 16(4): 790–796.

38. Barnes, P. M., B. Bloom, R. L. Nahin, and U.S. National Center for Health Statistics. 2008. *Complementary and Alternative Medicine Use Among Adults and Children: United States, 2007.* Hyattsville, MD: U.S. Department of Health and Human Services, Centers for Disease Control and Prevention, National Center for Health Statistics.

39. Marra, M. V. and A. P. Boyar. Dec 2009. Position of the American dietetic association: Nutrient supplementation. *Journal of the American Dietetic Association* 109(12): 2073–2085.

40. Dwyer, J. T., D. B. Allison, and P. M. Coates. May 2005. Dietary supplements in weight reduction. *Journal of the American Dietetic Association* 105(5 Suppl 1): S80–S86.

41. Kingston, R. L. and S. W. Borron. Sep 2, 2003. The relative safety of *Ephedra* compared with other herbal products. *Annals of Internal Medicine* 139(5 Pt 1): 385; author reply 386–387.

42. National Center for Complementary and Alternative Medicine, National Institutes of Health. 2011. Dietary and herbal supplements. http://nccam.nih.gov/health/supplements/ (Accessed: February 24, 2011).

43. Hursel, R., W. Viechtbauer, and M. S. Westerterp-Plantenga. 2009. The effects of green tea on weight loss and weight maintenance: A meta-analysis. *International Journal of Obesity (2005)* 33(9): 956–961. doi:10.1038/ijo.2009.135

44. Phung, O. J., W. L. Baker, L. J. Matthews, M. Lanosa, A. Thorne, and C. I. Coleman. 2010. Effect of green tea catechins with or without caffeine on anthropometric measures: A systematic review and meta-analysis. *The American Journal of Clinical Nutrition* 91(1): 73–81. doi:10.3945/ajcn.2009.28157

45. Pittler, M. H. and E. Ernst. 2004. Dietary supplements for body-weight reduction: A systematic review. *The American Journal of Clinical Nutrition* 79(4): 529–536.

46. Pittler, M. H., K. Schmidt, and E. Ernst. 2005. Adverse events of herbal food supplements for body weight reduction: Systematic review. *Obesity Reviews: An Official Journal of the International Association for the Study of Obesity* 6(2): 93–111. doi:10.1111/j.1467-789X.2005.00169

47. U.S. Department of Health and Human Services, U.S. Department of Agriculture. 2008. *Physical Activity Guidelines for Americans. 2008.* Washington, DC: U.S. Government Printing Office.

48. National Institute of Diabetes and Digestive and Kidney Diseases. Physical activity and weight control. Weight Control Information Network [database online]. 2010. http://www.nal.usda.gov/fnic/pubs/bibs/topics/weight/consumer.pdf (Accessed: February 24, 2011).

49. Centers for Disease Control and Prevention. Physical activity for a healthy weight. 2011. http://www.cdc.gov/healthyweight/physical_activity/index.html (Accessed: February 24, 2011).

50. Tremblay, A., E. Doucet, and P. Imbeault. 1999. Physical activity and weight maintenance. *International Journal of Obesity* (Suppl) 23(3): S50–S54.

51. Weight control information network. U.S. Department of Health and Human Services, National Institutes of Health [database online]. 2010. http://win.niddk.nih.gov/publications/prescription.htm (Accessed: February 26, 2011).

52. Connolly, H. M., J. L. Crary, M. D. McGoon, D. D. Hensrud, B. S. Edwards, W. D. Edwards, and H. V. Schaff. 1997. Valvular heart disease associated with fenfluramine–phentermine. *The New England Journal of Medicine* 337(9): 581–588. doi:10.1056/NEJM199708283370901

53. Perry, C. D., M. M. Hutter, D. B. Smith, J. P. Newhouse, and B. J. McNeil. 2008. Survival and changes in co-morbidities after bariatric surgery. *Annals of Surgery* 247(1): 21.

54. American Society for Metabolic and Bariatric Surgery. 2009. *Fact Sheet: Metabolic & Bariatric Surgery.* www.asbs.org/Newsite07/media/asbs_presskit.html (Accessed: March 9, 2011).

55. NIH conference. Gastrointestinal surgery for severe obesity. Consensus development conference panel Dec 15, 1991. *Annals of Internal Medicine* 115(12): 956–961.

56. Leff, D. R. and D. Heath. Sep 22, 2009. Surgery for obesity in adulthood. *BMJ (Clinical Research Ed.)* 339: b3402.

57. Colquitt, J. L., J. Picot, E. Loveman, and A. J. Clegg. 2009. Surgery for obesity. *Cochrane Database of Systematic Reviews Issue 2*: CD003641. doi:10.1002/14651858. CD003641.pub3

58. Flum, D. R. and E. P. Dellinger. Oct 2004. Impact of gastric bypass operation on survival: A population-based analysis. *Journal of the American College of Surgeons* 199(4): 543–551.

59. Sjostrom, L., A. K. Lindroos, M. Peltonen, J. Torgerson, C. Bouchard, B. Carlsson, S. Dahlgren et al. Dec 23, 2004. Lifestyle, diabetes, and cardiovascular risk factors 10 years after bariatric surgery. *The New England Journal of Medicine* 351(26): 2683–2693.

60. Heber, D., F. L. Greenway, L. M. Kaplan, E. Livingston, J. Salvador, C. Still, and Endocrine Society. Nov 2010. Endocrine and nutritional management of the post-bariatric surgery patient: An endocrine society clinical practice guideline. *The Journal of Clinical Endocrinology and Metabolism* 95(11): 4823–4843.

61. Magro, D. O., B. Geloneze, R. Delfini, B. C. Pareja, F. Callejas, and J. C. Pareja. Jun 2008. Long-term weight regain after gastric bypass: A 5-year prospective study. *Obesity Surgery* 18(6): 648–651.

62. Sjostrom, L., K. Narbro, C. D. Sjostrom, K. Karason, B. Larsson, H. Wedel, T. Lystig et al. Aug 23, 2007. Effects of bariatric surgery on mortality in Swedish obese subjects. *The New England Journal of Medicine* 357(8): 741–752.

63. Richardson, D. W. and A. I. Vinik. Mar 2005. Metabolic implications of obesity: Before and after gastric bypass. *Gastroenterology Clinics of North America* 34(1): 9–24.

64. Schauer, P. R., B. Burguera, S. Ikramuddin, D. Cottam, W. Gourash, G. Hamad, G. M. Eid et al. Oct 2003. Effect of laparoscopic roux-en Y gastric bypass on type 2 diabetes mellitus. *Annals of Surgery* 238(4): 467, 484; discussion 84–85.

65. Hinojosa, M. W., J. E. Varela, B. R. Smith, F. Che, and N. T. Nguyen. Apr 2009. Resolution of systemic hypertension after laparoscopic gastric bypass. *Journal of Gastrointestinal Surgery: Official Journal of the Society for Surgery of the Alimentary Tract* 13(4): 793–797.

66. Zlabek, J. A., M. S. Grimm, C. J. Larson, M. A. Mathiason, P. J. Lambert, and S. N. Kothari. Nov–Dec 2005. The effect of laparoscopic gastric bypass surgery on dyslipidemia in severely obese patients. *Surgery for Obesity and Related Diseases: Official Journal of the American Society for Bariatric Surgery* 1(6): 537–542.

67. Kolasa, K. M., C. Kay, S. Henes, and C. Sullivan. Jul–Aug 2006. The clinical nutritional implications of obesity and overweight. *North Carolina Medical Journal* 67(4): 283–287.

68. White House Task Force on Childhood Obesity. 2010. *Solving the Problem of Childhood Obesity Within a Generation.* Washington, DC: White House Task Force on Childhood Obesity, Office of the U.S. President.

69. U.S. Department of Health and Human Services. 2010. *Healthy People 2020.* Washington, DC: Office of Disease Prevention and Health Promotion.

70. U.S. Department of Health and Human Services. 2010. *U.S. Preventive Services Task Force (USPSTF).* Rockville, MD: Agency for Healthcare Research and Quality.

6 Exercise Management of the Obese Patient

Joshua Lowndes, MA and
Theodore J. Angelopoulos, PhD, MPH

CONTENTS

INTRODUCTION

It is beyond question that the performance of regular physical activity directly contributes to better health outcomes. These benefits, which have been previously described, are great enough to warrant public health agencies issuing recommendations on the amount and type of physical activity individuals should be performing. However, consideration also has to be paid to the inherent risk that is present for the performance of all forms of physical activity. A comprehensive discussion of these risks is beyond the scope of this text; instead, the focus of this chapter will be those specific aspects of risk to which the obese patient may be more prone and what steps can be taken to mitigate these risks with specific attention paid to the risk of suffering an acute coronary event.

PREPARATION: KNOW YOUR PATIENT

The risks associated with physical activity are not uniform throughout the entire population. For instance, a competitive high school cross-country runner is not at the same level of risk as is a middle-aged, obese, hypertensive male with a family history of heart disease. Due to the level of deconditioning and the extra weight being carried, the latter will have to take more precautions to protect against the development of exercise-induced injuries (i.e., musculoskeletal injury, heart). How likely it is for an acute coronary event is to be provoked by physical activity depends on the prevalence of cardiac disease within the population of interest. Correctly identifying the population to which a patient belongs is therefore of critical importance, and it should be understood that the obese patient should be thought of not as part of a homogeneous "at-risk" population but as an individual for whom the risks associated with physical activity are determined by a multitude of individual factors. One of the primary responsibilities of the physician or health-care professional working with an obese patient wishing to begin a regime of physical activity is to correctly identify the specific population to which the individual belongs and the risk associated with that determination. All decisions on pre-exercise screening and recommendations for exercise will be based on this determination of risk.

DETERMINING RISK

The American College of Sports Medicine (ACSM) has laid out guidelines to help exercise professionals and health and fitness facilities determine the risk an individual poses. One of the primary tools available for this purpose is a self-reported health history questionnaire such as the Physical Activity Readiness Questionnaire (ParQ) or the American Heart Association (AHA)/ACSM Health/Fitness Facility Preparticipation Screening Questionnaire. On the basis of the responses given, the exercise facility/health professional will determine the appropriateness of allowing the individual to begin utilizing their services without further medical clearance.

The physician may see obese patients who have gone through this process and had it indicated that they needed physician clearance to begin exercise, or they may see patients who have not yet even had this initial level of screening. Regardless, the physician's first step should be to obtain values for the necessary clinical measures, even for those who reported knowing them on the ParQ. The accuracy of a patient's recall is questionable, but also even accurately recalled values are subject to change since the time they were last measured. The list of measures obtained is at the discretion of the physician, but at a minimum should include every risk factor for the development of coronary artery disease (CAD) as determined by ACSM (Table 6.1).

In addition to these clinical measures, ACSM lists positive family history (myocardial infarction or acute coronary death younger than 55 years in a first-degree male relative or 65 in a female first-degree relative), cigarette smoking (smoked within the past 6 months), and physical inactivity (failure to meet the surgeon

TABLE 6.1
Clinically Determined Risk Factors for the Development of Coronary Artery Disease

Clinical Measure of Interest	Thresholds
Body mass index	Obesity • BMI > 30 kg/m^2 • Waist circumference > 102 cm (M) or 88 cm (F)
Resting blood pressure	Target • SBP < 140 mm Hg • DBP < 90 mm Hg
Fasting blood glucose	Target • <100 mg/dL
Fasting blood lipids[a]	Target • Total cholesterol < 200 mg/dL • Low-density lipoprotein < 130 mg/dL • High-density lipoprotein ≥ 45 mg/dL

[a] Positive blood lipid values may be discounted if HDL ≥ 60.

general's recommendations—accumulation of 30 min of moderate-intensity physical activity on most if not all days of the week) as other CAD risk factors that should be identified as part of a basic medical history.

This information, coupled with the clinical assessment described earlier, allows the physician to determine the risk the individual presents for suffering an acute cardiac event as a result of physical activity according to the criteria in Table 6.2. The level of screening that is appropriate prior to the initiation of an exercise program and how that exercise is managed will be determined in large part by this assessment.

TABLE 6.2
ACSM Risk Stratification Categories

Risk Group	Definition
Low	Men < 45 and women < 55 years No more than two risk factors
Moderate	Men ≥ 45 and women ≥ 55 years Two or more risk factors
High	Signs or symptoms of cardiovascular disease[a] or known cardiovascular, pulmonary, or metabolic disease

[a] See Table 6.3.

APPROPRIATE LEVELS OF PRE-EXERCISE SCREENING

APPARENTLY HEALTHY AND LOW RISK

According to the criteria already discussed, a young (male < 45 or female < 50 years) obese individual with no family history of heart disease and no other risk factors would be considered at low risk of acute cardiovascular problems during a bout of physical activity. However, for the purposes of this chapter, the focus is on individuals who are looking to begin an exercise program and are therefore currently classified as sedentary. This reference patient would automatically be regarded as moderate risk due to the presence of two risk factors (obesity and sedentary lifestyle). However, a brief comment on the obese low-risk patient is warranted. An example of such a patient would be someone who accumulates sufficient physical activity but who is preparing to increase the amount and intensity of their activity regime. While appropriate care would need to be taken to progress the exercise sensibly and productively, nothing in the way of pre-exercise screening would be required for this patient.

APPARENTLY HEALTHY BUT MODERATE RISK

It is typical for many of the principal risk factors for the development of chronic disease to cluster within an individual. Due to the direct role that obesity plays in insulin resistance, which in turn can directly contribute to the development of other risk factors, such risk factor clustering is even more likely in obese individuals. As such, even in the absence of clear evidence of disease, it is more likely that an obese patient is going to be considered moderate risk and thus will require a little more care than already described in preparing them for exercise. Also, in the context of this chapter, in which presently inactive patients are seeking to begin exercising, as has already been mentioned, it can be assumed that all obese patients meet at least this level of risk.

Exercise Stress Test with ECG Monitoring

The ECG exercise stress test is the cornerstone of clearing participants to exercise who are rated as more than minimal risk. Clinicians will be familiar with this test in the context of trying to reproduce symptoms of ischemia (typical angina) of which the patient has previously complained, and/or trying to quantify the level of physical activity that can be performed before these symptoms occur. However, the patients who meet the criteria discussed in this section are not presenting with chest pain and therefore are a different proposition when it comes to the ECG stress test.

For these people, an exercise stress test with ECG monitoring might not be considered an absolutely essential component of providing clearance to begin exercise, especially as they do not present as the typical stress-test patient, but performing the test still can provide some valuable information. At the very least, it can provide some provisional information about the individual's cardiorespiratory fitness, which may be of benefit in providing the initial exercise prescription. However, members of this group are still classified as being at a greater risk than the minimal level, and so additional confidence that high-intensity activity can be performed without cardiovascular complications can be important for peace of mind. ACSM provides guidelines indicating that while moderate-risk individuals need not have a pre-screening ECG stress test before beginning an exercise program, all those who wish to participate in vigorous activity should be tested [1]. This is possibly more relevant due to the growing appreciation of the efficacy of high-intensity, even supramaximal interval training for conditioning, improvements in markers for chronic disease, and even, possibly, weight loss [2–8]. These studies have used a variety of populations, some even more at risk than the population of focus, suggesting that on average, such an approach to exercise could be appropriate for these patients. However, an ECG stress test, taken all the way to age-predicted maximal heart rate (HR) or volitional fatigue resulting in normal findings, would be appropriate for someone from this population initiating this form of activity.

Given the slightly different goal of this test for this population, it is important to understand the benefits that may be achieved from a slightly modified approach to testing. Many clinicians, when dealing with the symptomatic patients with whom they are most familiar, are satisfied when achieving 85% of age-predicted maximal HR—the presumption being that the vast majority of activities that such an individual might encounter are insufficient in their metabolic demand to cause any cardiovascular complications. That presumption has already been made about an individual in this population prior to the test being performed, and so stopping the test at this level of effort will provide no additional information than was already known prior to the performance of the test. Instead, the end point should be the attainment of 100% maximal HR or preferably higher if the patient has the capacity to continue, especially in younger participants. Of course, in the unlikely event that the test elicits signs or symptoms of ischemia, the termination of the test should be handled in the same way as with any other patient (Table 6.3).

A second beneficial modification to the approach might be a change in protocol. The sort of protocols that most clinicians in this setting are most familiar with (Bruce, modified Bruce, and Ellestad) are those that provide the opportunity for the patient to achieve a physiological steady state. The advantage of this is that it allows better identification and quantification of the ischemic threshold. However, this provides

---

TABLE 6.3

Signs and Symptoms Suggestive of Cardiovascular Disease

Sign or Symptom

Pain, discomfort (or other angina equivalent) in the chest, neck, jaw, arms, or other areas that may result in ischemia

Shortness of breath at rest or with mild exertion

Dizziness or syncope

Orthopnea or paroxysmal nocturnal dyspnea

Ankle edema

Palpitations or tachycardia

Intermittent claudication

Known heart murmur

Unusual fatigue or shortness of breath with usual activities

no benefit when testing a population we are confident will not experience ischemia. Instead, a protocol that is designed to more accurately determine cardiorespiratory fitness would be beneficial. Such a protocol would be referred to as "ramped" (rather than "staged") where the increases in intensity happen so frequently that the participant never achieves a physiological steady state. With sufficient computer-controlled systems, these increases in exercise intensity can be minute and occur continuously throughout the protocol. Even without computer-controlled systems, exercise intensity can be manually increased every 15 or 30s to achieve the same end. The advantage of this type of protocol is that participants do not unduly fatigue themselves at challenging but submaximal workloads and are not shocked by relatively large increases in intensity when already performing at near-maximal effort. This may be especially beneficial if gas exchange measurements are being made for the direct measurement of VO2max simultaneously with ECG monitoring.

In summary, clinicians can use their best judgment, based on their pretest assessment, and if this assessment concludes that the patient is unlikely to produce signs or symptoms of ischemia during the test, some modifications can be made. If exercise capacity is the primary goal, a ramped protocol would be most beneficial. If the identification and quantification of ischemia are the primary goals, a staged protocol might be best. In either case, in the absence of signs of ischemia, benefits will be achieved from extending the test beyond the 85% of maximal HR threshold and for as long as the participant can tolerate.

Testing Protocols

The advantage of ramped protocols over staged protocols has already been covered; however, this is not the only consideration. It has been observed that a test that is completed between 6 and 12 min gives the highest VO2 peak values [9]. It should seem obvious that asking a young, obese, but otherwise healthy, man who runs several times per week to perform the first two stages of the modified Bruce protocol is unnecessary. Similar considerations should be made to match the characteristics of the chosen protocol to the individual patient, which in part comes back to the ability of the clinician to gather the necessary information during the *getting-to-know-your-patient* phase.

Ramped protocols can be more individualized than the more famous staged protocols. The Bruce protocol is pictured in the following:

Bruce Protocol (Submaximal Table)

Stage	Minutes	% Grade	MPH	METS
1	3	10	1.7	4.7
2	6	12	2.5	7.0
3	9	14	3.4	10.1
4	12	16	4.2	12.9
5	15	18	5.0	15.0
6	18	20	5.5	16.9
7	21	22	6.0	19.1

As can be seen, the patient would start out at 4.7 METS and still be working at this intensity by the end of the third minute. If the Bruce protocol is deemed suitably challenging for the patient, but a ramped protocol is preferred, a sample progression would be as follows*:

Stage	Seconds	% Grade	MPH	METS
1	30	0	1.3	2.0
2	60	2.5	1.4	2.6
3	90	4.0	1.6	3.1
4	120	5.0	1.8	3.6
5	150	6.0	2.0	4.2
6	180	6.5	2.2	4.7

As can be seen, this progression starts at a lower level and, over the course of five equal jumps every 30 s, ends up at the same intensity level as the Bruce protocol by the end of the third minute (Table 6.4).

If, based on the personal history obtained from the patient, it is deemed that a subject with a high physical capacity is being dealt with, increasing the size of the incremental increases at the same frequency might be a suitable approach. A convenient solution would be to devise three standardized ramped protocols: a low-tolerance protocol with jumps leading to a lesser demand than the Bruce protocol (66% of Bruce = 23.3 mL by end of minute 9), a moderate tolerance protocol that replicates the demands of the Bruce protocol (Table 6.4), and an athlete protocol that is even more aggressive than the Bruce protocol (133% of Bruce = 47 mL by end of minute 9).

Modifications of ECG Measurement

When performing an ECG stress test, it is a common practice to relocate the right and left leg electrodes immediately superior to the right and left iliac crests and the right and left arm electrodes to the chest immediately inferior to the clavicle on the respective side of the chest. This minimizes the artifact that would be produced by the movement of the limbs with exercise while maintaining the appropriate vectors of the six limb leads (not to mention the improved safety of not having leads dangling by the feet of a walking patient). However, the obese patient, especially one with considerable abdominal fat accumulation, presents several unique problems. First, electrodes placed on the right and left suprailiac will move more during exercise on an obese individual than on a normal-weight individual; thus, greater artifact is produced. Secondly, the additional fat mass of this site blunts the signal magnitude. This combination of factors means that poor-quality signals will often be produced in leads II, III, and aV_F. In our lab, we have found that improved clarity of these leads can be achieved by instead placing the right and left leg electrodes on the small of the back. This modification, just like the standard modified electrode placement for exercise testing, improves the clarity of the signal in the respective leads while maintaining the same vectors between the electrodes.

---

* An extended version of the protocol is shown in Table 6.4.

TABLE 6.4
Sample Ramped Exercise Protocol

Stage	Seconds	% Grade	MPH	METS*
1	30	0	1.3	2.0
2	60	2.5	1.4	2.6
3	90	4.0	1.6	3.1
4	120	5.0	1.8	3.6
5	150	6.0	2.0	4.2
6	180	6.5	2.2	4.7
7	210	7.0	2.4	5.2
8	240	7.5	2.5	5.5
9	270	8.0	2.6	5.9
10	300	8.5	2.7	6.2
11	330	9.0	2.8	6.6
12	360	9.5	2.9	7.0
13	390	10.0	3.1	7.6
14	420	10.5	3.2	8.1
15	450	11.0	3.3	8.5
16	480	11.5	3.4	9.0
17	510	12.0	3.5	9.5
18	540	12.5	3.6	10.0
19	570	13.0	3.8	10.7
20	600	13.5	3.9	11.2
21	630	14.0	3.9	11.5
22	660	14.5	4.0	12.1
23	690	15.0	4.0	12.3
24	720	15.0	4.2	12.9

*METs = ((0.1 * MPH * 26.8) + (1.8 * MPH ** 26.8 * Grade/100) + 3.5)/3.5.
Obtained from Appendix D of reference 1.

HIGH RISK AND KNOWN DISEASE

The predominant factor that determines the approach with patients who fall into this category is not that they are obese but that they are high risk or have known disease. The process of clearing these patients for exercise and the subsequent management of that exercise obviously require more caution than for previously described groups of patients. However, these patients present as the typical patient a clinician sees for an exercise stress test, and so despite the added complications, the familiarity the clinician has with this patient may make them an easier case.

For previous groups, it was stated that a preclearance exercise stress test was beneficial if not absolutely necessary. With these patients, it would be unwise to allow them to being exercising without first having gone through this test. In previously described cases, the ECG monitoring of the patient during the stress test was a consideration secondary to getting information about cardiorespiratory fitness. With patients who fall into the high risk and known disease category, those priorities are likely to be flipped. However, even within this category of patients, significant variation exists with respect to how dangerous a bout of challenging physical activity might be, and so the first role of the physician is to use the pretest patient history to make this judgment. Are there recent signs or symptoms that have not been ruled out as being because of occult disease? If there is known disease, how long has it been since the last event? What has the pattern of activity been like since that event and how well was that activity tolerated?

As was discussed previously, the more the test is focused on the effective ECG monitoring of the patient, the more affected the ability to accurately measure fitness. The lower the pretest risk of exercise to cause an acute event, more focus can be made toward assessing fitness. The higher the pretest risk, the more concessions will have to be made toward effective monitoring of the patient and the ability to quantify the exercise level required to elicit symptoms.

With lower-risk patients described previously, the main tool the clinician had in varying the approach to the stress test to match the specific goals of performing the test as determined by the patient history was the exercise protocol. Ramped protocols may be less likely to be used with the high-risk or known-disease population, but the consideration is still one to be made. In addition, whether or not the patient should be tested while on their medication will also be a relevant consideration. If the main goal is determining whether signs and symptoms are the result of CAD, it might be warranted to perform the test after weaning the patient off medications that may protect against the development of exercise-induced ischemia, thus reducing the risk of obtaining a false negative. In these cases, the diagnostic value of the test is primary, and the approach taken is designed to meet that goal. If a diagnosis is already known, or if an accurate gauge of the real-life (medicated) physical capacity of the patient is determined to be the priority, then it might be most beneficial to perform the test with their patient following the normal medication regime.

How the physician most appropriately balances these needs of measuring fitness with the need for accurate monitoring of the cardiovascular response may be different for every patient within this population. These decisions should therefore be made on a case-by-case basis after obtaining a thorough patient history and then determining the primary goal for conducting the test (Figure 6.1).

EXERCISE CONSIDERATIONS

The obese state creates a situation where the initiation of an exercise program needs to be undertaken carefully so that it is appropriate for the individual's goals and it is being done in a manner suitable for the level of risk the individual present. There are considerations that apply to all obese patients with additional levels of considerations based on the level of risk of the patient and the results of the pre-exercise screening.

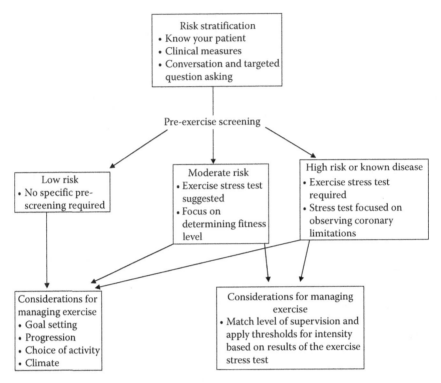

FIGURE 6.1   Decision tree.

CONSIDERATIONS APPLICABLE TO ALL

Goal Setting

While not necessary to receive much of the benefits of a regimen of physical activity, weight loss is likely to be a priority for the obese patient. This may be reflected by the overall exercise prescription. So far in this chapter, all mentions of public health recommendations for the amount of physical activity to be performed have referenced the surgeon general's recommendations—the accumulation of 30 min of moderate-intensity activity on most if not all days of the week [10]. However, these guidelines address the minimal amount required to lower the risk of developing chronic disease compared to sedentary people. Separate guidelines have been published to specifically address the issue of weight loss, and these recommend that a greater amount of physical activity be performed [11,12]. Exercise professionals with the appropriate certifications should be sought to help develop the program of physical activity that matches the needs to the individual.

Conservative Progression

For most people, it would not be prudent to go from being sedentary to performing a full 150 min of moderate-intensity activity a week (or more depending on one's goals). Instead, most people would benefit from easing into their new regime. This is addressed in most structured exercise prescriptions with the duration, frequency, and intensity of exercise to be performed gradually increased over the initial weeks of the adoption. Such an approach will generally help protect against musculoskeletal aches and pains and thus facilitate the long-term adoption of the exercise program. An obese person is going to be more prone to picking up these sorts of minor ailments during the initial phase of the program. As such, conservative progression toward the ultimate goal for duration, frequency, and intensity may be more important than for the normal-weight patient.

Choice of Activity

The general principle behind the aforementioned recommendation is that long-term adherence to the exercise program is vital for the benefits to be obtained. The same principle is what drives the next recommendation—"effectiveness of the activity is secondary to compliance." One of the most common questions an exercise professional will receive relates to whether one exercise "works" better than another. However, in the context of a sedentary, obese individual, the "best" choice of activity will be the one the individual is most likely to perform. Level of enjoyment (or tolerance), accessibility, and convenience should be more important considerations than the number of calories per minute different activities burn. As a result, portable activities, such as walking or other forms of activities that can be done anywhere at any time and without any equipment, should be seen as a good starting point. A focus on walking would also help minimize the musculoskeletal complications that come with adoption of a new form of activity compared to other more challenging activities that patients may feel compelled to start with.

There is a considerable amount of conflicting evidence on the role of resistance training in weight management. The weight of evidence suggests that improvements in lean mass are accrued [13,14] even in the absence of dietary changes. However, the likely diet-resistance training interaction likely explains much of the conflicting results. It does appear that if resistance training aids in weight management, then effect is small, and this is reflected in the low importance the various public health recommendations assign it [10–12]. However, increased strength, especially in those who are extremely deconditioned, may aid the adoption of a generally healthier lifestyle, which in turn will have positive health benefits. There is also evidence that, even in the absence of weight loss, improvements in markers of health may be achieved through resistance training, including improved lipid profile [15], insulin sensitivity [16], and resting blood pressure [17]. These benefits are sufficient to support the practice of resistance training in obese individuals as a supplement to energy-expending, cardiovascular exercise. Such a program should focus on compound movements requiring extensive use of the body's muscle mass, which can help achieve the necessary improvements in lean mass and strength in a time-efficient manner.

Climate

Exercise produces a competition for blood flow between the active tissues (to fuel activity) and the skin (to help regulate temperature). Generally, this competition can occur without untoward consequences. However, it is always prudent to be careful of extreme climates that might pose an additional challenge. This may be even more important in obese individuals, who run a greater risk of heat-related injuries from exercise because they generate more heat for a given level of exercise compared to normal-weight individuals. As such, a general recommendation would be if exercise is going to be performed outside, especially in hot and humid climates, the hottest time of the day should be avoided. In certain parts of the country, this may limit the hours in which exercise can safely be performed outside. So while walking was spoken about earlier as an *anywhere, anytime* activity, it may not be in the context of hot and humid weather. While many people may be turned off from the thought of joining a gym or fitness facility, or may simply view it as inconvenient, the advantage is that it allows exercise to be performed in a climate-controlled environment. This, or even the purchase of home indoor exercise equipment, provides the potential for expanded hours in several states, which may help adherence to the exercise regime especially in the summer months.

The challenge that exercise performed in the heat poses is partly related to the level of cardiorespiratory and metabolic conditioning of the individual. Conservative progression of frequency, duration, and intensity has already been mentioned, but this may be even more important for those who will be performing their exercise outside of a climate-controlled environment.

MODERATE RISK

The approach taken for patients in this category will be determined by the outcome of the exercise stress test and larger screening process. In the likely outcome that no coronary compromise was found, the patient may begin the exercise program with no further considerations than already discussed.

HIGH RISK OR KNOWN DISEASE

As already discussed, all previous considerations for the obese exercising patient apply. Additionally, the results of the exercise stress test should be used to develop a safe and effective plan of exercise for the patient, with an increased emphasis on safety, as defined by the specific outcome of the exercise stress test. Referrals to clinically supervised facilities may also be indicated.

An additional word on climate is appropriate for those at this elevated level of risk. Exercise in the heat for this population is particularly dangerous as even minor limitations in coronary blood flow (caused by diversion of blood flow to the skin) can prompt an acute coronary event. Those who will be exercising outside of a clinically supervised facility may warrant extra counseling about the dangers of exercise in the heat.

REFERENCES

1. *ACSM's Guidelines for Exercise Testing and Prescription* (7th edn). Lippincott Williams & Wilkins, Philadelphia, PA.
2. MacDonald MH, Currie KD. 2009. Interval exercise is a path to good health, but how much, how often and for whom? *Clinical Science* 116: 315–316.
3. Warburton DE, McKenzie DC, Haykowsky MJ et al. 2005. Effectiveness of high-intensity interval training for the rehabilitation of patients with coronary artery disease. *American Journal of Cardiology* 95: 1080–1084.

4. Wisløff U, Stoylen A, Loennechen JP et al. 2007. Superior cardiovascular effect of aerobic interval training versus moderate continuous training in heart failure patients: A randomized study. *Circulation* 115: 3086–3094.

5. Coppoolse R, Schols AM, Baarends EM et al. 1999. Interval versus continuous training in patients with severe COPD: A randomized clinical trial. *European Respiratory Journal* 14: 258–263.

6. Tjønna AE, Lee SJ, Rognmo O et al. 2008. Aerobic interval training versus continuous moderate exercise as a treatment for the metabolic syndrome: A pilot study. *Circulation* 118: 346–354.

7. Lutes LD, Winett RA, Barger SD et al. 2008. Small changes in nutrition and physical activity promote weight loss and maintenance: 3-month evidence from the ASPIRE randomized trial. *Annals Behavioral Medicine* 35: 351–357.

8. Hood MS, Little JP, Tarnopolsky MA, Myslik F, Gibala MJ. 2011. Low-volume interval training improves muscle oxidative capacity in sedentary adults. *Medicine and Science in Sports and Exercise* 43: 1849–1856.

9. Buchfuhrer MJ, Hansen JE, Robinson TE, Sue DY, Wasserman K, Whipp BJ. 1983. Optimizing the exercise protocol for cardiopulmonary assessment. *Journal of Applied Physiology* 55: 1558–1564.

10. United States Department of Health and Human Services: Physical activity and health: A report of the Surgeon General, 1996.

11. Donnelly JE, Blair SN, Jakicic JM, Manore MM, Rankin JW, Smith BK (American College of Sports Medicine). 2009. Appropriate physical activity intervention strategies for weight loss and prevention of weight regain for adults. *Medicine and Science in Sports and Exercise* 41: 459–471.

12. Saris WH, Blair SN, van Baak MA et al. 2003. How much physical activity is enough to prevent unhealthy weight gain? Outcome of the IASO 1st Stock Conference and consensus statement. *Obesity Reviews* 4: 101–114.

13. Hunter GR, Bryan DR, Wetzstein CJ, Zuckerman PA, Bamman MM. 2002. Resistance training and intra-abdominal adipose tissue in older men and women. *Medicine and Science in Sports and Exercise* 34: 1023–1028.

14. Hunter GR, Wetzstein CJ, Fields DA, Brown A, Bamman MM. 2000. Resistance training increases total energy expenditure and free living physical activity in older adults. *Journal of Applied Physiology* 89: 977–984.

15. Goldberg L, Elliot DL, Schutz RW, Kloster FE. 1984. Changes in lipid and lipoprotein levels after weight training. *Journal of the American Medical Association* 252: 504–506.

16. Ibanez J, Izquierdo M, Arguelles I, Forga L, Larrion JL, Garcia-Unciti M, Idoate F, Gorostiaga EM. 2005. Twice-weekly progressive resistance training decreases abdominal fat and improves insulin sensitivity in older men with type 2 diabetes. *Diabetes Care* 28: 662–667.

17. Kelley G. 1997. Dynamic resistance exercise and resting blood pressure in adults: A meta-analysis. *Journal of Applied Physiology* 82(5): 1559–1565.

7 Behavioral Management of the Obese Patient

Craig A. Johnston, PhD,
Jennette P. Moreno, PhD,
and John P. Foreyt, PhD

CONTENTS

INTRODUCTION

Despite countless diets, exercise regimens, drugs, and behavior modification strategies, the prevalence of obesity continues its relentless increase in both developed and developing nations [1]. Although many necessary components to treat obesity have been identified, behavior modification remains the bedrock of weight control programs [2]. Behavior modification strategies with the most success take a lifestyle change approach aimed at helping patients adhere to healthy diets and sensible physical activity regimens. These strategies involve a tailored problem-solving approach that includes self-monitoring, goal setting, contracting, problem solving, stimulus control, cognitive restructuring, stress management, and social support [3].

TABLE 7.1
Guide to Selecting Treatment

Treatment	BMI Category				
	25–26.9	27–29.9	30–34.9	35–39.9	≥40
Diet, physical activity, and behavior therapy	With comorbidities	With comorbidities	a	a	a
Pharmacotherapy		With comorbidities	a	a	a
Surgery				With comorbidities	

Source: Adapted from National Institutes of Health, *The Practical Guide: Identification, Evaluation, and Treatment of Overweight and Obesity in Adults*, NIH publication 00-4084, National Institutes of Health, Rockville, MD, 2000. http://www.nhlbi.nih.gov/guidelines/obesity/prctgd_c.pdf (accessed June 8, 2011).

a Treatment should be used regardless of the comorbidities. For individuals with a BMI of 25–29.9 without comorbidities, maintenance of weight through lifestyle intervention is recommended.

A guide to selecting treatments for obesity has been developed by the National Institutes of Health [4]. As can be seen in Table 7.1, behavior modification is recommended for all individuals receiving treatment for overweight and obesity. Although changes in diet and physical activity remain the goals of therapy, it is the behavioral strategies used that can help patients to overcome barriers that are associated with making these changes. Even in the case of bariatric surgery, behavioral therapy is needed to promote the lifestyle changes that are necessary for short- and long-term weight control.

BEHAVIORAL STRATEGIES

SELF-MONITORING

Self-monitoring is the core component of behavioral weight loss treatments [5]. Self-monitoring involves raising self-awareness through observing and recording behaviors such as food intake, physical activity, and weight [6]. At the outset of treatment, patients may be asked to simply observe and record without attempting to change their diet or physical activity habits. These records provide the clinician and the individual with important information that serves as a guide to treatment. In addition to recording food intake and energy expended in exercise, other variables may be recorded, such as the time of day the food is eaten, the type of exercise done, and the emotional state of the patient. The patient learns to recognize patterns of behavior (e.g., eating when bored or increasing sedentary behavior when depressed) that can then be the target of intervention. An example of food record is provided in Figure 7.1.

The feedback process of evaluating records both by the clinician and the patient is the most powerful aspect of self-monitoring. Several studies have demonstrated a correlation between self-monitoring of food intake and long-term weight loss [7]. Additionally, frequently self-monitoring one's weight is associated with improved weight loss and long-term weight maintenance [8–10]. These benefits of self-monitoring are found even though individuals tend to underestimate their

Name: _____   **Food Diary**   Date: _____

Meal	Food	Amount	Where?	With whom?	Mood	Time
Breakfast						
Snack						
Lunch						
Snack						
Dinner						
Snack						

FIGURE 7.1   Food diary.

food intake and overestimate their physical activity [11,12]. Even if inaccurate, the act of self-monitoring is still effective because it increases the individuals' awareness of their behaviors and serves as a persistent reminder of their weight-related goals.

We find that patients tend to not like self-monitoring. This task is often perceived as tedious and boring, leading to the abandonment of this important technique. In these situations, tailoring self-monitoring to meet the specific needs of a patient can be an excellent compromise. For example, most individuals have less difficulty managing their food intake during the morning and early afternoon; however, late afternoon, evenings, and weekends are times that patients have the most trouble with overeating. Once a specified time of overeating is identified, self-monitoring may be used only during this specific problem time. Focusing on a limited time period not only encourages the patient to use this important skill, but it also provides the clinician with needed information to track treatment progress.

GOAL SETTING

Once the individual gains greater self-awareness of areas for improvement, goal setting may be used to focus on measurable and attainable changes in behavior. Effective goal setting aids in keeping the individual focused and motivated. Goals should be both short and long term. Patients are generally encouraged to make most of their short-term goals about the process rather than the long-term goal of weight loss. Increasing fruit and vegetable intake is an example of a process goal, whereas losing 50 lb is an outcome goal. Process goals provide structure to treatment as the clinician may organize sessions around the identification and reduction of barriers to achieving these goals. Meeting initial program goals (e.g., increasing a daily walk by 5 min) can encourage long-term goal achievement (i.e., weight loss) [13]. Example goals are provided in Figure 7.2.

Look AHEAD and the Diabetes Prevention Program (DPP) are two programs that used a goal-based approach for weight loss [14,15]. These programs included a tailored approach so that individuals could achieve their goals using strategies most appropriate for their specific situations. Overall, individuals in both of these studies experienced significant weight loss, improved maintenance of weight loss, fitness, glycemic control, and a decrease in cardiovascular risk factors [14,15].

A focus on goal setting can significantly improve patient motivation as well. The establishment of small, measurable, and achievable goals at the beginning of treatment allows the patient to create positive momentum for future change. Many patients have tried multiple times to lose weight and feel that future attempts are unlikely to be successful. Small goals can help to foster a sense of accomplishment. Additionally, this allows the clinician an opportunity to discuss the positive changes being made creating a supportive atmosphere that encourages treatment adherence. Taking the time to praise and reinforce the small changes accomplished through goal setting is an essential part of successfully promoting weight change.

---

1. Keep accurate track of my calories and activity 7 days a week.
2. Eat no more than _____cal per day.
    Starting weight of 250 lb or less = 1200–1500 cal goal.
    Starting weight of more than 250 lb = 1500–1800 cal goal.
3. Use meal replacements for two meals and one snack 7 days a week.
4. Do a minimum of 175 min of moderate physical activity each week.
5. Lose _____ lb (Minimum of 3 lb if below 10% weight loss goal)
                                    OR
    Maintain current weight of _____lb. (If 10% weight loss goal achieved)
6. Reach 10,000 steps per day.
7. Send an email update to my clinician.
8. Talk with my family about ways that they can support the changes I am making.
9. Find a walking partner for the next week.

FIGURE 7.2   Example goals for weight management.

I,_____, agree to do_____
　　　　　　　(your name)　　　　　　　　　　　　　　　　　　　　　　*(activity or goal)*

for or by _____ . I will monitor my progress by
　　　　　(how long, how often, by when)

_____. I will evaluate my progress every
　　(the specific method you will use)

_____with my support person_____
　　　　　(how often)　　　　　　　　　　　　　　　　　　　　　　　　　*(name)*

I will reward myself with _____
　　　　　　　　　　　　　　　(something realistic yet motivating)

Signed_____Witnessed _____Date_____

Notes:

FIGURE 7.3 Behavioral contract.

CONTRACTING

Contracting is a useful strategy for motivating short-term behavioral changes that can be used in combination with goal setting [16]. Contracting involves a patient selecting one or more behavioral goals to perform between sessions. These behaviors should be easy and realistic to accomplish. For example, an individual might decide to limit eating out to one less meal a week or walk for 10 extra minutes a day. In session, the patient writes down the behavior(s) to be performed and signs a document to make the agreement official. An example of a contract is provided in Figure 7.3.

Developing a contract is a concrete way of defining expectations and responsibilities. Many patients may look to an expert to create changes in their lives. Although clinicians play a significant role in weight loss efforts, it is important that patients understand their responsibilities in making change happen. The process of writing down expectations for the patient can provide an opportunity to explicitly discuss what will be required of the patient in order for treatment to be successful. For many patients, contracts also result in increased motivation to engage in treatment, especially in the short term.

PROBLEM SOLVING

Problem solving entails identifying barriers to adopting a healthy lifestyle and implementing strategies to overcome these barriers. Problem solving is an important part of the goal-setting process. Once patients have set goals, they are taught to identify potential problems that may hinder achievement of these goals and brainstorm possible solutions. This process can increase individuals' confidence in their ability to achieve their goals and prepare the individual to effectively tackle potential obstacles.

Given the obesogenic nature of our modern environment, foreseeing potential problems and brainstorming solutions are critical for long-term maintenance of weight loss. Problem solving is an ongoing process where individuals monitor progress toward goals, determine the effectiveness of implemented solutions, and identify new solutions if necessary. Problem solving has been shown to be an integral skill needed for weight loss and maintenance [17].

A common problem in obesity treatment is patient attrition. Failure to return to the clinic may occur for many different reasons. For example, we have experienced multiple cases in which the patient did not return for their next appointment because of weight gain or not meeting a goal. This may be due to a patient's desire to be seen in a positive light. Although this trait can assist with a patient's adherence to treatment, it can lead to avoidance of the clinician when treatment is not going well. Taking a problem-solving approach from the beginning of treatment can help to alleviate this issue by acknowledging that "setbacks" are a normal part of the treatment process. Using a problem-solving approach, the clinician and patient can develop a plan that can be implemented when setbacks occur.

Stimulus Control

Stimulus control is another important component of weight management. Stimulus control refers to techniques that are intended to alter and manage cues in the environment in order to facilitate behavior change [18]. The goal of stimulus control as it relates to weight management is to manipulate environmental cues that may trigger adaptive or maladaptive patterns of exercise and eating. As part of the self-monitoring, goal setting, and problem-solving process, the patient and clinician might evaluate cues in the environment that support goals for behavior change. For example, keeping a gym bag in the car may increase the likelihood of engaging in physical activity after work, and keeping unhealthy snacks out of plain sight may assist in decreasing caloric consumption. Another important example of stimulus control focuses on controlling the setting in which actual eating occurs, which, in turn, affects patterns of intake. Eating only at the kitchen table and preparing your plate before you sit down, as opposed to serving foods placed at the center of the table, are examples of methods used to create an adaptive setting in which to eat. Making changes to the immediate environment to support healthy lifestyle changes is one of the keys to successful weight management.

Stimulus control may be a particularly important component as shifts in our environment lead to the promotion of excessive food intake and the discouragement of physical activity [19]. For example, the number of fast-food restaurants has increased significantly especially in lower-income neighborhoods [20]. Portion sizes have been steadily increasing over the past several decades [21]. Americans spend an average of 7.7 h a day (55% of their waking hours) in sedentary behaviors, the amount of time spent watching television and using a computer appears to be continuing to rise [22], and only a small proportion of people are engaged in regular physical activity even if their neighborhood has free access to exercise facilities [23]. These issues have led some to term our current environment as obesogenic [24]. Given the nature of our environment, the need to establish environmental changes that promote health through stimulus control is critical.

Meal replacements and partial meal replacements are a specific form of stimulus control that have received considerable attention. This form of stimulus control reduces cues to overeat by providing exact portions and decreasing exposure to certain foods that may trigger overeating in an individual. Studies incorporating meal replacements into lifestyle change interventions have shown excellent results. These studies typically replace one or two meals per day with portion-controlled, vitamin- and mineral-fortified low-energy meals. Typically, meal replacements include drinks and shakes, meal bars, and frozen entrees. Meal replacements also have been shown to be a safe and effective strategy for weight loss and long-term maintenance [25–27].

COGNITIVE RESTRUCTURING

With cognitive restructuring, a clinician assists patients in identifying dysfunctional thinking patterns that may undermine weight loss and teaches them to restructure their thoughts to be of a more beneficial nature (e.g., Refs. [28,29]). Cognitive techniques are commonly used to deal with setbacks regarding weight loss. When dealing with setbacks, patients may be prone to black and white thinking (e.g., Ref. [28]). For example, eating a high-fat dessert or failing to exercise when intended may be viewed by some individuals as completely derailing their weight loss attempts, and they may be tempted to abandon their efforts altogether. Conversely, patients may use denial when dealing with setbacks and tell themselves that overeating or taking a week off from exercise is nothing to be concerned about. These types of thoughts may impede long-term weight loss. In these instances, cognitive restructuring would have patients recognize that the thoughts about their behaviors were rather extreme. Patients would then describe their behavior in a manner that was more realistic and more encouraging of progress toward weight loss.

Cognitive restructuring also helps individuals recognize and manage unrealistic expectations about weight loss. It is not uncommon to encounter obese patients who believe that losing weight will remedy problems in multiple facets of their lives. Cognitive restructuring can aid individuals in recognizing and accepting a more realistic vision of what weight loss can and cannot alter in their life.

STRESS MANAGEMENT

Stress can be a significant factor that interferes with behavioral change [16]. Further complicating matters, some patients report that the lifestyle changes add to their level of stress. It is unlikely that individuals with high levels of stress will have the psychological resources needed to make meaningful changes in their lives. Stress management techniques include progressive muscle relaxation, meditation, and physical activity. Managing stress levels not only makes the transition toward a healthier lifestyle easier but also increases the likelihood that these changes are maintained.

SOCIAL SUPPORT

Support from others has been shown to be important for both weight loss and for long-term maintenance [2]. The changes needed for weight loss are often viewed as difficult and demanding, and the support of other important individuals can make these changes appear less daunting. In terms of long-term maintenance, individuals without social support are more likely to slowly return to their pretreatment behaviors. Engaging the entire family in lifestyle change is an ideal way to naturalistically include a social support component in obesity treatment. Support groups may also consist of friends or any other individuals with similar goals. Social support provides many benefits including role modeling, assisting with problem solving, and serving as an emotional outlet for issues that may be experienced during weight loss treatments.

SUMMARY OF BEHAVIORAL COMPONENTS

The behavioral strategies discussed are typically used as a collective "package" (e.g., Ref. [30]), and the individual contribution of each is not known. Long-term dismantling studies are needed to determine the relative impact of individual components. On the whole, these strategies have been shown to be effective in yielding short-term weight loss (e.g., Ref. [30]). Despite initial weight loss, most patients receiving behavioral treatment remain overweight, and approximately 50% regain these losses 1 year after the intervention ends. At 2 year follow-up, 66% regain their losses. Weight regain has become a focus of newer programs that add extended behavioral intervention programs to help prevent continued weight gain after initial treatment ends.

SUPPORTING COMPLIANCE

The promise of behavior modification has always been that inappropriate lifestyle behaviors could be self-controlled after patients receive training in the use of these techniques. If behavioral techniques are successful, they should be self-reinforcing because they would lead to weight loss and a sense of self-control [31]. Patients who undergo behavioral training do lose weight, typically around 8% during 6 months of intervention but do not continue weight loss following treatment. Without continued treatment, patients tend to regain their lost weight over time. Compliance to weight loss suggestions is typically due to social pressure associated with clinician contact or by peer pressure from group members. The primary success of behavioral treatment is due to its emphasis on specific eating and exercise changes.

Intensity of treatment. It seems that many patients fail to use their self-control strategies when they are experiencing high levels of stress or other strong emotions. Behavioral training does not improve "willpower." For many, the behavioral strategies oftentimes are seen as a burden, and some patients resist the use of them. The best strategy for weight losses is treatment intensity, both in frequency and duration of clinician contact. Continued contact with a clinician, support group, or program is required for maintenance [31].

Encourage self-reinforcing behaviors. Encouraging behaviors that may be self-reinforcing would help negate the need for self-control or willpower. Dieting is not self-reinforcing; it is punishing to patients because there is a sense of deprivation. Aerobic exercise appears to be self-reinforcing for many individuals, and it does have habit forming effects for some. Putting a strong emphasis on aerobic exercise, starting slowly and then building to a sustainable level, has been shown to increase feelings of well-being, along with improving many health parameters. Clinically, it appears helpful to encourage physical activity for many reasons, and put less emphasis on highly restrictive dieting [32].

Reduce the stress of losing weight. Physical activity reduces stress reactivity and should be used as a first-line strategy for helping patients manage stressful life events. Other forms of stress management include strategies such as increasing meditation and progressive relaxation. Meditation is a relatively easy strategy for patients to learn and practice in their daily lives to increase their feeling of self-control. Like aerobic exercise, meditation appears to be habit forming for some individuals. Progressive relaxation and other stress-reduction approaches have been shown to help patients maintain lower levels of stress during weight loss and maintenance.

Focus on realistic management goals. Clinically, 5%–10% weight loss is a realistic goal for patients to achieve. It is often helpful for the clinician to focus on not just the weight loss but on improvements in health, energy, and fitness that frequently occur with these modest losses. For example, a weight loss of just 5% or 10% will often-times improve a patient's sense of well-being and self-esteem. We have noticed that many of our patients feel more in control and have improved mood and appearance. Likewise, functional and recreational activities may increase with weight losses at this level. Patients may be better able to play with their children, walk up a flight of stairs without being out of breath, or even be able to tie their shoes with less difficulty. Focusing on these small changes in lifestyle may help patients become aware of improvements in their health and may lessen their focus on losing unrealistically large amounts of weight.

Emphasize the key elements of weight loss and maintenance. For a clinician, the key elements of weight loss and maintenance include helping patients raise their level of awareness of physical activity and caloric intake. Then gradually increasing physical activity and gradually reducing dietary fat should make it relatively easy for patients to lose weight at a safe rate of about 0.5 kg/week. By doing so, patients will avoid feelings of food deprivation. Social support groups, as an adjunct to the clinician's intervention, should be encouraged. The overriding principle for the clinician is to maintain social scrutiny as long as possible. In our experience, patients tend to maintain their losses significantly better as long as they believe that they are under scrutiny, either from the clinician, support groups, or supportive family members or friends. Thus, increasing social support through asking patients to join like-minded groups or enlisting help from family or friends can promote long-term weight maintenance [5,33].

Relapse prevention. Finally, relapse prevention is important to help patients handle situations in which they regain weight or fall back into old unhealthy habits [16]. Patients are taught strategies for preventing relapse such as making plans for how to deal with the holidays, social situations, and the influence of friends and family members. Patients are also taught cognitive strategies to assist them in dealing with their thoughts when transgressions may occur.

EXAMPLE OF A BEHAVIORAL LIFESTYLE INTERVENTION

The Look AHEAD study is an intensive lifestyle intervention for overweight and obese adults with type 2 diabetes, which incorporates the behavioral modification techniques discussed earlier [34]. The principal goal of the lifestyle intervention was to achieve sustained weight loss (minimum weight loss of 7% of their initial body weight) through a combination of dietary modification and increased physical activity [35]. The dietary intervention utilized meal replacements as a form of portion control. Participants were given a daily calorie goal that varied (1200–1800 cal. a day) depending on the individual's calorie needs. During the initial phase of treatment, participants were encouraged to replace two meals a day with a liquid shake and one snack with a bar, as well as increase intake of fruits and vegetables. After month 7, calorie goals were adjusted based on weight loss during the first 6 months and individuals' future weight loss goals. A gradual shift of replacing one meal and one snack a day with a shake or bar and increasing consumption of low-energy-dense foods was a long-term goal of this program. The physical activity intervention was structured to increase participants' physical activity to 175 min weekly by the end of 6 months.

Incorporating goal setting. Goal setting was ingrained in all aspects of the Look AHEAD study. Participants set goals for overall weight loss, caloric intake, and physical activity. In order to achieve the larger goals of the program (i.e., 175 min of physical activity a week), participants set smaller goals to make manageable changes. For example, the physical activity goal during the first month was to walk for 50 min a week, and the amount of minutes gradually increased over time. Because participants in this study were seen over an extended time period, the establishment of differing goals to accomplish a similar outcome was important to lessen the monotony of constantly working toward the same goal. In order to accomplish this, participants were further encouraged to engage in physical activity by setting goals to increase their daily step count to reach 10,000 steps a day. Framing goals in different ways is important to allow individuals to choose goals that are most meaningful to them.

Incorporating self-monitoring. Self-monitoring was used in Look AHEAD in a variety of ways. Specifically, participants recorded their daily food intake totaling calories consumed and monitored physical activity by recording minutes of activity and step count. Weekly weighing was also conducted at each meeting in order to provide participants' feedback about their progress and to increase motivation. Although all of the self-monitoring techniques used in this study were strongly correlated with one another, the strongest correlate of weight loss at 1 year was self-reported physical activity [36]. Increased self-monitoring was also related to greater treatment attendance. It was not possible to conclude that physical activity increased or diet improved in this study because self-reported adherence instead of actual changes in diet and activity was measured. This lends further support to the importance of self-monitoring. Even though participants in this study may not have accurately reported their behavioral changes, self-monitoring, especially of physical activity, was still associated with weight loss.

Incorporating lifestyle changes. The importance of encouraging changes that can easily be implemented throughout a "regular" day cannot be overstated. Although methods that "add to" an individual's day (e.g., going to the gym) may help to meet specific goals, these changes are easy to abandon if not incorporated into a daily or weekly ritual. In the Look AHEAD study, the focus was to provide individuals with at-home exercises that could be incorporated into their daily routine. These strategies included taking the stairs instead of the elevator, walking to a colleague's office instead of sending an email, and parking at the back of the parking lot instead of in the closest spot. Providing clients with manageable changes to their current lifestyle is more likely to promote sustainability than changes that are not consistent with a person's typical day.

Incorporating social support. During the initial phase of the intervention, participants attended weekly sessions (three group sessions and one individual session monthly). The group sessions were designed to increase social support among participants. Participants also were encouraged to seek social support from family members, other participants, and friends. For example, participants recruited walking partners to help keep them on track with their physical activity goals. Forming a close bond with other intervention participants helped to promote a sense of accountability for reaching weight loss goals. Additionally, techniques to support the relationship between the participants and research staff, such as the use of elements of motivational interviewing, were implemented to increase the social support provided by the treatment provider.

Outcomes associated with lifestyle intervention. Overall, individuals randomized to the intensive lifestyle intervention of the Look AHEAD trial succeeded in losing an average of 8.6% of their initial body weight by 1 year [37]. Improvements in weight at year 1 were associated with improved glycemic control and cardiovascular disease risk factors, as well as reduced use of lipid and glucose lowering medications [37]. Four-year results demonstrated that while the differences in weight change between treatment and control decreased, the treatment group experienced greater improvements in weight, fitness, glycemic control, and several cardiovascular risk factors [38]. Patients receiving the intensive lifestyle intervention have shown additional improvements in symptoms of sleep apnea [39], participation in physical activity, cardiorespiratory fitness [40], physical functioning in patients with knee pain [41], body image [42], and health-related quality of life [43].

ADDITIONAL CONSIDERATIONS

Several other factors can impact treatment outcomes and should be taken into account by the clinician. For example, individuals with reduced income may be more averse to changing their eating habits if this results in an increased monthly food bill. They also may have less access to safe locations to engage in physical activity. Clinicians should assist individuals with problem solving in order to deal with these limitations. Low-income individuals may be limited in their access to health care and preventative care. Clinicians have attempted to address this issue by using churches, schools, and other community locations as accessible and familiar outlets for weight management programs. Using community-based resources also decreases barriers for individuals with limited resources or access to transportation. Engaging the entire family may be also useful in low-income areas with there often being a number of family members responsible for food preparation and grocery shopping. Gaining support of other members of the household is an excellent example of increasing social support.

Cultural differences are also very important considerations for clinicians. Aspects of culture such as perceptions of weight, lifestyle issues, and language can also serve as barriers to healthy weight status. Language barriers often limit access to information about improving health or nutrition, thus providing materials in the appropriate language and teaching individuals strategies to overcome the language barriers can be helpful (e.g., identifying important information on food labels). Treating patients as experts in their culture and asking them to teach the clinician about their traditional foods, lifestyle, and activities can be useful. For example, clinicians may assist individuals with incorporating traditional foods and pastimes into a healthy lifestyle. Overall, tailoring strategies to the individual is important in making behavioral strategies successful.

OTHER MEDIUMS

Traditionally weight loss interventions have been provided in a clinic-based setting. However, traveling to clinics for treatment can result in significant costs for individuals in terms of time and money. This can present a barrier to attendance for an extended period of time. Maintaining contact is important in order to keep patients motivated and focused on their weight loss goals. Continued contact is beneficial both during the intervention, especially during high-risk periods such as holidays, and as part of maintenance efforts once the initial intervention has ended. However, maintaining in-person contact may be difficult; thus, alternatives to in-person meetings, such as the Internet, telephone, and other technological platforms, have been examined for efficacy.

The Internet. One of the most promising approaches for the delivery of low-cost clinical weight management interventions is the Internet [5]. Among the many possibilities that the Internet offers is its convenience, compared with the traditional need for patients to trek to an inconveniently located site for in-person intervention. A number of studies have examined the efficacy of delivering weight management interventions online [44]. The Internet has been used as a tool for education, self-monitoring of eating and physical activity, and as a way to get feedback from clinicians.

The telephone. The telephone has been used in a number of studies to help augment clinical weight management interventions. Telephone calls have been used to improve adherence to diet and physical activity and to increase long-term adherence to exercise (e.g., Refs. [45,46]). Phone calls during holidays have been shown to improve adherence to self-monitoring and to help individuals manage their weight during this high-risk period [47]. Telephone calls have also been used to increase adherence to a walking program. For example, one study reported that 63% of individuals who received frequent telephone calls continued their walking program after

6 months, compared with 22%–26% of those who received infrequent phone calls, and only 4% who received no phone calls [45].

Cell phones and PDAs. Studies have also examined the efficacy of using cell phones and wireless personal digital assistants (PDAs). Cell phones and PDAs allow users to interact with health-care providers through text messaging and can facilitate self-monitoring and goal setting through auditory prompts that are easily programmed into these devices. One study evaluated whether a text-message-based intervention was effective at promoting weight loss [48]. In the text-message-based intervention, participants were sent several SMS (short message service) and MMS (multimedia message service) messages on a daily basis. Additionally, they received print materials and brief monthly phone calls from a trained health counselor. All of these strategies combined resulted in significantly more weight loss than an intervention delivered with only face-to-face contact. Research is needed to test the long-term use of mobile forms of communication in weight management programs.

Emerging technologies. The increasing prevalence of smart phones and tablet computers suggests that these are promising mediums through which to facilitate continued contact with the patient. These highly portable devices make Internet access easy and convenient. Further, application software, or "apps," has become increasingly sophisticated yet easier to create and use, which suggests that weight loss software may be easily developed by researchers and accessed with little difficulty by patients. These devices are promising tools for self-monitoring, and their remote data connection allows for immediate feedback from the clinician. To date, few studies have examined the efficacy of smart phones, and tablet computers have yet to be examined. It is a worthy endeavor to determine the viability of these platforms and to find the most user-friendly and effective interfaces for weight loss software on these devices.

EMERGING OPTIONS FOR CLINICAL WEIGHT MANAGEMENT: BEHAVIORGENOMICS

Nutrigenomics, the study of the way specific genes and bioactive food components interact, has enormous potential for helping weight management clinicians prevent and treat diet-related diseases [49,50]. Likewise, behaviorgenomics has similar potential for aiding the clinician in managing obesity and related diseases. In the future, we believe that patients will be able to come to a nutritional genomics clinician and receive a specific nutrition, exercise, and lifestyle prescription that will minimize the risk of cardiovascular diseases. The clinician will be able to scan the patient's electronic genome card for the individual's genetic profile with respect to lifestyle-related genes. Using this information, the clinician will be able to provide the patient with a perspective on the intersection of the patient's diet, physical activity, and lifestyle with their genes and provide the individual with precise, tailored, targeted recommendations [49,50]. The clinician will be able to prescribe the optimal amount of calories, the correct macro- and micronutrient content of the diet, the specific type and amount of physical activity, and the most appropriate behavioral changes needed. The future of clinical weight management is undoubtedly intertwined with nutrigenomics, exergenomics, and behaviorgenomics.

CONCLUSION

A solid foundation for the treatment of obesity has been laid with behavioral change strategies playing a prominent role. These strategies are critical in assisting patients to make lifestyle changes. Much work has been done recently to find new and inventive ways of incorporating these strategies, but significant research is required to improve weight-based outcomes. This is especially true for long-term maintenance of weight loss. Although some of these improvements are likely to come in the form of advances in technology and scientific discovery, the management of behaviors associated with obesity will continue to play an integral role in the treatment of this disease.

ACKNOWLEDGMENTS

We would like to thank the USDA/ARS Children's Nutrition Research Center for their support.

REFERENCES

1. Flegal, K. M., Carroll, M. D., Ogden, C. L., and L. R. Curtin. 2010. Prevalence and trends in obesity among US adults, 1999–2008. *Journal of the American Medical Association* 303:235–241.
2. Foreyt, J. P., and V. R. Pendleton. 2000. Management of obesity. *Primary Care Report* 6:19–30.
3. Poston, W. S. C., and J. P. Foreyt. 2000. Successful management of the obese patient. *American Family Physician* 61:3615–3622.
4. National Institutes of Health. 2000. *The Practical Guide: Identification, Evaluation, and Treatment of Overweight and Obesity in Adults.* NIH publication 00-4084. Rockville, MD: National Institutes of Health. http://www.nhlbi.nih.gov/guidelines/obesity/prctgd_c.pdf, (Accessed June 8, 2011).
5. Berkel, L. A., Poston, W. S. C., Reeves, R. S., and J. P. Foreyt. 2005. Behavioral interventions for obesity. *Journal of the American Dietetic Association* 105:S35–S43.
6. Kanfer, F. H. 1970. Self-monitoring: Methodological limitations and clinical applications. *Journal of Consulting and Clinical Psychology* 35:148–152.
7. Williamson, D. A., Anton, S. D., Han, H. et al. 2010. Early behavioral adherence predicts short and long-term weight loss in the POUNDS LOST study. *Journal of Behavioral Medicine* 33:305–314.
8. Epstein, L. H., Valoski, A., Vara, L. S. et al. 1995. Effects of decreasing sedentary behavior and increasing activity on weight change in obese children. *Health Psychology* 14:109–115.
9. Israel, A. C., Guile, C. A., Baker, J. E., and W. K. Silverman. 1994. An evaluation of enhanced self-regulation training in the treatment of childhood obesity. *Journal of Pediatric Psychology* 19:737–749.
10. Wing, R. R., Tate, D. F., Gorin, A. A., Raynor, H. A., and J. L. Fava. 2006. A self-regulation program for maintenance of weight loss. *The New England Journal of Medicine* 355:1563–1571.
11. Trabulsi, J., and D. A. Schoeller. 2001. Evaluation of dietary assessment instruments against doubly labeled water, a biomarker of habitual energy intake. *American Journal of Physiology, Endocrinology and Metabolism* 281:E891–E899.
12. Lichtman, S. W., Pisarska, K., Berman, E. R. et al. 1992. Discrepancy between self-reported and actual caloric intake and exercise in obese subjects. *The New England Journal of Medicine* 327:1893–1898.

13. The Diabetes Prevention Program Research Group. 2004. Achieving weight and activity goals among diabetes prevention program lifestyle participants. *Obesity Research* 12:1426–1434.
14. Knowler, W. C., Fowler, S. E., Hamman, R. F. et al. 2009. 10-year follow-up of diabetes incidence and weight loss in the Diabetes Prevention Program Outcomes Study. *Lancet* 374:1677–1686.
15. Pi-Sunyer, X., Blackburn, G., Brancati, F. L. et al. 2007. Reduction in weight and cardiovascular disease risk factors in individuals with type 2 diabetes: One-year results of the Look AHEAD trial. *Diabetes Care* 30:1374–1383.
16. Foreyt, J. P. 2005. Need for lifestyle intervention: How to begin. *American Journal of Cardiology* 96:11E–14E.
17. Perri, M. G., Nezu, A. M., McKelvey, W. F., Shermer, R. L., Renjilian, D. A., and B. J. Viegener. 2001. Relapse prevention training and problem-solving therapy in the long-term management of obesity. *Journal of Consulting and Clinical Psychology* 69:722–726.
18. Brownell, K. D. 2000. *The LEARN Program for Weight Management 2000*. Dallas, TX: American Health Publishing Co.
19. French, S. A., Story, M., and R. W. Jeffery. 2001. Environmental influences on eating and physical activity. *Annual Review of Public Health* 22:309–335.
20. Powell, L. M., Chaloupka, F. J., and Y. Bao. 2007. The availability of fast-food and full-service restaurants in the United States: Associations with neighborhood characteristics. *American Journal of Preventative Medicine* 33:S240–S245.
21. Young, L. R., and M. Nestle. 1995. Portion sizes in dietary assessment: Issues and policy implications. *Nutrition Reviews* 53:149–158.
22. Matthews, C. E., Chen, K. Y., Freedson, P. S. et al. 2008. Amount of time spent in sedentary behaviors in the United States, 2003–2004. *American Journal of Epidemiology* 167:875–881.
23. French, S. A., Jeffery, R.W., and J. A. Oliphant. 1994. Facility access and self-reward as methods to promote physical activity among healthy sedentary adults. *American Journal of Health Promotion* 8:257–262.
24. Lake, A., and T. Townshend. 2006. Obesogenic environments: Exploring the built and food environments. *The Journal of the Royal Society for the Promotion of Health* 126:262–267.
25. Heymsfield, S. B., van Mierlo, C. A. J., van der Knaap, H. C. M., Heo, M., and H. I. Frier. 2003. Weight management using meal replacement strategy: Meta and pooling analysis from six studies. *International Journal of Obesity* 27:537–549.
26. Flechtner-Mors, M., Boehm, B. O., Wittmann, R., Thoma, U., and H. H. Ditschuneit. 2010. Enhanced weight loss with protein-enriched meal replacements in subjects with the metabolic syndrome. *Diabetes/Metabolism Research and Reviews* 26:393–405.
27. Flechtner-Mors, M., Ditschuneit, H. H., Johnson, T. D., Suchard, M. A., and G. Adler. 2000. Metabolic and weight loss effects of long-term dietary intervention in obese patients: Four-year results. *Obesity Research* 8:399–402.
28. Fabricatore, A. N. 2007. Behavior therapy and cognitive-behavioral therapy of obesity: Is there a difference? *Journal of the American Dietetic Association* 107:92–99.
29. Wadden, T. A., and G. D. Foster. 2000. Behavioral treatment of obesity. *Medical Clinics of North America* 84:441–461.
30. Wadden, T. A., and M. L. Butryn. 2003. Behavioral treatment of obesity. *Endocrinology Metabolism Clinics of North America* 32:981–1003.
31. Foreyt, J. P., Goodrick, G. K., and A. M. Gotto. 1981. Limitations of behavioral treatment of obesity: Review and analysis. *Journal of Behavioral Medicine* 4:159–174.
32. Foreyt, J. P., and G. K. Goodrick. 1994. *Living Without Dieting*. New York: Warner Books.
33. Jeffery, R. W., Drewnowski, A., Epstein, L. H. et al. 2000. Long-term maintenance of weight loss: Current status. *Health Psychology* 19(supplement):5–16.

34. The Look AHEAD Research Group. 2006. The Look AHEAD Study: A description of the lifestyle intervention and the evidence supporting it. *Obesity* 14:737–752.

35. The Look AHEAD Research Group. 2003. Look AHEAD (Action for Health in Diabetes): Design and methods for a clinical trial of weight loss for the prevention of cardiovascular disease in type 2 diabetes. *Controlled Clinical Trials* 24:610–628.

36. Wadden, T. A., West, D. S., Neiberg, R. H. et al. (Look AHEAD Research Group). 2009. One-year weight losses in the Look AHEAD study: Factors associated with success. *Obesity (Silver Spring)* 17(4):713–722.

37. The Look AHEAD Research Group. 2007. Reduction in weight and cardiovascular disease risk factors in individuals with type 2 diabetes. *Diabetes Care* 30(6) (June):1374–1383.

38. The Look AHEAD Research Group. 2010. Long-term effects of a lifestyle intervention on weight and cardiovascular risk factors in individuals with type 2 diabetes mellitus. *Archives of Internal Medicine* 170:1566–1575.

39. The Look AHEAD Research Group. 2009. A randomized study on the effect of weight loss on obstructive sleep apnea among obese patients with type 2 diabetes. *Archives of Internal Medicine* 169:1619–1626.

40. The Look AHEAD Research Group. 2009. Effect of a lifestyle intervention on change in cardiorespiratory fitness in adults with type 2 diabetes: Result from the Look AHEAD Study. *International Journal of Obesity* 33:305–316.

41. The Look AHEAD Research Group. 2011. Intensive lifestyle intervention improves physical function among obese adults with knee pain: Findings from the Look AHEAD Trail. *Obesity* 19:83–93.

42. Stewart, T. M., Bachand, A. R., Han, H. et al. 2011. Body images changes associated with participation in an intensive lifestyle weight loss intervention. *Obesity* 19:1290–1295.

43. The Look AHEAD Research Group. 2009. Impact of a weight management program on health-related quality of life in overweight adults with type 2 diabetes. *Archives of Internal Medicine* 169:163–171.

44. Tate, D. F., Wing, R. R., and R. A. Winett. 2001. Using Internet technology to deliver a behavioral weight loss program. *Journal of American Medical Association* 285:1172–1177.

45. Lombard, D. N., Neubauer Lombard, T., and R. A. Winett. 1995. Walking to meet health guidelines: The effect of prompting frequency and prompt structure. *Health Psychology* 14:164–170.

46. Jeffery, R. W., Sherwood, N. E., Brelje, K. et al. 2003. Mail and phone interventions for weight loss in a managed-care setting: Weigh-To-Be one-year outcomes. *International Journal of Obesity* 27:1584–1592.

47. Boutelle, K. N., Kirschenbaum, D. S., Baker, R. C., and M. E. Mitchell. 1999. How can obese weight controllers minimize weight gain during the high risk holiday season? By self-monitoring very consistently. *Health Psychology* 18:364–368.

48. Patrick, K., Raab, F., Adams, M. A. et al. 2009. A text message-based intervention for weight loss: Randomized controlled trial. *Journal of Medical Internet Research* 11(1) (January): e1.

49. DeBusk, R. M., Fogarty, C. P., Ordovas, J. M., and K. S. Kornman. 2005. Nutritional genomics in practice: Where do we begin? *Journal of American Dietetic Association* 105:589–598.

50. Trujillo, E., Davis, C., and J. Milner. 2006. Nutrigenomics, proteomics, metabolomics, and the practice of dietetics. *Journal of American Dietetic Association* 106:403–413.

8 Managing Childhood Obesity

Craig A. Johnston, PhD and
Jennette P. Moreno, PhD

CONTENTS

The prevalence of childhood obesity has steadily increased over the last decades with approximately 35% of children aged 6–19 classified as overweight or obese [1]. Recently, a plateau in the increasing rates of obesity has been observed [2]. Despite this leveling off, overweight and obese children are heavier than they have ever been, putting them at increased risk for consequences associated with obesity [1]. If left unabated, obesity will become the most common cause of preventable death in adults [3]. Given the implications of childhood obesity, there is a pressing need for health professionals to possess a clear understanding of this epidemic. This chapter will present information on the definition, assessment, consequences, and treatment of childhood obesity.

DEFINITION

Body mass index (BMI) is commonly used in epidemiologic studies to indicate adiposity in adults. However, children are growing, and growth rates differ depending on gender and age. Because of this, BMI in children should be compared with gender- and age-specific values from a reference population. A variety of reference data sets are available and range from using representative data from a specific country to others using data on children from around the world. In the United States, reference values are based on representative data from the 2000 Centers for Disease Control and Prevention (CDC) growth charts [4].

A variety of terms have been used to describe high BMI-for-age categories in children. While the terminology may vary, expert committees have consistently recommended using two cutoff values: the 85th and 95th percentiles of BMI-for-age. These two cutoff points are based on varying levels of health risks. A child with a BMI at or above the 95th percentile will likely have high levels of body fat, as opposed to high lean body mass, and increased health risks. BMI at the 85th to the 94th percentiles includes children with excess body fat as well as those with high lean body mass. Therefore, this cutoff denotes varying susceptibility to health risks depending on factors such as family history and body composition. Current expert committee recommendations refer to a BMI-for-age ≥85th and <95th percentiles as "overweight" and BMI values at or above the 95th percentile as "obese" [5,6]. This proposed terminology is a change from previous recommendations, which referred to BMI-for-age ≥85th and <95th percentiles as "at risk for overweight" and BMI-for-age at or above the 95th percentile as "overweight" [7]. The Institute of Medicine, one of the agencies responsible for the new recommendations, explained this proposed change in terminology as a response to the grave nature of the problem of childhood obesity. "The term 'obese' more effectively conveys the seriousness, urgency, and medical nature of this concern than does the term 'overweight,' thereby reinforcing the importance of taking immediate action" [5].

In addition to the cutoffs at the 85th and 95th percentiles, a third cutoff has been proposed to designate an extreme level of obesity in children. Some data suggest that BMI-for-age values ≥99th percentile are strongly associated with an increased frequency of biochemical abnormalities and are highly predictive of adult obesity [8]. It has been suggested that this percentile may be used to indicate children who need more aggressive treatments. However, a 99th percentile cutoff point is not currently offered on the growth charts. Further, the cutoff value of the 99th percentile does not have the same level of unified agreement as the 85th and 95th percentiles. For example, the 97th percentile or ≥120% of the 95th percentile is sometimes used in the literature to indicate a severe level of obesity [9].

While the terminologies discussed earlier are appropriate for use in the literature and for documentation and risk assessment, these terms may not be appropriate for use in the clinician's office. It has been recommended that more neutral terms be used, such as "weight," "excess weight," and "BMI," in clinical settings. Careful language such as this may help to reduce weight-based stigmatization and discrimination [10].

ASSESSMENT

Body mass Index. While the strict medical definition of obesity is excess body fat, it is difficult to directly measure adiposity. Thus, BMI is widely used as a proxy for fatness in order to assess obesity among children aged 2 and older. BMI is used to denote weight adjusted for height and is calculated with the equation weight (kg) divided by height squared (m^2). Although this provides a measure of excess body weight (i.e., overweight status) and not fat, BMI is used to identify both overweight and obesity because it correlates well with excess adiposity, is easy to obtain, and is cost effective. Once BMI is calculated, it should be plotted on the CDC growth charts in order to obtain a percentile. This percentile is used to categorize a child's weight status (e.g., BMI ≥ 95th percentile is obese). Other methods used to assess body fat, such as skinfold thickness, waist circumference, and dual-energy x-ray absorptiometry are often used in research settings but are not currently recommended for routine clinical use. Issues such as costs and level of difficulty involved in learning to properly use these methods have precluded their recommendation [6,10].

Health risks. Once a diagnosis of overweight or obesity has been made, steps should be taken to rule out underlying causes (if suspected). For example, those with Prader–Willi and Cohen syndromes present with physical characteristics, such as dysmorphic features, developmental delay, or poor linear growth that should prompt further testing. If it is determined that obesity is not secondary to other conditions, the level of health risks should be identified. Determining health risks may be done by assessing medical history, diet and physical activity habits, body fat distribution, and laboratory tests. These assessments are important in determining the level of intervention required. For example, a child who is classified as overweight may be found to have little body fat and no family history of obesity-related illnesses. Further, diet and activity records may reveal that the child is involved in team sports and generally eats a well-balanced diet. Such a child may be deemed healthy by the clinician, which would result in an emphasis on prevention methods rather than treatment.

Diet and physical activity history. As stated earlier, determining lifestyle habits via diet and activity assessments can help to clarify level of health risks. Additionally, evaluating eating and physical activity can identify modifiable behaviors, and the assessment process can be used as an opportunity to evaluate readiness to change. Depending on the age of the patient, these assessments may be done on the child alone or with a parent. However, it may be most beneficial to include both parent and child regardless of the child's age. The assessment should identify the child's and family's typical patterns of eating and activity and identify any barriers to adopting a healthier lifestyle. Food and activity diaries, 24 h food recalls, and food frequency questionnaires are methods often used for assessment in research settings. A healthcare professional may find it more practical to ask questions directly related to specific modifiable behaviors, such as "How many fruits and vegetables do you eat each day?" and "How much time do you spend watching television or playing video games?" Several tools are available to guide the practitioner in rapidly assessing modifiable behaviors, such as the WAVE (weight, activity, variety, excess) questionnaire and the REAP (rapid eating and activity assessment for participants) questionnaire [11,12].

CONSEQUENCES

There are numerous physiological and psychosocial consequences associated with childhood obesity. These consequences are positively correlated with BMI; thus, as BMI increases, so do the risks of developing comorbidities and negative social outcomes. Many of these negative consequences present in childhood. Additionally, risks of developing comorbidities in adulthood increase as there is a high likelihood that an obese child will become an obese adult. It has also been demonstrated that there is an increased risk of multiple comorbidities in adulthood even if pediatric obesity does not persist [13].

Insulin resistance, dyslipidemia, hypertension, gallstones, obstructive sleep apnea, and orthopedic complications are some of the physiological consequences of childhood obesity. Psychological and social consequences may be even more common than physical comorbidities. These include reduced quality of life, body dissatisfaction, a decreased self-concept, and increased depressive symptomology. While depression may result in behaviors that promote obesity, negative social outcomes that result from obesity may increase symptoms of depression. Obese children report more adverse social conditions than normal weight children, such as teasing by peers and family members and social isolation. Pediatric obesity has also been shown to be linked with poorer grades and decreased performance on standardized tests. This decreased performance in the academic realm may result in harmful social consequences that persist into adulthood. For example, heavier adolescent girls have been shown to have decreased educational attainment, which negatively impacted their occupational attainment [14].

TREATMENT

Given the numerous consequences associated with pediatric obesity, the prevention and treatment of this condition beginning in childhood is clear. However, prevention programs have yet to show promising results [15,16]. This is concerning as the incidence and prevalence of this condition is expected to increase once again in the United States and worldwide [2,17].

An expert committee was formed to develop recommendations for the treatment of pediatric obesity [10]. This committee developed a stepwise approach for the treatment and prevention of obesity in children. This approach proposes that certain stages should be followed with differing goals based on the child's age, weight status, and other related factors. A total of four stages are presented. Children in the normal weight range (5th–84th BMI percentile) should follow recommendations for a healthy lifestyle, but it is not until children become overweight (≥85th percentile) that this multistage process begins. The overall goal for children who are normal weight is to engage in healthy eating and activity lifestyle habits that maintain their BMI status. These habits recommended by the expert committee include the following behaviors:

1. Limiting consumption of sugar-sweetened beverages
2. Encouraging the consumption of fruits and vegetables
3. Limiting television and other forms of screen time

4. Eating breakfast daily
5. Limiting eating out at restaurants
6. Encouraging family meals
7. Limiting portion size

In the prevention plus stage (stage 1), children who are overweight are encouraged to focus on these healthy habits and gradually improve BMI status. Families and care providers are encouraged to work together to identify health behaviors that most impact the child's energy balance. Once agreement has been reached on specific health behaviors, small and measurable steps should be taken to make changes. If the child has not made improvements in 3–6 months, stage 2, structured weight management, is encouraged. In this stage, children and families receive more structure and support for their targeted behavior change. Some of the main differences for this stage are providing the family with a planned diet, incorporating structured meals, and planned physical activity.

Stages 3 (comprehensive multidisciplinary intervention) and 4 (tertiary care intervention) are suggested after stages 1 and 2 have been attempted and do not appear intensive enough to curb the velocity of the child's weight gain. Some of the primary components of stage 3 include a structured behavior modification program, systematic evaluation of body measurements and behavior change, and frequent appointments (weekly). Stage 4 is the final stage offered to some severely obese youth. This stage would include the possible incorporation of medications, a very low-calorie diet, or surgery. The remainder of this chapter focuses primarily on stage 3 interventions and provides an overview of techniques and settings in which these interventions may be provided.

In terms of efficacious interventions, numerous programs have been developed to address childhood obesity [16]. Most treatments take a multidisciplinary approach to improve eating behaviors, physical activity, and sedentary behaviors [18]. The studies with the greatest efficacy are also based in the principles of behavior modification [19,20]. Behavior modification in obesity treatment involves modifying behavioral and environmental factors in order to support a healthier lifestyle [18,19].

BEHAVIORAL COMPONENTS

Behavior modification procedures form the foundation of the treatment of obesity in both adults and children [21,22]. Commonly used techniques in behavioral counseling sessions include self-monitoring, goal setting, and reinforcement [23]. One of the most important behavioral techniques to teach the patient is self-monitoring. Self-monitoring raises awareness through completion of daily records about health behaviors such as food intake and/or physical activity. Although young children may have difficulty recording their food intake, children are encouraged to be involved as much as possible in the self-monitoring process. This information can be used to further structure the counseling session. Specifically, feedback on records is provided, and goals for behavior change are made. The key to successful goal setting is to set small, achievable goals. Small successes create behavioral momentum for children to continue to make behavioral changes. Finally, reinforcement of behavior change increases the likelihood of maintaining these behaviors as lifestyle changes.

Other behavioral techniques that are used outside of the behavioral counseling session include stimulus control, modeling, and social support. Stimulus control involves identifying the situations in which a child is likely to engage in behaviors that contribute to weight gain and making changes to the environment to reduce the likelihood of engaging in those behaviors. Examples might include avoiding buffets, ridding the house of unhealthy foods, eating only at the dinner table, and putting one's fork down between bites. Modeling can be defined as a way of learning in which individuals determine how to act based on observing others. Children naturally learn by watching others in their environment. Parents, teachers, and other children can be powerful role models for children. Similarly, the support of these individuals is also important for maintaining behavioral changes. The overall goal of behavior change is not to make short-term changes in health behaviors, but to create changes that can be maintained throughout the life span (i.e., lifestyle changes). Chapter 7 provides an in-depth discussion of these behavioral components.

FAMILY-BASED BEHAVIORAL INTERVENTIONS

Parents and families play a critical role in the development of childhood obesity. For example, children are more likely to be overweight or obese when they have overweight parents [24–26]. Parents are extremely influential in modeling eating patterns and physical activity habits. Parents help to create a home environment to be either prohibitive or conducive to overeating and exercise and provide reinforcement for certain diet and physical activity patterns. Further, parenting practices and the emotional climate of the home environment also affect the development of childhood obesity. For these reasons, including parents is thought to be important in the treatment of childhood obesity.

The efficacy of family-based interventions for overweight children has been replicated over the last 25 years [27]. Family-based approaches have traditionally targeted both the parent and child [28], although some interventions have had success exclusively targeting parents as the sole agent of change [29,30]. In fact, one study demonstrated that an intervention targeting the parents exclusively was more successful than an intervention targeting the child as the sole agent of change [29]. Most recent interventions not only address health-related behaviors of the family, but also general family functioning [31,32]. Family-based interventions have targeted the extended family as well in an effort to be more culturally relevant (e.g., interventions targeting Hispanic children) [33].

There are many common elements implemented in different family-based interventions, such as the use of behavioral techniques, nutrition education, and physical activity. The behavioral components used in these programs are, for the most part, consistent. For example, programs often use self-monitoring, stimulus control, and contingency management (i.e., reinforcement). Parents are also trained to use behavioral strategies with their children in order to improve diet and physical activity. Parents are taught to be aware of and model appropriate behaviors, to not use food as a reward, and various other techniques to induce behavior change in their children.

While family-based treatments that incorporate behavioral strategies have been shown to be superior to education alone, the independent contribution of each behavioral technique is currently unknown. More specifically, dismantling studies have not been conducted to determine the relative impact that each strategy has on weight loss or weight maintenance in children. Whereas the aforementioned strategies have consistently been shown to be efficacious, several additional components have not been shown to improve outcomes. For example, problem solving does not appear to add to the effectiveness of treatment beyond standard family-based treatment [34]. Additionally, cognitive interventions do not appear to improve outcomes compared to behavioral interventions [35].

Family-based intervention studies have demonstrated positive long-term results with sustained weight loss for up to 10 years following treatment [36]. Due to the importance attributed to the role of the family in the treatment for pediatric obesity, recommendations for best practice indicate that the family should also be involved in school and community interventions in order to augment and maintain results [18,21].

Despite the strong evidence supporting family-based treatments, most research-based programs have yet to be translated into "real-world" interventions. To further complicate this matter, issues related to cost-effectiveness and parental attendance still need to be addressed. For example, school- and community-based studies have had difficulty obtaining access to parents [33]. This is likely due to many factors including a lack of parental resources and time to attend interventions. Finding ways to more fully incorporate parents appears integral.

SCHOOL-BASED INTERVENTIONS

Schools have been a popular setting for interventions aimed at combating the obesity epidemic. The school environment has been deemed advantageous for various reasons. For example, children spend approximately 20% of their waking hours and eat up to two meals a day at school. Further, schools provide a preexisting structure of policies, personnel, and curricula that lends itself to health-related programs. Despite the many advantages to conducting weight-management studies in school settings, few have demonstrated actual decreases in weight-based outcomes [37,38]. Nonetheless, school-based interventions remain promising as they have often demonstrated positive changes in measures of diet, physical activity, and sedentary behaviors [16].

Considerable variability is found in school-based studies. Not only do the interventions vary in terms of methodology, but they also differ in terms of overall focus and aims. For example, the method of delivery ranges from the use of school personnel to dedicated intervention staff. In terms of focus, many school-based programs center on environmental changes throughout the entire school, whereas others aim for a very specific change (e.g., foods offered in the school cafeteria). Several school-based interventions address only physical activity or diet, while others are more comprehensive in scope. The heterogeneity of approaches has made it difficult to assess which components are necessary to produce the most effective school-based interventions in terms of changes in weight. However, several salient features of effective interventions have been identified and include the following: (1) parental involvement, (2) increased intensity and duration, (3) encompassing both physical activity and dietary instruction, (4) a behavioral underpinning, (5) cultural tailoring, and (6) the use of dedicated intervention staff [38,39].

Of the factors listed, parental involvement may be the most difficult to modify. While a representative survey of U.S. households found that the public cited schools more often than health-care providers and the government as having a "lot of responsibility" to curb childhood obesity [40], attempts to involve parents in school-based interventions have been largely unsuccessful [33]. Finding ways to increase parental involvement will aid interventions in achieving long-term success.

Increasing intensity and duration may also be difficult unless dedicated intervention staff are used. Some weight-management programs in schools have been limited by their reliance on administrators, teachers, and staff to provide nutrition/health training in addition to their primary academic duties [41]. This often inhibits the intensity with which program components are delivered. Programs that rely solely on teachers to achieve these goals will likely overburden their schedules and prove to be unrealistic. Using trained staff may be necessary to successfully implement the treatment with the recommended intensity. However, finding ways to effectively use teachers and school staff is still a worthy endeavor as this may ultimately prove a more practical option to translate into "real-world" interventions.

While few school-based studies have proven to be efficacious in decreasing weight, there are a few quality studies that have demonstrated success [33,42–44]. One study group has demonstrated decreases in BMI standardized for age and gender (zBMI) at 6 months, 1 year, and 2 years for Mexican American children randomized to an intensive healthy lifestyle program compared to children in a self-help condition [33]. This study is promising because of the lack of school-based studies reporting long-term results (e.g., >1 year). Another research group demonstrated that after 9 months, students enrolled in a lifestyle-focused, fitness-oriented gym class significantly decreased body fat, increased cardiovascular fitness, and improved fasting glucose compared to children in a standard gym class [42]. While the number of studies demonstrating efficacy is few, these studies suggest that schools may provide a promising infrastructure through which to address childhood obesity.

Understanding the factors that make school-based programs effective is important because schools provide an ideal setting for impacting children's health habits. Developing more effective school-based interventions may be especially important for certain minority communities. A lack of resources, such as money and transportation, may preclude some minorities and low-income families from seeking help in clinic-based settings. School-based interventions offer certain groups the opportunity to receive treatment to which they may not otherwise have access. Further, finding the combination of components that are most effective may help in creating more efficient and financially feasible programs, thus turning research into a "real-world" option.

COMMUNITY-BASED INTERVENTIONS

Community-based programs generally seek to utilize preexisting community resources to deliver intervention components. Community settings include community centers, neighborhoods, low-cost health clinics, churches, and after-school programs. While school-based interventions are a form of community intervention, they are usually discussed separately in the literature due to their unique structure.

Communities and schools have been identified as the best settings for implementing multidimensional strategies (e.g., multicomponent programs, programs that intervene on multiple levels of the environment) [45].

While there are many school-based obesity treatment programs for children and adolescents, there are a limited number of interventions in community settings. This may be due, in part, to greater issues with recruitment and attrition. Community interventions have attempted various strategies to address these issues. For example, the participatory research model has become increasingly popular. Participatory research, which seeks to incorporate community stakeholders, has now become a part of many community-based programs. Community-based participatory research attempts to involve the public in every phase of the research process "by incorporating their public views in the prioritization, review, and translation and dissemination of research" [46]. Involving the input of those who are members of the community can aid in assessing a program's potential for acceptance and integration in the community. Additionally, this model may increase participation and boost the likelihood that study components and principles will be adopted by the community well after the intervention has ended. Finally, such community programs may be beneficial for reaching immigrant and minority communities as fewer minority participants enroll in clinical trials or go to clinic-based programs.

SPECIAL POPULATIONS

INTERVENTIONS AIMED AT ETHNIC MINORITIES

Many ethnic groups are disproportionately affected by obesity and its associated comorbidities. Approximately 39% of Mexican American, 36% of Black, and 40% or more of American Indian children are considered to be overweight or obese [1,47]. However, very few interventions have been developed to treat obesity in these minority groups [48–51]. Unfortunately, studies examining treatments for minority children are often plagued by lack of experimental rigor and/or small sample sizes. While many interventions appear promising, they have not been shown to be more effective than control at reducing weight-based outcomes (e.g., Refs. [52–57]). Only a few quality studies have been shown to be efficacious with Hispanic and Black populations (e.g., Refs. [33,58,59]).

The tailoring of interventions to be culturally appropriate for the intended population is important [60]. Despite many within-group differences [61], some common cultural values can be seen within ethnic and racial groups. For example, the Hispanic culture emphasizes the value of collectivism, specifically, *familismo*, which incorporates the commitment to support family members both emotionally and financially, reliance on family for help, and deferring to family for how one should think or behave [62]. The promotion of *simpatía* or positive emotions among groups and *educación* or education is of great importance in this culture [62]. Because of the importance of the family, positive interactions, and the education of the family in Hispanic culture, interventions should focus on improving family functioning and educating individuals about ways to improve the health of the family as a whole instead of the individual alone.

Black culture also has several cultural values that should be incorporated into treatment. For example, Blacks typically find a larger body size to be ideal [63]. At times this may be thought to interfere with weight loss; however, this perspective may be helpful in terms of promoting healthy lifestyles rather than the pursuit of an unrealistic body size.

The Native American culture emphasizes the importance of cooperation, collectivism, and learning through storytelling and active play [64]. As a result, stories reinforcing the history of healthful eating and activity practices in the American culture may be of importance. Additionally, tailoring traditional games to increase physical activity and reinforce healthy messages may also be effective. Overall, the health disparities in these minority groups indicate a clear need for effective yet culturally relevant interventions targeting minority populations.

SOCIOECONOMIC STATUS

Research is also needed to determine effective treatments for children in low-income families. Given the increased risk of overweight and obesity in lower socioeconomic populations (e.g., Ref. [65]), interventions that specifically address the needs of these families need to be developed. A paucity of information is available on this topic. A major critique of family-based behavioral treatments for pediatric overweight is their lack of inclusion of lower-income groups. Low-income families present unique challenges to treatment. For example, these families may live in multifamily and multigenerational households, which make stimulus control difficult. In these situations, it is even more important to enlist the support of the entire family, although it may be difficult to coordinate efforts to include the entire family. Meal replacements, a form of stimulus control, may be one possible option for low-income families. Although nutritious home-prepared meals are ideal for children, the convenience and potentially low cost of meal replacements may be a viable option and serve as an adjunct to standard treatments [66].

ADJUNCTS TO TREATMENT

MEAL REPLACEMENTS

Weight-reduction programs featuring meal replacements have demonstrated significant weight loss in overweight adolescents. A study by Ball et al. [67] found that overweight adolescents on a low-glycemic-index (GI) meal replacement plan requested additional food later than those adolescents on a high-GI meal replacement plan. The authors concluded that the prolonged satiety, as seen with the low-GI meal replacements, may be an effective method for reducing caloric intake, which is important for achieving long-term weight control. The limited research on this subject also suggests that meal replacements may prove to be most beneficial for very overweight adolescents.

PHARMACOTHERAPY

Pharmacotherapy in conjunction with lifestyle modifications (e.g., Refs. [68–70]) has shown results in weight reduction among obese and severely obese pediatric patients.

However, experts suggest that pharmacotherapy should only be considered for extremely obese children with severe comorbidities after dietary and lifestyle modifications alone have proven insufficient (e.g., Refs. [68,70]). In addition, the potential risks of a pharmacotherapeutic treatment need to be taken into account and weighed against the potential weight loss benefits, and patients need to be closely monitored by experienced clinicians for any potential adverse reactions [68].

Currently, orlistat, a gastrointestinal lipase inhibitor, is the only form of pharmacotherapy approved for use in adolescents [71]. Several studies have demonstrated the safety and efficacy of orlistat on weight loss in obese adults (e.g., Refs. [72–74]). Fewer studies have evaluated the use of orlistat in children and adolescents, though it has been shown to be safe and effective when used in combination with diet, exercise, and behavior modification in both children and adolescents [69]. Children on orlistat treatment should take a daily multivitamin supplement due to the potential interference of the drug with fat-soluble vitamins such as vitamins A, D, E, and K [75].

BARIATRIC SURGERY

Although bariatric surgery is not the focus of this chapter, considerable attention has been given to implications of these procedures in children. For obese children and adolescents, weight loss has many benefits and is important to improving health and cardiovascular risks and lowering long-term mortality risk [76]. However, this situation is complicated by the increased risk of nutritional deficiencies, which might affect children's growth and development [77]. Taking into account the risk, side effects, invasiveness, and costs, O'Brien [78] suggests that bariatric surgery should be treated as the last therapeutic option, after lifestyle changes and pharmacotherapy have failed. The current patient selection criteria for bariatric surgery include physical maturity (completing 95% of adult stature or at least over age 12), psychological maturity, BMI ($\geq$35 with major comorbidities and $\geq$40 with other comorbidities), ability to comply with pre- and postoperative treatment regimens, and previous interventions to control their weight [79]. There are several surgical procedures available, with the most recent, safest, and least invasive one being adjustable gastric banding (AGB), which has been demonstrated to induce satiety [80]. However, AGB has not been approved by the U.S. Food and Drug Administration for patients under 18 years old [81]. Additional known surgical procedures in order of recommendation include Roux-en-Y gastric bypass, sleeve gastrectomy, and open and laparoscopic biliopancreatic diversion [78]. Biliopancreatic diversion is less ideal for adolescents considering the risk of malnutrition and malabsorptive consequences [82]. Both gastric bypass and AGB are relatively safe and have led to larger percent of excess weight loss and resolution of metabolic syndrome comparing to nonsurgical therapies [78]. Even though the short- and median-term outcomes of bariatric surgery are superior to nonsurgical procedures, there are few long-term studies on the effectiveness of bariatric surgery in adolescents [83]; therefore, opponents of bariatric surgery are often concerned with issues such as whether adolescents can take on the lifetime responsibility of dietary and lifestyle changes after the operation in order to maintain the weight loss [84].

FUTURE DIRECTIONS

A firm foundation for the treatment of pediatric obesity has been established. However, a great deal of work remains to be done in this area, given that children who receive treatment typically remain overweight and long-term maintenance of weight loss is not typically demonstrated. Furthermore, the interventions discussed earlier have yet to demonstrate consistent positive results with very overweight children and economically and culturally diverse families. However, the body of knowledge in treating childhood obesity in these populations is steadily growing. In fact, this review indicates that there are a multitude of interventions in disparate settings that show great promise. Advances in this field will come as researchers and practitioners create new interventions and/or enhance currently existing treatments for use with diverse groups and with new technologies.

ACKNOWLEDGMENTS

We would like to thank the USDA/ARS Children's Nutrition Research Center for their support.

REFERENCES

1. Ogden, C. L., Carroll, M. D., Curtin, L. R., Lamb, M. M., and K. M. Flegal. 2010. Prevalence of high body mass index in US children and adolescents, 2007–2008. *Journal of the American Medical Association* 303(3):242–249.
2. Rokholm, B., Baker, J. L., and T. I. Sørensen. 2010. The levelling off of the obesity epidemic since the year 1999—A review of evidence and perspectives. *Obesity Reviews* 11(12):835–846.
3. U.S. Department of Health and Human Services. 2001. *The Surgeon General's Call to Action to Prevent and Decrease Overweight and Obesity.* Rockville, MD: U.S. Department of Health and Human Services, Public Health Service, Office of the Surgeon General.
4. Kuczmarski, R. J., Ogden, C. L., Guo, S. S. et al. 2000. CDC growth charts for the United States: Methods and development. National Center for Health Statistics. *Vital and Health Statistics* 11(246) (June):1–190.
5. Committee on Prevention of Obesity in Children and Youth. 2005. *Preventing Childhood Obesity: Health in the Balance*, Appendix B, eds. J. P. Koplan, C. T. Liverman, and V. A. Kraak, p. 336, Washington, DC: The National Academies Press.
6. Krebs, N. F., Himes, J. H., Jacobson, D., Nicklas, T. A., Guilday, P., and D. Styne. 2007. Assessment of child and adolescent overweight and obesity. *Pediatrics* 120(Suppl. 4):S193–S228.
7. Himes, J. H., and W. H. Dietz. 1994. Guidelines for overweight in adolescent preventive services: Recommendations from an expert committee: The Expert Committee on Clinical Guidelines for Overweight in Adolescent Preventive Services. *The American Journal of Clinical Nutrition* 59:307–316.
8. Freedman, D. S., Mei, Z., Srinivasan, S. R., Berenson, G. S., and W. H. Dietz. 2007. Cardiovascular risk factors and excess adiposity among overweight children and adolescents: The Bogalusa Heart Study. *Journal of Pediatrics* 150:12–17.
9. Flegal, K. M., Wei, R., Ogden, C. L., Freedman, D. S., Johnson, C. L., and L. R. Curtin. 2009. Characterizing extreme values of body mass index-for-age by using the 2000 Centers for Disease Control and Prevention growth charts. *The American Journal of Clinical Nutrition* 90:1314–1320.

10. Barlow, S. E., and Expert Committee. 2007. Expert committee recommendations regarding the prevention, assessment, and treatment of child and adolescent overweight and obesity: Summary report. *Pediatrics* 120(Suppl. 4):S164–S192.

11. Isasi, C. R., Soroudi, N., and J. Wylie-Rosett. 2006. Youth WAVE screener: Addressing weight-related behaviors with school-age children. *The Diabetes Educator* 32(3):415–422.

12. Segal-Isaacson, C. J., Wylie Rosett, J., and K. M. Gans. 2004. Validation of a short dietary assessment questionnaire: The Rapid Eating and Activity and Assessment for Participants short version (REAP-S). *The Diabetes Educator* 30:774–778.

13. Must, A., Jacques, P. F., Dallal, G. E., Bajema, C. J., and W. H. Dietz. 1992. Long-term morbidity and mortality of overweight adolescents: A follow-up of the Harvard Growth Study of 1922 to 1935. *The New England Journal of Medicine* 327:1350–1355.

14. Glass, C. M., Hass, S. A., and E. N. Reither. 2010. The skinny on success: Body mass, gender and occupational standing across the life course. *Social Forces* 88(4):1777–1806.

15. Kamath, C. C., Vickers, K. S., Ehrlich, A. et al. 2008. Clinical review: Behavioral interventions to prevent childhood obesity: A systematic review and metaanalyses of randomized trials. *Journal of Clinical Endocrinology & Metabolism* 93(12):4606–4615.

16. Summerbell, C. D., Ashton, V., Campbell K. J., Edmunds, L., Kelly, S., and E. Waters. 2003. Interventions for treating obesity in children. *The Cochrane Database of Systematic Reviews* 3:CD001872.

17. Wang, Y., Beydoun, M. A., Liang, L., Caballero, B., and S. K. Kumanyika. 2008. Will all Americans become overweight or obese? Estimating the progression and cost of the US obesity epidemic. *Obesity (Silver Spring)* 16(10):2323–2330.

18. Kelly, S. A., and B. M. Melnyk. 2008. Systematic review of multicomponent interventions with overweight middle adolescents: Implications for clinical practice and research. *Worldviews on Evidence-Based Nursing* 5(3):113–135.

19. Artinian, N. T., Fletcher, G. F., Mozaffarian, D. et al. 2010. Interventions to promote physical activity and dietary lifestyle changes for cardiovascular risk factor reduction in adults: A scientific statement from the American Heart Association. *Circulation* 122(4):406–441.

20. Oude Luttikhuis, H., Baur, L., Jansen, H. et al. 2009. Interventions for treating obesity in children. *Cochrane Database Systematic Reviews* 1:CD001872.

21. American Dietetic Association. 2006. Position of the American Dietetic Association: Individual-, family-, school-, and community-based interventions for pediatric overweight. *Journal of the American Dietetic Association* 106:925–945.

22. Epstein, L. H., Wing, R. R., Sternachack, L., Dickson, B., and J. Michelson. 1980. Comparison of family-based behavior modification and nutrition education for childhood obesity. *Journal of Pediatric Psychology* 5:25–36.

23. Jelalian, E., Wember, Y. M., Bungeroth, H., and V. Birmaher. 2007. Practitioner review: Bridging the gap between research and clinical practice in pediatric obesity. *Journal of Child Psychology and Psychiatry, and Allied Disciplines* 48:115–127.

24. Charney, E., Goodman, H. C., McBride, M. et al. 1976. Childhood antecedents of adult obesity—Do chubby infants become obese adults? *The New England Journal of Medicine* 295:6–9.

25. Garn, S. M., Sullivan, T. V., and V. M. Hawthorne. 1989. Fatness and obesity of the parents of obese individuals. *American Journal of Clinical Nutrition* 50:1308–1313.

26. Grilo, C. M., and M. F. Pogue-Geile. 1991. The nature of environmental influences on weight and obesity: A behavior genetic analysis. *Psychological Bulletin* 110(3):520–537.

27. Epstein, L. H., Paluch, R. A., Roemmich, J. N., and M. D. Beecher. 2007. Family-based obesity treatment, then and now: Twenty-five years of pediatric obesity treatment. *Health Psychology* 26:381–391.

28. Epstein, L. H., Mckenzie, S. J., Valoski, A., Klein, K. R., and R. R. Wing. 1994. Effects of mastery criteria and contingent reinforcement for family-based child weight control. *Addictive Behaviors* 19(2):135–145.

29. Golan, M., and S. Crow. 2004. Targeting parents exclusively in the treatment of childhood obesity: Long-term results. *Obesity Research* 12:357–361.

30. West, F., Sanders, M. R., Cleghorn, G. J., and P. S. W. Davies. 2010. Randomised clinical trial of a family-based lifestyle intervention for childhood obesity involving parents as the exclusive agents of change. *Behaviour Research and Therapy* 48:1170–1179.

31. Kitzmann, K. M., and B. M. Beech. 2006. Family-based interventions for pediatric obesity: Methodological and conceptual challenges from family psychology. *Journal of Family Psychology* 20:175–189.

32. Nowicka, P., and C. Flodmark. 2008. Family in pediatric obesity management: A literature review. *International Journal of Pediatric Obesity* 3:44–50.

33. Johnston, C. A., Tyler, C., Fullerton, G. et al. 2010. Effects of a school-based weight maintenance program for Mexican American children: Results at 2 years. *Obesity* 18:542–547.

34. Epstein, L. H., Paluch, R. A., Gordy, C. C., Saelens, B. E., and M. M. Ernst. 2000. Problem solving in the treatment of childhood obesity. *Journal of Consulting and Clinical Psychology* 68:717–721.

35. Herrera, E. A., Johnston, C. A., and R. G. Steele. 2004. A comparison of cognitive and behavioral treatments for pediatric obesity. *Children's Health Care* 33:151–167.

36. Epstein, L. H., Valoski, A., Wing, R. R., and J. McCurley. 1994. Ten-year outcomes of behavioral family-based treatment for childhood obesity. *Health Psychology* 13(5):373–383.

37. Shaya, F. T., Flores, D., Gbarayor, C. M., and J. Wang. 2008. School-based obesity interventions: A literature review. *The Journal of School Health* 78(4):189–196.

38. Zenzen, W., and S. Kridli. 2009. Integrative review of school-based childhood obesity prevention programs. *Journal of Pediatric Health Care* 23(4):242–258.

39. Katz, D. L. 2009. School-based interventions for health promotion and weight control: Not just waiting on the world to change. *Annual Review of Public Health* 30:253–272.

40. Evans, W. D., Finkelstein, E. A., Kamerow, D. B., and J. M. Renaud. 2005. Public perceptions of childhood obesity. *American Journal of Preventive Medicine* 28(1):26–32.

41. Koplan J. P., Liverman C. T., and V. I. Kraak. 2005. *Preventing Childhood Obesity: Health in the Balance*. Washington, DC: National Academies Press.

42. Carrel, A. L., Clark, R. R., Peterson, S. E., Nemeth, B. A., Sullivan, J., and D. B. Allen. 2005. Improvement of fitness, body composition, and insulin sensitivity in overweight children in a school-based exercise program: A randomized, controlled study. *Archives of Pediatrics & Adolescent Medicine* 159(10):963–968.

43. Lange, D., Wahrendorf, M., Siegrist, J., Plachta-Danielzik, S., Landsberg, B., and M. J. Müller. 2011. Associations between neighbourhood characteristics, body mass index and health-related behaviours of adolescents in the Kiel Obesity Prevention Study: A multilevel analysis. *European Journal of Clinical Nutrition* 65(6):711–719.

44. Graf, C., Rost, S. V., Koch, B. et al. 2005. Data from the STEP TWO programme showing the effect on blood pressure and different parameters for obesity in overweight and obese primary school children. *Cardiology in the Young* 15(3):291–298.

45. Flynn, M. A. T., McNeil, D. A., Maloff, B. et al. 2006. Reducing obesity and related chronic disease risk in children and youth: A synthesis of evidence with 'best practice' recommendations. *Obesity Reviews* 7:7–66.

46. Institute of Medicine. 2003. *Engaging the Public in the Clinical Research Enterprise*. Washington, DC: National Academy of Sciences.

47. Zephier, E., Himes, J. H., Story, M., and X. Zhou. 2006. Increasing prevalences of overweight and obesity in northern plains American Indian children. *Archives of Pediatrics & Adolescent Medicine* 160:34–39.

48. Branscum, P., and M. Sharma. 2010. A systematic analysis of childhood obesity prevention interventions targeting Hispanic children: Lessons learned from the previous decade. *Obesity Reviews* 2:1–8.

49. Halpern, P. 2007. Obesity and American Indians/Alaska Natives. U. S. Department of Health and Human Services, Assistant Secretary for Planning and Evaluation, http://aspe.hhs.gov/hsp/07/ai-an-obesity/report.pdf (accessed April 7, 2011).

50. Hudson, C. E. 2008. An integrative review of obesity prevention in African American children. *Issues in Comprehensive Pediatric Nursing* 31:147–170.

51. Stevens, C. J. 2010. Obesity prevention interventions for middle school-age children of ethnic minority: A review of the literature. *Journal for Specialists in Pediatric Nursing* 15:233–243.

52. Caballero, B., Himes, J., Lohman, T. et al. 2003. Pathways: A school-based, randomized controlled trial for the prevention of obesity in American Indian schoolchildren. *American Journal of Clinical Nutrition* 78:308–312.

53. Colchico, K., Zybert, P., and C. E. Basch. 2000. Effects of after-school physical activity on fitness, fatness, and cognitive self-perceptions: A pilot study among urban, minority adolescent girls. *American Journal of Public Health* 90:977–978.

54. Klesges, R. C., Obarzanek, E., Kumanyika, S. et al. 2010. The Memphis Girls' health Enrichment Multi-site Studies (GEMS): An evaluation of the efficacy of a 2-year obesity prevention program in African American girls. *Archives of Pediatrics & Adolescent Medicine* 164:1007–1014.

55. Resnicow, K., Yaroch, A. L., Davis, A. et al. 2000. GO GIRLS!: Results from a nutrition and physical activity program for low-income, overweight African American adolescent females. *Health Education & Behavior* 27:616–631.

56. Robinson, T. N., Matheson, D. M., Kraemer, H. C. et al. 2010. A randomized controlled trial of culturally tailored dance and reducing screen time to prevent weight gain in low-income African American girls: Stanford GEMS. *Archives of Pediatrics & Adolescent Medicine* 164:995–1004.

57. Story, M., Sherwood, N. E., Himes, J. H. et al. 2003. An after-school obesity prevention program for African-American girls: The Minnesota GEMS pilot study. *Ethnicity and Disease* 13:S54–S64.

58. Coleman, K. J., Tiller, C. L., Sanchez, J. et al. 2005. Prevention of the epidemic increase in child risk of overweight in low-income schools: The El Paso coordinated approach to child health. *Archives of Pediatrics & Adolescent Medicine* 159:217–224.

59. Fitzgibbon, M. L., Stolley, M. R., Schiffer, L., Van Horn, L., KauferChristoffel, K., and A. Dyer. 2005. Two-year follow-up results for Hip-Hop to Health Jr.: A randomized controlled trial for overweight prevention in preschool minority children. *Journal of Pediatrics* 146:618–625.

60. Daniels, S. R., Jacobson, M. S., McCrindle, B. W., Eckel, R. H., and B. McHugh Sanner. 2009. American Heart Association childhood obesity research summit report. *Journal of the American Heart Association* 119:489–517.

61. Centrella-Nigro, A. 2009. Hispanic children and overweight: Causes and interventions. *Pediatric Nursing* 35:352–356.

62. Marin, G., and B. Marin. 1991. *Research with Hispanic Populations*. Newbury Park, CA: Sage Publications.

63. Baskin, M. L., Ahluwalia, H. K., and K. Resnicow. 2001. Obesity intervention among African-American children and adolescents. *Pediatric Clinics of North America* 48:1027–1039.

64. Davis, S. M., Going, S. B., Helitzer, D. L. et al. 1999. Pathways: A culturally appropriate obesity-prevention program for American Indian schoolchildren. *American Journal of Clinical Nutrition* 69:796S–802S.

65. Gordon-Larsen, P., Adair, L. S., and B. M. Popkin. 2003. The relationship of ethnicity, socioeconomic factors, and overweight in US adolescents. *Obesity Research* 11:121–129.

66. Berkel, L. A., Poston, W. S., Reeves, R. S., and J. P. Foreyt. 2005. Behavioral interventions for obesity. *Journal of the American Dietetic Association* 105:S35–S43.

67. Ball, S. D., Keller, K. R., Moyer-Mileur, L. J., Ding, Y. W., Donaldson, D., and W. D. Jackson. 2003. Prolongation of satiety after low versus moderately high glycemic index meals in obese adolescents. *Pediatrics* 111:488–494.
68. August, G. P., Caprio, S., Fennoy, I. et al. 2008. Prevention and treatment of pediatric obesity: An endocrine society clinical practice guideline based on expert opinion. *Journal of Clinical Endocrinology & Metabolism* 93:4576–4599.
69. Chanoine, J. P., Hampl, S., Jensen, C., Boldrin, M., and J. Hauptman. 2005. Effect of orlistat on weight and body composition in obese adolescents: A randomized controlled trial. *Journal of the American Medical Association* 293:2873–2883.
70. Dunican, K. C., Desilets, A. R., and J. K. Montalbano. 2007. Pharmacotherapeutic options for overweight adolescents. *The Annals of Pharmacotherapy* 41(9):1445–1455.
71. Butryn, M. L., Wadden, T. A., Rukstalis, M. R., Bishop-Gilyard, C., Xanthopoulos, M. S., Louden, D., and R. I. Berkowitz. 2010. Maintenance of weight loss in adolescents: Current status and future directions. *Journal of Obesity* 24(3):306–313.
72. Finer, N., James, W. P., Kopelman, P. G., Lean, M. E., and G. Williams. 2000. One-year treatment of obesity: A randomized, double-blind, placebo-controlled, multicentre study of orlistat, a gastrointestinal lipase inhibitor. *International Journal of Obesity and Related Metabolic Disorders* 24:306–313.
73. Rössner, S., Sjöström, L., Noack, R., Meinders, A. E., and G. Noseda. 2000. Weight loss, weight maintenance, and improved cardiovascular risk factors after 2 years treatment with orlistat for obesity. European Orlistat Obesity Study Group. *Obesity Research* 8:49–61.
74. Torgerson, J. S., Hauptman, J., Boldrin, M. N., and L. Sjöström. 2004. XENical in the prevention of diabetes in obese subjects (XENDOS) study: A randomized study of orlistat as an adjunct to lifestyle changes for the prevention of type 2 diabetes in obese patients. *Diabetes Care* 27:155–161.
75. Singhal, V., Schwenk, W. F., and S. Kumar. 2007. Evaluation and management of childhood and adolescent obesity. *Mayo Clinic Proceedings* 82:1258–1264.
76. Leslie, D. B., Kellogg, T. A., and S. Ikramuddin. 2009. The surgical approach to management of pediatric obesity: When to refer and what to expect. *Reviews in Endocrine Metabolic Disorders Journal* 10:215–229.
77. Inge, T. H., Xanthakos, S. A., and M. H. Zeller. 2007. Bariatric surgery for pediatric extreme obesity: Now or later? *Obesity* 31(1):1–14.
78. O'Brien, P. E. 2010. Bariatric surgery: Mechanisms, indications, and outcomes. *Journal of Gastroenterology and Hepatology* 25(8):1358–1365.
79. Pratt, J. S. A., Lenders, C. M., Dionne, E. A. et al. 2009. Best practice updates for pediatric/adolescent weight loss surgery. *Obesity* 17(5):901–910.
80. Dixon, A. F., Dixon, J. B., and P. E. O'Brien. 2005. Laparoscopic adjustable gastric banding induces prolonged satiety: A randomized blind crossover study. *Journal of Clinical Endocrinology & Metabolism* 90:813–819.
81. Inge, T. H., Krebs, N. F., Garcia, V. F. et al. 2004. Bariatric surgery for severely overweight adolescents: Concerns and recommendations. *Pediatric* 114(1):217–223.
82. Inge, T. H., Zeller, M. H., Lawson, L., and S. R. Daniels. 2005. A critical appraisal of evidence supporting a bariatric surgical approach to weight management for adolescents. *Journal of Pediatrics* 147(1):10–19.
83. Daniels, S. R., Jacobson, M. S., McCrindle, B. W., Eckel, R. H., and B. M. Sanner. 2009. American Heart Association childhood obesity research summit: Executive summary. *Circulation* 119:2114–2123.
84. Hyman, B., Kool, K., and D. Ficklen. 2008. Bariatric surgery in adolescents. *Journal of School Health* 78(8):452–454.

9 Drug Treatment of Obesity

Raymond E. Bourey, MD
and Charles P. Lambert, PhD

CONTENTS

INTRODUCTION

Drug treatment of obesity has had a history of minor successes and expensive failures. In October 2010, there seemed little reason to write this chapter as the Food and Drug Administration (FDA) removed sibutramine (Meridia) from the market and rejected new applications for lorcaserin (APD-356, Lorqess), and a combination of phentermine and topiramate (Qnexa). These setbacks followed a recent FDA committee vote to reject rimonabant, a cannabinoid-1 receptor antagonist, in 2007. Therefore, after close to 2000 years of drug treatment of obesity, currently available treatment has been restricted to one long-term medication, orlistat (Xenical), approved by the FDA in 1999, and a handful of sympathomimetics, which are controlled substances approved only for short-term use. As short-term therapy of obesity results in weight regain or rebound (Bray 1993), drug treatment of obesity has been effectively reduced to a single, marginally effective medication with potential for socially unacceptable side effects (see the following). As one anonymous researcher in the treatment of obesity tried to summarize this chapter, "Nothing works."

In this context, it is not surprising that drug treatment of obesity has become relatively rare in spite of the high prevalence of obesity and associated morbidity and mortality. A recent study of 4.2 million Blue Cross Blue Shield subscribers found a drop in already low use of antiobesity medication from 1% in 2002 to 0.7% in 2005 (Bolen et al. 2010). Of those patients for whom antiobesity medication was prescribed, most (74%–79%) took medication for less than 12 weeks. These figures support the premise that available medications are both ineffective and poorly tolerated. In addition, this study found many physicians undertook inappropriate prescription of medications for obesity. Up to 17% of patients filled prescriptions for sympathomimetics longer than the recommended 3 months (Bolen et al. 2010). In addition, more than 50% of patients trying to undertake weight loss through medication also took narcotic analgesics, which could blunt effectiveness.

There is hope, however, that effective drug treatment of obesity is on the near horizon. To date, almost all medications identified for potential use in obesity have been discovered through serendipity. When medications designed for use in narcolepsy, epilepsy, or other conditions were found to have a significant side effect of weight loss, research often turned toward potential use as therapy for obesity. With improved understanding of physiological mechanisms responsible for metabolic efficiency and storage of unused caloric intake as fat, pharmacological development has targeted specific pathways of energy metabolism. In view of the multiplicity of mechanisms involved in the development and maintenance of human obesity, future medications will likely target simultaneously and effectively multiple mechanisms that contribute to adiposity. Specific causes of obesity, such as those associated with atypical antischizophrenic medication, nicotine cessation, sleep deprivation, or endocrine disruptors, might soon have specific treatment. With improved genetic testing and identification of specific mechanisms contributing to obesity in individual patients or kindreds, development of custom therapies should follow.

Slim margins between effectiveness and safety have plagued all medications for obesity used to date. At doses required to produce significant effects on body weight, intolerable side effects often occur. This has led the FDA and European Medicines Agency (EMEA) to recommend more rigorous criteria for efficacy and safety. Given the ineffectiveness of short-term treatment of obesity, since 1996, the FDA has recommended long-term (2 year) studies for safety and efficacy and to limit treatment to patients with body mass index (BMI) greater than 30 (or greater than 27 with comorbidity). In a 2007 draft guidance, the FDA specifically recommended a benchmark of efficacy of 5% weight loss beyond placebo in greater than 35% of subjects after 1 year treatment (Food and Drug Administration Center for Drug Evaluation and Research 2007). In addition, to assure fat loss, a subset of subjects must undergo body composition analysis by dual energy x-ray absorptiometry (DEXA) or equivalent technique. EMEA guidelines are similar and require 10% weight loss from baseline over 1 year and, again, greater than 5% above weight loss beyond placebo. The EMEA also has an optimistic secondary goal of absence of weight regain after cessation of medication (European Medicines Agency 2008), a goal achieved by no therapy for obesity developed to date, but one that might be achieved in the near future.

Any medication that achieves both weight loss and absence of weight regain after cessation of medication must address the loss of lean mass and drop in metabolic rate associated with prolonged negative caloric balance. As discussed in more detail elsewhere in this volume, unexercised muscle tends to be metabolized as a source of fuel during negative caloric balance. The obvious solution, exercise, is not always a viable option for patients suffering orthopedic and cardiovascular consequences of chronic, morbid obesity. Consequently, this chapter emphasizes development of new drugs for treatment of obesity that enhance or preserve muscle mass.

HIGHLIGHTS IN THE HISTORY OF DRUG TREATMENT OF OBESITY

Sudden death is more common in those who are naturally fat than in the lean.

—*Hippocrates* (**Littré 1839**)

This quote was provided in an excellent overview of the history of obesity by Bray (2009). Bray also noted that ancient Greeks had described infrequent menses and infertility in obese women. This description of what might now constitute polycystic ovarian syndrome might have been the first to counter the widespread belief among ancient peoples that obesity was a sign of fertility.

Other than use of cathartics (described by Soranus, a Greek physician in the second century), ancient therapies for obesity were primarily behavioral until Sangye Gyamtso recommended in a seventeenth century Tibetan medical treatise, entitled *The Blue Beryl,* that obesity be treated by eating the gullet, hair, and flesh of a wolf (Bray 2009). This might be the first description of thyroid therapy for obesity.

Little occurred in drug treatment of obesity until hyperthermic illnesses of some munition workers during the First World War brought widespread identification and use of dinitrophenol as a means to increase metabolic rate in treatment of obesity (Dunlop 1934). In 1924, Lisser in the United States (Lisser 1924) and Mason in Canada (Mason 1924) described successful use of thyroid in treatment of obesity and encouraged colleagues to more aggressively pursue a diagnosis of underlying metabolic disease in obese patients. In what might be historically interpreted as ill-advised or desperate practice, dinitrophenol and thyroid were used in a somewhat dangerous combination to increase metabolic rate and treat severe obesity, especially in the setting of myxedema (Dunlop 1934).

After weight loss was noted with early attempts to treat of narcolepsy, Benzedrine and other amphetamines were used for treatment of obesity in the late 1930s. Early use and possible effects of amphetamines on metabolic rate, muscle activity, and appetite were described in 1947 (Harris et al. 1947). That same year, the FDA approved use of amphetamines for weight loss.

The 1960s saw an increase in the use of amphetamines and other medications as "diet pills." In an early recognition of the importance of affecting multiple metabolic mechanisms to achieve weight loss, combinations of multiple medications included amphetamines, thyroid, laxatives, diuretics, digitalis, and narcotics or barbiturates. These treatments were quite popular, and benefits seemed to outweigh obvious risks until patients died. Deaths attributed to these treatments were well publicized by the lay press and led to Senate hearings in 1968 led by Senator Hart of Michigan, chairman of the Judiciary Subcommittee on Antitrust and Monopoly. These hearings culminated in a resolution critical of amphetamine "trafficking" as diet pills.

Phentermine has been one of the most widely prescribed and studied drugs for weight loss in the modern era. Phentermine, an amphetamine-like stimulant, was first approved by the FDA in 1959. It found its most popular use in combination with fenfluramine, a serotonin reuptake inhibitor approved in 1973 (fen–phen). Weight reduction with this combination was described in an extensive publication in 1992 (Weintraub 1992). Although FDA approval of dexfenfluramine (Redux) was associated with much fanfare in 1996, by 1997, data supporting a relationship between this combination of medications and both pulmonary hypertension and cardiac valvular disease (Connolly et al. 1997) became strong enough to result in an FDA request for removal from the market and subsequent liability of pharmaceutical companies and providers estimated at over $14 billion in total costs.

Amphetamines and central nervous system stimulants have been gradually removed from the market due to safety concerns. Phenylpropanolamine was withdrawn due to increased risk of stroke. Similarly, ephedra was removed from the U.S. market in 2004 due to hypertension and reported stroke and cardiac events. Ephedrine alkaloids, in general, were in the same year restricted to use for respiratory symptoms only and effectively banned for use in obesity.

MEDICATIONS CURRENTLY APPROVED
FOR TREATMENT OF OBESITY

In spite of the relatively minimal effects on weight loss required by the FDA (see Introduction), as of January 2011, physicians in the United States are limited to use of orlistat (Xenical), approved for long-term use, and a handful of class III–IV sympathomimetics approved only for short-term use, and thereby of extremely limited or nil efficacy. We will provide here a practical approach to use of pharmacological agents available for treatment of obesity as of January 2011. These agents are listed in Table 9.1.

ORLISTAT

Although effects of orlistat on weight are modest (see Effectiveness) and side effects are notorious, orlistat is available in the United States, European Union, and Australia for sale without prescription. In the United States, its patent expired in 2009 but continues as of this date to be sold exclusively under the trade names Xenical (120 mg, prescription only) and Alli (60 mg, nonprescription). Internationally, it is available from many companies, but there have been recent concerns about safety and efficacy of generic preparations as nine of nine preparations recently failed purity tests and two of nine were not soluble (Taylor et al. 2010).

Pharmacology

Orlistat (tetrahydrolipstatin or (S)-((S)-1-((2S,3S)-3-hexyl-4-oxooxetan-2-yl)tridecan-2-yl) 2-formamido-4-methylpentanoate, Xenical) is a stable, hydrated, derivative of lipstatin, a potent, nCatural, inhibitor of pancreatic lipase that is isolated from *Streptomyces toxytricini* (Hauptman et al. 1992). The FDA approved its use for treatment of obesity in adults in 1997 and for treatment of obesity in adolescents (aged 12–18 years) in 2003. At clinically prescribed doses of 120 mg three times daily, it reversibly inhibits gastric and pancreatic lipases through covalent binding of an active serine and reduces fat absorption from the gut by about 30%. There is minimal increase in effectiveness in doses beyond 400 mg daily.

Bioavailability is less than 1% with 97% excreted in feces with 83% of fat unchanged.

Indications and Recommended Use

Orlistat is indicated for obesity management in patients with BMI $\geq$ 30 kg/m^2 or BMI $\geq$ 27 kg/m^2 in the presence of other metabolic risk factors (e.g., hypertension, diabetes, and dyslipidemia) when used in conjunction with reduced calorie diet (Roche Laboratories 2010). Orlistat is also indicated to reduce risk for weight regain after prior weight loss. In addition to medication, patients should be instructed on hypocaloric (−20%), low-fat (30%) diet and exercise. Due to effects on fat-soluble vitamins, daily use of a multivitamin should be "strongly encouraged" (Roche Laboratories 2010).

TABLE 9.1

Drugs Approved for Treatment of Obesity

Drug	Other Names	Category	Mechanism	IUPAC Name	Duration of Use	Controlled Substance Act Classification
Orlistat	Tetrahydrolipstatin Xenical	Lipase inhibitor	Blocks absorption of dietary fat	(S)-((S)-1-((2S,3S)-3-Hexyl-4-oxooxetan-2-yl)tridecan-2-yl) 2-formamido-4-methylpentanoate	Long-term use	
Amfepramone	Diethylcathinone Diethylpropion Anorex Linea Nobesine Prefamone Regenon Tepanil Tenuate	Sympathomimetic	Anorexia/norepinephrine releasing agent	(RS)-2-Diethylamino-1-phenylpropan-1-one	Short-term use	IV
Benzphetamine	Didrex	Sympathomimetic	Anorexia/norepinephrine– dopamine releasing agent	(2S)-N-Benzyl-N-methyl-1-phenylpropan-2-amine	Short-term use	III

Mazindol	Mazanor Sanorex	Sympathomimetic	Anorexic norepinephrine, dopamine, and serotonin releasing agent	(±)-5-(4-Chlorophenyl)-3,5-dihydro-2H-imidazo[2,1-a]isoindol-5-ol	Short-term use	IV
Phendimetrazine	Bontril Adipost Anorex-SR Appecon Melfiat Obezine Phendiet Plegine Prelu-2 Statobex	Sympathomimetic	Anorexia/norepinephrine–dopamine releasing agent	3,4-Dimethyl-2-phenylmorpholine	Short-term use	III
Phentermine	Phenyl-tertiary-butylamine Ionamin Adipex-P Twenty-four other trade names	Sympathomimetic	Anorexia/norepinephrine–epinephrine–dopamine–serotonin releasing agent	2-Methyl-1-phenylpropan-2-amine	Short-term use	IV

Effectiveness

Meta-analyses of 16 similar placebo-controlled trials of orlistat (120 mg three times daily) in addition to behavioral therapies for obesity in adults greater than 18 years of age (n = 10,631) demonstrated reduction in body mass of 2.9 kg (CI = 2.5–3.2 kg) from a mean mass of 104 kg (−2.7%) (Hauptman et al. 1992; Padwal et al. 2003, 2004). Average attrition rate was approximately 30% at 1 year. During weight "maintenance" phase, orlistat and placebo arms demonstrated similar amounts of weight regain, but the weight differential obtained during the weight loss phase was preserved. Meta-analyses of related studies demonstrated small reduction in cholesterol but not triglycerides, and small but significant reductions in systolic and diastolic blood pressure reductions of 1.5 and 1.4 mm of mercury (Hauptman et al. 1992; Padwal et al. 2003, 2004).

Although weight loss was relatively small (−5.8 kg in treatment group and −3.0 kg in placebo group), one 4 year study of 3304 patients found reduction in the development of diabetes mellitus-2 from 9.0% to 6.2% (hazard ratio 0.63, 95% CI = 0.46–0.86) with majority of effect in patients with impaired glucose tolerance at baseline (Torgerson et al. 2004). Unfortunately, this study also reported an attrition rate of 40%. There have been no reports of improved cardiovascular morbidity or mortality to date. When evaluated by Framingham score, improvement in 10 year cardiovascular risk after 12 months of treatment with orlistat (n = 170) was identical to that of placebo (n = 169) (Swinburn et al. 2005).

Side Effects and Warnings

Orlistat is contraindicated in patients with chronic malabsorption syndrome, cholestasis, or known hypersensitivity (Roche Laboratories 2010). Orlistat is associated with significant gastrointestinal side effects. During its development, some researchers dubbed this medication *fatabuse*, an allusion to Antabuse (disulfiram), a medication used as aversion therapy for chronic alcoholism by causing acute nausea and headache when alcohol is consumed. Similarly, if subjects taking Xenical try to enjoy a high-fat meal, they will incur severe fat malabsorption, abdominal cramping, steatorrhea, bloating, and other unpleasant side effect. In the meta-analyses of Padwal et al. (2003, 2004; Hauptman et al. 1992), 80% of orlistat-treated patients experienced at least one gastrointestinal side effect with absolute frequency 24% higher than placebo (95% CI 20%–29%; 14 studies). Most commonly reported problems were fatty stool, urgency, and oily spotting. Five percent of orlistat-treated patients discontinue therapy due to gastrointestinal side effects (2% higher than placebo, 12 studies). Fecal incontinence was reported as 6% above that of patients on placebo. Due to its mechanism of action, mild reduction in fat-soluble vitamins has been found, but no study reported occurrence of clinically significant deficiency. Safety and effectiveness have not been reported beyond 4 years.

Twelve foreign and one U.S. postmarketing reports of severe liver injury and hepatic failure of undetermined etiology (13 cases between 1999 and August 2009 included 5 cases of liver failure) prompted recommendation for label change by the FDA in 2009 (FDA 2010). Extremely rare pancreatitis has also been reported in postmarketing surveillance, although no causal relationship or mechanism has been proposed.

Elevated urinary oxalate and rare nephropathy have also been reported and have been subjects of concern (Ahmed 2010; Karamadoukis et al. 2008; Singh et al. 2007).

Although metabolism of warfarin is not affected, decreased intake or absorption of vitamin K can increase potency of warfarin (MacWalter et al. 2003). Orlistat might have direct effects on absorption of levothyroxine (Madhava and Hartley 2005), amiodarone (Zhi et al. 2003), and cyclosporine (Zhi et al. 2002). Current labeling recommends levothyroxine administration 4 h before or after administration of orlistat (Roche Laboratories 2010). Although it is recommended that the daily multivitamin be taken 2 h before or after administration of orlistat, direct effects of orlistat on absorption of supplemental fat-soluble vitamins have not been reported (Roche Laboratories 2010).

Orlistat is currently not recommended for use in pregnancy or while nursing. It is listed as category B for teratogenic effects. Safety and effectiveness have not been established for patients over 65 years of age or for any patients beyond 4 years of treatment (Roche Laboratories 2010). In the United States, six pages of information approved by the FDA should be provided by the pharmacist to the patient on filling the first prescription (Roche Laboratories 2010).

Pediatric Use

Adult obesity and morbidity has its roots in pediatric obesity, and many physicians and policy makers have targeted treatment of childhood obesity to prevent obesity in adulthood. Current guidelines suggest consideration of drug treatment for overweight children with severe comorbidity, or obese children, only after failure of a formal, intense program of lifestyle modification (August et al. 2008). As of January 2011, only three medications have been reported to reduce BMI in adolescents: (1) sibutramine, no longer approved for use by the FDA or EMEA; (2) metformin, approved only for use in diabetes mellitus; (3) and orlistat, approved for use after age 12.

The FDA approved orlistat for use in adolescents (12–18 years) in December 2003. Studies are based on selection for BMI greater than $2 kg/m^2$ above reference value for 95th percentile based on age and gender. Approval and recommendations were based on a 12 month study of 539 adolescents aged 12–16 years, which demonstrated decrease in BMI by $0.6 kg/m^2$ in the treatment group and $0.3 kg/m^2$ in the placebo group with attrition rate of 35% (Chanoine et al. 2005). Effectiveness and safety seem similar to that of treatment in adults (Roche Laboratories 2010).

Sympathomimetic Agents

As of January 2011, this group includes amfepramone, benzphetamine, phendimetrazine, and phentermine (Table 9.1). Due to significant safety concerns, this group of medications has seen significant regulatory attrition (see Section Highlights in the History of Drug Treatment of Obesity). They demonstrate significant tachyphylaxis and tolerance as well as potential for abuse, and are therefore controlled substances approved only for short-term use. They have no role in long-term treatment of obesity and weight maintenance. In the face of these limitations and absence of patent protection, it is not surprising that there have been no significant outcome studies on individual agents since 1975 (Bray 2010).

In view of lack of efficacy after discontinuation, known risks, and regulatory limitations associated with these medications, they should not be recommended for routine treatment of obesity. In spite of this, physicians continue to prescribe these medications for long periods of time and in combination with other medications that increase risk and liability (Bolen et al. 2010; Hendricks et al. 2009). In the medical–legal environment of 2011, use of these medications might be considered in conjunction with aggressive diet and exercise in a short-term (usually defined as 3 months), life-saving effort for patients with morbid obesity and no contraindications. These medications are contraindicated in patients with atherosclerosis, cardiovascular disease, hypertension, hyperthyroidism, glaucoma, hypersensitivity to sympathetic medications, history of agitated state, or history of drug abuse. They should not be used with other medications with sympathomimetic effects. We recommend documentation of informed consent over the signature of the patient and physician.

DRUG COMBINATION AWAITING FINAL APPROVAL BY FDA

NALTREXONE/BUPROPION (CONTRAVE)

Treatment with naltrexone, a μ-receptor antagonist and analog of naloxone, might affect appetite through blockade of action of endogenous opioids including β-endorphin. Naloxone reduces short-term feeding behavior in rats (Holtzman 1979), but naltrexone does not generally result in significant effect on weight loss in man (Atkinson et al. 1985; Lee and Fujioka 2009; Malcolm et al. 1985; Plodkowski et al. 2009; Spiegel et al. 1987). Bupropion inhibits reuptake of 5-HT, dopamine, and norepinephrine and has been marketed for treatment of major depressive order since 1985 and smoking cessation since 1987. In data provided in labeling, 9% of patients on bupropion gained weight, but 28% of patients lost 5 lb or more. As effects on weight loss are weak, this drug would also not be considered suitable for monotherapy. Furthermore, reports of hypertension with use of bupropion might further limit its usefulness in treatment in which improvement of cardiovascular risk was a secondary goal.

On December 7, 2010, the FDA Endocrinologic and Metabolic Drugs Advisory Committee voted 13-7 for approval of combination of naltrexone (μ-receptor antagonist) and bupropion (SSRI/SNRI) to be marketed as Contrave, for treatment of obesity and weight management. Although the FDA usually follows the advice of its committees, discussion reported in the lay press suggests approval will not be automatic. Specific concerns included lack of long-term data, lack of data on cardiovascular mortality and morbidity, and risk of hypertension. At the proposed daily maintenance dose of 32 mg naltrexone/360 mg bupropion, beneficial effects of weight loss on blood pressure and heart rate were attenuated when compared to placebo, and placebo responders had the most favorable changes in blood pressure and heart rate (Coleman 2010).

The FDA analyzed four phase III trials of approximately 4500 subjects (Coleman 2010). The total daily maintenance a dose of two tablets of 8 mg naltrexone/90 mg bupropion by mouth twice daily is reached after 3 weeks of gradual increase in dose from one daily. Placebo-subtracted weight change from baseline to week 56 was −3.3% to −4.8% in 3 trials of 3200 subjects. There were minimal improvements in HDL cholesterol and triglycerides and, in a diabetic study, glycohemoglobin.

When gauged by standards of the 2007 draft guidance of the FDA (see Introduction), data at the maintenance dose did not satisfy mean efficacy criterion.

The most frequent adverse event in one study of the combination was nausea (naltrexone 32 mg plus bupropion, 29.8%; naltrexone 16 mg plus bupropion, 27.2%; placebo, 5.3%) (Smith 2011). Headache, constipation, dizziness, vomiting, and dry mouth were also more frequent in the naltrexone plus bupropion groups (Smith 2011). Problems with attention, memory, and sleep might further limit use of this medication. If approved, there will undoubtedly be a repeat of the boxed warnings for bupropion, and its use will be contraindicated in patients with history of seizures, serious neuropsychiatric events, depression, suicidal ideation, or suicide attempt.

Note: On 1 February 2011, the FDA declined to approve Contrave and told the drug maker that approval would require long-term study to demonstrate the drug does not increase risk of cardiac events.

DEVELOPMENT OF NEW DRUGS FOR TREATMENT OF OBESITY

Early drug treatment of obesity generally followed serendipity. Medications were developed for obesity only after weight loss was noted as a toxic effect (dinitrophenol) or side effect to drug treatment for other conditions such as hypothyroidism, narcolepsy (amphetamines), depression (bupropion, sibutramine, rimonabant), Alzheimer's disease (tesofensine), seizure (topiramate), and diabetes. Perhaps we should not be surprised that the sole survivor for long-term treatment of obesity is orlistat, a medication designed specifically for weight loss. Most medications currently in development are products of new knowledge of physiology of weight control and are specifically designed for treatment of obesity. Most target one mechanism, but some newer drugs and combinations are designed to effect changes through more than one metabolic pathway. This approach acknowledges the presence of redundant, physiological mechanisms that assure metabolic efficiency and secure energy storage as depots of fat—mechanisms on which our very existence as a species depended only a brief evolutionary period ago.

Unfortunately, attempts to disrupt or modulate one metabolic pathway usually disrupt or modulate others. Agents targeting the central nervous system are especially likely to cause effects in undesired if not unpredictable ways. Neuromodulation of metabolism is intimately associated not only with appetite, satiety, and metabolic rate, but also sleep, locomotion, emotion, and reproduction. We should not be surprised, therefore, when an agent, aimed at central mechanisms of appetite, also produces untoward effects of insomnia, periodic limb movement disorder, restless legs, suicidal ideation, movement disorders, and decreased libido. In reviewing the history of modern drug treatment of obesity, one is constantly reminded of the slim margin between efficacy and undesirable effects. Medications to date have produced very modest results with often great expense.

Any medication that achieves both weight loss and absence of weight regain after cessation of medication must address the loss of lean mass and drop in metabolic rate associated with prolonged negative caloric balance. As discussed in more detail elsewhere in this volume, unexercised muscle tends to be metabolized as a source of fuel during negative caloric balance. As exercise is not always an option in the morbidly

TABLE 9.2

Selected Drugs in Development for Treatment of Obesity

Mechanism of Action	Drug
Intestinal lipase inhibitors	Cetilistat
Monoamine receptor targets	Tesofensine
Atypical anticonvulsants	Zonisamide
	Topiramate
GLP-1 analogs	Exenatide
	Liraglutide
	Oxyntomodulin
Amylin analogs	Pramlintide
Leptin analogs	Metreleptin
Combination therapies	Bupropion/naltrexone (Contrave)
	Zonisamide SR/bupropion SR (Empatic)
	Pramlintide/metreleptin
	Pramlintide/estradiol
	Phybrids
	Chimeras
Skeletal muscle anabolics	β_2-adrenergic agonists
	Growth hormone
	Androgens
	SARMs
	Myostatin antagonists

obese, medications that maintain or enhance muscle mass in the face of weight loss are needed. Ironically, medications currently in consideration for treatment of cachexia, where maintenance of muscle mass is also critical, might be useful in treatment of obesity. Table 9.2 contains a list of selected drugs currently in development.

INTESTINAL LIPASE INHIBITOR

Cetilistat

This intestinal lipase inhibitor is in phase 3 trials in Japan. It appears to have similar action, effectiveness, and side effects to orlistat (Kopelman et al. 2007).

DRUGS WITH MONOAMINE TARGETS

5-Hydroxytryptamine$_{2C}$ Receptors

5-HT or serotonin receptors are a group of seven families of neural receptors. 5-HT$_{2C}$ receptors are excitatory G_q/G_{11}-protein-coupled receptors that act via phosphoinositol hydrolysis. The finding that *HTR2C* knockout mice were hyperphagic and suffered early obesity and type-2 diabetes suggested activation of this receptor might suppress food intake (Nonogaki et al. 1998). Up until recently, this receptor has generated some excitement. Anorexic effects seem to be exerted through 5-HT$_{2C}$ receptors on proopiomelanocortin (POMC) neurons in the arcuate nucleus of the hypothalamus, which, in turn, increases α-melanocyte-stimulating hormone (α-MSH), an agonist of the MC_4 receptor (Xu et al. 2008). Anorexic effects of fenfluramine and dexfenfluramine are likely mediated through 5-HT_{2C} receptors (Vickers et al. 1999, 2001). Unfortunately, cross-reactivity of the active metabolite at the 5-HT_{2B} receptor can be associated with valvulopathy (Fitzgerald et al. 2000) and primary pulmonary hypertension (Launay et al. 2002)—reasons for withdrawal of these medications from the market. In view of these studies, however, attempts have been made to develop selective 5-HT_{2C} receptor agonists. Unfortunately, in spite of promising results in clinical trials, the first of these highly selective 5-HT_{2C} receptor agonists, lorcaserin, was rejected by the FDA over safety concerns that overshadowed the drug's modest effectiveness, and further development of drugs in this class might be blunted.

Tesofensine

Tesofensine is a norepinephrine, dopamine, and serotonin reuptake inhibitor that might also indirectly stimulate cholinergic activity (Kennett and Clifton 2010; Thatte 2001). It was originally targeted at treatment of Alzheimer's disease and Parkinson's disease, but in an otherwise unsuccessful trial, persistent weight loss was evident (Astrup et al. 2008b). Meta-analysis of initial trials suggests FDA and EMEA criteria for efficacy might be met, but as with other monoamine reuptake inhibitors, this efficacy might be at the expense of increased heart rate and blood pressure (Astrup et al. 2008a,b). Phase III testing is now underway at the lower two of three doses.

Atypical Anticonvulsants

Zonisamide (Zonegran)

Zonisamide is a sulfonamide antiepileptic medication that is thought to exert its therapeutic effects by blockade of T-type calcium channels and voltage-gated sodium channels. It also functions as a carbonic anhydrase inhibitor. Mechanism of action is unknown, but as with topiramate (see the following section), a contribution to its effects on weight loss through effects of carbonic anhydrase inhibition on taste or lipogenesis has been discussed (De Simone et al. 2008). In rodents, there is some evidence that zonisamide can increase extra neuronal monoamines including dopamine, norepinephrine, and serotonin (Yamamura et al. 2009).

The medication has significant side effects and has been associated with loss of appetite, nausea, dizziness, vomiting, incoordination accidental injury, oligohidrosis and hyperthermia, suicidal behavior, metabolic acidosis, adverse cognitive and neuropsychiatric events, somnolence, and nephrolithiasis. It is teratogenic in animals. Although studies continue to evaluate use of a sustained-release form of this medication for obesity, in December 2010, the Medicaid Fraud Control Units and Office of Inspector General entered into multimillion-dollar corporate integrity agreements, and criminal and civil fines totaling $224 million were assessed for improper promotional activities including marketing for obesity among low-income and foster children. As with topiramate (see the following section), side effects will likely preclude use of this medication as monotherapy. Even if a dose can be found that meets criteria for both effectiveness and expectations for minimal side effects, political hurdles might prove limiting to attempts at approval for an indication for treatment of obesity.

Topiramate

Like zonisamide, topiramate is thought to exert anticonvulsant action through voltage-gated sodium channel blockade and blockade of T-type calcium channels. Also similar to zonisamide, topiramate is a potent inhibitor of carbonic anhydrase II. There is also some evidence in rodents that topiramate can increase extra neuronal monoamines including dopamine, norepinephrine, and serotonin (Yamamura et al. 2009). Meta-analysis of efficacy demonstrated 6.5% weight loss beyond placebo at doses between 96 and 196 mg per 24 weeks (Li et al. 2005).

Unfortunately, side effect profile is similar to that of zonisamide and includes dizziness, memory impairment, insomnia, somnolence, depression, and paresthesias and altered taste. It has also been shown to be teratogenic in animals. These side effects have precluded development of this medication as monotherapy and may have influenced the FDA in recent rejection of its use for obesity in combination with phentermine in October 2010.

GASTROINTESTINAL AND NEURAL PEPTIDES FOR TREATMENT OF OBESITY

Glucagon-Like Peptide-1 Analogs

Glucagon-like peptide-1 (GLP-1) is cleaved from proglucagon along with glucagon and glicentin. The latter gives rise to oxyntomodulin, which can act through both the glucagon receptor and GLP-1 receptor. GLP-1 receptors are found both centrally and peripherally and appear to be involved in modulation of feeding, gastric motility, and glucose-stimulated insulin release. After GLP-1 was noted to effect reduction in food intake in rodents, similar effects with short-term infusions were noted in normal, obese (Gutzwiller et al. 1999b; Naslund et al. 1999), and diabetic (Gutzwiller et al. 1999a) men. A subsequent 5 day study established that prandial, subcutaneous injections of GLP-1 resulted in decreased food intake and weight loss in nondiabetic, obese subjects (Naslund et al. 2004). This effect was not seen with continuous administration (Naslund et al. 2004). Stable analogs GLP-1 were found and developed for use in diabetes. These include exenatide (Byetta) and liraglutide (Victoza), which currently have approval from the FDA for treatment of diabetes mellitus-2. They have drawn interest for potential treatment of obesity as they remain the only medications currently in use for diabetes mellitus-2 to cause significant and sustained weight loss.

Exenatide

Exenatide (exendin-4) was found in salivary gland of *Heloderma suspectum* (Gila monster) and has 50% homology with GLP-1. As a peptide, it must be parenterally administered. Unlike native GLP-1, exenatide is resistant to diaminopeptidyl peptidase-4, and it has a half-life of 2.4 h. It is eliminated predominantly by glomerular filtration with subsequent proteolytic degradation.

The main side effect is nausea. Labeling currently requires a boxed warning for risk of pancreatitis. Its effects on obesity are modest. Eight, 16 to 52 weeks, randomized studies of diabetic patients demonstrated mean weight loss between 1.6 and 4.2 kg (Bradley et al. 2010). A randomized, 24 week trial of exenatide in 152 obese, nondiabetic subjects found placebo-subtracted difference in percent weight reduction of $-3.3\% \pm 0.5\%$ ($P < 0.001$) (Rosenstock et al. 2010). Weight loss, even at maximal doses of this medication, is modest, and, therefore, exenatide might not meet FDA or EMEA criteria as a medication for weight loss. Furthermore, long-term safety in nondiabetic subjects has not been established. This medication might find a role in treatment of obesity when combined with another modality such as laparoscopic gastric banding (Rothkopf et al. 2009) or in combination with another medication.

Liraglutide

Liraglutide is a GLP-1 analog with 97% homology to human GLP-1. It has a long half-life of about 13 h and has been approved for once daily administration by subcutaneous injection for treatment of diabetes mellitus. It causes a dose-dependent weight loss and has been studied in nondiabetic patients as a treatment for obesity. In a randomized, 20 week study of 564 subjects analyzed by intention to treat, mean weight loss at the highest dose of liraglutide (3.0 mg/day) was 4.4 kg greater than placebo (Astrup et al. 2009). At that dose, 76% of subjects lost greater than 5% of their weight as compared with the placebo-treated group, in which 30% lost more than 5% of baseline weight. Side effects are generally tolerable. Three percent of the placebo group withdrew due to adverse events, and the overall withdrawal rate was 19%. This compares favorably with liraglutide at the highest dose, in which 5% of the individuals withdrew due to adverse events and the overall withdrawal rate was 12% (Astrup et al. 2009). There were also improvements in secondary outcomes including blood pressure, glucose tolerance, and insulin resistance. Long-term studies of liraglutide are underway.

Oxyntomodulin

Oxyntomodulin is secreted by intestinal L cells. It was found to delay gastric emptying and reduce feeding in rodents (Dakin et al. 2001, 2004). Short studies in man suggest potential utility in treatment of obesity. Treatment with oxyntomodulin seems to be associated with both decreased food intake and increased food expenditure (Cohen et al. 2003; Wynne and Bloom 2006; Wynne et al. 2005, 2010). Analogs are under study (Liu et al. 2010).

Amylin Analogs

Amylin is a 37-amino-acid peptide synthesized in beta cells of pancreatic islets and cosecreted with insulin. Amylin acts to inhibit gastric emptying, food intake, and glucagon secretion. Receptors are hetero marriage complexes of the calcitonin receptor, a G-protein-coupled receptor (family B), and receptor activity-modifying proteins (RAMPs). There are currently three subtypes numbered by the associated RAMP1, 2, or 3.

Pramlintide is an analog of amylin approved for premeal therapy of diabetes mellitus in combination with insulin. In healthy subjects, the half-life of pramlintide is approximately 48 min, and it is metabolized primarily by the kidneys. Des-lys[1] pramlintide, the primary metabolite, has similar half-life and biological activity, at least in rodents. Due to its effects on gastric emptying, most adverse events are gastrointestinal in nature.

In a 24 week study, pramlintide at current maximal clinical dose provided only 1.5% weight loss beyond the placebo group (Aronne et al. 2010). Addition of phentermine or sibutramine to pramlintide improved results by another 7% weight loss (Aronne et al. 2010). In a study that used pramlintide at twice the highest recommended dose for use in diabetes (360 mg twice daily), a more impressive 8% weight loss was found at 20 weeks (Ravussin et al. 2009). Unfortunately, this study was not placebo controlled, but it does suggest that higher doses might be necessary but better tolerated for treatment of obesity in nondiabetic patients.

Leptin Analogs

Leptin is a cytokine synthesized predominantly in white adipose tissue but also in many other tissues. Receptors are widespread. Leptin can produce satiety through binding of neuropeptide Y neurons in the arcuate nucleus. It can also increase activity of neurons expressing α-MSH. Recent studies suggest that leptin might also contribute to increased metabolic rates recognition sympathetic nervous system and perhaps are some direct effects on liver and skeletal muscle metabolism. Like other neural modulators of metabolism, it appears to be important not only for appetite, satiety, and metabolic rate but also for reproduction.

When it was discovered that animals with inadequate leptin or leptin receptor were obese, and that leptin therapy reversed the obesity, it was hoped that leptin therapy might have application in the treatment of human obesity as well (Heymsfield et al. 1999). Unfortunately, obesity is associated with higher leptin levels, and the concept of leptin resistance has been used to explain the lack of efficacy of leptin therapy.

Metreleptin is an analog of leptin (methionyl recombinant leptin) that has been developed for multiple uses including treatment of obesity. As a single agent in a 24 week trial for treatment of obesity, metreleptin at a dose of 5 mg twice daily was similar in efficacy to pramlintide alone with mean of 8% weight loss (Ravussin et al. 2009).

THERAPIES AIMED AT MULTIPLE MECHANISMS

Evolutionary pressure toward metabolic efficiency and efficient storage of excess energy as fat resulted in a complex interaction of psychological and physiological mechanisms to maintain body weight. Active weight loss is met with counter-regulatory mechanisms to reduce energy expenditure and improve energy intake and storage. Combination therapies have always been popular dating back at least to combination of dinitrophenol and thyroid (Dunlop 1934), but new understanding of mechanisms for weight regulation, as well as improved statistical methods, has allowed a more targeted approach (Roth et al. 2010). Although we will not review them here, combinations of catecholaminergic, opioidergic, or GABA/AMPA/kainate are currently in various stages of industrial development (Gadde and Allison 2009; Greenway et al. 2009). In this section, we present some of the more promising combinations that are well into the regulatory pipeline in touch on promising novel concepts.

Combination Therapy

Bupropion/Naltrexone (Contrave)

Naltrexone was chosen as a complement to bupropion in order to block compensating mechanisms that attempt to prevent long-term, sustained weight loss. This medication is currently awaiting final approval by the FDA, and it was addressed in detail earlier (see Drug Combination Awaiting Final Approval by FDA).

Pramlintide/Leptin

As noted earlier, neither pramlintide nor leptin is a good candidate for monotherapy. Following studies that suggested that amylin treatment could restore leptin-mediated signaling in leptin-resistant rats (Roth et al. 2008), studies of combination therapy were undertaken. In combination with pramlintide, significantly greater weight loss (13%) was obtained than with either pramlintide (8%) or metreleptin alone (8%) (Ravussin et al. 2009). Mild to moderate nausea was common, but improved with time.

Although similar effectiveness was seen in studies of combinations of pramlintide with sibutramine and pramlintide with phentermine, both combinations were associated with increased heart rate and blood pressure (Aronne et al. 2010). In view of potential for adverse cardiovascular events, these combinations are unlikely to proceed toward approval for use.

Zonisamide SR/Bupropion SR (Empatic)

This combination approach is designed to promote hypothalamic POMC activity (appetite reduction and stimulation of energy expenditure) while blocking a parallel compensatory pathway (agouti-related peptide or AgRP). A small 12 week open-label study of zonisamide 400 mg at bedtime in combination with bupropion 200 mg every morning demonstrated 7.5% weight loss, which compared favorably with zonisamide alone at 3.1% weight loss (Gadde et al. 2007). Even more impressive results were reported on a larger study of 623 patients presented in abstract form at the *Obesity Society Annual Scientific Meeting* in 2007 (Fujioka et al. 2007). Treatment of obesity with combination of zonisamide 360 mg with bupropion 360 mg resulted in weight loss (analyzed by intention to treat) of 7.5% greater than the placebo group over the course of 24 weeks. There was a near-linear increase in weight loss that increased with dose of study medication. At the highest dose, 17% of subjects discontinued the medication due to adverse events as compared to 9% of the placebo group. The most common adverse events were nausea, insomnia, dry mouth, and anxiety (Fujioka et al. 2007). Unfortunately, effects on blood pressure were not noted. As of January 2011, this medication has not started phase III trials.

Pramlintide/Estradiol

In females, estrogen maintains energy homeostasis via estrogen receptor$_\alpha$ and estrogen receptor$_\beta$, by suppressing energy intake and lipogenesis, enhancing energy expenditure, and ameliorating insulin secretion and sensitivity (Mauvais-Jarvis 2011). Not surprisingly, marked increases in weight occur with menopause, and menopausal women comprise the majority of morbidly obese patients (BMI $\geq$ 40 kg/m^2) in whom weight loss agents are indicated for use (Flegal et al. 2010). In preclinical studies, Trevaskis et al. (2010) demonstrated that chronic amylin treatment of ovariectomized mice inhibited usual weight gain, an effect that might be amplified by estradiol (Lutz 2011). These findings follow demonstration of additive effects or estradiol on decrease in meal size mediated by CCK (Geary 2001) or glucagon (Geary and Asarian 2001). Although early in development, combinations of estrogens and incretin hormones seem especially promising for treatment of obesity in the context of menopause.

Custom Molecules with Multiple Mechanisms

Phybrids

One strategy to combine dual pharmacological mechanisms is through chemical link of two peptides. In the absence of significant steric hindrance, peptide hybrids (phybrids) might act as dual agonists by activating distinct receptors to produce complementary pharmacological effects. In a proof of concept study (with data on file at Amylin Corp., San Diego, CA), an amylin/PYY_{3-36} phybrid demonstrated additive effects that were similar to those of the combination therapy with separate peptides (Roth et al. 2010).

Chimeras

Chimeras are molecules designed as dual- or coagonist compounds. The first successful chimera to reach active exploration for drug development combined agonists for glucagon receptor and GLP-1 receptor and has successfully treated obesity in rodents (Day et al. 2009; Pocai et al. 2009). In addition, collaboration between the University of Cincinnati and Indiana University has also produced a promising GLP-1/GIP dual agonist (MAR701 and MAR709, Marcadia Biotech, Carmel, IN) and, most recently, an estrogen/GLP-1 dual agonist (Finan et al. 2011).

Drugs Anabolic to Skeletal Muscle in the Treatment of Obesity

Importance of Muscle Mass to Resting Energy Expenditure

As will be described later, skeletal muscle mass is important for maintaining metabolic rate. Resting metabolic rate is typically the largest portion of the energy expenditure side of the energy balance equation. Therefore, anything significantly increasing or decreasing the resting energy expenditure can have a profound effect on weight gain or loss.

Much of what we know about the effects of muscle mass on resting metabolic rate comes from aging studies. Tzankoff and Norris (1977) reported that decline in muscle mass with aging correlated very closely with decline in the resting metabolic rate. These investigators reported that muscle mass, as measured by 24 h creatinine excretion, declined with increasing age after 45 years and that the relationship between resting oxygen consumption and muscle mass was very strong (r = 0.644). Bosy-Westphal et al. (2003) reported a Pearson correlation coefficient of 0.75 between fat-free mass measured by DEXA and resting metabolic rate in individuals with a wide range of body compositions. Fat-free mass contains bone, skin, blood, and organs, in addition to muscle, but appears to be an excellent surrogate to estimate muscle in relation to resting energy expenditure. Thus, from these results, we can conclude that there is a significant, linear relationship between skeletal muscle mass and metabolic rate.

Effects of Weight Loss on Fat-Free Mass and Metabolic Rate

Clearly a portion of the weight loss occurring as result of caloric restriction is fat-free mass. For example, Friedlander et al. (2005) studied 3 weeks of caloric restriction in normal weight young men. These investigators induced a reduction of energy intake by 40% and found that over the 21 days there was a ~5% reduction of body weight and 2.5% or roughly half of the weight was fat-free mass. With this 2.5% reduction of fat-free mass, there was a 15% reduction in resting metabolic rate. Martin et al. (2007) reported a strong relationship between the resting metabolic rate and fat-free mass in individuals undergoing caloric restriction by 25%, those who expended excess calories by caloric restriction (12.5%) and by exercise (12.5%), and those on a low calorie supplement (890 kcal/day) all groups over 6 months. The R^2 for this relationship was −0.77. A ~25% reduction in fat-free mass corresponded to a ~20% reduction in resting metabolic rate. Thus, from these two studies, it is clear that there is reduction in resting metabolic rate with weight loss and that this is mirrored by a reduction in fat-free mass. From the previous section, it is clear that there is a relationship between the reduction in fat-free mass and the reduction in resting metabolic rate.

Physical Frailty: Another Reason to Maintain Muscle Mass in Obesity

In addition to metabolic complications of obesity such as diabetes and coronary artery disease, another manifestation of obesity is often physical frailty. Physical frailty might manifest itself in difficulty climbing stairs or rising from a chair. In the nonobese elderly, this occurs from insufficient muscle strength due, at least in part, to relatively low muscle mass. In the obese, physically frail, it is not simply low muscle strength and/or muscle mass, but it is due to the fact that non-force-producing tissue, fat mass, is abundant relative to muscle strength/mass. Thus, the problem in the obese physically frail is a low muscle strength/body weight ratio. As previously described by Villareal et al. (2006), weight loss is an effective strategy for improving physical frailty in the obese as typically a person loses more fat mass than muscle mass and therefore the ratio of muscle mass/body weight improves. Another effective strategy is resistance training, which increases muscle strength/mass and therefore also improves the muscle strength/body weight ratio (Villareal et al. 2006). It appears that an ideal combination would be combining resistance exercise training with weight loss. Interestingly, exercise training (combined resistance and aerobic exercise) is more efficacious in increasing anabolic signals and decreasing catabolic signals (mRNAs) in skeletal muscle than weight loss (Lambert et al. 2008).

Exercise is an Anabolic Stimulus to Skeletal Muscle

One obvious result of the loss of muscle mass and reduced resting energy expenditure that accompanies the loss of muscle mass is a positive energy balance and deposition of fat. This would not be a beneficial adaptation. It is clear that acute exercise, such as a resistance exercise bout, can increase resting energy expenditure after the bout of exercise. In addition, the addition of muscle mass as a result of resistance exercise training should result in increase in resting energy expenditure. Campbell et al. (1994) addressed this hypothesis. These investigators reported 12 weeks of resistance training in older adults (56–80 years of age), resulted in a 1.4 kg increase in fat-free mass and a 6.8% increase in energy expenditure equivalent to an extra 4.6 kcal/h, 40,186 kcal/year, and, given that 3,500 kcal is 1 lb of fat, the expenditure of 11.5 lb of fat/year. The calorie burning effect of resistance training through its effect on the addition of muscle mass is therefore not trivial. As a result, it appears that a practically significant increase in resting energy expenditure, and as a result body fat loss, can be achieved by older individuals undertaking a resistance exercise training protocol. Additionally, during the period of resistance exercise training, there was a 2.2% drop in the body fat level. Thus, resistance exercise predominately through the addition of muscle mass appears to be an excellent way to expend energy (calories).

Utility of Resistance Exercise during Diet-Induced Weight Loss

Resistance exercise training during weight loss induced by energy restriction typically results in maintenance of lean body mass (Ballor et al. 1988; Bryner et al. 1999), while aerobic exercise training during diet-induced weight loss does not (Bryner et al. 1999). This is important as lean body mass is very metabolically active and thus combusts a large amount of energy. In contrast, aerobic exercise is better for inducing a caloric deficit for weight loss than resistance exercise training since aerobic exercise training burns more energy than resistance exercise of equal duration. It would appear to maximize fat losses and maintain lean body mass; a combination of aerobic and resistance exercise training should be undertaken during diet-induced weight loss.

Caloric Restriction, Effects on Circulating Androgens, Fat-Free Mass, and Role of Increased Protein Intake

As described earlier, we know that weight loss through energy restriction (caloric restriction) results in a loss of fat-free mass. Interestingly, caloric restriction also has an effect on androgens. Long-term caloric restriction in humans reduces total and free testosterone and appears independent of the amount of adipose tissue present (Cangemi et al. 2010). Fontana et al. (2008) have proposed that it is not caloric restriction per se but a lower than normal protein intake that causes this reduction in androgens. They found that reducing protein intake from 1.67 to 0.95 g/kg of body weight for 3 weeks in individuals undergoing caloric restriction resulted in a ~22% reduction in circulating insulin-like growth factor-I (IGF-I). This finding by Fontana et al. (2008) may provide a mechanism for the findings that an increased protein intake of ~1.5 g/kg body weight compared to ~0.8 g/kg body weight results in 1.4 times greater loss of fat-free mass in middle-aged women (Layman et al. 2003). Similarly, findings have been reported by Mettler et al. (2010) in young men, who reduced caloric intake by 60%. One group ate 2.3 g/kg body weight of protein (roughly 2.9× the RDA), and the other group ate 1.0 g/kg body weight of protein. The group that ate 1.0 g/kg protein/day lost roughly 5.3 times more fat-free mass than the group that ate 2.3 g/kg body weight of protein per day. By ingesting extra protein one might reduce the amount of fat-free mass (i.e., muscle mass) lost as a result of a weight loss diet.

Pharmacological Agents for Increasing Muscle Mass

Testosterone

Clearly, in the aging male ($\geq$45 years), low-circulating testosterone concentrations are related to increased total fat mass (Couillard et al. 2000; Zumoff et al. 1990) and increased visceral fat mass (Nielsen et al. 2007). Therefore, from the standpoint of an endocrine treatment of obesity, administration of testosterone to normalize testosterone concentrations in men with low testosterone would appear to be a logical first step. From the literature, it is clear that favorable changes in body composition are observed as a result of testosterone administration in individuals with low testosterone (please see recent review: Bassil et al. 2009). However, in perimenopausal and postmenopausal women, the picture on the role of androgens and body fat is far from clear. Casson et al. (2010) have reported that high-serum testosterone concentrations were related to reduced body fat levels in postmenopausal women, while others indicate that higher testosterone is related to higher visceral fat mass in postmenopausal women (Janssen et al. 2010) and a higher propensity for developing type II diabetes (Kalyani et al. 2009). The reasons for these equivocal results in older women need to be elucidated. To our knowledge, the administration of testosterone has not been combined with diet and weight loss.

Growth Hormone

The seminal study of Yarasheski et al. (1995) does not support a role for growth hormone in skeletal muscle anabolism, but growth hormone was beneficial in the loss of fat mass. In addition to the lack of efficacy with regard to changes in skeletal muscle mass, the administration of growth hormone resulted in side effects such as carpal tunnel syndrome and sleep apnea. To our knowledge, the effects of growth hormone in combination with caloric restriction on fat loss have not previously been evaluated.

β_2-Adrenergic Agonists

For many years, members of the β_2-adrenergic agonist drug family have been used to favorably alter body composition of animals such as poultry and livestock to improve their palatability to consumers (Gonzalez et al. 2010). Only recently have human studies been undertaken. In one such study, Uc et al. (2003) reported that salbutamol (albuterol) at a dose of 16 mg/day increased muscle mass by ~5%, without the addition of exercise, when given to Parkinson's disease patients for 12 weeks. In a yet to be published follow-up study to examine the mechanism of action, Lambert et al. (unpublished observations) found a 90% increase in mixed muscle skeletal muscle protein synthesis in healthy elderly men and women as a result of 10 days of salbutamol administration (16 mg/day). Clearly, salbutamol at the dose of 16 mg/day is anabolic to skeletal muscle. However, salbutamol in addition to stimulating the β2-receptor also has β1-receptor cross-reactivity and therefore stimulates cardiac muscle. Therefore, one potential drawback of β_2-adrenergic agonists is cardiac hypertrophy. This potential negative effect of the β_2-adrenergic agonists needs to be sorted out with long-term clinical trials.

Selective Androgen Receptor Modulators

Testosterone is a potent anabolic agent in skeletal muscle; however, this hormone has side effects that curtail its widespread exogenous administration. Potentially, the most detrimental side effect of testosterone is the fact that this hormone binds to the prostate and can induce prostate hypertrophy and potentially prostate cancer. As a result, selective androgen receptor modulators (SARMs) have been developed. Generally speaking, there are two large classes of SARMs: (1) steroidal SARMs in which the testosterone molecule is altered and (2) nonsteroidal SARMs (Bhasin et al. 2006). These drugs theoretically show great promise for the maintenance and/or an increase in muscle mass with age or during weight loss of different types (Mauvais-Jarvis 2011), and are currently in preclinical and clinical trials. Time will tell.

Myostatin Blockade

Growth differentiation factor-8 (GDF-8) or myostatin is a member of the transforming growth factor-β family. Myostatin is a negative regulator of muscle growth and differentiation. It was reported by McPherron et al. (1997) that knocking out the gene for myostatin in mice resulted in heavily muscled "mighty mice." Also in 1997, Kambadur et al. (1997) reported that impaired myostatin expression resulted in "double-muscled" cows, which were of the Belgian Blue and Piedmontese varieties. Thus, clearly, myostatin is a potent inhibitor of muscle growth, and modulating myostatin expression and function can have profound effects on muscle hypertrophy and atrophy. This theoretically is a potentially fruitful area of scientific inquiry for maintenance of muscle mass, and compounds are currently in development for prevention and treatment of obesity.

SUMMARY

Long-term drug treatment of obesity has been effectively reduced to a single, marginally effective medication with significant gastrointestinal side effects (Table 9.1). It is no wonder that frustrated patients and physicians turned to unsafe or unproven practices. Fortunately, improved understanding of mechanisms responsible for weight gain and maintenance in a physically inactive and nutritionally replete society has created new and more specific targets for drug treatment of obesity. Combination therapies with effects on both energy intake and disposal might prove especially effective. Drug development will likely target specific populations at risk for obesity including those on atypical antipsychotic medications, menopausal women, and children with multiple risk factors. Genetic therapy or customized drug therapy for families with identifiable genetic predisposition to obesity might follow.

The EMEA now has an optimistic secondary goal of absence of weight regain after cessation of medication (European Medicines Agency 2008), a goal achieved by no drug therapy for obesity developed to date. Although exercise can fill this role, many morbidly obese patients are incapable of sufficient physical activity. In theory, muscle-sparing or muscle-enhancing drugs might maintain or increase metabolic rate sufficiently to produce long-term effects after cessation of medication.

Ironically, much of the background on use of these drugs comes from studies of cachexia with cancer, inactivity of aging, and chronic disease. Nonetheless, drugs such as selective β_2-adrenergic agonists, SARMs, and myostatin inhibitors show promise in this promising field of drug development.

REFERENCES

Ahmed, M. H. 2010. Orlistat and calcium oxalate crystalluria: An association that needs consideration. *Ren Fail* 32 (8):1019–1021.

Aronne, L. J., A. E. Halseth, C. M. Burns, S. Miller, and L. Z. Shen. 2010. Enhanced weight loss following coadministration of pramlintide with sibutramine or phentermine in a multicenter trial. *Obesity (Silver Spring)* 18 (9):1739–1746.

Astrup, A., S. Madsbad, L. Breum, T. J. Jensen, J. P. Kroustrup, and T. M. Larsen. 2008a. Effect of tesofensine on bodyweight loss, body composition, and quality of life in obese patients: A randomised, double-blind, placebo-controlled trial. *Lancet* 372 (9653):1906–1913.

Astrup, A., D. H. Meier, B. O. Mikkelsen, J. S. Villumsen, and T. M. Larsen. 2008b. Weight loss produced by tesofensine in patients with Parkinson's or Alzheimer's disease. *Obesity (Silver Spring)* 16 (6):1363–1369.

Astrup, A., S. Rossner, L. Van Gaal, A. Rissanen, L. Niskanen, M. Al Hakim, J. Madsen, M. F. Rasmussen, M. E. Lean, and N. N. Study Group. 2009. Effects of liraglutide in the treatment of obesity: A randomised, double-blind, placebo-controlled study. *Lancet* 374 (9701):1606–1616.

Atkinson, R. L., L. K. Berke, C. R. Drake, M. L. Bibbs, F. L. Williams, and D. L. Kaiser. 1985. Effects of long-term therapy with naltrexone on body weight in obesity. *Clin Pharmacol Ther* 38 (4):419–422.

August, G. P., S. Caprio, I. Fennoy, M. Freemark, F. R. Kaufman, R. H. Lustig, J. H. Silverstein, P. W. Speiser, D. M. Styne, and V. M. Montori. 2008. Prevention and treatment of pediatric obesity: An endocrine society clinical practice guideline based on expert opinion. *J Clin Endocrinol Metab* 93 (12):4576–4599.

Ballor, D. L., V. L. Katch, M. D. Becque, and C. R. Marks. 1988. Resistance weight training during caloric restriction enhances lean body weight maintenance. *Am J Clin Nutr* 47 (1):19–25.

Bassil, N., S. Alkaade, and J. E. Morley. 2009. The benefits and risks of testosterone replacement therapy: A review. *Ther Clin Risk Manag* 5 (3):427–448.

Bhasin, S., O. M. Calof, T. W. Storer, M. L. Lee, N. A. Mazer, R. Jasuja, V. M. Montori, W. Gao, and J. T. Dalton. 2006. Drug insight: Testosterone and selective androgen receptor modulators as anabolic therapies for chronic illness and aging. *Nat Clin Pract Endocrinol Metab* 2 (3):146–159.

Bolen, S. D., J. M. Clark, T. M. Richards, A. D. Shore, S. M. Goodwin, and J. P. Weiner. 2010. Trends in and patterns of obesity reduction medication use in an insured cohort. *Obesity (Silver Spring)* 18 (1):206–209.

Bosy-Westphal, A., C. Eichhorn, D. Kutzner, K. Illner, M. Heller, and M. J. Muller. 2003. The age-related decline in resting energy expenditure in humans is due to the loss of fat-free mass and to alterations in its metabolically active components. *J Nutr* 133 (7):2356–2362.

Bradley, D. P., R. Kulstad, and D. A. Schoeller. 2010. Exenatide and weight loss. *Nutrition* 26 (3):243–249.

Bray, G. A. 1993. Use and abuse of appetite-suppressant drugs in the treatment of obesity. *Ann Intern Med* 119 (7 Pt 2):707–713.

Bray, G. A. 2009. History of obesity. In *Obesity: Science to Practice*, G. Williams and G. Frühbeck, eds. Chichester, U.K.: John Wiley & Sons, Ltd.

Bray, G. A. 2010. Medical therapy for obesity. *Mt Sinai J Med* 77 (5):407–417.

Bryner, R. W., I. H. Ullrich, J. Sauers, D. Donley, G. Hornsby, M. Kolar, and R. Yeater. 1999. Effects of resistance vs. aerobic training combined with an 800 calorie liquid diet on lean body mass and resting metabolic rate. *J Am Coll Nutr* 18 (2):115–121.

Campbell, W. W., M. C. Crim, V. R. Young, and W. J. Evans. 1994. Increased energy requirements and changes in body composition with resistance training in older adults. *Am J Clin Nutr* 60 (2):167–175.

Cangemi, R., A. J. Friedmann, J. O. Holloszy, and L. Fontana. 2010. Long-term effects of calorie restriction on serum sex-hormone concentrations in men. *Aging Cell* 9 (2):236–242.

Casson, P. R., M. J. Toth, J. V. Johnson, F. Z. Stanczyk, C. L. Casey, and M. E. Dixon. 2010. Correlation of serum androgens with anthropometric and metabolic indices in healthy, nonobese postmenopausal women. *J Clin Endocrinol Metab* 95 (9):4276–4282.

Chanoine, J. P., S. Hampl, C. Jensen, M. Boldrin, and J. Hauptman. 2005. Effect of orlistat on weight and body composition in obese adolescents: A randomized controlled trial. *JAMA* 293 (23):2873–2883.

Cohen, M. A., S. M. Ellis, C. W. Le Roux, R. L. Batterham, A. Park, M. Patterson, G. S. Frost, M. A. Ghatei, and S. R. Bloom. 2003. Oxyntomodulin suppresses appetite and reduces food intake in humans. *J Clin Endocrinol Metab* 88 (10):4696–4701.

Coleman, E. 2010. FDA Briefing Document, NDA 200063, Contrave (Naltrexone 4 mg, 8 mg/Bupropion HCL 90 mg extended release tablet).

Connolly, H. M., J. L. Crary, M. D. McGoon, D. D. Hensrud, B. S. Edwards, W. D. Edwards, and H. V. Schaff. 1997. Valvular heart disease associated with fenfluramine–phentermine. *N Engl J Med* 337 (9):581–588.

Couillard, C., J. Gagnon, J. Bergeron, A. S. Leon, D. C. Rao, J. S. Skinner, J. H. Wilmore, J. P. Despres, and C. Bouchard. 2000. Contribution of body fatness and adipose tissue distribution to the age variation in plasma steroid hormone concentrations in men: The HERITAGE Family Study. *J Clin Endocrinol Metab* 85 (3):1026–1031.

Dakin, C. L., I. Gunn, C. J. Small, C. M. Edwards, D. L. Hay, D. M. Smith, M. A. Ghatei, and S. R. Bloom. 2001. Oxyntomodulin inhibits food intake in the rat. *Endocrinology* 142 (10):4244–4250.

Dakin, C. L., C. J. Small, R. L. Batterham, N. M. Neary, M. A. Cohen, M. Patterson, M. A. Ghatei, and S. R. Bloom. 2004. Peripheral oxyntomodulin reduces food intake and body weight gain in rats. *Endocrinology* 145 (6):2687–2695.

Day, J. W., N. Ottaway, J. T. Patterson, V. Gelfanov, D. Smiley, J. Gidda, H. Findeisen et al. 2009. A new glucagon and GLP-1 co-agonist eliminates obesity in rodents. *Nat Chem Biol* 5 (10):749–757.

De Simone, G., A. Di Fiore, and C. T. Supuran. 2008. Are carbonic anhydrase inhibitors suitable for obtaining antiobesity drugs? *Curr Pharm Des* 14 (7):655–660.

Dunlop, D. M. 1934. The use of 2:4-dinitrophenol as a metabolic stimulant. *Br Med J* 1 (3820):524–527.

European Medicines Agency, Committee for Medicinal Products for Human Use. 2008. Guidance on clinical evaluation of medicinal products used in weight control, London, U.K.

FDA. 2010. FDA Drug Safety Communication: Completed safety review of Xenical/ Alli (orlistat) and severe liver injury. http://www.fda.gov/Drugs/DrugSafety/ PostmarketDrugSafetyInformationforPatientsandProviders/ucm213038.htm (Last Accessed: January 9, 2012).

Finan, B., R. DiMarchi, V. Gelfanov, N. Ottaway, D. Perez-Tilve, P. Pfluger, M. Tschöp, and B. Yang. 2011. Estrogen conjugates of GLP-1 demonstrate enhanced efficacy in DIO mice. Paper read at *Keystone Symposium on Diabetes*, January 15, 2011, Keystone, CO.

Fitzgerald, L. W., T. C. Burn, B. S. Brown, J. P. Patterson, M. H. Corjay, P. A. Valentine, J. H. Sun et al. 2000. Possible role of valvular serotonin 5-HT(2B) receptors in the cardiopathy associated with fenfluramine. *Mol Pharmacol* 57 (1):75–81.

Flegal, K. M., M. D. Carroll, C. L. Ogden, and L. R. Curtin. 2010. Prevalence and trends in obesity among US adults, 1999–2008. *JAMA* 303 (3):235–241.

Fontana, L., E. P. Weiss, D. T. Villareal, S. Klein, and J. O. Holloszy. 2008. Long-term effects of calorie or protein restriction on serum IGF-1 and IGFBP-3 concentration in humans. *Aging Cell* 7 (5):681–687.

Food and Drug Administration Center for Drug Evaluation and Research. 2007. Draft. Guidance for Industry. Developing products for weight management. http://www.fda. gov/cder/guidance/index.htm (Last Accessed: January 9, 2012).

Friedlander, A. L., B. Braun, M. Pollack, J. R. MacDonald, C. S. Fulco, S. R. Muza, P. B. Rock et al. 2005. Three weeks of caloric restriction alters protein metabolism in normal-weight, young men. *Am J Physiol Endocrinol Metab* 289 (3):E446–E455.

Fujioka, K., F. L. Greenway, M. A. Cowley, M. Guttadauria, J. Robinson, R. Landbloom, A. A. McKinney, and G. D. Tollefson. 2007. Dose ratio optimization with zonisamide SR and bupropion SR for weight loss. Paper read at *NAASO, The Obesity Society Annual Scientific Meeting*, New Orleans, LA.

Gadde, K. M., and D. B. Allison. 2009. Combination therapy for obesity and metabolic disease. *Curr Opin Endocrinol Diabetes Obes* 16 (5):353–358.

Gadde, K. M., G. M. Yonish, M. S. Foust, and H. R. Wagner. 2007. Combination therapy of zonisamide and bupropion for weight reduction in obese women: A preliminary, randomized, open-label study. *J Clin Psychiatry* 68 (8):1226–1229.

Geary, N. 2001. Estradiol, CCK and satiation. *Peptides* 22 (8):1251–1263.

Geary, N., and L. Asarian. 2001. Estradiol increases glucagon's satiating potency in ovariectomized rats. *Am J Physiol Regul Integr Comp Physiol* 281 (4):R1290–R1294.

Gonzalez, J. M., S. E. Johnson, A. M. Stelzleni, T. A. Thrift, J. D. Savell, T. M. Warnock, and D. D. Johnson. 2010. Effect of ractopamine-HCl supplementation for 28 days on carcass characteristics, muscle fiber morphometrics, and whole muscle yields of six distinct muscles of the loin and round. *Meat Sci* 85 (3):379–384.

Greenway, F. L., M. J. Whitehouse, M. Guttadauria, J. W. Anderson, R. L. Atkinson, K. Fujioka, K. M. Gadde et al. 2009. Rational design of a combination medication for the treatment of obesity. *Obesity (Silver Spring)* 17 (1):30–39.

Gutzwiller, J. P., J. Drewe, B. Goke, H. Schmidt, B. Rohrer, J. Lareida, and C. Beglinger. 1999a. Glucagon-like peptide-1 promotes satiety and reduces food intake in patients with diabetes mellitus type 2. *Am J Physiol* 276 (5 Pt 2):R1541–R1544.

Gutzwiller, J. P., B. Goke, J. Drewe, P. Hildebrand, S. Ketterer, D. Handschin, R. Winterhalder, D. Conen, and C. Beglinger. 1999b. Glucagon-like peptide-1: A potent regulator of food intake in humans. *Gut* 44 (1):81–86.

Harris, S. C., A. C. Ivy, and L. M. Searle. 1947. The mechanism of amphetamine-induced loss of weight: A consideration of the theory of hunger and appetite. *J Am Med Assoc* 134 (17):1468–1475.

Hauptman, J. B., F. S. Jeunet, and D. Hartmann. 1992. Initial studies in humans with the novel gastrointestinal lipase inhibitor Ro 18-0647 (tetrahydrolipstatin). *Am J Clin Nutr* 55 (1 Suppl):309S–313S.

Hendricks, E. J., R. B. Rothman, and F. L. Greenway. 2009. How physician obesity specialists use drugs to treat obesity. *Obesity (Silver Spring)* 17 (9):1730–1735.

Heymsfield, S. B., A. S. Greenberg, K. Fujioka, R. M. Dixon, R. Kushner, T. Hunt, J. A. Lubina et al. 1999. Recombinant leptin for weight loss in obese and lean adults: A randomized, controlled, dose-escalation trial. *JAMA* 282 (16):1568–1575.

Holtzman, S. G. 1979. Suppression of appetitive behavior in the rat by naloxone: Lack of effect of prior morphine dependence. *Life Sci* 24 (3):219–226.

Janssen, I., L. H. Powell, R. Kazlauskaite, and S. A. Dugan. 2010. Testosterone and visceral fat in midlife women: The Study of Women's Health Across the Nation (SWAN) fat patterning study. *Obesity (Silver Spring)* 18 (3):604–610.

Kalyani, R. R., M. Franco, A. S. Dobs, P. Ouyang, D. Vaidya, A. Bertoni, S. M. Gapstur, and S. H. Golden. 2009. The association of endogenous sex hormones, adiposity, and insulin resistance with incident diabetes in postmenopausal women. *J Clin Endocrinol Metab* 94 (11):4127–4135.

Kambadur, R., M. Sharma, T. P. Smith, and J. J. Bass. 1997. Mutations in myostatin (GDF8) in double-muscled Belgian Blue and Piedmontese cattle. *Genome Res* 7 (9):910–916.

Karamadoukis, L., L. Ludeman, and A. J. Williams. 2008. Is there a link between calcium oxalate crystalluria, orlistat and acute tubular necrosis? *Nephrol Dial Transplant* 23 (5):1778–1779.

Kennett, G. A., and P. G. Clifton. 2010. New approaches to the pharmacological treatment of obesity: Can they break through the efficacy barrier? *Pharmacol Biochem Behav* 97 (1):63–83.

Kopelman, P. A., A. Bryson, R. Hickling, A. Rissanen, S. Rossner, S. Toubro, and P. Valensi. 2007. Celistat (ATL-962), a novel lipase inhibitor: A 12-week randomized, placebo-controlled study of weight reduction in obese patients. *Int J. Obes (Lond.)* 31(3):494–499.

Lambert, C. P., N. R. Wright, B. N. Finck, and D. T. Villareal. 2008. Exercise but not diet-induced weight loss decreases skeletal muscle inflammatory gene expression in frail obese elderly persons. *J Appl Physiol* 105 (2):473–478.

Launay, J. M., P. Herve, K. Peoc'h, C. Tournois, J. Callebert, C. G. Nebigil, N. Etienne et al. 2002. Function of the serotonin 5-hydroxytryptamine 2B receptor in pulmonary hypertension. *Nat Med* 8 (10):1129–1135.

Layman, D. K., R. A. Boileau, D. J. Erickson, J. E. Painter, H. Shiue, C. Sather, and D. D. Christou. 2003. A reduced ratio of dietary carbohydrate to protein improves body composition and blood lipid profiles during weight loss in adult women. *J Nutr* 133 (2):411–417.

Lee, M. W., and K. Fujioka. 2009. Naltrexone for the treatment of obesity: Review and update. *Expert Opin Pharmacother* 10 (11):1841–1845.

Li, Z., M. Maglione, W. Tu, W. Mojica, D. Arterburn, L. R. Shugarman, L. Hilton et al. 2005. Meta-analysis: Pharmacologic treatment of obesity. *Ann Intern Med* 142 (7):532–546.

Lisser, H. 1924. The frequency of endogenous endocrine obesity and its treatment by glandular therapy. *Calif West Med* 22 (10):509–514.

Littré, E. 1839. *Hippocrates. Oeuvres Complètes d'Hippocrate: Traduction nouvelle avec le texte grec*. Paris, France: JB Baillière.

Liu, Y. L., H. E. Ford, M. R. Druce, J. S. Minnion, B. C. Field, J. C. Shillito, J. Baxter, K. G. Murphy, M. A. Ghatei, and S. R. Bloom. 2010. Subcutaneous oxyntomodulin analogue administration reduces body weight in lean and obese rodents. *Int J Obes (Lond)* 34 (12):1715–1725.

Lutz, T. A. 2011. Amylin may offer (more) help to treat postmenopausal obesity. *Endocrinology* 152 (1):1–3.

MacWalter, R. S., H. W. Fraser, and K. M. Armstrong. 2003. Orlistat enhances warfarin effect. *Ann Pharmacother* 37 (4):510–512.

Madhava, K., and A. Hartley. 2005. Hypothyroidism in thyroid carcinoma follow-up: Orlistat may inhibit the absorption of thyroxine. *Clin Oncol (R Coll Radiol)* 17 (6):492.

Malcolm, R., P. M. O'Neil, J. D. Sexauer, F. E. Riddle, H. S. Currey, and C. Counts. 1985. A controlled trial of naltrexone in obese humans. *Int J Obes* 9 (5):347–353.

Martin, C. K., L. K. Heilbronn, L. de Jonge, J. P. DeLany, J. Volaufova, S. D. Anton, L. M. Redman, S. R. Smith, and E. Ravussin. 2007. Effect of calorie restriction on resting metabolic rate and spontaneous physical activity. *Obesity (Silver Spring)* 15 (12):2964–2973.

Mason, E. H. 1924. The Treatment of Obesity. *Can Med Assoc J* 14 (11):1052–1056.

Mauvais-Jarvis, F. 2011. Estrogen and androgen receptors: Regulators of fuel homeostasis and emerging targets for diabetes and obesity. *Trends Endocrinol Metab* 22 (1):24–33.

McPherron, A. C., A. M. Lawler, and S. J. Lee. 1997. Regulation of skeletal muscle mass in mice by a new TGF-beta superfamily member. *Nature* 387 (6628):83–90.

Mettler, S., N. Mitchell, and K. D. Tipton. 2010. Increased protein intake reduces lean body mass loss during weight loss in athletes. *Med Sci Sports Exerc* 42 (2):326–337.

Naslund, E., B. Barkeling, N. King, M. Gutniak, J. E. Blundell, J. J. Holst, S. Rossner, and P. M. Hellstrom. 1999. Energy intake and appetite are suppressed by glucagon-like peptide-1 (GLP-1) in obese men. *Int J Obes Relat Metab Disord* 23 (3):304–311.

Naslund, E., N. King, S. Mansten, N. Adner, J. J. Holst, M. Gutniak, and P. M. Hellstrom. 2004. Prandial subcutaneous injections of glucagon-like peptide-1 cause weight loss in obese human subjects. *Br J Nutr* 91 (3):439–446.

Nielsen, T. L., C. Hagen, K. Wraae, K. Brixen, P. H. Petersen, E. Haug, R. Larsen, and M. Andersen. 2007. Visceral and subcutaneous adipose tissue assessed by magnetic resonance imaging in relation to circulating androgens, sex hormone-binding globulin, and luteinizing hormone in young men. *J Clin Endocrinol Metab* 92 (7):2696–2705.

Nonogaki, K., A. M. Strack, M. F. Dallman, and L. H. Tecott. 1998. Leptin-independent hyperphagia and type 2 diabetes in mice with a mutated serotonin 5-HT2C receptor gene. *Nat Med* 4 (10):1152–1156.

Padwal, R., S. K. Li, and D. C. Lau. 2003. Long-term pharmacotherapy for obesity and overweight. *Cochrane Database Syst Rev* (4):CD004094.

Padwal, R., S. K. Li, and D. C. Lau. 2004. Long-term pharmacotherapy for obesity and overweight. *Cochrane Database Syst Rev* (3):CD004094.

Plodkowski, R. A., Q. Nguyen, U. Sundaram, L. Nguyen, D. L. Chau, and S. St Jeor. 2009. Bupropion and naltrexone: A review of their use individually and in combination for the treatment of obesity. *Expert Opin Pharmacother* 10 (6):1069–1081.

Pocai, A., P. E. Carrington, J. R. Adams, M. Wright, G. Eiermann, L. Zhu, X. Du et al. 2009. Glucagon-like peptide 1/glucagon receptor dual agonism reverses obesity in mice. *Diabetes* 58 (10):2258–2266.

Ravussin, E., S. R. Smith, J. A. Mitchell, R. Shringarpure, K. Shan, H. Maier, J. E. Koda, and C. Weyer. 2009. Enhanced weight loss with pramlintide/metreleptin: An integrated neurohormonal approach to obesity pharmacotherapy. *Obesity (Silver Spring)* 17 (9):1736–1743.

Roche Laboratories. 2010. Xenical (orlistat) Label Update December 17, 2010.

Rosenstock, J., L. J. Klaff, S. Schwartz, J. Northrup, J. H. Holcombe, K. Wilhelm, and M. Trautmann. 2010. Effects of exenatide and lifestyle modification on body weight and glucose tolerance in obese subjects with and without pre-diabetes. *Diabetes Care* 33 (6):1173–1175.

Roth, J. D., B. L. Roland, R. L. Cole, J. L. Trevaskis, C. Weyer, J. E. Koda, C. M. Anderson, D. G. Parkes, and A. D. Baron. 2008. Leptin responsiveness restored by amylin agonism in diet-induced obesity: Evidence from nonclinical and clinical studies. *Proc Natl Acad Sci U S A* 105 (20):7257–7262.

Roth, J. D., J. L. Trevaskis, V. F. Turek, and D. G. Parkes. 2010. "Weighing in" on synergy: Preclinical research on neurohormonal anti-obesity combinations. *Brain Res* 1350:86–94.

Rothkopf, M. M., M. L. Bilof, L. P. Haverstick, and M. J. Nusbaum. 2009. Synergistic weight loss and diabetes resolution with exenatide administration after laparoscopic gastric banding. *Surg Obes Relat Dis* 5 (1):128–131.

Singh, A., S. R. Sarkar, L. W. Gaber, and M. A. Perazella. 2007. Acute oxalate nephropathy associated with orlistat, a gastrointestinal lipase inhibitor. *Am J Kidney Dis* 49 (1):153–157.

Smith, S. R. 2011. Naltrexone–buproprion causes weight loss in overweight and obese adults. *Evid Based Med* 16:53–54.

Spiegel, T. A., A. J. Stunkard, E. E. Shrager, C. P. O'Brien, M. F. Morrison, and E. Stellar. 1987. Effect of naltrexone on food intake, hunger, and satiety in obese men. *Physiol Behav* 40 (2):135–141.

Swinburn, B. A., D. Carey, A. P. Hills, M. Hooper, S. Marks, J. Proietto, B. J. Strauss, D. Sullivan, T. A. Welborn, and I. D. Caterson. 2005. Effect of orlistat on cardiovascular disease risk in obese adults. *Diabetes Obes Metab* 7 (3):254–262.

Taylor, P. W., I. Arnet, A. Fischer, and I. N. Simpson. 2010. Pharmaceutical quality of nine generic orlistat products compared with Xenical(r). *Obes Facts* 3 (4):231–237.

Thatte, U. 2001. NS-2330 (Neurosearch). *Curr Opin Investig Drugs* 2 (11):1592–1594.

Torgerson, J. S., J. Hauptman, M. N. Boldrin, and L. Sjostrom. 2004. XENical in the prevention of diabetes in obese subjects (XENDOS) study: A randomized study of orlistat as an adjunct to lifestyle changes for the prevention of type 2 diabetes in obese patients. *Diabetes Care* 27 (1):155–161.

Trevaskis, J. L., V. F. Turek, C. Wittmer, P. S. Griffin, J. K. Wilson, J. M. Reynolds, Y. Zhao, C. M. Mack, D. G. Parkes, and J. D. Roth. 2010. Enhanced amylin-mediated body weight loss in estradiol-deficient diet-induced obese rats. *Endocrinology* 151 (12):5657–5668.

Tzankoff, S. P., and A. H. Norris. 1977. Effect of muscle mass decrease on age-related BMR changes. *J Appl Physiol* 43 (6):1001–1006.

Uc, E. Y., C. P. Lambert, S. I. Harik, R. L. Rodnitzky, and W. J. Evans. 2003. Albuterol improves response to levodopa and increases skeletal muscle mass in patients with fluctuating Parkinson disease. *Clin Neuropharmacol* 26 (4):207–212.

Vickers, S. P., P. G. Clifton, C. T. Dourish, and L. H. Tecott. 1999. Reduced satiating effect of d-fenfluramine in serotonin 5-HT(2C) receptor mutant mice. *Psychopharmacology (Berl)* 143 (3):309–314.

Vickers, S. P., C. T. Dourish, and G. A. Kennett. 2001. Evidence that hypophagia induced by d-fenfluramine and d-norfenfluramine in the rat is mediated by 5-HT2C receptors. *Neuropharmacology* 41 (2):200–209.

Villareal, D. T., M. Banks, D. R. Sinacore, C. Siener, and S. Klein. 2006. Effect of weight loss and exercise on frailty in obese older adults. *Arch Intern Med* 166 (8):860–866.

Weintraub, M. 1992. Long-term weight control: The National Heart, Lung, and Blood Institute funded multimodal intervention study. *Clin Pharmacol Ther* 51 (5):581–585.

Wynne, K., and S. R. Bloom. 2006. The role of oxyntomodulin and peptide tyrosine–tyrosine (PYY) in appetite control. *Nat Clin Pract Endocrinol Metab* 2 (11):612–620.

Wynne, K., B. C. Field, and S. R. Bloom. 2010. The mechanism of action for oxyntomodulin in the regulation of obesity. *Curr Opin Investig Drugs* 11 (10):1151–1157.

Wynne, K., A. J. Park, C. J. Small, M. Patterson, S. M. Ellis, K. G. Murphy, A. M. Wren et al. 2005. Subcutaneous oxyntomodulin reduces body weight in overweight and obese subjects: A double-blind, randomized, controlled trial. *Diabetes* 54 (8):2390–2395.

Xu, Y., J. E. Jones, D. Kohno, K. W. Williams, C. E. Lee, M. J. Choi, J. G. Anderson et al. 2008. 5-HT2CRs expressed by pro-opiomelanocortin neurons regulate energy homeostasis. *Neuron* 60 (4):582–589.

Yamamura, S., T. Hamaguchi, K. Ohoyama, Y. Sugiura, D. Suzuki, S. Kanehara, M. Nakagawa et al. 2009. Topiramate and zonisamide prevent paradoxical intoxication induced by carbamazepine and phenytoin. *Epilepsy Res* 84 (2–3):172–186.

Yarasheski, K. E., J. J. Zachwieja, J. A. Campbell, and D. M. Bier. 1995. Effect of growth hormone and resistance exercise on muscle growth and strength in older men. *Am J Physiol* 268 (2 Pt 1):E268–E276.

Zhi, J., R. Moore, L. Kanitra, and T. E. Mulligan. 2002. Pharmacokinetic evaluation of the possible interaction between selected concomitant medications and orlistat at steady state in healthy subjects. *J Clin Pharmacol* 42 (9):1011–1019.

Zhi, J., R. Moore, L. Kanitra, and T. E. Mulligan. 2003. Effects of orlistat, a lipase inhibitor, on the pharmacokinetics of three highly lipophilic drugs (amiodarone, fluoxetine, and simvastatin) in healthy volunteers. *J Clin Pharmacol* 43 (4):428–435.

Zumoff, B., G. W. Strain, L. K. Miller, W. Rosner, R. Senie, D. S. Seres, and R. S. Rosenfeld. 1990. Plasma free and non-sex-hormone-binding-globulin-bound testosterone are decreased in obese men in proportion to their degree of obesity. *J Clin Endocrinol Metab* 71 (4):929–931.

10 Surgical Treatment of Obesity

Dong Wook Kim, MD and
Caroline M. Apovian, MD, FACN, FACP

CONTENTS

INTRODUCTION

Weight loss surgery (referred to as "bariatric surgery") has been used to treat severe obesity that has not responded to behavior modification, dietary therapy, exercise, and drug therapy. The word "bariatric" originates from a Greek word "baros" and "iatrikos" meaning "weight" and "medicine," respectively. Bariatric surgery includes a variety of procedures, which are performed on those who are obese, for the purpose of losing weight and improving or resolving comorbidities. Currently, this surgery provides the greatest degree of sustained weight loss for obese patients.

The prototype of bariatric procedures is the jejunoileal bypass, which was originated in 1953 and 1954 initially for the management of hyperlipidemia. This procedure dominated bariatric surgery for more than 20 years [1,2]. Weight loss with the jejunoileal bypass was an opportune development, but it led to significant complications such as gas-bloat syndrome, diarrhea, electrolyte imbalance, hepatic fibrosis and failure, nephrolithiasis, cutaneous eruptions, febrile states, and impaired mentation [2]. Therefore, it was eventually abandoned. Currently, the most commonly performed bariatric procedure is the Roux-en-Y gastric bypass (RYGB), which was developed in the late 1970s and found to have similar weight losses as the jejunoileal bypass but with much lower risk of complications [3]. The laparoscopic adjustable gastric band has been gaining in popularity since its introduction into the marketplace because of its facility of placement and low complication rate. It has supplanted the need for the vertical banded gastroplasty (VBG), which is not performed any longer. The more aggressive procedures include the biliopancreatic

---

TABLE 10.1
Types of Bariatric Surgical Procedures

Predominantly restrictive procedures
- VBG
- Adjustable gastric band
- Sleeve gastrectomy

Predominantly malabsorptive procedures
- Jejunoileal bypass
- BPD

Mixed procedures
- Gastric bypass surgery
- BPD/DS

---

diversion (BPD) and biliopancreatic diversion with duodenal switch (BPD/DS). A newer procedure called the sleeve gastrectomy is also gaining in popularity, with weight losses in between the laparoscopic adjustable band and the RYGB.

There are three broad categories of bariatric procedures: (1) restrictive, limiting the amount of food ingested; (2) malabsorptive, limiting the amount of nutrients absorbed and bypassing a portion of the intestine; and (3) a combination of both (Table 10.1). The choice of procedure is guided by multiple factors, including the degree of patients' obesity, age, comorbid conditions, cost of the operation, and the choice of the patients and surgeons. This chapter will review the indications and contraindications of surgery, type of surgery, its outcome, and complications.

INDICATIONS

Patients should be carefully selected for any bariatric surgical procedure. Indications for surgical management in cases of extreme obesity were first outlined by the National Institutes of Health (NIH) Consensus Development Panel in 1991, which continues to represent generally accepted guidelines to date [4]. The selection criteria for bariatric surgery starts with a diagnosis of obesity based on body mass index (BMI) of $40\,kg/m^2$ or greater, or greater than or equal to $35\,kg/m^2$ in patients with the presence of comorbid conditions such as severe sleep apnea, obesity-related cardiomyopathy, obesity hypoventilation syndrome, diabetes mellitus, or severe osteoarthritis.

In February 2011, the Food and Drug Administration (FDA) expanded approval of a particular brand of adjustable gastric band to patients with BMI of greater than or equal to $35\,kg/m^2$ or over $30\,kg/m^2$ with one weight-related medical condition such as diabetes or sleep apnea (Table 10.2). However, as with the more aggressive procedures, adjustable gastric banding should be utilized only after less invasive methods such as diet and behavior modification have failed.

TABLE 10.2
Criteria for Consideration of Bariatric Surgery

Weight- and obesity-associated comorbidities
- BMI $\geq 40\,kg/m^2$ (BMI $\geq 35\,kg/m^2$, adjustable gastric banding) without obesity-associated comorbid conditions (e.g., sleep apnea, obesity-related cardiomyopathy, obesity hypoventilation syndrome, diabetics mellitus, and obesity-induced disability)
- BMI $\geq 35\,kg/m^2$ (BMI $\geq 30\,kg/m^2$, adjustable gastric banding) with obesity-associated comorbid conditions

Weight loss history
- Failure of previous nonsurgical weight loss attempts

Medical and psychological conditions
- Without reversible endocrine or other disorder that can cause obesity (e.g., Cushing's syndrome and hypothalamic obesity syndrome)
- Without severe coexisting medical condition (e.g., unstable angina and advanced liver disease)
- Without active substance abuse
- Without uncontrolled psychiatric illness

CONTRAINDICATIONS

Contraindications to bariatric surgery include patients with severe psychiatric illness, active substance abuse, defined noncompliance with previous medical care, or severe preexisting medical conditions. Eating disorders should be carefully treated before considering surgery, because bariatric procedures, especially ones that alter the size of stomach to restrict food intake, may exacerbate bulimia or anorexia nervosa. Prior to undergoing a bariatric procedure, patients should be aware of risks, expected benefits, alternative outcomes, and lifestyle changes required with bariatric surgery. Mental or cognitive impairment limits patients' ability to understand the procedure and thus precludes informed consent [5,6].

Bariatric procedures are not recommended for patients with reversible endocrine or other disorders that can cause obesity such as Cushing syndrome or hypothalamic obesity syndrome [7].

General contraindications for bariatric surgery are the same as those for any elective abdominal operation. For example, very severe coexisting medical conditions, such as unstable coronary artery disease or advanced liver disease with portal hypertension, will significantly increase the risks of surgery [5]. Pregnancy should be delayed until the body weight stabilizes, generally 12–24 months after surgery; therefore, effective contraception is strongly encouraged during this period [8,9].

MECHANISMS OF WEIGHT LOSS

Restriction of intake and malabsorption of nutrients are two generally recognized mechanisms of weight loss after bypass surgery. Restrictive procedures limit caloric intake by reducing the stomach's reservoir capacity via resection, bypass, or creation of a proximal gastric outlet. VBG and laparoscopic adjustable gastric banding (LAGB) are purely restrictive procedures. The induction of satiety and satiation after gastric banding has been demonstrated in a prospective blinded crossover study as being a key factor in achieving weight loss [10].

Malabsorptive procedures decrease the effectiveness of nutrient absorption by shortening the length of functional small intestine, either through bypass of the small bowel absorptive surface area or diversion of the biliopancreatic secretions that facilitate absorption. The jejunoileal bypass, sleeve gastrectomy, and the BD with and without duodenal switch operations are examples of malabsorptive procedures.

The RYGB is a combination of restrictive and malabsorptive procedures. Enterohormonal changes, which contribute to weight loss and diabetes control, are currently being intensely investigated and are now believed to be crucial to the success of RYGB surgery and the other malabsorptive procedures. The enterohormonal axis involves communication directly to the central nervous system to regulate feeding behavior, and bariatric surgery generates alterations in liver, adipose, muscle, and pancreatic physiology. There are two competing hypotheses that have been popularized as the potential mechanism of these effects after malabsorptive bariatric surgery. The "hindgut" hypothesis is based on the substantial changes in incretin and other enteroendocrine responses from more direct nutrient delivery to the distal intestine [11]. The importance of early nutrient delivery to the distal small bowel is clearly supported by ileal transposition experiments, in which a segment of the ileum is moved proximally to the duodenal–jejunal junction, leading to reduced food intake and weight loss without fat malabsorption and associated with increased glucagon-like peptide-1 (GLP-1), peptide YY, and preproglucagon levels [12]. These changes are seen with only a relatively short segment of upper intestine bypassed in the typical RYGB surgery, and, so far, the major incretin hormone accentuated in studies seems to be GLP-1, but other potential candidate mediators could be operative as well.

The "foregut" hypothesis proposes that stimulation of the proximal bowel with nutrients would trigger a counterregulatory signal that controls the enhancement of insulin secretion and action induced by incretins in normal individuals. Therefore, surgical exclusion of ingested nutrients from the duodenum and proximal small intestine may exert antidiabetic and weight-reducing effects possibly by an as yet unknown putative signal. In a series of surgical experiments, Rubino et al. demonstrated glycemic improvement with duodenal–jejunal bypass compared with gastrojejunostomy on sham-operated nonobese diabetic rats [13]. In this experiment, if the "hindgut hypothesis" played a dominant role, gastrojejunostomy and duodenal–jejunal bypass should have been equally effective in improving glucose tolerance since they equivalently expedite nutrient delivery to the hindgut. This study, which strongly supports the "foregut" hypothesis, shows that the exclusion of the proximal small intestine plays a major role in the beneficial effect of gastrointestinal bypass surgery on type 2 diabetes.

PREOPERATIVE PREPARATION

To be considered for weight loss surgery, patients should undergo a multidisciplinary evaluation to assess medical fitness as well as nutritional, behavioral, and psychological evaluations. Giusti et al. performed a prospective cohort study to evaluate the impact of preoperative teaching. This study shows that preoperative education on eating behaviors, psychological implications, and risks and disadvantages of bariatric surgery led 9% of patients to opt out of bariatric surgery and 15% of patients to opt from one type of surgery to another. Moreover, preoperative teaching is effective in clarifying doubts and defining surgical expectations in 99% of patients [14]. Therefore, preoperative training by a multidisciplinary team, with an obesity medicine specialist, dietitian, psychiatrist or psychologist, and bariatric surgeon, is a necessary step in helping patients understand the surgical procedures and preparing the patient prior to bariatric surgery.

Studies show that a preoperative weight loss of $\geq 5\%$ is associated with a decrease in operative time and a potential reduction in surgical risk [15]. Patients who followed a very-low-energy diet before surgery also had a significant decrease in liver volume [16]. A reduction in liver size prior to bariatric surgery has been recommended to decrease surgical difficulty and help prevent conversions from laparoscopic to open procedures [17,18]. Therefore, preoperative weight loss of 5%–10% of initial body weight is recommended for patients, especially with BMI of greater than 50 (kg/m^2) [19].

Preoperatively, vitamin and trace mineral deficiencies, especially vitamin D (40%), zinc (Zn) (28%), and iron (Fe) (14%), are common [20]. Nutritionally, it is very important to monitor deficiencies in vitamin D, thiamine, calcium, Fe, vitamin B12, and folic acid and to replete as indicated before and after surgery [19]. Smoking is associated with difficulty in postoperative weaning from a ventilator and increases the risk of postoperative marginal ulceration [21,22]. Therefore, smoking cessation preoperatively is also highly recommended.

TYPES OF CURRENT BARIATRIC SURGERY

GASTRIC BYPASS SURGERY

Gastric bypass surgery has undergone numerous technical refinements since the first description by Mason in 1967 to its current form, the RYGB [23]. Now, it is the most common bariatric procedure performed in the United States and is considered to be the gold standard among bariatric procedures. The gastric bypass is considered a hybrid of restrictive and malabsorptive procedures. It involves stapling of the stomach to create a small (≤30.0 mL) upper gastric pouch. The small intestine is then divided at the midjejunum, and the distal portion (called the alimentary, or Roux, limb) is anastomosed to the gastric pouch. The distal portion of the stomach and proximal small intestine (the biliopancreatic limb) are anastomosed. Food comes into contact with pancreatic and biliary secretions only below this anastomosis (Figure 10.1).

The first laparoscopic RYGB series was reported by Wittgrove et al. in 1994 in the United States [24]. In a randomized study of outcomes after laparoscopic and open gastric bypasses, Nguyen and colleagues presented a 155-patient series

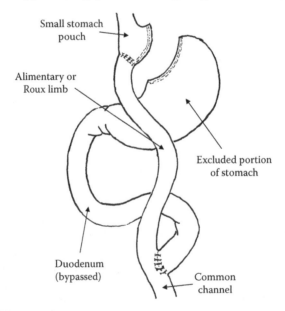

FIGURE 10.1   Roux-en-Y gastric bypass surgery.

(79 laparoscopic, 76 open) with 2 years of follow-up in 2001 [25]. The percent excess body weight loss (EBWL) during the first year was similar in two groups: 68% in the laparoscopic group and 62% in the open group. The mean operative time for the laparoscopic operation exceeded that of the open operation. The late anastomotic stricture rate was 11.4% in the laparoscopic group, as compared to 2.6% in the open group. However, the laparoscopic group had less complications, specifically postoperative leak, wound infection, and incisional hernia [25]. Another randomized controlled trial showed significantly higher rates of anastomotic stricture (4.7% vs. 0.7%), gastrointestinal bleeding (1.9% vs. 0.6%), and late postoperative bowel obstruction (3.1% vs. 2.1%) in the laparoscopic group [26]. The length of hospital stay is typically shorter in the laparoscopic versus open bypass.

A large prospective multi-institutional trial involving 2975 laparoscopic RYGB procedures showed a 0.2% 30 day postoperative mortality rate [27]. Patients aged 65 years and older have a nearly threefold increase in the risk of mortality after surgery; however, this is still a viable option for older patients since the overall mortality rate is so low [28]. In a retrospective series of 1067 patients undergoing RYGB, men had more than a threefold higher mortality rate than women, even after controlling for BMI differences [29]. Surgeon and hospital procedural volume is inversely associated with early postoperative death and adverse outcomes following bariatric surgery. A retrospective review covering 4685 cases shows that surgeons who performed fewer than 10 procedures per year had a 28% risk of adverse outcome and a 5% risk of death, compared to 14% (P < .05) and 0.3%, respectively, for high-volume surgeons [30]. Therefore, adverse outcomes are significantly lower when gastric bypass is performed by higher-volume surgeons. The creation of Centers of Excellence for Bariatric Surgery in the United States, with credentialing of surgeons, hospitals, and the bariatric team, has assisted in reducing the mortality and complication rates of these procedures.

LAPAROSCOPIC ADJUSTABLE GASTRIC BANDING

LAGB is a purely restrictive procedure (Figure 10.2). The laparoscopic gastric band has become popular in the United States over the past 10 years and has a highly acceptable safety risk profile, making it attractive for less obese patients as an alternative to medical therapy. Recently, the FDA expanded approval for the LAP-BAND device (ALLERGAN) to patients with BMI of greater than or equal to 35 kg/m^2 or over 30 kg/m^2 with one weight-related medical condition such as diabetes or obstructive sleep apnea.

LAGB does not require division of the stomach or intestinal resection. As a result, it has the lowest mortality rate (0%–0.5%) among all bariatric procedures [27,31]. The mean percent EBWL after LAGB in published series is 46%, and the mean resolution of diabetes is 56%, both substantially lower than rates after RYGB surgery [32]. Moreover, complications associated with band and port such as band slippage, band erosion, balloon failure, port malposition, band and port infections, and esophageal dilatation are not uncommon. In fact, retrospective reviews show that 16%–50% of patients, which is about twice the rate seen in the other bariatric operations, will require reoperation due to various complications and inadequate weight loss [33–35].

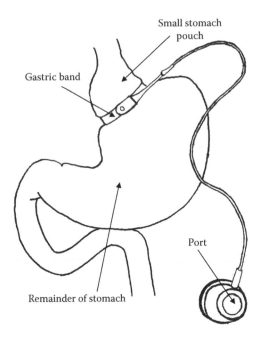

Small stomach
pouch

Gastric band

Port

Remainder of stomach

FIGURE 10.2   Laparoscopic adjustable gastric banding.

VERTICAL BANDED GASTROPLASTY

VBG is a purely restrictive procedure. Mason introduced a vertical gastroplasty with a Marlex mesh band wrapped around the outlet channel through a gastric window constructed with the end-to-end stapler in 1980 [36] (Figure 10.3). A reduction of caloric intake of solid food causes weight loss. The EBWL is greater in patients who underwent VBG (EBWL of 58%) than in patients who underwent adjustable gastric banding procedure (EBWL of 42%) after 12 months [37]. However, after 10 years, only 20% of the patients who underwent VBG lost and maintained 50% excess weight loss [38]. VBG was a popular bariatric procedure in the 1980s. However, with time, it became apparent that mesh band–related complications including erosion and stenosis were common with VBG. A prospective study documented that as many as 49.7% of VBG patients ultimately sought a revisional surgery [37]. The majority of revisions were required due to staple line disruption, stomal stenosis, band erosion, band disruption, pouch dilatation, vomiting, and gastroesophageal reflux disease. Due to a combination of these complications and inadequate weight loss and weight regain, VBG has been replaced largely by the LAGB and other procedures and is rarely performed today.

SLEEVE GASTRECTOMY

Sleeve gastrectomy, a relatively new surgical approach, was initially introduced as a restrictive component of BPD/DS in the era of open bariatric surgery. The stomach is reduced to about 25% of its original size, by surgical removal of a large portion of the stomach, following the major curve. The greater curvature of the stomach is

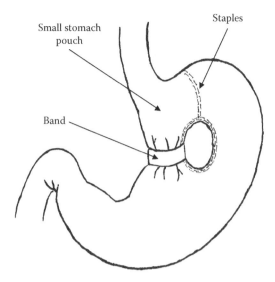

FIGURE 10.3   Vertical banded gastroplasty.

resected, producing a narrow, tubular stomach with the size and shape of a banana (Figure 10.4). Sleeve gastrectomy is technically easier than RYGB because it does not require gastrointestinal anastomosis or intestinal bypass. It also avoids implantation of an artificial device around the stomach compared to VBG and LAGB [39]. Weight loss following sleeve gastrectomy is achieved by both restriction and hormonal modulation. Ghrelin levels consistently decrease after sleeve gastrectomy.

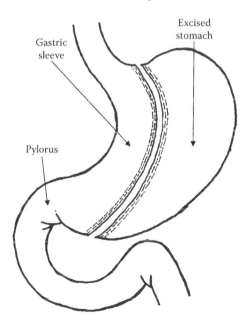

FIGURE 10.4   Sleeve gastrectomy.

Gastric resection and removal of ghrelin-secreting tissue are the major differences between sleeve gastrectomy and other restrictive procedures that do not lower ghrelin levels. A prospective comparison shows ghrelin reduction from the first month to 12 months after sleeve gastrectomy but increased ghrelin proportionate to weight loss after LAGB [40]. A prospective randomized controlled trial showed that weight loss and loss of feeling of hunger after 1 year and 3 years are greater after sleeve gastrectomy than LAGB but that the severity of complications appears higher with the sleeve gastrectomy [41]. Sleeve gastrectomy may be offered to patients as a definitive procedure for obesity or as a first step in a staged surgical approach for patients with very high BMI ($>60\,kg/m^2$) [42].

BILIOPANCREATIC DIVERSION/DUODENAL SWITCH

BPD, which is also known as the Scopinaro procedure, was first reported in 1979 [43]. The procedure consists of a partial horizontal gastrectomy with a closure of duodenal stump, gastrojejunostomy with a long Roux limb, and anastomosis of the long biliopancreatic limb to the ileum at a distance of 50 cm proximal to the ileocecal valve (Figure 10.5).

Contrary to the jejunoileal bypass, BPD does not defunctionalize any small bowel and, consequently, minimizes risk of liver injury (see Section Jejunoileal Bypass).

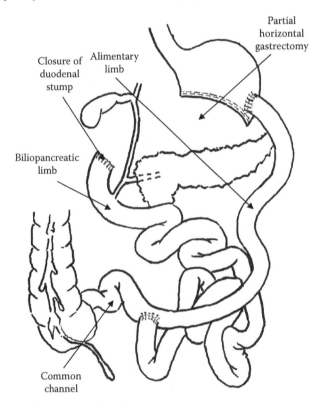

FIGURE 10.5   Biliopancreatic diversion.

In a review of 3000 original types of BPD operations, the initial excess weight loss after 1 year was about 70% and was maintained for 25 years [44]. However, BPD is associated with a risk of severe protein calorie malnutrition (9.8%) and marginal ulcers (10.6%) requiring hospitalization and parenteral nutrition support [45,46]. Moreover, patients who undergo BPD can have dumping syndrome similar to patients who undergo RYGB surgery [45]. The dumping syndrome will be further discussed under the complication section.

In 1993, the BPD/DS was first introduced in order to decrease the side effects of BPD while preserving a significant weight loss [47].

BPD/DS is a hybrid of restrictive and malabsorptive procedures. The restrictive portion of the surgery involves a partial sleeve gastrectomy with preservation of the pylorus, and the malabsorptive portion of the surgery involves creation of a Roux limb with a short common channel. The common channel is the portion of small intestine, usually 75–150 cm long, in which the contents of the digestive path mix with the bile from the biliopancreatic loop before emptying into the large intestine. The BPD/DS procedure differs from BPD in the portion of the stomach that is removed, as well as preservation of pylorus [3]. BPD also differs from jejunoileal bypass in that no intestinal limb is excluded from flow, thus avoiding creation of a blind loop (see Section Jejunoileal Bypass) (Figures 10.5 and 10.6). Initial excess weight loss at

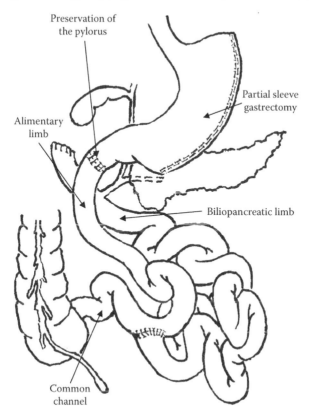

FIGURE 10.6 Biliopancreatic diversion with duodenal switch.

24 months was over 80%, using a common channel of 50–100 cm, and 75% excess weight loss at 11 years after surgery has been reported [45,48]. Because the pyloric valve between stomach and small intestine is preserved, those who have undergone BPD/DS do not experience the dumping syndrome common with those who have undergone the RYGB bypass surgery or standard BPD [49]. The number of marginal ulcers is reduced from 3% occurring after standard BPD to 0.3% in the BPD/DS [45]. This procedure provides superior weight loss in high-BMI patients (BMI ≥ 50 kg/m²) compared with gastric bypass. Successful weight loss (EBWL > 50%) was significantly greater in patients following BPD/DS than gastric bypass (36 months, 84.2% vs. 59.3%) [50]. However, it is technically more demanding and invasive than other bariatric procedures. It is not widely accepted as a first-line surgical treatment for less severe obesity because of concerns regarding the risks of long-term malabsorption.

Jejunoileal Bypass

Jejunoileal bypass was a surgical weight loss procedure performed from the 1950s through the 1970s. Jejunoileal bypass involved joining the proximal jejunum to the distal ileum, bypassing a large segment of the nutrient-absorbing small bowel.

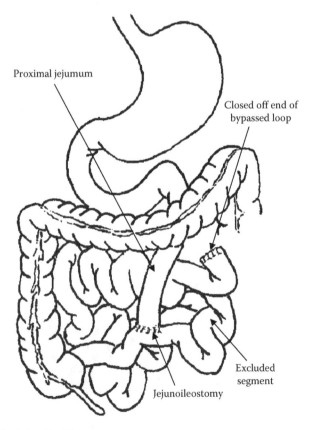

Proximal jejumum

Closed off end of bypassed loop

Excluded segment

Jejunoileostomy

FIGURE 10.7 Jejunoileal bypass.

Jejunoileal bypass is a classic example of a malabsorptive weight loss procedure (Figure 10.7). However, although excess weight loss was excellent, jejunoileal bypass was associated with multiple complications, such as severe diarrhea, electrolyte imbalances, oxalate renal stones, vitamin deficiencies, malnutrition, arthritis, and hepatic failure [51]. Notably, progressive hepatic structural abnormalities occurred in 29% of the patients, and there was a 7% incidence of cirrhosis [52]. As a consequence of all these complications, jejunoileal bypass is no longer a recommended bariatric surgical procedure.

OUTCOMES AND EFFECTIVENESS AFTER BARIATRIC SURGERY

The purpose of bariatric surgery is to induce substantial clinically important weight loss that is sufficient to reduce obesity-related morbidities. The loss of fat mass, particularly visceral fat, is associated with improved insulin sensitivity and glucose disposal, reduced flux of free fatty acids, increased adiponectin levels, and decreased interleukin-6, tumor necrosis factor-α, and high-sensitivity C-reactive protein levels. Loss of visceral fat also reduces intra-abdominal pressure, and this change may result in improvements in urinary incontinence, gastroesophageal reflux, systemic hypertension, pseudotumor cerebri, venous stasis disease, and hypoventilation [7]. It is now clear that bariatric surgery significantly decreases overall mortality in severely obese patients [53,54].

The fastest rate of weight loss occurs during the first 3 months postoperatively when dietary intake remains very restrictive. This rapid weight loss decreases by 6–9 months [7]. A maximum weight loss was observed after 1–2 years in patients undergoing gastric bypass [53]. After 15 years of follow-up in the Swedish Obese Subjects (SOS) study, the mean weight remained within ±2% of baseline weight in medically managed subjects, while the mean weight loss was 27% ± 12%, 18% ± 11%, and 13% ± 14% in patients undergoing gastric bypass surgery, VBG, and banding surgery, respectively [53]. A sustained weight loss differentiates surgery from other medical treatments for obesity.

Many studies also demonstrate that bariatric surgery is effective in reducing obesity-related comorbidities. Buchwald et al. performed a meta-analysis about the impact of bariatric surgery on weight loss and four obesity comorbidities (diabetes, hyperlipidemia, hypertension, and obstructive sleep apnea). This study included a total of 131 studies and 22,094 patients. It showed that 78.1% of diabetic patients had a complete resolution, and diabetes was improved or resolved in 86.6% of patients after bariatric procedures of all kinds. Diabetes resolution was the greatest for patients undergoing BPD/DS (95.1% resolved), followed by gastric bypass (80.3%), gastroplasty (79.7%), and LAGB (56.7%) [32]. Hyperlipidemia was significantly improved (over 70%) after bariatric procedures of all types. The maximum improvements in hyperlipidemia by meta-analysis occurred with the BPD or BPD/DS (99.1%) and with gastric bypass surgery (96.9%). Hypertension and obstructive sleep apnea were also significantly improved across all surgical procedures [55].

It has been reported that development of type 2 diabetes could be prevented by bariatric surgery. LAGB was also associated with decreased insulin resistance and a dramatic reduction in fulfillment of the criteria for the metabolic syndrome [56].

Weight loss after RYGB surgery in patients with impaired glucose tolerance prevents the progression to diabetes by more than 30-fold [57].

MORTALITY

Mortality from surgery is usually determined by calculating the mortality rate from all causes within 30 days of the operation. In meta-analyses, operative mortalities were 0.1% for the purely restrictive procedures (0%–0.1% LAGB, 0.15% VBG), 0.2%–0.5% for gastric bypass, and 0.8%–1.1% for BPD or DS [27,55,58]. In a multi-institutional consecutive cohort study, the overall complication rate was 3.2%, and the 30 day mortality rate was 0% for restrictive procedures such as VBG or gastric banding. For gastric bypass procedures, the overall complication rate was 16%, and the 30 day mortality rate was 0.4% [59]. In a review of 13,871 bariatric surgical procedures (6,122 adjustable gastric banding, 4,215 vertical banded gastroplasties, 1,106 gastric bypasses, 1,988 BPDs, 303 biliointestinal bypasses, and 137 various procedure), pulmonary embolism represented the most common cause of death, and cardiac failure, intestinal leak, and respiratory failure are other common causes of mortality [58].

Factors that have been found to contribute to increased postsurgical mortality include a lack of experience of surgeons, advanced patient age (over the age of 65), male gender, severe obesity (BMI $\geq$ 50), and coexisting conditions [28,60].

POSTOPERATIVE COMPLICATIONS

There are various complications following bariatric surgery, and they can be grouped based upon the type of procedure performed. In general, the rate of complications can be as high as 40% [61]. A study of insurance claims of 2522 patients, who had undergone bariatric surgery (2395, gastric bypass; 127, banding or gastroplasty), showed 21.9% rate of complications during the initial hospital stay and a total of 40% in the subsequent 6 months. Overall, 18.2% of the patients had some type of postoperative visit to the hospital with complications (through readmission, outpatient hospital visit, or emergency room visit) within 180 days [62].

Surgical complications are also classified as early and late complications. Early complications that occur less than 30 days after surgery include bleeding, leaks, internal hernia, and cardiovascular and pulmonary complications. Late complications of bariatric surgery include cholelithiasis and various nutritional deficiencies.

ANASTOMOTIC LEAK

Anastomotic leak is a potentially fatal complication and one of the most challenging complications of gastric bypass surgery or BPD/DS. It is reported to occur in up to 5% of RYGB procedures [7,63,64]. Gastrografin studies or CT scanning should be performed for the initial diagnostic evaluation of anastomotic leak. Exploratory laparoscopy or laparotomy is recommended for clinically unstable patients with a high suspicion of anastomotic leak. After the diagnosis of anastomotic leak, emergent surgical reexploration is usually necessary, either laparoscopically or with an open procedure [7].

BLEEDING

The incidence of early postoperative gastrointestinal hemorrhage is 0.8%–4.4% [65,66]. In the early postoperative period (within 72 h), significant bleeding is usually due to an intraoperative complication or anastomotic ischemia. From 72 h to 1 week, erosions and ulcerations occur at band sites or anastomosis (marginal ulcer) [67]. Intraluminal bleeding is most common, but extraluminal bleeding also occurs occasionally. Major intraluminal bleeding can lead to transient obstruction from clotting at the distal (jejunojejunal) anastomosis, which increases the risk of perforation at the proximal (gastrojejunal) anastomosis or the gastric remnant [67]. Common presentations of postoperative gastrointestinal bleeding include melena, large blood output from drains, tachycardia, hypotension, oliguria, and a decrease in hematocrit. Most cases respond to conservative therapy, and reoperation is rarely indicated. Failure of conservative management requires operative intervention, such as enteroscopy and laparotomy [66].

INTERNAL HERNIA

Common sites of internal hernia are Petersen's space, mesocolon window, and at an enteroenterostomy mesenteric defect [68]. If a patient is suspected to have an internal hernia as etiology of abdominal pain, urgent surgical exploration is indicated because this complication can be missed with upper gastrointestinal studies and CT scans [7]. A strangulated hernia may require extensive small bowel resection and potentially result in the development of short bowel syndrome [69].

CARDIOVASCULAR COMPLICATIONS

Morbidly obese patients have a high prevalence of known and unknown cardiopulmonary diseases. Cardiac failure and myocardial infarction are one of the most common causes (12.5%–16.7% of all mortalities) of mortality after bariatric surgery along with respiratory complications and technical complications such as intestinal leak or bleeding [58,70]. Therefore, preoperative coronary evaluations are recommended for patients with cardiac history and/or ECG abnormalities. Patients with known coronary artery disease should be managed in an intensive care unit setting for the first 24–48 h after bariatric surgery. Medications used in managing coronary artery disease or hypertension should be administered parenterally while patients remain without oral intake. This approach is especially important for beta adrenergic blocking agents because their abrupt discontinuation can be associated with increased risks of cardiac complications such as acute coronary syndrome [7].

PULMONARY EMBOLISM AND OTHER PULMONARY COMPLICATIONS

The incidence of pulmonary embolism in patients who have undergone bariatric surgical procedures has been reported to be up to 2%. It is the most common unexpected cause of mortality after bariatric surgery and can occur any time during the immediate postoperative period [7]. Generally, obese patients are less active than nonobese patients due to degenerative disk and joint disease. Particularly, superobese patients may be confined to bed or chair, which causes venous stasis disease such as underlying deep vein thrombosis [71].

Standard diagnostic tests for pulmonary embolism such as a nuclear lung scan, CT-angiography, pulmonary angiography, and lower extremity duplex scan may not be physically feasible in extremely obese patients. Therefore, a diagnosis of pulmonary embolism in severely obese patients can be challenging. Anticoagulation therapy should be started immediately for patients for whom there is a high level of clinical suspicion.

Hypoxemia and apneic episodes are frequently observed in sedated patients with or without a preexisting diagnosis of obstructive sleep apnea. Atelectasis is the most common cause of fever and tachycardia during the first 24 h after bariatric surgery [71]. Pulmonary management after bariatric surgery includes aggressive pulmonary toilet and incentive spirometry for prevention of atelectasis [7].

WOUND COMPLICATIONS

Wound complications after open bariatric surgery are common, and their incidence is significantly diminished by a laparoscopic approach [71]. The incidence of wound infections can be decreased by preoperative administration of antibiotics [72]. For treatment of wound infections, aggressive management with incision, drainage, and orally administered antibiotics are important. Partial opening of the incision in several locations is usually necessary for adequate drainage of subcutaneous infection [71]. Major wound infections are extremely rare with laparoscopic procedures [7].

STOMAL STENOSIS

Stomal stenosis is common (6%–12%) and results from a restricted size of gastric pouch and associated edema [73]. This complication is more common after laparoscopic versus open gastric bypass surgery [26]. Most strictures appear during the first 3 months after surgery, and patients usually present with nausea, vomiting, dysphagia, gastroesophageal reflux, and intolerance of oral intake [74]. Endoscopy is a preferred method for evaluating stomal obstruction because it can be used for a diagnosis and treatment with transendoscopic balloon dilation [75].

MARGINAL ULCERATION

Marginal ulceration after gastric bypass surgery is a well-recognized complication. The incidence of marginal ulceration varies between 1% and 27% [76,77]. Marginal ulcers between the stomach pouch and small intestine are a frequent source of epigastric pain, blood loss, and Fe deficiency. The common causes of marginal ulcers are poor tissue perfusion due to tension, gastrogastric fistulas, helicobacter pylori infection, smoking, and medications such as nonsteroidal anti-inflammatory agents, aspirin, and cyclooxygenase-2 inhibitors [78,79]. Prior to surgery, smoking cessation and treatment of helicobacter pylori infection are recommended. The treatment of helicobacter pylori significantly reduces the incidence of postoperative marginal ulcers [80].

Diarrhea/Constipation

Diarrhea and steatorrhea are common complications after malabsorptive procedures, especially after jejunoileal bypass surgery, BPD, or BPD/DS. The causes of post–bariatric surgery diarrhea include malabsorption/maldigestion, bile salt diarrhea, dumping syndrome, exacerbation of preexisting subclinical lactose intolerance, and bacterial overgrowth [67]. Regardless of the cause of diarrhea, chronic diarrhea or steatorrhea can cause nutritional and metabolic complications. Therefore, chronic or persistent diarrhea should be evaluated and treated after bariatric surgery.

Conversely, constipation is more common after gastric banding or VBG [81]. During the first few months after bariatric surgery, dehydration, which is the primary cause of constipation, results from decreased water consumption associated with postoperative loss of appetite and breakdown of water during active lipolysis and fat mobilization [67]. Daily fluid intake is encouraged for patients with post–bariatric surgery constipation.

Cholelithiasis

Cholelithiasis is common after significant weight loss and is related to the rate of weight loss. It develops in as many as 38% of patients within 6 months of surgery [82]. A prospective randomized controlled trial showed that a high frequency of cholelithiasis can be reduced to as low as 2% with a 6 month course of ursodeoxycholic acid given prophylactically after weight loss surgery [83]. There is no consensus regarding the need to perform cholecystectomy at the time of bariatric operations. Currently, it is accepted to perform prophylactic cholecystectomy if a patient has symptomatic gallstones preoperatively [7]. However, cholecystectomy has been shown to increase the operative time and the length of hospital stay [84].

Dumping Syndrome

Clinically significant dumping syndrome can occur in up to 10% of gastric surgery patients when high levels of simple carbohydrates are ingested [85]. The syndrome is usually precipitated with ingestion of high-sugar foods. It is caused by rapid emptying of food into the jejunum where the hyperosmolarity of intestinal contents results in an influx of fluid and subsequent intestinal distension, which causes abdominal pain or diarrhea. Additionally, the release of vasoactive substances, including serotonin, bradykinin, and vasoactive intestinal peptide, leads to hypotension and consequent sensations of nausea, lightheadedness, tachycardia, flushing, and syncope [86]. Management and prevention of dumping syndrome include avoidance of foods that are high in simple sugar content and replacing them with a diet consisting of high fiber, complex carbohydrate, and protein-rich foods. Behavioral modification, such as eating small, frequent meals and separating solids from liquid intake by 30 min, are also recommended. Generally, dumping syndrome is self-limited and resolves within 7–12 weeks [85].

METABOLIC AND NUTRITIONAL DERANGEMENTS

PROTEIN CALORIE MALNUTRITION

Protein calorie malnutrition is a very uncommon complication after gastric bypass surgery and pure restrictive surgery. Although rare, protein calorie malnutrition remains the most severe form of macronutrient complication and is associated with a high degree of postoperative mortality and morbidity. A retrospective study showed a very high mortality rate (18%) in patients with protein calorie malnutrition after gastric bypass surgery, and hospitalization was required in 54.4% of the cases [87].

The risks of protein calorie malnutrition are highest in patients with a short common channel (less than 150 cm) in malabsorptive procedures and with severe intolerance of protein-rich foods after bariatric surgery [88]. Intolerance of protein-rich foods such as meat products is common within a year after bariatric surgery. Therefore, many people (17% of patients) experience persistent intolerance of protein-rich foods and limit their intake of protein to less than 50% of the recommended amount [89].

In cases of severe protein calorie malnutrition, enteral or parenteral nutrition therapy may be necessary. Mild to moderate cases usually respond to dietary counseling and increased compliance with clinical follow-up visits. Prevention involves regular assessment of protein intake, encouragement of protein-rich food ingestion (>60 g/day), and use of modular protein supplements. Therefore, more frequent monitoring may be necessary for patients with risks of protein calorie malnutrition especially from the dietitian on the bariatric team [7,90].

VITAMIN B12

Vitamin B12 plays an important role in DNA synthesis and neurological function. In a normal healthy stomach, acid and peptic hydrolysis help liberate vitamin B12. In the duodenum, vitamin B12 binds to an intrinsic factor that is released from parietal cells. The vitamin B12-intrinsic factor complex is then absorbed in the terminal ileum. Impairment of vitamin B12 absorption after gastric bypass surgery results from a decrease in digestion of protein-bound cobalamins and impaired formation of intrinsic factor vitamin B12 complexes required for absorption [86]. Moreover, many postsurgical patients are unable to tolerate meat and dairy products, which are good sources of vitamin B12. After RYGB, more than 30% of patients develop this deficiency within 1–9 years [91].

Vitamin B12 deficiency is usually defined at a level less than 200 pg/mL in the bloodstream. Measurements of serum methylmalonic acid and homocysteine concentrations are more sensitive in screening for vitamin B12 deficiency than measuring serum vitamin B12 concentrations, as it can distinguish between vitamin B12 and folate deficiency [90].

Optimal dosing of oral, sublingual, or intranasal forms of vitamin B12 supplementation has not been well studied. However, initiation of vitamin B12 supplementation is recommended within 6 months postoperatively. After gastric bypass surgery, oral supplementation with crystalline vitamin B12 at a dosage of greater than 350 µg daily may be used to maintain the appropriate vitamin levels [7]. The incidence of vitamin B12 deficiency can be reduced by intramuscular vitamin B12 (1000 μg) injections every 3 months [92].

FOLATE

Folate is a generic term for a water-soluble B-complex vitamin that exists in many different forms and is an essential cofactor in metabolic pathways, especially amino acid conversion and DNA synthesis, and is necessary for erythrocyte formation and growth. Folate deficiency is not common because folate absorption occurs throughout the entire small bowel. Thus, deficiency is unlikely if patients are taking a daily multivitamin (usually containing approximately 1 mg of folate) as instructed. Therefore, biomarker monitoring is not necessary [7]. Folate replacement is important in women who become pregnant postoperatively, as it is in women in general before pregnancy, to avoid neural tube defects.

THIAMINE

Thiamine is a water-soluble vitamin of the B complex, which is a coenzyme in the catabolism of sugars and amino acids. Thiamine deficiency is one of the recognized deficiencies after bariatric surgery although it is rare compared to vitamin B12 deficiency.

Thiamine stores in the human body usually last 3–6 weeks, and these stores can be exhausted after an unbalanced increased intake of carbohydrate. It occurs due to marked emesis and/or malabsorption after bariatric surgery. Clinical symptoms vary from cardiac beriberi (wet beriberi) to neurological beriberi (dry beriberi), which can present with peripheral neurological symptoms or central neurological symptoms such as Wernicke's syndrome [93]. Wernicke's encephalopathy (ocular disorders with nystagmus, ataxia, and mental disturbances and confusion) after bariatric surgery usually occurs between 4 and 12 weeks postoperatively. It can occur as early as 2 weeks or as late as 18 months [94]. Aggressive parenteral thiamine is a treatment of choice for Wernicke's syndrome, and it should be continued for 7–14 days [89].

A multivitamin supplement is usually adequate in preventing thiamine deficiency. If thiamine deficiency occurs, it should be treated with parenteral thiamine of 50–200 mg/day until symptoms clear, and 10–100 mg by mouth daily [90]. Thiamine deficiency should be treated as soon as possible before permanent neurological sequelae ensue.

LIPID-SOLUBLE VITAMINS

In contrast to water-soluble vitamin deficiencies, which occur quickly postsurgically, fat-soluble nutrient deficiencies develop more slowly based on the extent of progressive fat malabsorption [95].

Vitamin A deficiency after bariatric surgery results from poor nutritional intake, maldigestion, malabsorption, and impaired hepatic release of vitamin A. Vitamin A has numerous biochemical roles within the body, and it is vital for ocular metabolism, including maintenance of conjunctival and corneal epithelial surfaces as well as retinal phototransduction and pigment epithelial viability. The prevalence of vitamin A deficiency is up to 69% in patients 4 years after malabsorptive bariatric surgeries (BPD and BPD/DS) [96]. Symptoms of vitamin A deficiency include ocular xerosis and night blindness. Oral supplementation of vitamin A of 5,000–10,000 IU/day is recommended until the serum vitamin A level normalizes.

Vitamin E deficiency can lead to anemia, ophthalmoplegia, and peripheral neuropathy. Preexisting vitamin E deficiency has been reported in up to 23% of RYGB patients [97]. Neuropathy has been reported in association with vitamin E deficiency after gastrectomy for gastric cancer [98]. However, symptomatic deficiencies after bariatric surgery have not been reported.

Vitamin D is needed for both skeletal and extraskeletal functions including immune function, cancer prevention, and cardiovascular health. Deficiencies are further compounded postsurgically by limited intake of dairy products due to dietary intolerance and bypassing of the primary absorption sites of calcium and vitamin D, namely, duodenum and proximal jejunum, and jejunum and ileum, respectively. To compensate for inadequate intake, insufficient absorption, and increased excretory losses of calcium after bariatric surgery, the body is induced into a state of secondary hyperparathyroidism. Further, malabsorptive procedures that stimulate hyperparathyroidism cause bone demineralization (elevated bone resorption) with a concurrent increase in serum alkaline phosphatase and increase the risk of pathologic fractures [96]. Calcium citrate is recommended in doses ranging from 0.5 to 1.5 g/day. Vitamin D dosage recommendations range from 400 to 800 IU/day [99].

Vitamin K is not stored in the body to any significant degree. Sources of vitamin K are either through diet or bacterial production in colon, both of which can be affected after bariatric surgical procedures. Vitamin K supplementation is recommended for patients with increased INR [100].

TRACE ELEMENT DEFICIENCY

Iron Deficiency

Fe deficiency is commonly found in patients who have undergone RYGB and is a major cause of anemia among this population. Fe deficiency has been reported in 20%–49% of gastric bypass patients, with a greater incidence in menstruating women [101]. Several factors account for low Fe levels post–bariatric surgery, which include decreased production of hydrochloric acid in the stomach that is necessary for dietary Fe in the ferric form to be converted to ferrous state, reduced intake of meat due to intolerance, and reduced intestinal Fe absorption capacity due to bypassing of the primary sites of Fe, namely, the duodenum and proximal jejunum, during bariatric procedures. A Fe supplement of 80–100 mg/day is recommended, and taking Fe supplements between meals with food containing vitamin C will enhance absorption [99,102].

Zinc Deficiency

Common symptoms of Zn deficiencies are hair loss, diarrhea, emotional disorders, weight loss, intercurrent infection, dermatitis, and hypogonadism in males. Zn is absorbed in the duodenum and proximal jejunum, and Zn is lost in the feces;

therefore, patients with chronic diarrhea are at risk for Zn deficiency [7]. Zn deficiency has been reported in up to 42% of gastric bypass patients [103]. Neve et al. reported significant hair loss in about one-third of their patients after VBG, which was reversed by supplementation of 600 mg of Zn sulfate daily [104].

Copper Deficiency

Copper is essential for production of red blood cells and for maintenance of the structure and functioning of the nervous system. Copper absorption is thought to take place in the upper gastrointestinal tract, but the precise location and mechanisms have not been understood completely. Copper deficiency is more common in patients who have undergone BPD than RYGB [105]. Despite the proximal gut being bypassed in gastric bypass surgery, copper deficiency remains relatively uncommon. However, up to 16% of published cases of myelopathy associated with copper deficiency were related to bariatric surgery [106].

Copper deficiency can induce anemia (normocytic or macrocytic) and neurological symptoms, which are very similar to symptoms of vitamin B12 deficiency [107]. A high level of serum Zn has been suggested as a possible contributor and has been associated with copper deficiency [108]. Therefore, injudicious supplementation with Zn can lead to copper deficiency [109]. Copper deficiency should be monitored in post–gastric bypass patients, who develop neurological symptoms despite the adequate level of vitamin B12, unexplained anemia, and a low ceruloplasmin level.

PREGNANCY

Pregnancy should be discouraged in the first year after bariatric surgery since it is associated with the most rapid weight loss, and pregnancies that occur during this time are associated with higher rates of miscarriage and preterm labor [110]. The ideal timing for conception is unknown, but evidence supports waiting for 12–18 months after the surgery before conceiving [9]. Postoperative patients desiring pregnancy should be counseled to adhere with their nutritional regimen, including use of micronutrient supplements. Folic acid and vitamin B12 status should be monitored for these patients during pregnancy and breastfeeding period [7].

SUMMARY

Since the introduction of the prototype of bariatric procedure (jejunoileal bypass) in 1953, surgical procedures for weight loss have changed dramatically and evolutionally. Currently, laparoscopic RYGB is the most commonly performed procedure in the United States due to a combination of two main mechanisms (restriction and malabsorption) of weight loss, which maximize the weight loss and durable long-term weight loss with less complications than the other more aggressive procedures. LA is becoming increasingly popular in the United States due to its simplicity in technique, adjustability, reversibility, and very low perioperative mortality.

Bariatric procedures are very effective in reducing not only mortality but also resolving or preventing obesity-related comorbidities such as type 2 diabetes, hypertension, sleep apnea, and hyperlipidemia. Surgical treatment of obesity has been recommended by the World Health Organization (WHO) as the most effective way of reducing weight and maintaining weight loss in severely obese patients.

Any bariatric procedure requires long-term dietary changes, behavioral modification, and medical supervision. All procedures have the potential for lifelong postoperative complications such as nutritional deficiencies. Therefore, the commitment of patients and health-care providers to a long-term follow-up is essential to the success of obesity surgery. Patients should have access to a multidisciplinary team of health professionals, including a physician, psychologist, dietitian, and exercise physiologist.

REFERENCES

1. Buchwald H, Rucker RD. The rise and fall of jejunoileal bypass. In: Nelson RL, Nyhus LM, eds. *Surgery of the Small Intestine*. Norwalk, CT: Appleton Century Crofts; 1987, pp. 529–541.
2. Kremen AJ, Linner LH, Nelson CH. An experimental evaluation of the nutritional importance of proximal and distal small intestine. *Ann Surg*. 1954; 140:439–444.
3. Buchwald H. Overview of bariatric surgery. *J Am Coll Surg*. 2002 Mar;194(3):367–375.
4. NIH conference. Gastrointestinal surgery for severe obesity. Consensus Development Conference Panel. *Ann Intern Med*. 1991 Dec 15; 115(12):956–961.
5. DeMaria EJ. Bariatric surgery for morbid obesity. *N Engl J Med*. 2007 May 24; 356(21):2176–2183.
6. Yermilov I, McGory ML, Shekelle PW, Ko CY, Maggard MA. Appropriateness criteria for bariatric surgery: Beyond the NIH guidelines. *Obesity (Silver Spring)*. 2009; 17(8):1521.
7. Mechanick JI, Kushner RF, Sugerman HJ et al. American Association of Clinical Endocrinologists, The Obesity Society, and American Society for Metabolic & Bariatric Surgery medical guidelines for clinical practice for the perioperative nutritional, metabolic, and nonsurgical support of the bariatric surgery patient. *Obesity (Silver Spring)*. 2009 Apr; 17 Suppl 1:S1–S70.
8. Choban PS, Jackson B, Poplawski S, Bistolarides P. Bariatric surgery for morbid obesity: Why, who, when, how, where, and then what? *Clevel Clin J Med*. 2002 Nov; 69(11):897–903.
9. Maggard MA, Yermilov I, Li Z et al. Pregnancy and fertility following bariatric surgery: A systematic review. *JAMA*. 2008; 300:2286–2296.
10. Dixon AF, Dixon JB, O'Brien PE. Laparoscopic adjustable gastric banding induces prolonged satiety: A randomized blind crossover study. *J Clin Endocrinol Metab*. 2005; 90:813–819.
11. McLaughlin T, Peck M, Holst J, Deacon C. Reversible hyperinsulinemic hypoglycemia after gastric bypass: A consequence of altered nutrient delivery. *J Clin Endocrinol Metab*. 2010; 95:1851–1855.
12. Strader AD, Vahl TP, Jandacek RJ, Woods SC, D'Alessio DA, Seeley RJ. Weight loss through ileal transposition is accompanied by increased ileal hormone secretion and synthesis in rats. *Am J Physiol Endocrinol Metab*. 2005; 288:E447–E453.
13. Cohen RV, Schiavon CA, Pinheiro JS, Correa JL, Rubino F. Duodenal-jejunal bypass for the treatment of type 2 diabetes in patients with body mass index of 22–34 kg/m²: A report of 2 cases. *Surg Obes Relat Dis*. 2007; 3:195–197.
14. Giusti V, De Lucia A, Di Vetta V et al. Impact of preoperative teaching on surgical option of patients qualifying for bariatric surgery. *Obes Surg*. 2004; 14:1241–1246.
15. Alami RS, Morton JM, Schuster R et al. Is there a benefit to preoperative weight loss in gastric bypass patients? A prospective randomized trial. *Surg Obes Relat Dis*. 2007; 3:141–145.

16. Colles SL, Dixon JB, Marks P, Strauss BJ, O'Brien PE. Preoperative weight loss with a very-low energy diet: Quantitation of changes in liver and abdominal fat by serial imaging. *Am J Clin Nutr*. 2006; 84:304–331.

17. Fris RJ. Preoperative low energy diet diminishes liver size. *Obes Surg*. 2004; 14:1165–1170.

18. Schwartz ML, Drew RL, Chazin-Caldie M. Laparoscopic Roux-en-Y gastric bypass: Preoperative determinants of prolonged operative times, conversion to open gastric bypasses, and postoperative complications. *Obes Surg*. 2003; 13:734–738.

19. Apovian CM, Cummings S, Anderson W et al. Best practice updates for multidisciplinary care in weight loss surgery. *Obesity (Silver Spring)*. 2009 May; 17(5):871–879. Epub 2009 Feb 19.

20. Madan AK, Whitney SO, Tichansky DS, Ternovits CA. Vitamin and trace mineral levels after laparoscopic gastric bypass. *Obes Surg*. 2006; 16:603–606.

21. Livingston EH, Langert J. The impact of age and Medicare status on bariatric surgical outcomes. *Arch Surg*. 2006; 141:1115–1120.

22. Wilson JA, Romagnuolo J, Byrne TK, Morgan K, Wilson FA. Predictors of endoscopic findings after Roux-en-Y gastric bypass. *Am J Gastroenterol*. 2006; 101:2194–2199.

23. Mason EE, Ito C. Gastric bypass. *Ann Surg*. 1969 Sep; 170(3):329–339.

24. Wittgrove AC, Clark GW, Tremblay LJ. Laparoscopic gastric bypass, Roux-en-Y: Preliminary report of five cases. *Obes Surg*. 1994; 4(4):353.

25. Nguyen NT, Goldman C, Rosenquist J et al. Laparoscopic versus open gastric bypass: A randomized study of outcomes, quality-of-life, and costs. *Ann Surg*. 2001; 234:279–291.

26. Podnos YD, Jimenez JC, Wilson SE, Stevens CM, Nguyen NT. Complications after laparoscopic gastric bypass: A review of 3464 cases. *Arch Surg*. 2003 Sep; 138(9):957–961.

27. Longitudinal Assessment of Bariatric Surgery (LABS) Consortium. Perioperative safety in the longitudinal assessment of bariatric surgery. *N Engl J Med*. 2009; 361:445–454.

28. Flum DR, Salem L, Elrod JA, Dellinger EP, Cheadle A, Chan L. Early mortality among Medicare beneficiaries undergoing bariatric surgical procedures. *JAMA*. 2005; 294:1903–1908.

29. Livingston EH, Huerta S, Arthur D, Lee S, De Shields S, Heber D. Male gender is a predictor of morbidity and age a predictor of mortality for patients undergoing gastric bypass surgery. *Ann Surg*. 2002; 236:576.

30. Courcoulas A, Schuchert M, Gatti G, Luketich J. The relationship of surgeon and hospital volume to outcome after gastric bypass surgery in Pennsylvania: A 3-year summary. *Surgery*. 2003; 134:613.

31. O'Brien PE, Dixon JB. Lap-band: Outcomes and results. *J Laparoendosc Adv Surg Tech A*. 2003; 13(4):265.

32. Buchwald H, Estok R, Fahrbach K, Banel D, Jensen MD, Pories WJ, Bantle JP, Sledge I. Weight and type 2 diabetes after bariatric surgery: Systematic review and meta-analysis. *Am J Med*. 2009 Mar; 122(3):248–256.

33. Kothari SN, DeMaria EJ, Sugerman HJ, Kellum JM, Meador J, Wolfe L. Lap-band failures: Conversion to gastric bypass and their preliminary outcomes. *Surgery*. 2002; 131(6):625.

34. Michalik M, Lech P, Bobowicz M, Orlowski M, Lehmann A. A 5-year experience with laparoscopic adjustable gastric banding-focus on outcomes, complications, and their management. *Obes Surg*. 2011 November, 21(11):1682–1686.

35. Himpens J, Cadière GB, Bazi M, Vouche M, Cadière B, Dapri G. Long-term outcomes of laparoscopic adjustable gastric banding. *Arch Surg*. 2011 Jul; 146:802–807. Epub 2011 Mar 21.

36. Mason EE. Vertical banded gastroplasty. *Arch Surg*. 1982; 117:701–706.

37. Miller K, Pump A, Hell E. Vertical banded gastroplasty versus adjustable gastric banding: Prospective long-term follow-up study. *Surg Obes Relat Dis.* 2007 Jan–Feb; 3(1):84–90. Epub 2006 Nov 20.

38. Balsiger B, Poggio JL, Mai J et al. Ten and more years after vertical banded gastroplasty as primary operation for morbid obesity. *J Gastrointest Surg.* 2000; 4(6):598–660.

39. Frezza EE. Laparoscopic vertical sleeve gastrectomy for morbid obesity: The future procedure of choice? *Surg Today.* 2007; 37(4):275–281.

40. Langer FB, Reza Hoda MA, Bohdjalian A, Felberbauer FX, Zacherl J, Wenzl E, Schindler K, Luger A, Ludvik B, Prager G. Sleeve gastrectomy and gastric banding: Effects on plasma ghrelin levels. *Obes Surg.* 2005; 15:1024–1029.

41. Himpens J, Dapri G, Cadière GB A prospective randomized study between laparoscopic gastric banding and laparoscopic isolated sleeve gastrectomy: Results after 1 and 3 years. *Obes Surg.* 2006; 16(11):1450.

42. Shi X, Karmali S, Sharma AM, Birch DW. A review of laparoscopic sleeve gastrectomy for morbid obesity. *Obes Surg.* 2010; 20:1171–1177.

43. Scopinaro N, Gianetta E, Civalleri D. Biliopancreatic bypass for obesity, II: Initial experiences in man. *Br J Surg.* 1979; 66:618–620.

44. Scopinaro N. Biliopancreatic diversion: Mechanisms of action and long-term results. *Obes Surg.* 2006 Jun; 16(6):683–689.

45. Hess DS, Hess DW, Oakley RS. The biliopancreatic diversion with the duodenal switch: Results beyond 10 years. *Obes Surg.* 2005 Mar; 15(3):408–416.

46. Cossu ML, Fais E, Meloni GB et al. Impact of age on long-term complications after biliopancreatic diversion. *Obes Surg.* 2004 Oct; 14(9):1182–1186.

47. Marceau P, Biron S, Bourque RA, Potvin M, Hould FS, Simard S. Biliopancreatic diversion with a new type of gastrectomy. *Obes Surg.* 1993 Feb; 3(1):29–35.

48. Hess DW, Hess DS. Biliopancreatic diversion with a duodenal switch. *Obes Surg.* 1998; 8:267–282.

49. Woodward BG. Bariatric surgery options. *Crit Care Nurs Q.* 2003 Apr–Jun; 26(2):89–100.

50. Prachand VN, Davee RT, Alverdy JC. Duodenal switch provides superior weight loss in the super-obese (BMI>or = 50 kg/m^2) compared with gastric bypass. *Ann Surg.* 2006; 244(4):611.

51. Salameh JR. Bariatric surgery: Past and present. *Am J Med Sci.* 2006 Apr; 331(4):194–200.

52. Hocking MP, Duerson MC, O'Leary JP, Woodward ER. Jejunoileal bypass for morbid obesity: Late follow-up in 100 cases. *N Engl J Med.* 1983; 308(17):995.

53. Sjöström L, Narbro K, Sjöström CD et al., for the Swedish Obese Subjects Study. Effects of bariatric surgery on mortality in Swedish obese subjects. *N Engl J Med.* 2007; 357:741–752.

54. Christou NV, Sampalis JS, Liberman M, Look D, Auger S, McLean AP, MacLean LD Surgery decreases long-term mortality, morbidity, and health care use in morbidly obese patients. *Ann Surg.* 2004; 240(3):416.

55. Buchwald H, Avidor Y, Braunwald E, Jensen MD, Pories W, Fahrbach K, Schoelles K. Bariatric surgery: A systematic review and meta-analysis. *JAMA.* 2004 Oct 13; 292(14):1724–1737.

56. O'Brien PE, Dixon JB, Laurie C et al. Treatment of mild to moderate obesity with laparoscopic adjustable gastric banding or an intensive medical program: A randomized trial. *Ann Intern Med.* 2006 May 2; 144(9):625–633.

57. Long SD, O'Brien K, MacDonald KG Jr, Leggett-Frazier N, Swanson MS, Pories WJ, Caro JF. Weight loss in severely obese subjects prevents the progression of impaired glucose tolerance to type II diabetes: A longitudinal interventional study. *Diabetes Care.* 1994 May; 17(5):372–375.

58. Morino M, Toppino M, Forestieri P, Angrisani L, Allaix ME, Scopinaro N. Mortality after bariatric surgery: Analysis of 13,871 morbidly obese patients from a national registry. *Ann Surg*. 2007 Dec; 246(6):1002–1007; discussion 1007–1009.

59. Nguyen NT, Silver M, Robinson M et al. Result of a national audit of bariatric surgery performed at academic centers: A 2004 University Health System Consortium Benchmarking Project. *Arch Surg*. 2006 May; 141(5):445–449; discussion 449–450.

60. Arterburn D, Livingston EH, Schifftner T, Kahwati LC, Henderson WG, Maciejewski ML. Predictors of long-term mortality after bariatric surgery performed in Veterans Affairs medical centers. *Arch Surg*. 2009; 144(10):914.

61. Encinosa WE, Bernard DM, Du D, Steiner CA. Recent improvements in bariatric surgery outcomes. *Med Care*. 2009; 47(5):531.

62. Encinosa WE, Bernard DM, Chen CC, Steiner CA. Healthcare utilization and outcomes after bariatric surgery. *Med Care*. 2006 Aug; 44(8):706–712.

63. Edwards MA, Jones DB, Ellsmere J, Grinbaum R, Schneider BE. Anastomotic leak following antecolic versus retrocolic laparoscopic Roux-en-Y gastric bypass for morbid obesity. *Obes Surg*. 2007; 17:292–297.

64. Fernandez AZ Jr, DeMaria EJ, Tichansky DS et al. Experience with over 3,000 open and laparoscopic bariatric procedures: Multivariate analysis of factors related to leak and related mortality. *Surg Endosc*. 2004; 18:193–197.

65. Higa K, Ho T, Boone KB. Laparoscopic Roux-en-Y gastric bypass: Technique and 3-year follow-up. *J Laparoendosc Adv Surg Tech*. 2001; 11:377–378.

66. Mehran A, Szomstein S, Zundel N, Rosenthal R. Management of acute bleeding after laparoscopic Roux-en-Y gastric bypass. *Obes Surg*. 2003; 13(6):842.

67. Kaplan LM. Gastrointestinal management of the bariatric surgery patient. *Gastroenterol Clin N Am*. 2005; 34:105–125.

68. Champion JK, Williams M. Small bowel obstruction and internal hernias after laparoscopic Roux-en-Y gastric bypass. *Obes Surg*. 2003 Aug; 13(4):596–600.

69. McBride CL, Petersen A, Sudan D, Thompson J. Short bowel syndrome following bariatric surgical procedures. *Am J Surg*. 2006 Dec; 192(6):828–832.

70. Gagner M, Milone L, Yung E, Broseus A, Gumbs AA. Causes of early mortality after laparoscopic adjustable gastric banding. *J Am Coll Surg*. 2008; 206(4):664.

71. Byrne TK. Complications of surgery for obesity. *Surg Clin N Am*. 2001; 81:1181–1193.

72. Pories WJ, van Rij AM, Burlingham BT, Fulghum RS, Meelheim D. Prophylactic cefazolin in gastric bypass surgery. *Surgery*. 1981; 90(2):426.

73. Schneider BE, Villegas L, Blackburn GL, Mun EC, Critchlow JF, Jones DB. Laparoscopic gastric bypass surgery: Outcomes. *J Laparoendosc Adv Surg Tech A*. 2003; 13(4):247.

74. Barba CA, Butensky MS, Lorenzo M, Newman R. Endoscopic dilation of gastroesophageal anastomosis stricture after gastric bypass. *Surg Endosc*. 2003; 17(3):416.

75. Sanyal AJ, Sugerman HJ, Kellum JM, Engle KM, Wolfe L. Stomal complications of gastric bypass: Incidence and outcome of therapy. *Am J Gastroenterol*. 1992; 87(9):1165.

76. Huang CS, Forse RA, Jacobson BC, Farraye FA. Endoscopic findings and their clinical correlations in patients with symptoms after gastric bypass surgery. *Gastrointest Endosc*. 2003; 58:859–866.

77. Sapala JA, Wood MH, Sapala MA, Flake TM Jr. Marginal ulcer after gastric bypass: A prospective 3-year study of 173 patients. *Obes Surg*. 1998; 8(5):505.

78. Dallal RM, Bailey LA. Ulcer disease after gastric bypass surgery. *Surg Obes Relat Dis*. 2006; 2(4):455.

79. Rasmussen JJ, Fuller W, Ali MR. Marginal ulceration after laparoscopic gastric bypass: An analysis of predisposing factors in 260 patients. *Surg Endosc*. 2007; 21(7):1090.

80. Schirmer B, Erenoglu C, Miller A. Flexible endoscopy in the management of patients undergoing Roux-en-Y gastric bypass. *Obes Surg*. 2002; 12(5):634.

81. Potoczna N, Harfmann S, Steffen R, Briggs R, Bieri N, Horber FF. Bowel habits after bariatric surgery. *Obes Surg.* 2008; 18(10):1287.

82. Shiffman ML, Sugerman HJ, Kellum JM, Brewer WH, Moore EW. Gallstone formation after rapid weight loss: A prospective study in patients undergoing gastric bypass surgery for treatment of morbid obesity. *Am J Gastroenterol.* 1991; 86(8):1000.

83. Sugerman HJ, Brewer WH, Shiffman ML, Brolin RE, Fobi MA, Linner JH, MacDonald KG, MacGregor AM, Martin LF, Oram-Smith JC. A multicenter, placebo-controlled, randomized, double-blind, prospective trial of prophylactic ursodiol for the prevention of gallstone formation following gastric bypass-induced rapid weight loss. *Am J Surg.* 1995; 169(1):91.

84. Hamad GG, Ikramuddin S, Gourash WF, Schauer PR. Elective cholecystectomy during laparoscopic Roux-en-Y gastric bypass: Is it worth the wait? *Obes Surg.* 2003; 13(1):76.

85. Ukleja A, Dumping syndrome: Pathophysiology and treatment. *Nutr Clin Pract.* 2005; 20(5):517.

86. Collene AL, Hertzler S. Metabolic outcomes of gastric bypass. *Nutr Clin Pract.* 2003 Apr; 18(2):136–140.

87. Faintuch J, Matsuda M, Cruz ME, Silva MM, Teivelis MP, Garrido AB Jr, Gama-Rodrigues JJ. Severe protein-calorie malnutrition after bariatric procedures. *Obes Surg.* 2004 Feb; 14(2):175–181.

88. Sugerman HJ, Kellum JM, DeMaria EJ. Conversion of proximal to distal gastric bypass for failed gastric bypass for superobesity. *J Gastrointest Surg.* 1997 Nov–Dec; 1(6):517–524; discussion 524–526.

89. Ziegler O, Sirveaux MA, Brunaud L, Reibel N, Quilliot D. Medical follow up after bariatric surgery: Nutritional and drug issues. General recommendations for the prevention and treatment of nutritional deficiencies. *Diabetes Metab.* 2009 Dec; 35(6 Pt 2):544–557.

90. Malinowski SS. Nutritional and metabolic complications of bariatric. *Am J Med Sci.* 2006 Apr; 331(4):219–225.

91. Kushner R. Managing the obese patient after bariatric surgery: A case report of severe malnutrition and review of the literature. *J Parenter Enteral Nutr.* 2000; 24:126–32.

92. Brolin RE, Leung M. Survey of vitamin and mineral supplementation after gastric bypass and biliopancreatic diversion for morbid obesity. *Obes Surg.* 1999; 9:150–154.

93. Angstadt JD, Bodziner RA. Peripheral polyneuropathy from thiamine deficiency following laparoscopic Roux-en-Y gastric bypass. *Obes Surg.* 2005; 15:890–892.

94. Singh S, Kumar A. Wernicki encephalopathy after obesity surgery: A systematic review. *Neurology.* 2007; 68:807–811.

95. Schweitzer DH, Posthuma EF. Prevention of vitamin and mineral deficiencies after bariatric surgery: Evidence and algorithms. *Obes Surg.* 2008 Nov; 18(11):1485–1488. Epub 2008 Mar 28.

96. Slater GH, Ren CJ, Siegel N, Williams T, Barr D, Wolfe B, Dolan K, Fielding GA. Serum fat-soluble vitamin deficiency and abnormal calcium metabolism after malabsorptive bariatric surgery. *J Gastrointest Surg.* 2004 Jan; 8(1):48–55.

97. Boylan LM, Sugerman HJ, Driskell JA. Vitamin E, vitamin B-6, vitamin B-12, and folate status of gastric bypass surgery patients. *J Am Diet Assoc.* 1988 May; 88(5):579–585.

98. Rino Y, Suzuki Y, Kuroiwa Y, Yukawa N, Saeki H, Kanari M, Wada H, Ino H, Takanashi Y, Imada T. Vitamin E malabsorption and neurological consequences after gastrectomy for gastric cancer. *Hepatogastroenterology.* 2007 Sep; 54(78):1858–1861.

99. Shankar P, Boylan M, Sriram K. Micronutrient deficiencies after bariatric surgery. *Nutrition.* 2010 Nov–Dec; 26(11–12):1031–1037. Epub 2010 Apr 3.

100. Stocker DJ. Management of the bariatric surgery patient. *Endocrinol Metab Clin N Am.* 2003; 32:437–457.

101. Brolin RE. Gastric bypass. *Surg Clin N Am.* 2001; 81:1077–1095.

102. Decker GA, Swain JM, Crowell MD, Scolapio JS. Gastrointestinal and nutritional complications after bariatric surgery. *Am J Gastroenterol.* 2007; 102:2571–2580.
103. Sallé A, Demarsy D, Poirier AL, Lelièvre B, Topart P, Guilloteau G, Bécouarn G, Rohmer V. Zinc deficiency: A frequent and underestimated complication after bariatric surgery. *Obes Surg.* 2010 Dec; 20(12):1660–1670.
104. Neve HJ, Bhatti WA, Soulsby C, Kincey J, Taylor V. Reversal of hair loss following vertical gastroplasty when treated with zinc sulphate. *Obes Surg.* 1996; 6:63–65.
105. Balsa JA, Botella-Carretero JI, Gómez-Martín JM, Peromingo R, Arrieta F, Santiuste C, Zamarrón I, Vázquez C. Copper and zinc serum levels after derivative bariatric surgery: Differences between Roux-en-Y gastric bypass and biliopancreatic diversion. *Obes Surg.* 2011 Jun; 21(6):744–750.
106. Jaiser SR, Winston GP. Copper deficiency myelopathy. *J Neurol.* 2010; 257:869–881.
107. Kumar N, Ahlskog JE, Gross JB Jr. Acquired hypocupremia after gastric surgery. *Clin Gastroenterol Hepatol.* 2004; 2:1074–1079.
108. Sandstead, HH. Zinc interference with copper metabolism. *JAMA.* 1978; 240:2188–2189.
109. Shahidzadeh R, Sridhar S. Profound copper deficiency in a patient with gastric bypass. *Am J Gastroenterol.* 2008 Oct; 103(10):2660–2662.
110. Murthy AS. Obesity and contraception: Emerging issues. *Semin Reprod Med.* 2010; 28:156–164.

11 Obesity and Health
Implications of Public Policy

Gregory W. Heath, DHSc, MPH, FACSM, FAHA

CONTENTS

INTRODUCTION

In light of the rapidly increasing obesity rates among adults and children/youth in the United States over the past 30 years,[1-5] and the failed attempts to curb this epidemic through individual-based approaches of behavior change,[6] communities have sought to implement more broad-based policy and environmental supports to address the energy-balance behaviors of healthy eating, active living, and decreased sedentary behavior (e.g., greater access to full-service grocery stores, affordable healthy foods, and access to safe places for physical activity and play).[7,8]

States and local communities appear to have had some success in developing and implementing a number of these environmental and policy supports for healthy eating and active living[9-12] and have provided public health decision makers and community leaders a growing evidence-base to draw from in addressing community-wide efforts to prevent obesity. However, there currently is a paucity of established measures with which to evaluate specific policy and environmental changes and their apparent impact on the energy-balance behaviors associated with this epidemic. To address this issue, the Centers for Disease Control and Prevention (CDC) recently published a set of Common Community Measures for Obesity Prevention.[13] The Common Community Measures report seeks to identify and recommend a set of obesity prevention strategies and corresponding suggested measurements that local governments and communities can use to plan, implement, and monitor initiatives to prevent obesity (see Table 11.1).

TABLE 11.1

Summary of Recommended Community Policy Strategies and Measurements to Prevent Obesity

Strategies to promote the availability of affordable healthy food and beverages

Strategy	*Communities should increase availability of healthier food and beverage choices in public service venues.*
Suggested measurement	A policy exists to apply nutrition standards that are consistent with the dietary guidelines for Americans [68] to all food sold (e.g., meal menus and vending machines) within local government facilities in a local jurisdiction or on public school campuses during the school day within the largest school district in a local jurisdiction.
Strategy	*Communities should improve availability of affordable healthier food and beverage choices in public service venues.*
Suggested measurement	A policy exists to affect the cost of healthier foods and beverages (as defined by the Institute of Medicine (IOM)[69] relative to the cost of less healthy foods and beverages sold within local government facilities in a local jurisdiction or on public school campuses during the school day within the largest school district in a local jurisdiction.
Strategy	*Communities should provide incentives for the production, distribution, and procurement of foods from local farms.*
Suggested measurement	Local government has a policy that encourages the production, distribution, or procurement of food from local farms in the local jurisdiction.

Strategies to support healthy food and beverage choices

Strategy	*Communities should restrict availability of less healthy foods and beverages in public service venues.*
Suggested measurement	A policy exists that prohibits the sale of less healthy foods and beverages (as defined by IOM [Institute of Medicine. *Preventing Childhood Obesity: Health in the Balance.* Washington, DC: The National Academies Press; 2005]) within local government facilities in a local jurisdiction or on public school campuses during the school day within the largest school district in a local jurisdiction.
Strategy	*Communities should institute smaller portion size options in public service venues.*
Suggested measurement	Local government has a policy to limit the portion size of any entree (including sandwiches and entrée salads) by either reducing the standard portion size of entrees or offering smaller portion sizes in addition to standard portion sizes within local government facilities within a local jurisdiction.
Strategy	*Communities should limit advertisements of less healthy foods and beverages.*
Suggested measurement	A policy exists that limits advertising and promotion of less healthy foods and beverages within local government facilities in a local jurisdiction or on public school campuses during the school day within the largest school district in a local jurisdiction.

TABLE 11.1 (continued)
Summary of Recommended Community Policy Strategies and Measurements to Prevent Obesity

Strategy	*Communities should discourage consumption of sugar-sweetened beverages.*
Suggested measurement	Licensed child care facilities within the local jurisdiction are required to ban sugar-sweetened beverages, including flavored/sweetened milk and limit the portion size of 100% juice.

Strategy to encourage breastfeeding

Strategy	*Communities should increase support for breastfeeding.*
Suggested measurement	Local government has a policy requiring local government facilities to provide breastfeeding accommodations for employees that include both time and private space for breastfeeding during working hours.

Strategies to encourage physical activity or limit sedentary activity among children and youth

Strategy	*Communities should require physical education in schools.*
Suggested measurement	The largest school district located within the local jurisdiction has a policy that requires a minimum of 150 min per week of PE in public elementary schools and a minimum of 225 min per week of PE in public middle schools and high schools throughout the school year (as recommended by the National Association of Sports and Physical Education).
Strategy	*Communities should increase the amount of physical activity in PE programs in schools.*
Suggested measurement	The largest school district located within the local jurisdiction has a policy that requires K–12 students to be physically active for at least 50% of time spent in PE classes in public schools.

Strategies to create safe communities that support physical activity

Strategy	*Communities should support locating schools within easy walking distance of residential areas.*
Suggested measurement	The largest school district in the local jurisdiction has a policy that supports locating new schools, and/or repairing or expanding existing schools, within easy walking or biking distance of residential areas.
Strategy	*Communities should enhance traffic safety in areas where persons are or could be physically active.*
Suggested measurement	Local government has a policy for designing and operating streets with safe access for all users, which includes at least one element suggested by the national complete streets coalition (http://www.completestreets.org).

Source: Adapted from CDC, *MMWR*, 58(RR-7), 1, 2009.

CDC defines measurement "as a single data element that can be collected through an objective assessment of policies or the physical environment and that can be used to quantify the performance of an obesity prevention strategy."[13] CDC defined community as "a social entity that can be classified spatially on the basis of where persons live, work, learn, worship, and play (e.g., homes, schools, parks, roads, and neighborhoods)."[13,14]

   The role of public policy and environmental supports in meting out effective public health programming and services has historically been part of the success of
efforts to address a number of public health challenges.[15] Those success stories where
policies have been combined with programmatic efforts, health services delivery,
and community promotion include vaccinations,[16] motor vehicle safety and prevention of injuries (CDC 1999c),[17] workplace safety,[18] prevention and control of infectious diseases,[19] promote healthy mothers and healthy babies,[20] ensure food satety,[21]
prevention of dental caries,[22] and the prevention of tobacco use.[23] The current chapter
seeks to outline a number of policies and policy-informed environmental supports
at various levels (e.g., national, state, and local), all of which have application for
promoting active living and healthy eating and the prevention of obesity. We first
examine agricultural and food supply policies, followed by health-care sector policies, educational and school-based policies, and finally address urban design/land-
use and transportation policies.

AGRICULTURE AND FOOD SUPPLY POLICIES
THAT SUPPORT HEALTHY EATING

At the federal level, the Food, Conservation, and Energy Act of 2008 (Farm Bill)
holds the most promise to affect the food supply in the United States. Over 50% of
the funds appropriated in this bill are allocated to nutrition/healthy eating programs.
This includes the national school meals programs, community food security, promotion of farmers' markets, fruit and vegetable promotion, and the Supplemental
Nutrition Assistance Program, which in the past was known as the Food Stamp program. The 2008 reauthorization of the Farm Bill allocates approximately 15% of its
funds to subsidize soybean and corn production.[24] These crops are less expensive
and are often used in food production thereby lowering the cost of many foods.
One consequence of this legislation is making such products as high-fructose corn
syrup more available for foods and sugared drinks. This product is an inexpensive
sweetener for sweetened drinks and has become more easily available in food stores
and eating establishments. It is significant to note that the percentage of adolescents
consuming carbonated sugary drinks (regular and low calorie) has risen by 48%
between 1977 and 1998[25] while among adults the rise has been 100% over the same
period of time.[26,27] Even more alarming is that carbonated sugared drinks account for
almost 14% of the total calorie intake per day for youth aged 12–19 years.[28]
   A significant breakthrough in the recent reauthorization of the Farm Bill is that
it provides $1.3 billion in new funding over 10 years for growing fruits, vegetables,
and nuts.[24] It also increases the funding of programs that support farmers' markets
and provides vouchers for low-income seniors to purchase fruits and vegetables from
local farmers.[24] At the state level, the Farm Bill provides about $500 million toward
the provision of fresh fruit and/or vegetable snacks in schools and allows schools to
have a greater variety of choices in buying foods from local farmers.[24]
   State and local efforts to enhance the consumption of healthier foods have
emerged, which include policies that affect lowering the cost of healthier foods and
drinks. Evidence exists that reducing the cost of healthier foods actually increases the

purchase of these foods.[29,30] For example, French et al.[31] demonstrated that the intake of fruits and carrots in high-school cafeterias increased after the price of these items was reduced. Similar results with an increase in the purchase of healthier foods were found when the price of low-fat snacks in vending machines in both school and work settings was lowered.[32,33] Further evidence supporting pricing reform is provided by Dong and Lin,[34] who demonstrated that a subsidized 10% price reduction on fruits and vegetables directly influenced low-income persons to increase their daily consumption of fruits vegetables. Additional studies have demonstrated similar results for interventions that use coupons redeemable for healthier foods and also price reduction incentives for purchasing healthier foods. These efforts have had the effect of increasing the purchase and consumption of healthier foods among a number of different population subgroups that include college students, participants in the Supplemental Nutrition Program for Women, Infants, and Children (WIC), and low-income older adults.[35–37] A more recent example of the successful use of vouchers among WIC participants was a community-based effort reported by Herman et al.,[38] where participants who received weekly $10 vouchers for fresh produce increased their consumption of fruits and vegetables compared with a control group with an effect lasting 6 months following the intervention.

It is commonly known that so-called supermarkets and full service grocery stores generally have a wider selection of fresh fruits and vegetables prices, which are lower than smaller grocery stores and convenience stores. Morland et al.[39] and Larson et al.[40] have independently shown that low-income, minority urban as well as rural communities have fewer full service grocery stores when compared with affluent suburban areas. Evidence also exists to support the notion that improved access to full service grocery stores positively impacts shoppers' selection of healthier foods and healthy eating.[40] A large population-based study consisting of over 10,000 respondents indicated that blacks who lived in neighborhoods with at least one full-service grocery store were more likely to eat five or more servings of fruits and vegetables compared with blacks living in neighborhoods without such grocery stores.[41] A recent study among over 70,000 adolescents established an association of BMI with food store availability.[42] Among these adolescents, controlling for socioeconomic status, greater access to grocery stores was associated with lower BMI while a higher concentration of convenience stores was associated with higher BMI.[42] Furthermore, evidence along these same lines is available that suggests that the availability of retail stores offering healthier food and drink choices is associated with both an increased intake of fruits and vegetables and a lower BMI.[43]

HEALTH CARE SERVICE POLICIES

At the national level, the National Committee for Quality Assurance (NCQA) starting in early 2006 approved the Healthcare Effectiveness Data and Information Set (HEDIS) measures of health plan performance regarding the measurement of physical activity and BMI as "vital signs" among adults, children, and adolescents. In addition, nutrition and physical activity assessment and counseling for adults, children, and adolescents were also recommended. Most U.S. health plans use HEDIS measures to monitor provider performance associated with patient care and services and report to providers, purchasers of health-care plans, and consumers on the quality of health care throughout the nation.[44] The new chronic disease prevention and obesity-related measures attempt to target improvements in providers' practice behaviors related to chronic disease and obesity prevention, care, and treatment. The launching of such chronic disease/obesity-related HEDIS measures demonstrates the role that a policy intervention can potentially impact health behavior change.

The Patient Protection and Affordable Care Act, often shortened to Affordable Care Act (ACA) of 2010, was signed into law on March 23, 2010. This attempted overhaul of the U.S. health-care delivery system is still being implemented and debated within the halls of Congress as well as within state legislatures and halls of justice. However, elements of the ACA will no doubt continue to be implemented. These elements include components within ACA that promise to have an impact on obesity prevention through the health-care delivery system itself.[45] Such components include increased Medicaid payments in fee-for-service and managed care for primary-care services provided by primary-care doctors (family medicine, general internal medicine, or pediatric medicine), including a 10% bonus payment to primary-care physicians in Medicare from 2011 to 2015.[45] These actions are intended to provide greater incentives for primary-care providers to integrate preventive care services into their practices. Included in ACA is the establishment of a National Prevention, Health Promotion and Public Health Council to coordinate federal prevention, wellness, and public health activities. This council will develop a national strategy to improve the nation's health, create a Prevention and Public Health Fund to expand and sustain funding for prevention and public health programs, and create working groups associated with the Clinical Preventive Services and Community Preventive Services Task Forces[46] to develop, update, and disseminate evidenced-based recommendations on the use of clinical and community prevention services. Further efforts will be made to provide coverage of preventive services that have been shown to be effective and further modification and possible elimination of cost-sharing for preventive services in Medicare and Medicaid. Finally, there will be an increase in Medicare payments for certain preventive services up to 100% of actual charges or fee schedule rates that are intended to include obesity prevention services.[45]

Examples of state-specific policies affecting preventive care include Act 1220, a state law passed in 2003 in Arkansas, which offers several strategies to address obesity in children and adolescents. The bill included the widespread measurement of BMI in all schoolchildren, limited vending machine access in public elementary schools, required reporting of vending machine profits by schools and reporting on contractual agreements with sugary drink companies. In addition, this legislation created specific regional/local advisory committees of parents, teachers, and local community leaders. Furthermore, Arkansas has established a law-based screening policy that will provide health monitoring information for the state, which includes the routine collection of state-specific and local data using the Youth Risk Behavior Surveillance System (YRBSS) and the Behavioral Risk Factor Surveillance System (BRFSS). In July 2004, the Centers for Medicare and Medicaid (CMS) established that obesity was a recognized disease in order to permit Medicare to consider covering payments for obesity-related treatments.[47] Despite Medicaid being a state administered program, the Medicare decision stimulated a number of states to extend their Medicaid programs' coverage of services to include both prevention and treatment of obesity. Examples include West Virginia[48] and Tennessee,[49] which offer both full and partial reimbursement for Weight Watchers programs.

EDUCATIONAL AND SCHOOL-BASED POLICIES

State and local education agencies are beginning to enforce newly adopted federal regulations, statutes, community planning guidelines, and active living guidelines that provide local communities guidance to improve school location sites, implement complete streets, regulate the nutritional value of foods and beverages available to students, and implement evidence-based physical education (PE) programming. For example, as of June 2008, a total of 25 states had established nutritional standards for "competitive foods," that is, foods and beverages available in schools but not approved for reimbursement under the National School Lunch Program.[50] Twenty-seven states had restricted the sale of competitive foods more tightly than did federal requirements, and 18 had adopted nutritional standards for in-school meals that were stricter than those required by the U.S. Department of Agriculture.[51]

School Siting

Walking and bicycling to and from school has been demonstrated to increase physical activity among children as part of active transport.[52]

The increased energy expenditure during active transport can potentially contribute to improved energy balance and the prevention of overweight and obesity. However, the proportion of students walking and/or bicycling to and from school has dropped precipitously over the past 40 years, in part because of the increased distance between children's homes and schools that has occurred over the same period of time.[53] Heath et al.[11] in their systematic review identified an evidence-base for community-scale urban design and land-use policies and practices that included locating schools, stores, workplaces, and recreation areas close to residential areas, thus promoting an increase in levels of physical activity among children and adults. An earlier simulation study identified school location and the quality of the built environment as producing a 13% increase in walking and biking to school.[54] Based on their findings, this same group proposed that the current trend of building larger schools associated with larger catchment areas should be replaced with an effort to locate schools within neighborhoods in order to facilitate decreased motorized transport, decreased air pollution, and increased active transport.[54] The decrease in walking to and from school has also been attributed to a poor walking environment, defined as a built environment that has low-population densities, little mixing of land uses, long blocks, and incomplete sidewalks.[54] This observation has been reinforced by evidence demonstrating that street-scale changes, such as mixed use, aesthetics, and continuity of sidewalks, lighting, and landscape increase physical activity and active transport.[11]

SCHOOL-BASED FOOD POLICIES

School-based policies that restrict access to sugary drinks (e.g., soda, juice drinks, energy, and sport drinks) may be an effective strategy to keep children and adolescents from over consuming calories. An example of such a strategy was carried out among American Indian high-school students where education to decrease the consumption of sugar-sweetened drinks was combined with an increased knowledge of diabetes risk factors through a youth-oriented fitness center.[55] The investigators demonstrated a substantial reduction in consumption of sugar-sweetened drinks over a 3 year period, which was accompanied by positive changes in glucose metabolism.[55] Further support for environmental interventions that seek to eliminate sugar-sweetened drinks is described by Ebbeling et al.,[56] where the intervention targeted homes of a diverse group of adolescents and demonstrated that, among heavier adolescents, exposure to the intervention resulted in a more significant decrease in BMI compared with controls. In addition to reducing access to sugary drinks, as an effective intervention to affect energy balance among children, increasing access to fresh fruits and vegetables has also proved to be effective in increasing consumption of such foods.[57,58] Another demonstration of increasing access to healthy foods to students consisted of a 2 year randomized control trial of a school-based environmental intervention that increased access to lower-fat foods in cafeteria à la carte areas and showed an increase in sales of lower-fat foods among those adolescents exposed to the intervention.[59]

SCHOOL-BASED PHYSICAL ACTIVITY POLICIES

A significant number of states mandate some level of PE in schools: 36 states mandate PE for elementary-school students, 33 states mandate PE for middle-school students, and 42 states mandate PE for high-school students.[60] Implementation of quality PE classes in schools has faced and continues to face major obstacles. These include the misconception of school administrators and teachers that PE classes compete with academic curricula and negatively influence academic performance. On the contrary, Kahn et al.,[61] in their systematic review that included 14 studies examining school-based PE, found that time spent in PE classes did not harm academic performance and was effective in increasing levels of physical activity and improving physical fitness. The review included studies of interventions that increased the amount of time spent in PE classes, the amount of time students are active during PE classes, or the amount of moderate or vigorous physical activity (MVPA) students engage in during PE classes. Increasing the amount of physical activity in school-based PE classes has also been demonstrated to be effective in increasing fitness among children.[61]

URBAN DESIGN, LAND-USE, AND TRANSPORTATION POLICIES FOR ACTIVE LIVING/HEALTHY EATING

Recent reviews have outlined the important role that access to places for physical activity and community-scale and street-scale environmental infrastructure can play in promoting physical activity and active living.[11,61] Ensuring the appropriate use and preservation of land, effective urban planning for active living, presence of efficient public transportation, and the availability of supportive infrastructure for active living are most adequately supported by appropriate policies and legislation. At the national level, the Transportation Bill, known as the Safe, Accountable Flexible Efficient Transportation Equity Act: A Legacy for Users (SAFETEA-LU), is a bill that, similar to the Farm Bill for nutrition, assures effective transportation policy at the national, state, and local levels. The bill, for example, has a section dedicated to metropolitan transportation planning, which is inclusive of all modes of transportation, including public transportation, walking, and bicycling. Besser and Dannenberg[62] demonstrated that 30% of persons who use public transportation achieve the recommended 150 min of physical activity per week by walking to and from public transportation from their homes and their jobs. The bill also contains funding support for bicycle lanes and pedestrian walkways, recreational trails, and the National Safe Routes to School Program, a federal initiative to promote children walking and bicycling to school.

Open space and outdoor recreational facilities provide space for people to participate in active living. These spaces include parks and green space, sports fields, walking and biking trails, public pools, and playgrounds. Accessibility of recreation facilities depends on a number of factors such as proximity to homes or schools, cost, hours of operation, and ease of access. Improving access to recreation facilities and places when combined with informational outreach has been shown to increase physical activity among children, adolescents, and adults.[61] In another comprehensive review of 108 studies, it was determined that access to facilities and programs for recreation near their homes, and time spent outdoors, correlated positively with increased physical activity among children and adolescents.[63] Enhancing infrastructure supporting bicycling includes creating bike lanes, shared-use paths, and routes on existing and new roads and providing bike racks in the vicinity of commercial and other public spaces. Improving bicycling infrastructure can be effective in increasing frequency of cycling for utilitarian purposes (e.g., commuting to work and school and bicycling for errands). Longitudinal intervention studies have demonstrated that improving bicycling infrastructure is associated with increased frequency of bicycling.[64,65]

Heath et al.[11] have reviewed the role of infrastructure in supporting walking and other forms of physical activity. Well-developed infrastructure supporting walking is an important element of the built environment and has been demonstrated to be associated with physical activity in adults and children.[11] Interventions aimed at supporting infrastructure for walking are included in street-scale urban design and land-use interventions that support physical activity in small geographic areas. These interventions can include improved street lighting, infrastructure projects to increase the safety of street crossings, use of traffic calming approaches (e.g., speed humps and traffic circles), and enhancing street landscaping.[11] These results comply with the guidelines for assessing effectiveness of community-based interventions from the Guide to Community Preventive Services, 2000. Intervention studies demonstrate the cost-effectiveness of enhanced walking infrastructure when combined with other strategies.[66] The evaluation of the Marin County Safe Routes to School program is an example where creating safe routes to school, together with educational components, increased the number of students walking to school.[65]

Zoning for mixed-use development is one type of community-scale land-use policy and practice that allows residential, commercial, institutional, and other public land uses to be located in close proximity to one another. Mixed-use development decreases the distance between destinations (e.g., home and shopping), which has been demonstrated to decrease the number of trips persons make by automobile and increase the number of trips persons make on foot or by bicycle. Heath et al.[11] identified mixed-use development and diversity of residential and commercial developments as examples of community-scale urban design and land-use policies and practices and showed that these characteristics increase physical activity. This evidence review identified street-scale urban design land-use policies and practices, which included interventions that sought to improve traffic safety and found that these practices were effective in increasing physical activity.[11] Included in these interventions were design characteristics that improved street lighting, infrastructure projects that increased pedestrian safety at street crossings, and use of traffic calming measures such as speed humps and round abouts.[11] Further support for the association of the role of the built environment on transport, physical activity, and obesity was recently reported by Durand et al.[67]

CONCLUSIONS

Evidence exists that policies at the national, state, and local levels can affect the energy-balance behaviors of active living and healthy eating. These policies appear most effective when addressing healthy food access and availability, health-care delivery systems that seek to integrate preventive strategies addressing healthy eating and active living, school-based access to healthy eating and active living, and a built environment that is supported by active living policies and practices. Such a comprehensive policy strategy can do much to support health-care providers in effectively assessing and counseling their patients in preventing weight gain and the associated outcomes of overweight, obesity, and attendant chronic diseases/conditions. In addition, such policies become the necessary scaffolding by which the normative health behaviors of eating and activity are shifted more toward healthy eating and active living. Thus, the recommendations and prescription from health-care providers for achieving and maintaining a healthy weight and improved body composition can be effectively reinforced with a greater likelihood of sustained benefits.

REFERENCES

1. Visscher TL, Seidell JC. 2001. The public health impact of obesity. *Annual Review of Public Health* 22:355–375.
2. Ogden CL, Carroll, MD, Curtin, LR et al. 2006. Prevalence of overweight and obesity in the United States, 1999–2004. *JAMA* 295:1549–1555.
3. Poirier P, Giles TD, Bray GA, Hong Y, Stern JS, Pi-Sunyer FX, Eckel RH. 2006. Obesity and cardiovascular disease: Pathophysiology, evaluation, and effect of weight loss: An update of the 1997 American Heart Association Scientific Statement on Obesity and Heart Disease from the Obesity Committee of the Council on Nutrition, Physical Activity, and Metabolism. *Circulation* 113:898–918.

4. Ogden CL, Carroll MD, Flegal KM. 2008. High body mass index for age among U.S. children and adolescents, 2003–2006. *JAMA* 299:2401–2405.

5. CDC. 2008. Prevalence of overweight, obesity, and extreme obesity among adults: United States, Trends 1976–80 through 2005–2006. Hyattsville, MD: U.S. Department of Health and Human Services, National Center for Health Statistics, CDC.

6. Lombard CB, Deeks AA, Teede HJ. 2009. A systematic review of interventions aimed at the prevention of weight gain in adults. *Public Health Nutr* 12:2236–2246.

7. U.S. Department of Health and Human Services. 2001. The Surgeon General's call to action to prevent and decrease overweight and obesity. Rockville, MD: U.S. Department of Health and Human Services, Public Health Service, Office of the Surgeon General.

8. Koplan J, Liverman CT, Kraak VI; Committee on Prevention of Obesity in Children and Youth. 2005. Preventing childhood obesity: Health in the balance: Executive summary. *J. Am. Diet. Assoc.* 105(1):131–138.

9. Hill JO, Peters JC. 1998. Environmental contributions to the obesity epidemic. *Science* 280:1371–1374.

10. Sallis JF, Glanz K. 2006. The role of built environments in physical activity, eating, and obesity in childhood. *Future Child* 16:89–108.

11. Heath GW, Brownson RC, Kruger J et al. 2006. The effectiveness of urban design and land use and transport policies and practices to increase physical activity: A systematic review. *Journal of Physical Activity and Health* 3(Suppl 1):S55–S76.

12. Sallis JF, Glanz K. 2009. Physical activity and food environments: Solutions to the obesity epidemic. *The Milbank Quarterly* 87:123–154.

13. CDC. 2009. Recommended community strategies and measurements to prevent obesity in the United States. *MMWR* 58(RR-7):1–29.

14. Keener D, Goodman K, Lowry A, Zaro S, Kettel Khan L. 2009. Recommended community strategies and measurements to prevent obesity in the United States: Implementation and measurement guide. Atlanta, GA: U.S. Department of Health and Human Services, Centers for Disease Control and Prevention.

15. Centers for Disease Control and Prevention (CDC). 1999. Ten great public health achievements—United States, 1900–1999. *MMWR* 48:241–243.

16. CDC. 1999. Impact of vaccines universally recommended for children—United States, 1990–1998. *MMWR* 48:243–248.

17. CDC. 1999. Motor-vehicle safety: A 20th century public health achievement. *MMWR* 48:369–374.

18. CDC. 1999. Improvements in workplace safety—United States, 1900–1999. *MMWR* 48:461–469.

19. CDC. 1999. Control of infectious diseases. *MMWR* 48:621–629.

20. CDC. 1999. Healthier mothers and babies. *MMWR* 48:849–857.

21. CDC. 1999. Safer and healthier foods. *MMWR* 48:905–913.

22. CDC. 1999. Fluoridation of drinking water to prevent dental caries. *MMWR* 48:933–940.

23. CDC. 1999. Tobacco use—United States, 1900–1999. *MMWR* 48:986–993.

24. Dietz WH, Benken DL, Hunter AS. 2009. Public health law and the prevention and control of obesity. *The Milbank Quarterly* 87:215–227.

25. French SA, Lin BH, Guthrie JF. 2003. National trends in soft drink consumption among children and adolescents age 6 to 17 Years: Prevalence, amounts, and sources, 1977/1978 to 1994/1998. *Journal of the American Dietetic Association* 103(10):1326–1331.

26. Enns C, Goldman J, Cook A. 1997. Trends in food and nutrient intakes by adults: NFCS 1977–78, CSFI 1989–91, and CSFII 1994–95. *Family Economics and Nutrition Review* 10(4):2–15.

27. Enns C, Mickle S, Goldman J. 2002. Trends in food and nutrient intakes by children in the United States. *Family Economics and Nutrition Review* 14(2):56–68.

28. Wang YC, Bleich SN, Gortmaker SL. 2008. Increasing caloric contribution from sugar-sweetened beverages and 100% fruit juices among U.S. children and adolescents, 1988–2004. *Pediatrics* 121:e1604–e1614.

29. French SA, Story M, Jeffrey RW. 2001. Environmental influences on eating and physical activity. *Annual Review of Public Health* 22:309–335.

30. Seymour JD, Yaroch AL, Serdula M et al. 2004. Impact of nutrition environmental interventions on point-of-purchase behavior in adults: A review. *Preventive Medicine* 39(Suppl 2):S108–S136.

31. French SA, Story M, Jeffery RW et al. 1997. Pricing strategy to promote fruit and vegetable purchase in high school cafeterias. *Journal of the American Dietetic Association* 97:1008–1010.

32. French SA, Jeffery RW, Story M et al. 2001. Pricing and promotion effects on low-fat vending snack purchases: The CHIPS Study. *American Journal of Public Health* 91:112–117.

33. French SA, Jeffery, RW, Story M et al. 1997. A pricing strategy to promote low-fat snack choices through vending machines. *American Journal of Public Health* 87:849–851.

34. Dong D, Lin B. 2009. Fruit and vegetable consumption by low-income Americans: Would a price reduction make a difference? Washington, DC: US Department of Agriculture, Economic Research Service.

35. Anderson JV, Bybee DI, Brown RM et al. 2001. Five a day fruit and vegetable intervention improves consumption in a low income population. *Journal of the American Dietetic Association* 101:195–202.

36. Cincirpini P. 1984. Changing food selections in a public cafeteria: An applied behavioral analysis. *Behavioral Modification* 8:520–539.

37. Jeffery RW, French SA, Raether C, Baxter JE. 1994. An environmental intervention to increase fruit and salad purchases in a cafeteria. *Preventive Medicine* 23:788–792.

38. Herman DR, Harrison GG, Afifi AA, Jenks E. 2008. Effect of a targeted subsidy on intake of fruits and vegetables among low-income women in the Special Supplemental Nutrition Program for Women, Infants, and Children. *American Journal of Public Health* 98:98–105.

39. Morland K, Wing S, Diez Roux A, Poole C. 2002. Neighborhood characteristics associated with the location of food stores and food service places. *American Journal of Preventive Medicine* 22:23–29.

40. Larson NI, Story MT, Nelson MC. 2008. Neighborhood environments: Disparities in access to healthy foods in the U.S. *American Journal of Preventive Medicine* 36:74–81.

41. Morland K, Wing S, Diez Roux A. 2002. The contextual effect of the local food environment on residents' diets: The atherosclerosis risk in communities study. *American Journal of Public Health* 92:1761–1767.

42. Powell LM, Auld MC, Chaloupka FJ et al. 2007. Associations between access to food stores and adolescent body mass index. *American Journal of Preventive Medicine* 33(Suppl):S301–S307.

43. Zenk SN, Schulz AJ, Hollis-Neely T et al. 2005. Fruit and vegetable intake in African Americans' income and store characteristics. *American Journal of Preventive Medicine* 29:1–9.

44. National Committee for Quality Assurance (NCQA). 2011. Performance Measures for Wellness and Healthy Promotion Accreditation. Available at http://www.ncqa.org/tabid/1255/Default.aspx (accessed March 3, 2011).

45. Henry J. Kaiser Foundation. 2010. Summary of New Health Reform Law. Available at http://www.kff.org/healthreform/upload/8061.pdf (accessed March 1, 2011).

46. Task Force on Community Preventive Services. 2000. Introducing the *Guide to Community Preventive Services*: Methods, first recommendations, and expert commentary. *American Journal of Preventive Medicine* 18(1S):1–142.

47. Centers for Medicaid and Medicare Services (CMS). 2004. *Treatment of Obesity*. MLN: M3502. Washington, DC: USDA.

48. Unicare. 2007. Lifestyle management: A wellness program that helps you take steps toward improving your health in key areas, such as: Losing weight, getting fit, eating healthier, managing stress and kicking cigarette. Available at http://www.unicare.com

49. Tenncare. 2005. Tenncare tackling obesity through Weight Loss Program with Weight Watchers. Media release. Available at http://tennessee.gov/tenncare/forms/151105.pdf

50. U.S. Department of Agriculture (USDA), Food and Nutrition Service. 2004. Measuring competitive foods in schools: Methods and challenges. Available at http://www.fns.usda.gov/oane/menu/published/CNP/FILES/CompFoodSum.pdf (accessed March 3, 2011).

51. Trust for America's Health. 2008. F as in Fat: How obesity policies are failing in America, 2008. Available at http://www.healthyamericans.org

52. Saelens B, Sallis J, Frank L. 2003. Environmental correlates of walking and cycling: Findings from the transportation, urban design, and planning literatures. *Annals of Behavioral Medicine* 25(2):80–91.

53. Ewing R, Cervero R. 2001. Travel and the built environment. *Transportation Research Record* 1780:87–114.

54. Environmental Protection Agency. EPA 231-R-03-004. 2003. Travel and environmental implications of school siting. Washington, DC: Environmental Protection Agency.

55. Ritenbaugh C, Teufel-Shone NI, Aickin MG et al. 2003. A lifestyle intervention improves plasma insulin levels among Native American high school youth. *Preventive Medicine* 36:309–319.

56. Ebbeling CB, Feldman HA, Osganian SK et al. 2006. Effects of decreasing sugar-sweetened beverage consumption on body weight in adolescents: A randomized, controlled pilot study. *Pediatrics* 117:673–680.

57. Faith MS, Fontaine KR, Baskin ML, Allison DB. 2007. Toward the reduction of population obesity: Macrolevel environmental approaches to the problems of food, eating, and obesity. *Psychological Bulletin* 133:205–226.

58. Jago R, Baranowski T, Baranowski JC. 2007. Fruit and vegetable availability: A micro environmental mediating variable? *Public Health Nutrition* 10:681–689.

59. French SA, Story M, Fulkesron JA, Hannan P. 2004. An environmental intervention to promote lower-fat food choices in secondary schools: Outcomes of the TACOS Study. *American Journal of Public Health* 94:1507–1512.

60. National Association for Sport and Physical Education and American Health Association (NASPE). 2006. Shape of the nation report: Status of physical education in the USA. Reston, VA: National Association for Sport and Physical Education.

61. Kahn EB, Ramsey LT, Brownson RC, Heath GW, Howze EH, Powell KE, Stone EJ, Rajab MW, Corso P. 2002. The effectiveness of interventions to increase physical activity. A systematic review. *American Journal of Preventive Medicine* 22(4 Suppl):73–107.

62. Besser LM, Dannenberg AL. 2005. Walking to public transit: Steps to help meet physical activity recommendations. *American Journal of Preventive Medicine* 29:273–280.

63. Sallis JF, Prochaska JJ, Taylor WC. 2000. A review of correlates of physical activity of children and adolescents. *Medicine & Science in Sports & Exercise* 32:963–975.

64. Macbeth AG. 1999. Bicycle lanes in Toronto. *ITE Journal* 69:38–46.

65. Staunton CE, Hubsmith D, Kallins W. 2003. Promoting safe walking and biking to school: The Marin County success story. *American Journal of Public Health* 93:1431–1434.

66. Wang G, Macera CA, Scudder-Soucie B, Schmid T, Pratt M, Buchner D. 2004. Cost effectiveness of a bicycle/pedestrian trail development in health promotion. *Preventive Medicine* 38(2):237–242.
67. Durand CP, Andalib M, Dunton GF, Wolch J, Pentz MA. 2011. A systematic review of built environment factors related to physical activity and obesity risk: Implications for smart growth urban planning. *Obesity Reviews* 10:67–78 [Epub ahead of print].
68. U.S. Department of Health and Human Services, U.S. Department of Agriculture 2005. *Dietary Guidelines for Americans*, 6th edn. Washington, DC: U.S. Government Printing Office.
69. Institute of Medicine. 2005. *Preventing Childhood Obesity: Health in the Balance.* Washington, DC: The National Academies Press.

Part II

Obesity and Specific
Medical Conditions

12 Obesity and Heart Disease

James M. Rippe, MD and
Theodore J. Angelopoulos, PhD, MPH

CONTENTS

The obesity epidemic in the United States and in many other industrialized countries has reached alarming proportions.[1,2] This epidemic has also reached global proportions impacting both industrialized and nonindustrialized countries.[3,4] Substantial increases in the prevalence of obesity have occurred in both genders and all age groups in the past 30 years.[5,6] While recent data suggest that the rate of increase in the prevalence of obesity may be slowing down,[7] the size of the epidemic remains staggering. In 2000–2008, the prevalence of obesity was 35.5% among adult women and 32.2% among adult men in the United States.[8]

Compounding this problem is a dramatic rise in obesity in children in the United States. The prevalence of obesity among children has tripled in the last 20 years.[9] Along with this shocking increase in childhood obesity comes a corresponding increase in risk factors for heart disease.[10]

The linkages between obesity and cardiovascular disease and its risk factors are well established. Not only is obesity linked to common risk factors for heart disease such as hypertension, diabetes, and dyslipidemias,[11–14] but, in addition, obesity represents a strong and independent risk factor for heart disease over and above its impact on risk factors.[15,16]

The purpose of this chapter is to review the cardiovascular effects of obesity as well as its association to various aspects of cardiovascular disease. In addition, we will review the effects of treatment on risk factors for heart disease and provide information on the clinical assessment of obese individuals with a particular emphasis on the cardiovascular system. We will also offer some suggestions for efficacious treatment of obesity and review the effects of such treatment on risk factors for cardiovascular disease.

In addition to its interaction with multiple risk factors for heart disease, obesity also adversely impacts with the hemodynamic profile of the entire cardiovascular system and is associated with a variety of cardiovascular complications[17] in addition to coronary heart disease (CHD) including heart failure and sudden death. Obesity is also associated with an increase in inflammatory markers[18–21] and a prothrombotic state,[22] both of which may exert negative influences on the cardiovascular system.

HEMODYNAMICS OF ADIPOSE TISSUE

It used to be thought that adipose tissue existed largely for storage purposes in the human body. However, research over the past two decades has shown that adipocytes, particularly in the abdominal region, are very metabolically active and supplied by an extensive capillary network. While the resting blood flow to adipose tissue is considerably less than skeletal muscle, it can increase dramatically after a meal.[23] The resting blood flow to adipose tissue is usually on the order of 2–3 mL/min/100 g of adipose tissue but may increase up to 10-fold after a meal.[24,25] (In contrast, skeletal muscle exhibits blood flow of 50–75 mL/min/100 g.) The overall increased blood flow observed in obese individuals cannot be explained completely by the capillary network of the adipose tissue, and this issue is an area of active investigation. Some investigators have suggested that the increase in lean muscle mass typically found in obese individuals may account for some of the increased cardiac output frequently observed in obese individuals.[26]

In addition to hemodynamic issues, adipose tissue represents a complex endocrine organ that excretes a variety of compounds into the bloodstream, which interact with the cardiovascular system. For example, adipose tissue is a significant source of leptin, adiponectin, insulin-like growth factor-1 (IGF-1), tumor necrosis factor-α (TNF-α), plasminogen activator inhibitor-1, lipoprotein lipase, and interleukin-6 (IL-6).[18–22] It has been estimated that approximately 30% of the circulating concentrations of IL-6 originate in adipose tissue.[27] This carries importance since IL-6 is involved in the modulation of CRP production in the liver and CRP appears to be a marker of a chronic inflammation that can trigger acute coronary syndromes.[28]

HEMODYNAMIC EFFECTS OF OBESITY

In many regards, obesity resembles high output or volume overload to the cardiovascular system.[29] Left ventricular filling pressures and volume are higher in obese individuals than in lean individuals. Total blood volume and cardiac output are also increased, thereby generating increased cardiac workload.[30] The combination of higher filling pressures and increased cardiac output may result in left ventricular dilatation[31] and ultimately congestive heart failure. Left atrial enlargement may also occur, which is thought to be a result of left ventricular diastolic dysfunction.[32] Atrial enlargement may contribute to the excess risk of atrial fibrillation observed in obese individuals. Ventricular hypertrophy is common in long-standing obesity and may be a result of systemic volume overload and/or hypertension.

Elevated cardiac filling pressures may also be present in obese individuals during exercise resulting from increased cardiac output and increased left ventricular filling pressures.[30] Some of these abnormalities may be partially ameliorated with weight loss.

EFFECTS ON LEFT VENTRICULAR FUNCTION

Long-standing obesity is associated with increased risk of left ventricular systolic dysfunction and impairment of left ventricular diastolic function.[33] In morbidly obese patients, eccentric left ventricular hypertrophy (LVH) is common, which can lead to both systolic and diastolic dysfunction. Fatty infiltration of the cardiac muscle can further compound these problems and exacerbate both left ventricular systolic and diastolic dysfunction.[34]

OBESITY AND CORONARY HEART DISEASE

Multiple studies have demonstrated that obesity correlates with established risk factors for CHD and also constitutes an independent risk.[35–38] In particular, there are well-established relationships between obesity, type 2 diabetes, hypertension, and dyslipidemias (particularly diminished HDL and elevated triglycerides). As illustrated in Figure 12.1, the relative risk of all of these relationships increases as body mass index (BMI) increases.[39]

As Figure 12.1 demonstrates, the relationship between obesity and risk factors for CHD is particularly strong for type 2 diabetes and hypertension.

In addition to its association with risk factors, obesity also has an independent relationship with increased risk of CHD.[35–38] As depicted in Figure 12.1, this relationship appears linear over a wide range of BMI values, suggesting that individuals of even average weight at mid-life are at substantial increased risk of CHD compared to leaner individuals. In addition to the well-established relationship between obesity and CHD, an independent and strong relationship exists with body fat distribution and CHD.[39] The increased risk of CHD associated with increased visceral

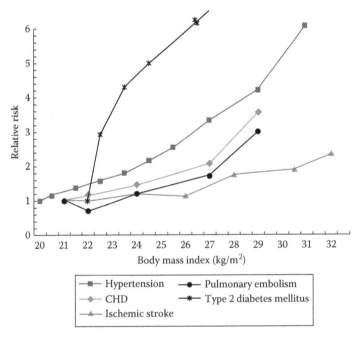

FIGURE 12.1 Relative risks for hypertension, CHD, ischemic stroke, pulmonary embolism, and diabetes, according to BMI up to 32 kg/m², after 14–16 years of follow-up, among women in the Nurses' Health study. Relative risks for type 2 diabetes are age adjusted. Relative risks for other conditions are adjusted for age, smoking status, menopausal status, postmenopausal hormone use, parental history of myocardial infarction, oral contraceptive use (for the outcomes of hypertension, ischemic stroke, and pulmonary embolism), and parity (for the outcomes of hypertension and pulmonary embolism). (Adapted from Bassuk, S.S. and Manson, J.E., *Am. J. Lifestyle Med.*, 2, 191, 2008.)

abdominal fat appears based on adverse metabolic consequences resulting from the highly lipolytic adipocytes in the abdominal region.[40–43]

PATHOGENESIS OF ATHEROSCLEROSIS

Multiple studies have demonstrated that the atherosclerotic process can be manifested in children as early as 5–10 years old as deposits of cholesterol in macrophage foam cells in the intima of large arteries (fatty streaks).[44,45] This, in turn, may cause endothelial cell dysfunction and inflammation of the vessel wall. It has been suggested that individuals at high risk for CHD could potentially be identified in childhood by measurement of carotid intima-medial thickness (IMT).[46] In adults, increase in carotid IMT is associated with multiple CHD risk factors including obesity.[47,48]

With age, atherosclerotic lesions become more complex. In one study involving postmortem examination of arteries in individuals 15–30 years old who died from suicides, homicides, or accidental injury, both fatty streaks and more advanced lesions were found in the right coronary artery and were associated with obesity.[49]

OBESITY AND RISK FACTORS FOR CORONARY HEART DISEASE

OBESITY AND HYPERTENSION

Observational studies have consistently demonstrated a direct association between weight and blood pressure.[11,12,17,50] The prevalence of hypertension is increased between two and fourfold in obese individuals. It has been estimated that more than one-third of cases of hypertension in the United States are associated with obesity.[51] Over half of all patients with high blood pressure are either overweight or obese.[52] High blood pressure is approximately six times more frequent in obese subjects compared to lean men and women.[52] In addition, weight gain is associated with an increased risk of developing hypertension. A 20 lb weight gain is associated with 3 mm/Hg higher systolic and 2.3 mm/Hg higher diastolic blood pressure, which results in an estimated 12% increased risk of CHD and 24% increase in stroke.[53]

A variety of mechanisms have been postulated to explain the link between obesity and hypertension. Elevated cardiac output and increased vascular resistance are both observed in obese individuals.[54] Additionally, insulin resistance and hyperinsulinemia, which frequently accompany obesity, increase sympathetic tone and renal sodium retention, which may both further contribute an increased risk of hypertension in the obese patient.[55–59]

OBESITY AND DIABETES/GLUCOSE INTOLERANCE

Body weight correlates strongly with both glucose intolerance and type 2 diabetes mellitus.[60,61] While not all of obese individuals are diabetic, most type 2 diabetics are obese. It has been estimated that at least 80% of all type 2 diabetics are obese. The link between obesity and type 2 diabetes, particularly abdominal obesity, is thought to be somewhat mediated by the resultant hyperinsulinemia,[62] which frequently accompanies obesity.[62]

As the prevalence of obesity has risen dramatically in the United States, so has the prevalence of diabetes. The prevalence of diabetes increased 61% from 1991 to 2001 in the United States.[60] In the Nurses' Health Trial, the risk of developing diabetes over 16 years of observation and follow-up was nearly 40-fold higher in women with a BMI ≥ 35 and 20-fold higher in women with a BMI 30.0–34.9 compared with women whose BMI ≤ 23.[61] Both the U.S. Male Health Professionals Follow-Up Study and NHANES data revealed similar trends with the prevalence of diabetes tracking strongly with increased BMI.[63]

Weight gain during adult years has also been associated with increased risk of diabetes in a number of observational studies. The increase in prevalence of developing diabetes varied from study to study from a 4- to 12-fold increased risk for individuals who gained between 5 and 20 kg during the adult years.[64,65] Since over 80% of individuals with diabetes die of CHD, the linkages to between diabetes and obesity are particularly worrisome because of the added risk of developing CHD.

Obesity and Dyslipidemias

Multiple different lipid abnormalities are associated with obesity. Higher triglyceride levels and lower HDL-cholesterol levels are related to BMI in both men and women in all age groups.[13,14,66] In addition, in men and women between the ages of 20 and 44, total cholesterol and LDL-cholesterol also correlate with BMI.[13,14] While the etiology of dyslipidemias associated with cholesterol is complex, it appears partially attributable to the lipolytic nature of adipocytes, particularly in the abdominal area, resulting in higher levels of free fatty acids that are released into the portal circulation and contribute to a wide range of metabolic derangements and hepatic dysfunction leading to a variety of dyslipidemias.[40]

Obesity and the Metabolic Syndrome*

The prevalence of the metabolic syndrome has increased dramatically in the United States in the past 20 years. It is now estimated that between 25% and 33% of adults in the United States have the metabolic syndrome.[67] The metabolic syndrome, which is a clustering of dyslipidemias (typically elevated triglycerides and depressed HDL), glucose intolerance, hypertension, and abdominal obesity, is thought to be driven largely through the metabolic derangements caused by excess abdominal fat.[68,69] The metabolic syndrome presents a significant risk factor for both diabetes and CHD. The NCEP Guidelines recommend that individuals with the metabolic syndrome be treated as though they already have CHD.[70]

Obesity and Vascular Disease

In addition to hypertension, a variety of other vascular diseases and/or conditions are frequently present in obesity. Pedal edema is common in obesity and may be related to elevated left and right ventricular filling pressures.[71] Venous thromboembolism is also more common in obese patients than in normal weight individuals,[72] including

---

* See also Chapter 14.

an increased risk for pulmonary embolism in obese women, although this complication is less clear for men.[73]

ARRHYTHMIAS

Obese individuals are at increased risk of arrhythmias and sudden cardiac death.[74,75] According to Framingham Study data, sudden cardiac death risk in obese men and women could be as much as more than 40 times higher than the nonobese population.[38,75]

A prolonged QT_c interval is found in approximately 30% of individuals with glucose intolerance or obesity.[76] A prolonged QT_c interval has been associated with a variety of cardiac arrhythmias.[77,78] In addition, alterations in the autonomic nervous system may play a role in arrhythmias and other cardiac complications related to obesity. Increased sympathetic tone leading to an increase in heart rate has been associated with increased body weight.[79]

INFLAMMATION

There is a strong correlation between obesity and markers of inflammation including IL-6 and CRP.[18,79] Obesity has been likened to total body, low-grade systemic inflammation. This inflammatory process may, in turn, play a role in multiple cardiac issues including endothelial dysfunction and hypertension.

SLEEP APNEA

A variety of respiratory complications may be present in obese individuals. Most prominent among these conditions is sleep apnea, which may be the result of respiratory insufficiency particularly in the supine state. It has been estimated that 40 million individuals have sleep disorders.[80] The prevalence of these increases substantially in obese individuals.[81] Sleep apnea can result in hypertension (both systolic and diastolic)[82] and is also associated with increased levels of CRP. Pulmonary hypertension may also accompany sleep apnea.

EFFECTS OF OBESITY TREATMENT ON RISK FACTORS FOR CORONARY HEART DISEASE

The effective treatment of obesity may result in a wide range of improvements in risk factors for CHD.[83,84] Typically, the amount of weight loss required to yield significant reduction in CHD risk factors is relatively modest—on the order of 5%–10% of loss of total body weight.[85]

EFFECTS OF WEIGHT LOSS ON HYPERTENSION

Weight loss has been reliably demonstrated to lower both systolic and diastolic blood pressure independent of other lifestyle factors.[86–88] The reports of the National High Blood Pressure Education Program Working Group on Primary Prevention of Hypertension[89] and the Joint National Committee on Prevention, Detection, Evaluation, and Treatment of High Blood Pressure (JNC VII)[90] have both recommended weight loss as a primary therapeutic modality for obese individuals with high blood pressure.

Four of the largest randomized trials of weight reduction utilizing lifestyle measures in adults with high-normal blood pressure have consistently showed that weight loss is the most effective lifestyle modality for lowering blood pressure in overweight or obese individuals.[86–88] Reductions in systolic and diastolic blood pressure on the order of 0.5–1 mm Hg for every kg of weight loss have been demonstrated. Clinically significant reductions in blood pressure comparable to results from many antihypertensive agents have been seen with weight loss of 5%–10% in overweight or obese individuals in body weight. Weight loss may also serve as adjunctive therapy to pharmacologic therapy to improve blood pressure control.

The exact mechanisms of blood pressure reduction in obese hypertensive individuals are not fully understood. Mechanisms that have been postulated include decreased vascular tone, decreased adrenergic tone, and decreased blood volume.[54]

EFFECTS OF WEIGHT LOSS ON TYPE 2 DIABETES AND GLUCOSE INTOLERANCE

Intervention studies in individuals with type 2 diabetes and also glucose intolerance have reliably shown that intentional weight loss in overweight or obese individuals— either alone or combined with physical activity—improves both glucose levels and insulin responsiveness.[91–93] The U.S. Diabetes Prevention Program, which was a 3 year randomized trial that enrolled 3234 men and women between the ages of 25 and 85 years old who had baseline impaired glucose tolerance (IGT), demonstrated a 58% reduction in progression to diabetes in the Lifestyle Intervention Group.[92] These individuals lost 5%–7% of their body weight and exercised an average of 30 min a day. The Finnish Diabetes Prevention Study, a research trial of 522 middle-aged overweight men and women with IGT, also demonstrated similar findings in the intensive lifestyle intervention group.[93] The Swedish Obese Subject study showed that over a 10 year period obese individuals without diabetes at baseline who achieved weight loss through bariatric surgery decreased their risk of developing diabetes by 75% when compared to matched obese controls.[84]

The precise mechanism by which weight loss improves glucose intolerance is not completely understood. Improvements in glucose intolerance may be somewhat impacted by calorie restriction per se in addition to the effects of weight loss.[84,92,93]

A large randomized control trial, the Look AHEAD (Action for Health in Diabetes) trial, should provide additional valuable information about the long-term effects of sustained weight loss through exercise and decreased calorie intake in obese individuals with diabetes on the risk of developing CVD.[94] Initial results from this trial are expected in 2012.

EFFECTS OF WEIGHT LOSS ON DYSLIPIDEMIAS

Weight loss has been demonstrated to yield a variety of beneficial effects on lipid profiles, although these benefits may be somewhat confounded by the nutritional components of lipid management. A meta-analysis of 70 trials of weight loss utilizing diet alone showed that weight loss resulted in significant decreases in total cholesterol, triglycerides, and LDL-cholesterol in individuals with dyslipidemia.[95]

Significant improvements in HDL-cholesterol were also achieved once individuals achieved reduced stabilized weight.

While results of weight loss on lipids are less consistent than in hypertension, several studies have suggested that lipid profiles can achieve meaningful improvements at weight loss levels less than 10% and that clinically relevant changes in cholesterol/ HDL ratios can occur with weight loss of 5%–10% of initial body weight.[95]

CARDIOPULMONARY BENEFITS OF WEIGHT LOSS

In addition to reduction of risk factors for CHD, intentional weight loss can improve aspects of the physiology of the cardiovascular system in obese individuals. Included in these potential benefits are improvement in left ventricular systolic and diastolic function, reduction in hemodynamic abnormalities from high output (including decreased blood volume, decreased stroke volume, and decreased cardiac output), decreased left ventricular mass,[96] decreased filling pressures of the right and left side of the heart, improvement or no change in systemic arterial resistance, decreased resting oxygen consumption, decreased heart rate, shortened QT_c interval, and increased heart rate variability.[96–98] All these factors may result in improved cardiovascular hemodynamics.

RISKS OF WEIGHT LOSS

While multiple benefits may accompany weight loss in obese individuals, it must be acknowledged that certain weight loss modalities result in increased cardiovascular risks. For example, very-low-calorie diets,[99] liquid protein diets,[100] and starvation[101] all have been associated with prolongation of the QT_c interval. Specifically, liquid protein diets have been associated with potentially life-threatening arrhythmias documented on 24 h Holter monitoring. These arrhythmias include ventricular tachycardia (torsades de pointes) and fibrillation. Unfortunately some of these diets remain in common use today. It is critically important to ensure micronutrient supplementation to ameliorate these adverse effects in patients who are following such diets.

Several medications that have been employed for weight loss including fenfluramine and dexfenfluramine have resulted in cardiac valve disorders and have been removed from the market.[102] Sibutramine hydrochloride has been associated with high blood pressure and should not be utilized in individuals with preexisting hypertension.[103] Several endocannabinoid receptor antagonists have been evaluated for obesity treatment but have not been approved for clinical use. The effects of these medications on cardiac structure and function are not known. A detailed discussion of pharmacologic therapies for obesity is found in Chapter 9.

DOES TREATMENT OF OBESITY DECREASE THE RISK OF CORONARY HEART DISEASE?

Much less information is currently available on the long-term effects of weight loss on CHD itself than on its risk factors. This is due to the high incidence of weight regain in clinical trials. It is hoped that the Look AHEAD trial will provide important information in this area related to obese patients with diabetes.[94]

In the Cancer Prevention study, a long-term follow-up study with over 750,000 women, those with obesity-related health conditions such as diabetes and hypertension who achieved intentional weight loss experienced a 9% reduction in CHD mortality.[104] However, in women without preexisting illness, these benefits were not achieved. The reductions in overall mortality came largely from reduced mortality from diabetes-related conditions as well as cancer-related conditions in addition to reductions in CHD mortality.

Clearly, large-scale prospective trials are required to resolve the issue of whether or not intentional weight loss positively affects CHD mortality. The clear association between intentional weight loss and reduced risk factors for CHD, however, should still provide impetus for clinicians to employ intentional weight loss as first line therapy for individuals with type 2 diabetes, hypertension, and/or dyslipidemias.

It is also important to note that controversy exists about cardiovascular risk related to numerous cycles of weight loss and regain (weight cycling). Data from the Framingham Study have suggested that individuals who weight cycle may increase their risk of heart disease[105]; however, a meta-analysis conducted by the National Task Force on the Prevention and Treatment of Obesity achieved the opposite conclusion that weight cycling did not increase the risk of CHD.[106]

ROLE OF ABDOMINAL OBESITY

Numerous studies have demonstrated that central (abdominal) obesity confers additional increased risk of CHD in addition to an elevated BMI.[107–109] Adipose tissue in the abdominal region is more metabolically active than in the hip, thigh, or buttocks. Abdominal fat accumulation is an important predictor in type 2 diabetes, dyslipidemias, hypertension, and CHD.

The underlying mechanism for increased CHD risk related to increased abdominal fat is not completely understood. However, abdominal fat cells appear to have increased sensitivity to lipolytic agents, which results in increased delivery of free fatty acids and glycerol to the liver, which may contribute to increased insulin resistance and dyslipidemia.[40,41] These derangements, in turn, may contribute to glucose intolerance and type 2 diabetes as well as hypertension in obese individuals.

Waist circumference has largely replaced waist to hip ratio as a means of estimating abdominal fat. Good correlations have been demonstrated between properly measured waist circumference and central fat documented by CT scan or MRI.[110] While there is a generally linear relationship between increased waist circumference and increased risk of CHD, circumferences greater than 35 in. in women and 40 in. in men are considered significant risk factors for CHD over and above increased total body fat.

Since increased abdominal fat is considered a core component of the metabolic syndrome,[67–69] issues related to the clustering of risk factors for CHD seen in metabolic syndrome constitute a potent synergistic risk in obese individuals (see also Chapter 14).

ROLE OF WEIGHT GAIN AS A RISK FACTOR
FOR CORONARY HEART DISEASE

While this chapter has focused largely on obesity and its association for both risk factors for CHD and CHD itself, it should also be noted that adult weight gain is also associated with CHD independently of obesity.[111] In the Nurses' Health Trial, weight gain between the age 18 and mid-life was associated on linear fashion with increased risk of CHD. Women who gained between 5 and 7.9 kg during this stage of life increased their risk of CHD by 1.25 times. Those who gained ≥20 kg increased their risk of CHD by 2.65 times. Significant weight gain after age 21 has also been correlated with increased risk of CHD in men in the U.S. Male Health Professionals Follow-Up Study.[63] Weight gain during adult years has also been correlated with increased risk of hypertension and stroke as well as adult-onset diabetes.[112]

The practical implication of this information to physicians is apparent. The first significant weight gain during adults years (greater than 10 lb) should result in counseling and other measures to prevent significant increase in the risk of CHD. A common finding in women, in particular, of weight gain following pregnancy should also be cause for increased scrutiny and counseling on the part of clinicians to prevent increased risk of CHD.

CHILDHOOD OBESITY

While the emphasis of this chapter is not on childhood obesity per se, as already noted, the earliest changes of atherosclerosis may be apparent as early as age 5 in obese children. Moreover, as the prevalence of childhood obesity has dramatically increased in the United States,[113] so have not only risk factors for CHD but also type 2 diabetes and the metabolic syndrome.[114] Thus, clinicians should be vigilant to offer early counseling in families where children are obese. These issues are discussed in much more detail in Chapter 8.

CLINICAL ASSESSMENT OF OBESE INDIVIDUALS*

HISTORY AND PHYSICAL EXAM

A careful history of weight should be taken in any obese individual to ascertain whether or not the individual was obese as a child or if weight gain occurred later in life. Physical examination may be challenging in an obese individual, and, thus, manifestations of cardiovascular pathology may be underestimated. Increased right heart filling pressure may be evident and may be either estimated through jugular venous distention or estimated by dorsal hand veins when the hand is lowered beneath the sternal angle. The arm is then gradually raised and on the dorsal veins observed. Heart sounds may be distant due to increased body mass, which may mask both cardiac murmurs and S1 and S2.

A more detailed discussion of the comprehensive history and physical examination of the overweight or obese individual can be found in Chapter 4.

---

* See also Chapter 4.

ELECTROCARDIOGRAM

The electrocardiogram (ECG) in obese individuals may be difficult to interpret because of increased distance between the electrodes and the heart due to excessive pannus.

A variety of changes in ECG may occur with increasing obesity. Low QRS voltage and left axis deviation as well as nonspecific ST and T wave flattening particularly in the inferior/inferolateral leads (attributed to diaphragmatic elevation and horizontal displacement of the heart)[115–117] and voltage criteria for either left atrial abnormality or LVH[118,119] are common findings. False-positive criteria for inferior myocardial infarction may also be present—also thought due to diaphragmatic elevation.[120] Some of these ECG parameters may change in obese individuals following weight loss, although these changes are not reliable findings.

ECHOCARDIOGRAPHY

Echocardiography may be particularly useful in obese individuals to help ascertain cardiac status.[121] Both chamber size and wall thickness as well as a variety of indices of left ventricular filling pressures may be derived from echocardiography and cardiac Doppler evaluation.

ASSESSMENT OF CHD WITH IMAGING TECHNIQUES

The use of imaging techniques to assess CHD may be very valuable in obese patients, particularly those with significant risk factors for CHD. Due to impaired exercise tolerance, dipyridamole thallium[122] or technetium perfusion scans[123] may be utilized for evaluation of the presence of ischemic heart disease.

Transesophageal echocardiography may also be useful but may be technically difficult in obese patients.

If cardiac catheterization is contemplated in an obese individual, use of the percutaneous radial approach may be most appropriate given difficulty of femoral access caused by volume of adipose tissue or the risk of bleeding complications resulting from this same issue.[124]

TREATMENT OF OBESITY IN CLINICAL PRACTICE

Physician recommendation for behavioral change has been demonstrated in a number of studies to result in significant clinical improvement, yet, in the area of obesity as a risk factor for cardiovascular disease, medical involvement appears to have been less than optimal. In a national survey of 2000 adults with BMI $\geq$ 25, only 23% of males and 39% of females ever received counseling about their weight.[125]

The reasons for lack of physician involvement in the important area of risk factor reduction for CHD in obese individuals may be multifactorial. Perhaps physicians underestimate the interaction between obesity and other risk factors for heart disease. Lack of reimbursement from insurance for counseling related to obesity has also been cited as a reason for physician lack of counseling efforts in this area.

It has also been argued that physician reluctance to treat obesity may be due to lack of demonstrated efficacy of long-term treatments for obesity. Furthermore, some physicians may unfortunately share in the negative stereotyping of obesity as a lack of self-discipline or will power. It is hoped that as scientific understandings of obesity as a chronic disease continue to develop, and the strong relationship between obesity and heart disease continues to be elucidated, more physician involvement in treating obesity to lower the risk of CHD will be accomplished.

The emerging science of how risk factors cluster in such conditions as the metabolic syndrome[67,68] may also stimulate physician interest in treating obesity to lower the risk of CHD. The opportunity to simultaneously reduce multiple risk factors for heart disease such as hypertension, dyslipidemias, and risk of type 2 diabetes through weight loss can serve as important reminders for reasons to attempt treatment for chronic obesity.

VITAL SIGNS OF OBESITY

Given the independent risk of both elevated BMI and waist circumference for CHD and its risk factors, it would appear reasonable to measure weight, BMI, and weight circumference in all overweight or obese individuals. The authors would advance the modest proposal of classifying these three factors as "vital signs" of obesity[126] and suggest that these weight-related vital signs should be taught to all medical students and house officers during training and measured by all physicians as part of routine office visits in overweight or obese individuals. For physicians who do not wish to compute BMI from height and weight data, multiple sources of convenient BMI tables are available (see also Chapter 4). The framework has been suggested for relating BMI to overall health risk and is found in Table 12.1.

Obtaining these three "vital signs" of obesity provides a basis for counseling for the overweight or obese individual and indicates that the physician is concerned about weight as a health issue.

TABLE 12.1
Health Risk Associated with BMI[a]

BMI Category	Health Risk Based on BMI	Risk Adjusted for Presence of Comorbid Conditions and/or Other Risk Factors
<25	Minimal	Low
25–27	Low	Moderate
27–30	Moderate	High
30–35	High	Very high
35–40	Very high	Extremely high
≥40	Extremely high	Extremely high

Source: Reprinted with permission from Shape Up America!, www.shapeup.org

[a] Metric values must be used for proper interpretation.

LIFESTYLE MANAGEMENT OF OBESITY

Lifestyle changes such as improved nutrition, increased physical activity, and behavior modification play important roles in the treatment of obesity. Despite the fact that in many patients the results of such interventions remain less than optimal, most research has indicated that a combination of all three of these modalities will act synergistically to improve the likelihood of loss and maintenance of weight loss.[127]

Caloric restriction remains the mainstay of nutritional approaches to weight loss. Recent controversies have arisen concerning whether or not macronutrient composition of weight loss diets matters in terms of their efficacy.[128] These and other issues related to the nutritional approach to weight loss are discussed in detail in Chapter 5.

Increased physical activity may confer further benefit in addition to nutritional interventions for both short- and long-term weight loss.[129] Physical activity is particularly important in the maintenance of weight loss and may play an important role in loss of abdominal fat as well as long-term adherence to loss strategies.[129] Physical activity may be particularly important in the area of prevention. Increases in physical activity lower the risk of CHD even if weight loss does not occur. All of these topics are discussed in detail in Chapter 6.

Behavioral strategies for weight loss have been clearly demonstrated to play a positive role in the overall approach to weight loss and maintenance of weight loss. Of course, nutritional practices and physical activity both represent examples of behavior; however, in addition to these strategies, multiple other strategies have been developed and demonstrated to be efficacious in weight loss particularly when combined with proper nutritional strategies and increased physical activity. Issues related to behavioral practices and weight management in adults are discussed in Chapter 7, and in children and adolescents in Chapter 8.

Issues related to weight regain are often misunderstood in the medical community. The National Weight Control Registry, a registry of over 5000 individuals who have lost significant amounts of weight and kept it off for at least 1 year, has demonstrated that individuals who adopt a daily strategy of monitoring their nutrition as well as participating in regular physical activity are highly successful in not only short-term weight loss but also maintenance of weight loss.[130] It is also critically important to emphasize that both increased physical activity and proper nutrition may convey benefits for reduction of risk of CHD independent of their role of weight loss and weight management. This fact alone provides justification for clinical intervention in these lifestyle-related areas for all patients but particularly for those who are overweight or obese as a way of reducing multiple components of CHD risk.

PHARMACOLOGIC THERAPY OF OBESITY

A limited number of pharmacologic modalities are available for the treatment of obesity. These are discussed in detail in Chapter 9. Pharmaceutical agents are invariably used in conjunction with lifestyle measures and appear to have synergistic effects with these practices. The history of cardiovascular problems associated with some pharmacologic agents utilized to treat obesity further complicates this area.

The FDA has recently rejected applications for several new antiobesity drugs based on central nervous system effects or lack of complete proof that no cardiovascular side effects were present.

CORONARY ARTERY DISEASE REVASCULARIZATION PROCEDURES IN OBESE INDIVIDUALS

Obese individuals tend to have a higher percentage of multivessel coronary artery disease but more no comorbidities than normal weight individuals when studied at heart catheterization.[131] Furthermore, obese patients have been shown to have a higher incidence of multiple postoperative complications following coronary artery bypass grafting (CABG) than lower-weight individuals.[132] They are particularly at high risk for thromboembolic disease, which may require an aggressive approach to deep venous thrombosis prophylaxis.[133] Of note, obesity is not associated with increased mortality rates or postoperative cerebrovascular accidents following CABG.[134,135] An increased incidence of complications such as wound infection and atrial dysrhythmias, however, has been documented.

BARIATRIC SURGERY

Bariatric surgery has been demonstrated to be highly efficacious for reducing the risk factors of heart disease and diabetes in individuals who are morbidly obese. Indications for bariatric surgery vary from institution to institution and have evolved over the last decade. These issues and other issues related to bariatric surgery are discussed in detail in Chapter 10.

CONCLUSIONS

There are strong and independent links between obesity and CHD. Obesity is also associated with multiple major risk factors for CHD including hypertension, dyslipidemias, type 2 diabetes, and the metabolic syndrome.

Clustering of risk factors that occurs in conditions such as the metabolic syndrome is common in individuals who develop obstructive atherosclerosis. Weight loss provides an attractive option for simultaneously treating multiple risk factors for CHD. Physicians should be aware of the multiple links between obesity and heart disease and emphasize not only treatment of obesity itself but also reduction in associated cardiac risk factors.

REFERENCES

1. World Health Organization. Obesity: Preventing and managing the global epidemic. [WHO Technical report series No. 894]. 2000. Geneva, Switzerland: World Health Organization.
2. Eckel RH, York DA, Rossner S, Hubbard V, Caterson I, St Jeor ST, Hayman LL, Mullis RM, Blair SN, American Heart Association. Prevention Conference VII: Obesity, a worldwide epidemic related to heart disease and stroke: Executive summary. *Circulation* 2004; 110:2968–2975.

3. Popkin BM. Global nutrition dynamics: The world is shifting rapidly toward a diet linked with noncommunicable diseases. *Am J Clin Nutr* 2006; 84:289–209.

4. Popkins BM, Conde W, Hou N, Monteiro C. Is there a lag globally in overweight trends for children compared with adults? *Obesity (Silver Spring)* 2006; 14:1846–1853.

5. Engeland A, Bjorge T, Sogaard AJ, Tverdal A. Body mass index in adolescence in relation to total mortality: 32-year follow-up of 227,000 Norwegian boys and girls. *Am J Epidemiol* 2003; 157:517–523.

6. Flegal KM, Carroll MD, Ogden CL, Curtin LR. Prevalence and trends in obesity among US adults, 1999–2008. *JAMA* 2010; 303(3):235–241.

7. Yanovski SZ, Yanovski JA. Obesity prevalence in the United States—Up, down, or sideways? *N Engl J Med* 2011; 364:987–989.

8. Ogden CL, Carroll MD, McDowell MA, Flegal KM. Obesity among adults in the United States—No change since 2003–2004. NCHS Data Brief No. 1. Hyattsville MD: National Center for Health Statistics, 2007.

9. Dietz W, Robinson T. Overweight children and adolescents. *N Engl J Med* 2005; 352:2100–2109.

10. Steinberger J, Daniels SR, Eckel RH, Hayman L, Lustig RH, McCrindle B, Mietus-Snyder ML. Progress and challenges in metabolic syndrome in children and adolescents: A scientific statement from the American Heart Association Atherosclerosis, Hypertension, and Obesity in the Young Committee of the Council on Cardiovascular Disease in the Young; Council on Cardiovascular Nursing; and Council on Nutrition, Physical Activity, and Metabolism. *Circulation* 2009; 119:628–647.

11. Stamler J. Epidemiologic findings on body mass and blood pressure in adults. *Ann Epidemiol* 1991; 4:347–362.

12. Fagerberg B, Berglund A, Anderson O, Bergland G. Weight reduction versus antihypertensive drug therapy in obese men with high blood pressure: Effects upon plasma insulin levels and association with changes in blood pressure and serum lipids. *J Hypertens* 1992; 10:1053–1061.

13. Denke MA, Sempos CT, Grundy SM. Excess body weight: An unrecognized contributor to high blood cholesterol levels in White American men. *Arch Intern Med* 1993; 153:1093–1103.

14. Denke MA, Seppos CT, Grundy SM. Excess body weight: An unrecognized contributor to high blood cholesterol levels in White American women. *Arch Intern Med* 1994; 154:401–410.

15. Poirier P, Giles TD, Bray GA et al. Obesity and cardiovascular disease: Pathophysiology, evaluation, and effect of weight loss: An update of the 1997 American Heart Association Scientific Statement on Obesity and Heart Disease from the Obesity Committee of the Council on Nutrition, Physical Activity, and Metabolism. *Circulation* 2006; 113(6):898–918.

16. Goldstein LB, Adams R, Alberts MJ et al. Primary prevention of ischemic stroke: A guideline from the American Heart Association/American Stroke Association Stroke Council: Cosponsored by the Atherosclerotic Peripheral Vascular Disease Interdisciplinary Working Group; Cardiovascular Nursing Council; Clinical Cardiology Council; Nutrition, Physical Activity, and Metabolism Council; and the Quality of Care and Outcomes Research Interdisciplinary Working Group. *Circulation* 2006; 113(24):e873–e923.

17. Poirier P, Martin J, Marceau P, Biron S, Marceau S. Impact of bariatric surgery on cardiac structure, function and clinical manifestations in morbid obesity. *Expert Rev Cardiovasc Ther* 2004; 2:193–201.

18. Wajchenberg BL. Subcutaneous and visceral adipose tissue: Their relation to the metabolic syndrome. *Endocr Rev* 2000; 21:697–738.

19. Hotamisligil GS, Arner P, Caro JF, Atkinson RL, Spiegelman BM. Increased adipose tissue expression of tumor necrosis factor-alpha in human obesity and insulin resistance. *J Clin Invest* 1995; 95:2409–2415.

20. Lundgren CH, Brown SL, Nordt TK, Sobel BE, Fujii S. Elaboration of type-1 plasminogen activator inhibitor from adipocytes: A potential pathogenetic link between obesity and cardiovascular disease. *Circulation* 1996; 93:106–110.

21. Yudkin JS, Stehouwer CD, Emeis JJ, Coppack SW. C-reactive protein in healthy subjects: Associations with obesity, insulin resistance, and endothelial dysfunction: A potential role for cytokines originating from adipose tissue? *Arterioscler Thromb Vasc Biol* 1999; 19:972–978.

22. Cigolini M, Targher G, Bergamo AI, Tonoli M, Agostino G, De Sandre G. Visceral fat accumulation and its relation to plasma hemostatic factors in healthy men. *Arterioscler Thromb Vasc Biol* 1996; 16:368–374.

23. Karpe F, Fielding BA, Ilic V, Humphreys SM, Frayn KN. Monitoring adipose tissue blood flow in man: A comparison between the (133)xenon washout method and microdialysis. *Int J Obes Relat Metab Disord* 2002; 26:1–5.

24. Lesser GT, Deutsch S. Measurement of adipose tissue blood flow and perfusion in man by uptake of 85Kr. *J Appl Physiol* 1967; 23:621–630.

25. Oberg B, Rosell S. Sympathetic control of consecutive vascular sections in canine subcutaneous adipose tissue. *Acta Physiol Scand* 1967; 71:47–56.

26. Collis T, Devereux RB, Roman MJ, de Simone G, Yeh J, Howard BV, Fabsitz RR, Welty TK. Relations of stroke volume and cardiac output to body composition: The strong heart study. *Circulation* 2001; 103:820–825.

27. Mohamed-Ali V, Goodrick S, Rawesh A, Katz DR, Miles JM, Yudkin JS, Klein S, Coppack SW. Subcutaneous adipose tissue releases interleukin-6, but not tumor necrosis factor-alpha, in vivo. *J Clin Endocrinol Metab* 1997; 82:4196–4200.

28. Ridker PM. Novel risk factors and markers for coronary disease. *Adv Intern Med* 2000; 45:391–418.

29. Alpert MA. Obesity cardiomyopathy; pathophysiology and evolution of the clinical syndrome. *Am J Med Sci* 2001; 321:225–236.

30. Kaltman AJ, Goldring RM. Role of circulatory congestion in the cardiorespiratory failure of obesity. *Am J Med* 1976; 60:645–653.

31. Ku CS, Lin SL, Wang DJ, Chang SK, Lee WJ. Left ventricular filling in young normotensive obese adults. *Am J Cardiol* 1994; 73:613–615.

32. Sasson Z, Rasooly Y, Gupta R, Rasooly I. Left atrial enlargement in healthy obese: Prevalence and relation to left ventricular mass and diastolic function. *Can J Cardiol* 1996; 12:257–263.

33. Alpert MA, Lambert CR, Panayiotou H, Terry BE, Cohen MV, Massey CV, Hashimi MW, Mukerji V. Relation of duration of morbid obesity to left ventricular mass, systolic function, and diastolic filling, and effect of weight loss. *Am J Cardiol* 1995; 76:1194–1197.

34. Montani JP, Carroll JF, Dwyer TM, Antic V, Yang Z, Dulloo AG. Ectopic fat storage in heart, blood vessels and kidneys in the pathogenesis of cardiovascular diseases. *Int J Obes Relat Metab Disord* 2004; 28(Suppl 4):S58–S65.

35. Wilson PW, D'Agostino RB, Sullivan L, Parise H, Kannel WB. Overweight and obesity as determinants of cardiovascular risk: The Framingham experience. *Arch Intern Med* 2002; 162:1867–1872.

36. Manson JE, Colditz GA, Stampfer MJ, Willett WC, Rosner B, Monson RR, Speizer FE, Hennekens CH. A prospective study of obesity and risk of coronary heart disease in women. *N Engl J Med* 1990; 322:882–889.

37. Hubert HB, Feinleib M, McNamara PM, Castelli WP. Obesity as an independent risk factor for cardiovascular disease: A 26-year follow-up of participants in the Framingham Heart Study. *Circulation* 1983; 67:968–977.

38. Rabkin SW, Mathewson FA, Hsu PH. Relation of body weight to development of ischemic heart disease in a cohort of young North American men after a 26 year observation period: The Manitoba Study. *Am J Cardiol* 1977; 39:452–458.

39. Bassuk S, Manson J. Lifestyle and risk of cardiovascular disease and type 2 diabetes in women: A review of the epidemiologic evidence. *Am J Lifestyle Med* 2008; 3:191–213.
40. Despres JP. Dyslipidemia and obesity. *Bailliere Clin Endocrinol Metab* 1994; 8:629–660.
41. Despres JP., Abdominal obesity as important component of insulin-resistance syndrome. *Nutrition* 1993; 4:452–459.
42. Prineas R, Folsom A, Kayes S. Central adiposity and increased risk of coronary artery disease mortality in older women. *Ann Epidemiol* 1993; 3:35–41.
43. Terry R, Page W, Haskell W. Waist/hip ratio, body mass index and premature cardiovascular mortality in US Army veterans during a 23 year follow up study. *Int J Obes* 1992; 16:417–423.
44. McGill HC Jr. Fatty streaks in the coronary arteries and aorta. *Lab Invest* 1968; 18:560–564.
45. Skalen K, Gustafsson M, Rydberg EK, Hulten LM, Wiklund O, Innerarity TL, Boren J. Subendothelial retention of atherogenic lipoproteins in early atherosclerosis. *Nature* 2002; 417:750–754.
46. Bots ML, Hofman A, Grobbee DE. Increased common carotid intima-media thickness: Adaptive response or a reflection of atherosclerosis? Findings from the Rotterdam Study. *Stroke* 1997; 28:2442–2447.
47. Heiss G, Sharrett AR, Barnes R, Chambless LE, Szklo M, Alzola C. Carotid atherosclerosis measured by B-mode ultrasound in populations: Associations with cardiovascular risk factors in the ARIC study. *Am J Epidemiol* 1991; 134:250–256.
48. Spence JD. Ultrasound measurement of carotid plaque as a surrogate outcome for coronary artery disease. *Am J Cardiol* 2002; 89:10B–15B.
49. McGill HC Jr, McMahan CA, Herderick EE, Malcom GT, Tracy RE, Strong JP. Origin of atherosclerosis in childhood and adolescence. *Am J Clin Nutr* 2000; 72:1307S–1315S.
50. Huang Z, Willett WC, Manson JE et al. Body weight, weight change, and risk for hypertension in women. *Ann Intern Med* 1998; 128(2):81–88.
51. MacMahon S, Cutler J, Brittain E, Higgins M. Obesity and hypertension: Epidemiological and clinical issues. *Eur Heart J* 1987; 8:57–70.
52. Stamler R, Stamler J, Riedlinger WF, Algera G, Roberts RH. Weight and blood pressure: Findings in hypertension screening of 1 million Americans. *JAMA* 1978; 240:1607–1610.
53. Clinical Guidelines on the Identification, Evaluation, and Treatment of Overweight and Obesity in Adults: The Evidence Report: National Institutes of Health. *Obes Res* 1998; 6(Suppl 2):51S–209S.
54. Stepniakowski K, Egan BM. Additive effects of obesity and hypertension to limit venous volume. *Am J Physiol* 1995; 268:R562–R568.
55. Muller DC, Elahi D, Pratley RE, Tobin JD, Andres R. An epidemiological test of the hyperinsulinemia–hypertension hypothesis. *J Clin Endocrinol Metab* 1993; 76:544–548.
56. Poirier P, Lemieux I, Mauriege P, Dewailly E, Blanchet C, Bergeron J, Despres JP. Impact of waist circumference on the relationship between blood pressure and insulin: The Quebec Health Survey. *Hypertension* 2005; 45:363–367.
57. Voors AW, Webber LS, Frerichs RR, Berenson GS. Body height and body mass as determinants of basal blood pressure in children: The Bogalusa Heart Study. *Am J Epidemiol* 1977; 106:101–108.
58. Johnson AL, Cornoni JC, Cassel JC, Tyroler HA, Heyden S, Hames CG. Influence of race, sex and weight on blood pressure behavior in young adults. *Am J Cardiol* 1975; 35:523–530.
59. Landsberg L, Troisi R, Parker D, Young JB, Weiss ST. Obesity, blood pressure, and the sympathetic nervous system. *Ann Epidemiol* 1991; 1:295–303.
60. Mokdad AH, Ford ES, Bowman BA et al. Prevalence of obesity, diabetes, and obesity-related health risk factors, 2001. *JAMA* 2003; 289(1):76–79.
61. Field AE, Coakley EH, Must A et al. Impact of overweight on the risk of developing common chronic diseases during a 10-year period. *Arch Intern Med* 2001; 161(13):1581–1586.

62. Seideli J, Gigolini M, Charzewska J, Ellsigner B, DiBiacs G. Fat distribution in European women: A comparison of anthropometric measurements in relation to cardiovascular risk factors. *Int J Epidemiol* 1990; 19:303–308.

63. Chan JM, Rimm EB, Colditz GA, Stampfer MJ, Willett WC. Obesity, fat distribution, and weight gain as risk factors for clinical diabetes in men. *Diabetes Care* 1994; 17:961–969.

64. Ford ES, Williamson DF, Liu S. Weight change and diabetes incidence: Findings from a national cohort of US adults. *Am J Epidemiol* 1997; 146(3):214–222.

65. Colditz GA, Willett WC, Rotnitzky A, Manson JE. Weight gain as a risk factor for clinical diabetes mellitus in women. *Ann Intern Med* 1995; 122(7):481–486.

66. Ashton WD, Nanchahal K, Wood DA. Body mass index and metabolic risk factors for coronary heart disease in women. *Eur Heart J* 2001; 22(1):46–55.

67. Ford ES, Giles WH, Dietz WH. Prevalence of the metabolic syndrome among US adults: Findings from the third National Health and Nutrition Examination Survey. *JAMA* 2002; 287(3):356–359.

68. Poirier P, Despres JP. Waist circumference, visceral obesity, and cardiovascular risk. *J Cardiopulm Rehabil* 2003; 23:161–169.

69. Hansen BC. The metabolic syndrome X. *Ann N Y Acad Sci* 1999; 892:1–24.

70. National Heart Lung and Blood Institute. Third report of the Expert Panel on Detection, Evaluation, and Treatment of High Blood Cholesterol in Adults (Adult Treatment Panel III), Washington, DC, 2004.

71. Nakajima T, Fujioka S, Tokunaga K, Matsuzawa Y, Tarui S. Correlation of intraabdominal fat accumulation and left ventricular performance in obesity. *Am J Cardiol* 1989; 64:369–373.

72. Hansson PO, Eriksson H, Welin L, Svardsudd K, Wilhelmsen L. Smoking and abdominal obesity: Risk factors for venous thromboembolism among middle-aged men: 'The study of men born in 1913.' *Arch Intern Med* 1999; 159:1886–1890.

73. Goldhaber SZ, Grodstein F, Stampfer MJ, Manson JE, Colditz GA, Speizer FE, Willett WC, Hennekens CH. A prospective study of risk factors for pulmonary embolism in women. *JAMA* 1997; 277:642–645.

74. Messerli FH, Nunez BD, Ventura HO, Snyder DW. Overweight and sudden death: Increased ventricular ectopy in cardiomyopathy of obesity. *Arch Intern Med* 1987; 147:1725–1728.

75. Kannel WB, Plehn JF, Cupples LA. Cardiac failure and sudden death in the Framingham Study. *Am Heart J* 1988; 115:869–875.

76. Brown DW, Giles WH, Greenlund KJ, Valdez R, Croft JB. Impaired fasting glucose, diabetes mellitus, and cardiovascular disease risk factors are associated with prolonged QTc duration: Results from the Third National Health and Nutrition Examination Survey. *J Cardiovasc Risk* 2001; 8:227–233.

77. Hirsch J, Leibel RL, Mackintosh R, Aguirre A. Heart rate variability as a measure of autonomic function during weight change in humans. *Am J Physiol* 1991; 261:R1418–R1423.

78. Eckel RH, Barouch WW, Ershow AG. Report of the National Heart, Lung, and Blood Institute–National Institute of Diabetes and Digestive and Kidney Diseases Working Group on the pathophysiology of obesity associated cardiovascular disease. *Circulation* 2002; 105:2923–2928.

79. Peterson HR, Rothschild M, Weinberg CR, Fell RD, McLeish KR, Pfeifer MA. Body fat and the activity of the autonomic nervous system. *N Engl J Med* 1988; 318:1077–1083.

80. Strollo PJ Jr, Rogers RM. Obstructive sleep apnea. *N Engl J Med* 1996; 334:99–104.

81. Vgontzas AN, Tan TL, Bixler EO, Martin LF, Shubert D, Kales A. Sleep apnea and sleep disruption in obese patients. *Arch Intern Med* 1994; 154:1705–1711.

82. Nieto FJ, Young TB, Lind BK, Shahar E, Samet JM, Redline S, D'Agostino RB, Newman AB, Lebowitz MD, Pickering TG. Association of sleep-disordered breathing, sleep apnea, and hypertension in a large community-based study. Sleep Heart Health Study. *JAMA* 2000; 283:1829–1836.

83. Backman L, Freyschuss U, Hallberg D, Melcher A. Cardiovascular function in extreme obesity. *Acta med Scand* 1973; 193:437–446.

84. Sjostrom L, Lindroos AK, Peltonen M et al., Swedish Obese Subjects Study Scientific Group. Lifestyle, diabetes, and cardiovascular risk factors 10 years after bariatric surgery. *N Engl J Med* 2004; 351:2683–2693.

85. Goldenstein DJ. Beneficial health effects of modest weight loss. *Int J Obes* 1992; 16:397–415.

86. Stamler R, Stamler J, Gosch F, Civinell J, Fishman J, McKeever P, McDonald A, Dyer A. Primary prevention of hypertension by nutritional-hygienic means: Final report of a randomized, controlled trial. *JAMA* 1989; 262:1801–1807.

87. Hypertension Prevention Trial Research Group. The hypertension prevention trial: Three year effects of dietary changes on blood pressure. *Arch Intern Med* 1990; 150:153–162.

88. Trials of Hypertension Prevention Collaborative Research Group. The effects of non-pharmacologic interventions on blood pressure of persons with high normal levels: Results of the Trials of Hypertension Prevention, phase I. *JAMA* 1992; 267:1213–1220.

89. National High Blood Pressure Education Program Working Group. National High Blood Pressure Education Program Working Group report on primary prevention of hypertension. *Arch Intern Med* 1993; 153:186–208.

90. Chobanian AV, Bakris GL, Black HR et al. The seventh report of the Joint National Committee on Prevention, Detection, Evaluation, and Treatment of High Blood Pressure: The JNC 7 report. *JAMA* 2003; 289:2560–2572.

91. Katzel L, Bleeker E, Colman E, Rogus E, Sorkin J, Goldberg A. Effects of weight loss vs aerobic exercise training on risk factors for coronary heart disease to healthy, obese, middle-aged and older men. *JAMA* 1995; 274:1915–1921.

92. Knowler WC, Barrett-Connor E, Fowler SE et al. Reduction in the incidence of type 2 diabetes with lifestyle intervention or metformin. *N Engl J Med* 2002; 346(6):393–403.

93. Tuomilehto J, Lindstrom J, Eriksson JG et al. Prevention of type 2 diabetes mellitus by changes in lifestyle among subjects with impaired glucose tolerance. *N Engl J Med* 2001; 344(18):1343–1350.

94. Ryan DH, Espeland MA, Foster GD et al. Look AHEAD (Action for Health in Diabetes): Design and methods for a clinical trial of weight loss for the prevention of cardiovascular disease in type 2 diabetes. *Control Clin Trials* 2003; 24(5):610–628.

95. Dattilo A, Kris-Etherton P. Effects of weight reduction on blood lipids and lipoproteins: A meta-analysis. *Am J Clin Nutr* 1992; 56:320–328.

96. MacMahon SW, Wilcken De, Macdonald GJ. The effect of weight reduction on left ventricular mass: A randomized controlled trial in young, overweight hypertensive patients. *N Engl J Med* 1986; 314:334–339.

97. Himeno E, Nishino K, Nakashima Y, Kuroiwa A, Ikeda M. Weight reduction regresses left ventricular mass regardless of blood pressure level in obese subjects. *Am Heart J* 1996; 131:313–319.

98. Tuck ML, Sowers J, Dornfeld L, Kledzik G, Maxwell M. The effect of weight reduction on blood pressure, plasma renin activity, and plasma aldosterone levels in obese patients. *N Engl J Med* 1981; 304:930–933.

99. Drenick EJ, Fisler JS. Sudden cardiac arrest in morbidly obese surgical patients unexplained after autopsy. *Am J Surg* 1988; 155:720–726.

100. Isner JM, Sours HE, Paris AL, Ferrans VJ, Roberts WC. Sudden, unexpected death in avid dieters using the liquid-protein-modified fast diet. Observations in 17 patients and the role of the prolonged QT interval. *Circulation* 1979; 60:1401–1412.

101. Pringle TH, Scobie IN, Murray RG, Kesson CM, Maccuish AC. Prolongation of the QT interval during therapeutic starvation: A substrate for malignant arrhythmias. *Int J Obes* 1983; 7:253–261.

102. From the Centers for Disease Control and Prevention. Cardiac valvulopathy associated with exposure to fenfluramine or dexfenfluramine: U.S. Department of Health and Human Services interim public health recommendations. *JAMA* 1997; 278:1729–1731.

103. McNeely W, Goa KL. Sibutramine: A review of its contribution to the management of obesity. *Drugs* 1998; 56:1093–1124.

104. Williamson D, Pamuk E, Thus M, Flanders D, Byers T, Heath C. Prospective study of intentional weight loss and mortality in never ending overweight US white women aged 40–64. *Am J Epidemiol* 1995; 141:1128–1141.

105. Hamm P, Shekelle R, Stamler J. Large fluctuations in body weight during young adulthood and 25 year risk of coronary death in men. *Am J Epidemiol* 1989; 129:312–318.

106. National Task Force on the Prevention and Treatment of Obesity. Weight cycling. *JAMA* 1994; 272:1196–1202.

107. Rexrode KM, Carey VJ, Hennekens CH et al. Abdominal adiposity and coronary heart disease in women. *JAMA* 1998; 280(21):1843–1848.

108. Zhang X, Shu XO, Yang G et al. Abdominal adiposity and mortality in Chinese women. *Arch Intern Med* 2007; 167(9):886–892.

109. Yusuf S, Hawken S, Ounpuu S et al. Obesity and the risk of myocardial infarction in 27,000 participants from 52 countries: A case-control study. *Lancet* 2005; 366(9497):1640–1649.

110. Pouliot MC, Despres JP, Lemieux S, Moorgani S, Bouchard C, Trembla A, Nadea A, Lupien P. Waist circumference and abdominal sagittal diabetes: Vest simple anthropometric indexes of abdominal visceral adipose tissue accumulation and related cardiovascular risk in men. *Am J Cardiol* 1994; 73:460–468.

111. Willett WC, Manson JE, Stampfer MJ et al. Weight, weight change, and coronary heart disease in women: Risk within the 'normal' weight range. *JAMA* 1995; 273(6):461–465.

112. Rexrode K, Hennekens CH, Willett WC, Colditz GA, Stampfer M, Rich-Edwards JW, Speizer EE, Manson JE. A prospective study of body mass index, weight change, and risk of stroke in women. *JAMA* 1997; 227:1539–1545.

113. Troiano RP, Flegal KM, Kuczmarksi RJ, Campbell SM, Johnson CL. Overweight prevalence and trends for children and adolescents: The National Health and Nutrition Surveys, 1963–1991. *Arch Pediatr Adolesc Med* 1995; 140:1085–1091.

114. Van Cleave J, Gortmaker SL, Perrin JM. Dynamics of obesity and chronic health conditions among children and youth. *JAMA* 2010; 303(7):623–630.

115. Eisenstein I, Edelstein J, Sarma R, Sanmarco M, Selvester RH. The electrocardiogram in obesity. *J Electrocardiol* 1982; 15:115–118.

116. Master AM, Oppenheimer ET. A study of obesity: Circulatory, roentgen-ray and electrocardiographic investigations. *JAMA* 1929; 92:1652–1656.

117. Alpert MA, Terry BE, Cohen MV, Fan TM, Painter JA, Massey CV. The electrocardiogram in morbid obesity. *Am J Cardiol* 2000; 85:908–910.

118. Casale PN, Devereux RB, Kligfield P, Eisenberg RR, Miller DH, Chaudhary BS, Phillips MC. Electrocardiographic detection of left ventricular hypertrophy: Development and prospective validation of improved criteria. *J Am Coll Cardiol* 1985; 6:572–580.

119. Abergel E, Tase M, Menard J, Chatellier G. Influence of obesity on the diagnostic value of electrocardiographic criteria for detecting left ventricular hypertrophy. *Am J Cardiol* 1996; 77:739–744.

120. Starr JW, Wagner GS, Behar VS, Walston A II, Greenfield JC Jr. Vectorcardiographic criteria for the diagnosis of inferior myocardial infarction. *Circulation* 1974; 49:829–836.

121. Alpert MA, Kelly DL. Value and limitations of echocardiography assessment of obese patients. *Echocardiography* 1986; 3:261–272.

122. Gal RA, Gunasekera J, Massardo T, Shalev Y, Port SC. Long-term prognostic value of a normal dipyridamole thallium-201 perfusion scan. *Clin Cardiol* 1991; 14:971–974.

123. Ferraro S, Perrone-Filardi P, Desiderio A, Betocchi S, D'Alto M, Liguori L, Trimigliozzi P, Turco S, Chiariello M. Left ventricular systolic and diastolic function in severe obesity: A radionuclide study. *Cardiology* 1996; 87:347–353.

124. McNulty PH, Ettinger SM, Field JM, Gilchrist IC, Kozak M, Chambers CE, Gascho JA. Cardiac catheterization in morbidly obese patients. *Catheter Cardiovasc Interv* 2002; 56:174–177.

125. X-Factor Study. New York: Louis Harris and Associates, Inc., 1997.

126. Rippe JM. Obesity as a risk factor for heart disease: An overview. *Nutr Clin Care* 1998; 1:3–14.

127. Lem M, Wing R, McGuire M, Seagle H, Hill J. A descriptive study of individuals successful at long-term maintenance of substantial weight loss. *Am J Clin Nutr* 1997; 66:239–346.

128. Sacks FM, Bray GA, Carey VJ et al. Comparison of weight-loss diets with different compositions of fat, protein, and carbohydrates. *N Engl J Med* 2009; 360:859–873.

129. U.S. Department of Health and Human Services. 2008 Physical Activity Guidelines for Americans. http://www.health.gov/ PAguidelines (accessed April 21, 2011).

130. The National Weight Control Registry. http://www.nwcr.ws/ (Accessed: September 26, 2011).

131. Gruberg L, Weissman NJ, Waksman R et al. The impact of obesity on the short-term and long-term outcomes after percutaneous coronary intervention: The obesity paradox? *J Am Coll Cardiol* 2002; 39:578–584.

132. Birkmeyer NJ, Charlesworth DC, Hernandez F, Leavitt BJ, Marrin CA, Morton JR, Olmstead EM, O'Connor GT. Obesity and risk of adverse outcomes associated with coronary artery bypass surgery: Northern New England Cardiovascular Disease Study Group. *Circulation* 1998; 97:1689–1694.

133. Marik P, Varon J. The obese patient in the ICU. *Chest* 1998; 113:492–498.

134. Ascione R, Angelini GD. Is obesity still a risk factor for patients undergoing coronary surgery? *Ital Heart J* 2003; 4:824–828.

135. Rockx MA, Fox SA, Stitt LW, Lehnhardt KR, McKenzie FN, Quantz MA, Menkis AH, Novick RJ. Is obesity a predictor of mortality, morbidity and readmission after cardiac surgery? *Can J Surg* 2004; 47:34–38.

13 Obesity and Diabetes

Ioannis G. Fatouros, PhD and
Asimina Mitrakou, MD, PhD

CONTENTS

It has long been recognized that obesity is linked to increased risk of developing type 2 diabetes (T2D) as well as cardiovascular diseases due to a dysregulation of various endocrine, neural, inflammatory, and cell-intrinsic mechanisms. Although in the recent years valuable information has been gathered on the interplay of these mechanisms, their concrete role in the pathogenesis of T2D is still obscure. These mechanisms are interrelated, and it is possible that their interplay may be implicated in the pathophysiology of insulin resistance and T2D. Understanding the relationship of these mechanisms linking obesity, insulin resistance, and/or T2D may contribute to the development of strategies toward the prevention and/or treatment of insulin resistance and the pathologies that are associated with it. This chapter aims at providing a general view of the mechanisms linking obesity to diabetes and the strategies that may contribute to the prevention and/or treatment of T2D in the obese.

PREVALENCE OF OBESITY PANDEMIC

OBESITY-ASSOCIATED MORBIDITY AND MORTALITY

Overweight and obesity are defined as excessive or abnormal fat accumulation that may impair health. Body mass index (BMI) is a simple index of weight for height that is commonly used in classifying overweight and obesity in adult populations and individuals. It is defined as the weight in kilograms divided by the square of the height in meters (kg/m^2). BMI provides the most useful population-level measure of overweight and obesity as it is the same for both sexes and for all ages of adults. However, it should be considered as a rough estimation because it may not correspond to the same degree of fatness in different individuals. The World Health Organization (WHO) defines "overweight" as a BMI equal to or more than 25 and "obesity" as a BMI equal to or more than 30. These cutoff points provide a benchmark for individual assessment, but there is evidence that risk of chronic disease in populations increases progressively from a BMI of 21. The new WHO Child Growth Standards, launched in April 2006, include BMI charts for infants and young children up to age 5. However, measuring overweight and obesity in children aged 5–14 years is a different issue because there is not a standard definition of childhood obesity applied worldwide. WHO is currently developing an international growth reference for school-age children and adolescents [1].

In 2007–2008, the age-adjusted prevalence of obesity was 33.8% (95% confidence interval [CI], 31.6%–36.0%) overall, 32.2% (95% CI, 29.5%–35.0%) among men, and 35.5% (95% CI, 33.2%–37.7%) among women. The corresponding prevalence estimates for overweight and obesity combined (BMI > 25) were 68.0% (95% CI, 66.3%–69.8%), 72.3% (95% CI, 70.4%–74.1%), and 64.1% (95% CI, 61.3%–66.9%). Over the 10 year period, obesity showed no significant trend among women (adjusted odds ratio [AOR] for 2007–2008 vs. 1999–2000, 1.12 [95% CI, 0.89–1.32]). For men, there was a significant linear trend (AOR for 2007–2008 vs. 1999–2000, 1.32 [95% CI, 1.12–1.58]); however, the three most recent data points did not differ significantly from each other [2].

The prevalence of obesity for adults aged 20–74 years increased by 7.9 percentage points for men and by 8.9 percentage points for women between 1976–1980 and

1988–1994, and subsequently by 7.1 percentage points for men and by 8.1 percentage points for women between 1988–1994 and 1999–2000 [3]. The sample size was sufficient to detect a linear increase of this magnitude. Between 1999–2000 and 2007–2008, there was an increase of 4.7 percentage points (95% CI, 0.5–9.0) for men and a nonsignificant increase of 2.1 percentage points (95% CI, −2.1–6.3) for women. For women, the prevalence of obesity showed no statistically significant changes over the 10 year period from 1999 through 2008. For men, there was a significant linear trend over the same period, but estimates for the periods 2003–2004, 2005–2006, and 2007–2008 did not differ significantly from each other. These data suggest that the increases in the prevalence of obesity previously observed between 1976–1980 and 1988–1994 and between 1988–1994 and 1999–2003 may not be continuing at a similar level over the period 1999–2008, particularly for women but possibly for men [2].

The estimates from the NHANES that have shown that the overall prevalence of obesity among both adults and children appears to have stabilized over the past 5–10 years seem to reflect the actual prevalence of obesity among adults and children in the United States [4]. One may interpret this stabilization as the result of increasing recognition by health-care professionals, researchers, schools, community organizations, industry, and governments of the health effects of obesity. This increased recognition may have led to changes that reduce the influence of environmental contributors to inappropriate weight gain, and, thus, we may have come to the point where most people who have a strong genetic susceptibility account for the ever-increasing number of adults with extreme obesity (BMI $\geq$ 40), while a resistant segment of the population remains lean despite our "toxic" environment. The distribution of BMI among adults and children in the United States has become increasingly skewed to the right. The stabilization of obesity rates among children and adolescents that appeared in the NHANES data does not seem to extend to the very heaviest boys (those with a BMI at or above the 97th percentile for their age), whose numbers continue to increase [5]. The prevalence of obesity remains unacceptably high, among some racial and ethnic minority populations. The effects of the current obesity epidemic on the physical, psychological, and economic health of the United States is extremely dangerous because the incidence of obesity-related diseases continues to increase among both adults and children [6,7]. Growing numbers of children now have diseases once considered to be diseases for only adults, such as T2D, nonalcoholic fatty liver disease, and hypertension. There is evidence that the onset of obesity-related diseases at an earlier age may be associated with more severe health consequences in adulthood. In addition, as the incidence of obesity-associated gestational diabetes increases, more fetuses are exposed to a potentially obesogenic intrauterine milieu that may have a significant effect on later risk for obesity, diabetes, and other metabolic disorders, possibly mediated by altered placental uptake of nutrients, which may lead to epigenetic changes and alterations in fetal neural programming. There comes then a vicious cycle of obesity and metabolic disorders that may adversely affect the health of the population for generations. Measures of overall and central adiposity have been strongly associated with the risk of incident diabetes in both men and women [8]. The authors of this study have used longitudinal measures of weight from midlife, at study entry, and over follow-up, and they were able to demonstrate that weight gain during midlife (after 50 years of age) and in late life (after 65 years of age) is an important risk factor for diabetes among older adults. Although the risk associated with weight gain appeared to wane with age, individuals in the highest category of BMI remained at twice the risk of diabetes compared with those in the lowest category among the participants of 75 years of age and older. Additional evidence suggests that high rates of weight gain during infancy may increase a person's later risk of obesity [9]. Thus, the trend toward stabilization of obesity rates could be temporary [10].

INSULIN RESISTANCE AND DIABETES: PATHOPHYSIOLOGY, SYMPTOMS, ASSESSMENT, AND ASSOCIATED COMPLICATIONS

OBESITY AND INSULIN RESISTANCE

Obesity-associated insulin resistance is a major risk factor for T2D and cardiovascular disease. A large number of endocrine, inflammatory, neural, and cell-intrinsic pathways have been shown to be dysregulated in obesity. Most of these factors are interdependent, and it is likely that their dynamic interplay underlies the pathophysiology of insulin resistance.

The influence of obesity on the risk of T2D is determined not only by the degree of obesity, meaning the increased total fat mass, but also by where fat accumulates. Increased upper body fat including visceral adiposity, as reflected in increased abdominal girth or waist-to-hip ratio, is associated with the metabolic syndrome, T2D, and cardiovascular disease [11,12]. Energy imbalance leads to storage of excess energy in adipocytes, which exhibit both hypertrophy and hyperplasia [13]. The processes of adipose hypertrophy and hyperplasia are associated with intracellular abnormalities of adipocyte function, particularly endoplasmic reticulum (ER) and mitochondrial stress. The result of intracellular and systemic consequences leads to adipocyte insulin resistance; production of adipokines, free fatty acids (FFAs), and inflammatory mediators; and promotion of systemic dysfunction that consequently leads to the clinical manifestations of obesity.

Fat tissue dysfunction in obesity is characterized by an altered capacity to store lipids, and enhanced adipose tissue inflammation plays a crucial role in the development of insulin resistance and T2DM [14]. Adipose tissue is supposed to serve as a metabolic buffer. Normally adipose tissue sequesters fatty acids in the postprandial state and releases them under fasting conditions. In abdominal obesity, this buffering action may be impaired, resulting in exposure of nonadipose tissues to excessive fluxes of lipids, promoting thus ectopic fat storage and subsequent development of insulin resistance and T2DM [15]. Under these conditions of energy imbalance that lead to obesity, adipose tissue is no longer regarded as a mere storage of fatty acid excess, but it regulates fatty acid handling as well [16].

Subcutaneous (sc) fat seems to lack the pathological effects of visceral fat or is simply a more neutral storage location, but this concept requires further studies. Beyond differences in body fat distribution, emerging evidence suggests that different subtypes of adipose tissue may be functionally distinct and may affect glucose homeostasis differentially. Adult humans have limited and variable numbers of brown fat cells [17], which play a role in thermogenesis and potentially influence energy expenditure and obesity susceptibility. Brown adipose tissue (BAT), in contrast to white adipose tissue (WAT), is involved in energy dissipation rather than storage [18] but was previously considered to have little physiological relevance in humans beyond early childhood. However, recent studies using ^{18}F-fluorodeoxyglucose (^{18}F-FDG) positron emission tomography–computed tomography (PET–CT) prove that BAT is present in adults, with an activity notably declining with increasing obesity [19]. Improved understanding of the function of different fat cell types and depots and their roles in metabolic homeostasis is a priority for investigation into the pathogenesis and complications of obesity.

Likewise, adipose tissue is composed of heterogeneous cell types. Immune cells within adipose tissue also contribute to systemic metabolic processes. As the study of adipose biology progresses, it will be important to consider whether additional subtypes of adipocytes or other cell types can be identified in order to refine our understanding of obesity complications and generate novel approaches to prevention.

Still, little is known regarding the mechanisms of the regulatory system in obesity, insulin resistance, and T2DM. Several mechanisms linking inflammation, ectopic fat disposition—mainly hepatic steatosis—and gut microbiota, and manipulation thereof by the prebiotic FOS, to adipose tissue dysfunction have been proposed [20,21].

It seems though that the main mechanisms that link obesity to insulin resistance and predispose to T2D are as follows: (1) increased production of adipokines/cytokines, including tumor necrosis factor-α (TNF-α), resistin, and retinol-binding protein 4 (RBP4), that contribute to insulin resistance as well as reduced levels of adiponectin [22–26]; (2) ectopic fat deposition, particularly in the liver and also in skeletal muscle, and the dysmetabolic sequelae [27,28]; and (3) mitochondrial dysfunction, evident by decreased mitochondrial mass and/or function [29]. Mitochondrial dysfunction could be one of the most important underlying defects linking obesity to diabetes, both by decreasing insulin sensitivity and by compromising β-cell function, which will be further elucidated in this chapter.

MECHANISMS OF PROGRESSIVE β-CELL DYSFUNCTION IN OBESE INDIVIDUALS

T2D and impaired glucose tolerance (IGT) have been identified as clinical entities sharing a deficit in both insulin secretion [30,31] and insulin sensitivity [32,33]. One of the main routes though which excess adiposity impairs glucose metabolism is the increased supply of fatty acids into the circulation [34–36]. As mentioned several times in this chapter, persistent positive energy balance is associated with increased storage of triglycerides. This expands the adipose depots and increases the proportion of hypertrophied adipocytes. Under conditions of normal insulin sensitivity, insulin suppresses the activity of hormone-sensitive lipase and thereby reduces lipolysis, which in turn limits the supply of fatty acids into the circulation. However, enlarged adipocytes become less sensitive to the antilipolytic action of insulin, causing an increase in the liberation and turnover of fatty acids. The fatty acids can then be taken up by liver and muscle where they are used in competition with glucose as a source of energy. Thus, the imbalance to the glucose–fatty acid Randle cycle [37] increases the availability of fatty acids and their oxidation and reduces the utilization of glucose. Fatty acid metabolites are also produced that impair the postreceptor pathway of intracellular insulin signaling and decrease insulin-stimulated glucose transport in muscle. Energy generated by fatty acid oxidation can be utilized by the liver in the production of glucose by gluconeogenesis, and fatty acid metabolites that impede insulin action that will inhibit the normal suppression of gluconeogenesis by insulin. Thus, disturbances of the glucose–fatty acid cycle enable increased fatty acids to exacerbate insulin resistance and notably hyperglycemia.

Hyperinsulinemia is the first response of the beta cell (β-cell) to obesity, and it reflects compensation by insulin-secreting β-cells to systemic insulin resistance [38]. A reduction in insulin action is accompanied by upregulation of insulin secretion so that normoglycemia can be maintained by a compensatory increase in insulin secretion [39]. Obese normoglycemic individuals have both increased β-cell mass and function [40–43]. Obesity-induced glucose intolerance reflects failure to mount one or more of these compensatory responses [44]. The reverse observation after weight loss of 10 kg confirms not only the role of obesity in the impairment of insulin secretion and in insulin resistance [45] but also the crucial role of lifestyle changes for obesity/diabetes treatment.

Factors predisposing to β-cell decompensation could also be primarily genetic or epigenetic. A clear, mechanistic basis for this decompensation remains still a matter of debate. Genome-wide association scans (GWAS) and candidate gene approaches now have identified more than 40 genes associated with T2D [46,47] mostly related to β-cell dysfunction and a similar number, of largely different genes, related to obesity. Many obesity gene variants appear to be involved in pathways affecting energy homeostasis. Although numerous diabetes- and obesity-associated genes have been identified, the known genes are estimated to predict only 15% of T2D and 5% of obesity risk. This low predictive power may reflect the serious importance of environmental factors. Less-frequent genetic variants with stronger effects, or gene–environment, gene–gene, and epigenetic interactions that have not yet been fully identified through methods based on population genetics, may play a role.

MECHANISMS LINKING OBESITY AND INSULIN RESISTANCE

INFLAMMATORY MEDIATORS IN OBESITY AND THEIR EFFECTS ON INSULIN SENSITIVITY

Adipose Tissue Macrophages: A Link between Obesity-Associated Inflammation and Insulin Resistance

It is generally accepted that overall adipocyte function represents an important regulator of systemic insulin sensitivity [48]. Adipocytes not only produce substantial amounts of proinflammatory cytokines and chemokines (also known as adipokines) such as TNF-α, interleukin-6 (IL-6), and monocyte chemotactic protein-1 (MCP-1), but they are also responsible for the systemic rise of TNF-α in the obese state [49], especially in the aged [50]. Characteristically, systemic inflammation was transmitted to lean animals when chronically inflamed adipocytes were transplanted from their obese counterparts [51]. The main contributor of inflammatory molecules to adipocytes is primarily macrophages, although other cells types (i.e., fat cells, endothelial cells, lymphocytes, etc.) may contribute [52]. It appears that obesity-induced inflammation results in a significant elevation of proinflammatory molecules (such as the inflammatory adipokines) production by the macrophages that accumulate in adipose tissue [53]. In agreement with these observations, a positive association between BMI and macrophages residing in adipose tissue in humans has been reported by Zeyda et al. [54]. Due to its considerable size, adipose tissue and its macrophages represent an important regulator of systemic inflammation and insulin sensitivity in the obese. Therefore, an augmented release of proinflammatory molecules such as the adipokines and cytokines by the adipose tissue macrophages may contribute considerably to insulin resistance in obese T2D individuals.

An important issue is the mechanism of macrophage infiltration into adipose tissue. Macrophages usually respond to signals concerning cellular damage or death. It appears that obesity-related fat cell hypertrophy results in adipocyte cell death, which then elicits an inflammatory response that includes an increased infiltration of adipose tissue by macrophage subpopulations in order to scavenge cellular debris and free lipid droplets [55]. This increase macrophage infiltration is seen in the adipose tissue of obese individuals but not in that of their lean counterparts [54]. It has been postulated that dying fat cells lack the ability to release chemokines due to metabolic disturbances at the level of ER suggesting that chemokine release should be attributed to other cell types such as the infiltrated macrophages [55]. The omental and subcutaneous adipose tissue (SAT) of obese animals or humans demonstrates increased protein levels and gene expression of various chemokines (i.e., MCP-1, MCP-2, MCP-3, MIP-1α, and RANTES) and their receptors as compared to their lean counterparts [56]. Transgenic animal studies have shown that chemokines released by adipose tissue may be related to macrophage attraction as well as impaired insulin sensitivity in the obese [57,58]. Among chemokines, CCR ligands (MCPs) appear to be responsible for macrophage attraction and infiltration into adipose tissue [59].

Although the mechanisms governing macrophage differentiation are unclear, it appears that the adipose tissue macrophages resemble phenotypically the anti-inflammatory subtype M2 [60,61]. Adipose tissue macrophages have been linked to uptake and removal of lipids, lipoproteins, hemoglobin, and apoptotic debris indicating that they contribute to the disposal of obesity-induced necrotic adipocytes [54,55]. Additionally, adipose tissue macrophages seem to be important sources of both anti-inflammatory (such as the IL-10) and proinflammatory cytokines (TNF-α, IL-1β, and IL-6) that contribute to adipose tissue dysfunction and metabolic dysregulation that is usually seen in the obese state [54]. Obesity appears to differentiate cytokine release patterns from adipose tissue macrophages, that is, from those usually secreted by the M2 subtype to those usually produced by the M1 subtype, contributing to a more proinflammatory milieu [61]. In contrast, weight loss has been associated with an M2 cytokine release pattern promoting a more anti-inflammatory profile [62]. However, it is unclear how obesity and other factors (e.g. nutrition and age) regulate the differentiation between the two macrophage subtypes (M1 and M2) and their cytokine release pattern. This is a critical question since a proinflammatory profile as the one induced by obesity is closely associated to insulin resistance. Indeed, obese humans and animals demonstrate increased circulating concentrations of proinflammatory cytokines, C-reactive protein (CRP), and adipokines [63,64], which may lead to insulin resistance [49,65]. It has been shown that in animal models insulin resistance is developed through intracellular signaling pathways that are activated by proinflammatory cytokines such as TNF-α [66]. Proinflammatory cytokines may also decrease insulin sensitivity by modifying the expression of genes encoding proteins such as the insulin receptor, the glucose transporter GLUT4, PPAR, and adiponectin or by altering insulin signaling–associated proteins [67]. It is believed that cytokines/chemokines promote insulin resistance by attracting macrophages into adipocytes. Then, once inside the adipose tissue, macrophages secrete proinflammatory molecules (such as MCP-1 or osteopontin) that may lead to further recruitment of macrophages. However, macrophages may not be the main source of inflammatory molecules, and cytokines-induced inflammation may not be the only cause of reduced insulin sensitivity in the obese state [68,69].

Toll-Like Receptor: Linking Obesity and Inflammation

The toll-like receptor 4 (TLR4) has been implicated as a potential link between obesity and diabetes. Obesity induces a marked elevation of FFA concentrations, which, in turn, may trigger an inflammatory response in cell types such as the macrophages and the adipocytes. In particular, saturated FFA may activate macrophage-like cells through the TLR4 pathway [48]. In fact, FFAs have been shown to activate nuclear factor kappa beta (NF-kB) intracellular signaling as well as cytokine production in macrophage-like cells [70]. However, this inflammatory signaling of FFA appears to disappear when TLR4 is nonfunctional or absent, indicating that this TLR4 on adipocytes and macrophages may act as a sensor of increased FFA levels that ultimately leads to an inflammatory response and insulin-desensitizing actions [48,71]. Characteristically, insulin resistance is prevented in animals not expressing TLR4 [71].

It has been proposed that TLR4 activation in insulin-resistant states may be induced by obesity-related endotoxemia as a result of a high-fat diet consumption. Endotoxins such as lipopolysaccharide (LPS) along with CD14 may be potent stimuli for TLR4 activation [72,73]. Gut-derived gram-negative bacteria produce endotoxins that enter the bloodstream by chylomicron transportation, which is greatly upregulated following high-fat meal consumption [74]. High-fat diets have been shown to upregulate endotoxemia in both animals and humans [75,76]. Furthermore, endotoxemia causes hepatic insulin resistance that results in fasting hyperglycemia and insulinemia as well as weight gain and adipose tissue inflammation [75]. Therefore, there is sufficient evidence to suggest that obesity-induced endotoxemia may induce insulin resistance through TLR4 activation.

Molecular Dysregulations Associated with Lipid Oversupply

T2D is associated with obesity-induced insulin resistance. Insulin resistance represents a state where peripheral tissues fail to increase whole-body glucose disposal in response to insulin action. Two of the most important peripheral tissues responsible for glucose clearance from the blood, liver and muscle, demonstrate reduced insulin-stimulated glucose uptake and metabolism contributing to the elevation of insulin resistance. This section will attempt to describe the molecular pathways responsible for the reduced insulin action when lipid supply is increased, as it is happening in obesity.

According to Randle's theory, accumulated fatty acids may hamper insulin-stimulated glucose uptake, especially in muscle [37]. Lipid oversupply leads to increased fat oxidation that elevates the mitochondrial ratio of acetyl coenzyme A to coenzyme A and NADH to NAD+ resulting in pyruvate dehydrogenase inactivation and citrate accumulation, thereby inhibiting phosphofructokinase and elevating intracellular levels of glucose-6-phosphate, (G6P) which, in turn, upregulate glycogen synthesis and hexokinase inhibition [37]. This cascade of events increases the intracellular glucose concentration that inhibits further glucose uptake by the tissue. Therefore, obesity-related lipid oversupply impairs intracellular glucose uptake and utilization by inactivating some key glycolytic enzymes. In support of this theory, when Perseghin et al. compared young, lean, and insulin-resistant adults with T2D with age- and weight-matched controls, they reported an inverse correlation between circulating fatty acid concentration and insulin sensitivity [77]. Other studies have shown an even stronger inverse association between insulin sensitivity and intramuscular lipid concentration (assessed either by magnetic resonance spectroscopy [MRS] or in muscle biopsies) [78–80]. If Randle's theory was right, insulin-resistant diabetics would have exhibited increased intramuscular concentrations of G6P and glycogen. However, studies that employed MRS revealed a reduced (>50%) insulin-stimulated glucose uptake, glycogen synthesis, and G6P concentration in muscle of type 2 diabetics as compared to healthy controls [81,82]. Similar findings have been reported from studies that elevated circulating plasma lipids in healthy individuals [83]. Hence, in contrast to the theory postulated by Randle and colleagues, increased lipid availability induces insulin resistance due to a defect in either glucose transport or phosphorylation (hexokinase step) but not due to glycolytic inhibition. Later studies revealed that insulin resistance is related not to a defect in the phosphorylation reaction catalyzed by hexokinase, but it appears that increased lipid availability blunts insulin-stimulated glucose transport [84]. Later studies revealed that insulin resistance due to increased lipid availability is related not to a defect in the phosphorylation reaction catalyzed by hexokinase but to a defective insulin-stimulated glucose transport [84] probably due to an impairment in insulin-mediated GLUT4 translocation to sarcolemmal membrane of the muscle cell [85].

Therefore, accumulation of fatty acids and their metabolites such as the diacylglycerols (DAG) leads to insulin resistance due to impaired glucose transport across the cell plasma membrane of peripheral tissues such as skeletal muscle. Indeed, inhibition of lipid accumulation in muscle cells by various methods (blockage of fat transport, lipoprotein lipase removal, and upregulation of energy expenditure) prevents insulin resistance [86]. However, obesity-related insulin resistance may not be prevented by merely shifting oxidation in muscle without increasing total energy expenditure [87]. The fact that the *ob/ob* adiponectin transgenic mouse that is leptin deficient (*ob/ob*) and overexpresses adiponectin (that improves insulin sensitivity) exhibits lower levels of triglycerides and DAG in the liver and higher insulin sensitivity and a larger body weight supports the DAG hypothesis [88]. Although endurance athletes and MCK-DGAT1 mice (overexpress DAG acyltransferase that transfers a fatty acid from a fatty acyl coenzyme A to DAG to make a triglyceride) exhibit high triglyceride concentration in their muscles, they do not demonstrate muscle insulin resistance [89]. What these two different species have in common? They both have a low intramuscular DAG concentration providing further support to the DAG hypothesis [90]. Therefore, obesity may induce insulin resistance through a mechanism related to increased accumulation of DAGs due to increased lipid availability and reduced capacity of peripheral tissues to oxidize fatty acids (probably due to reduced mitochondrial content) and/or convert DAGs to triacylglycerols (TAG) [91,92]. But how increased lipids in general and DAGs in specific reduce insulin sensitivity?

Insulin resistance in peripheral tissues and especially skeletal muscle may be caused by either impaired GLUT4 translocation or impaired insulin signaling. The fact that stimuli other than insulin, such as muscle contraction and hypoxia, promote glucose transport and uptake in obese insulin-resistant state via a distinctly different signaling pathway, suggests that the glucose transport mechanism is not hampered in an insulin-resistant state [93,94]. On the other hand, it has been shown that the early steps of the insulin signaling mechanism (i.e., autophosphorylation of the insulin receptor, phosphorylation of insulin receptor substrate 1 [IRS-1], activation of phosphatidylinositol 3-kinase, and the insulin-receptor tyrosine kinase activity) in the insulin-resistant state are depressed compared to the healthy state probably due to insulin receptor phosphorylation on serine and threonine residues [95,96]. So, what causes this phosphorylation?

Protein kinase C (PKC) phosphorylates and inhibits the insulin receptor, thereby inducing resistance [97]. Well-performed experiments have shown that, out of eight PKC isoforms, PKC-β is elevated in skeletal muscle of obese insulin-resistant individuals as compared to their lean noninsulin-resistant counterparts [96]. Experimentation with human skeletal muscle strips revealed that activation of PKC induces insulin resistance by reducing glucose transport while its inhibition upregulates insulin-mediated glucose transport, suggesting that the specific enzyme has a critical role in insulin signaling [98]. Same results were obtained when insulin resistance was induced following a lipid oversupply model (lipid–heparin infusion) in animals and humans, suggesting that fat accumulation provides a strong stimulus for PKC activation [99,100]. Therefore, PKC stimulation due to lipid oversupply may induce insulin resistance by impairing the insulin signaling pathway. However, is there a direct association between DAG accumulation and PKC activation?

Evidence suggests that DAG, fatty acyl-coenzyme A (CoA), ceramides, and other intramuscular lipid metabolic intermediates depress some early steps in the insulin signaling pathway [101]. For example, DAG and fatty acyl-CoA have been shown to activate PKC in numerous various tissues [101,102], while ceramides stimulate a phosphatase that dephosphorylates the akt/protein kinase B that ultimately depresses GLUT4 translocation and glucogenesis [103]. Furthermore, lipid oversupply elevates intramuscular fatty acyl-CoA concentration and activates PKC either directly or indirectly since these molecules are metabolic precursors for DAG synthesis [101]. Moreover, in insulin-resistant states, elevated DAG levels directly stimulate PKC [104].

A critical question here is: What causes the intracellular fat accumulation in peripheral tissues such as skeletal muscle? It has to do with either a depression of fatty acid oxidation and/or elevated FFA transport into the cells. Earlier studies have shown that these two alternatives may be valid in obesity-induced insulin resistance [105,106]. As it was shown by Hulver et al. [106], FFA oxidation is reduced, and fatty acyl-CoA concentration in skeletal muscle is substantially higher in moderately and severely obese individuals as compared to their healthy counterparts. However, the fact that in that study fatty acyl-CoA levels were increased despite that muscle's capacity for fat oxidation was intact and that skeletal muscle insulin resistance was comparable in moderately and severely obese individuals suggests that a depression of FFA oxidation is not necessary for fatty acyl-CoA accumulation inside the cells. Therefore, an increased FFA uptake may be responsible for the accumulation of FFA intermediates in the cells of peripheral tissues. Obesity has been shown to increase the levels of circulating lipids, a condition that may predispose to an increased FFA clearance by peripheral tissues such as the skeletal muscle in insulin-resistance states [107].

It seems that obesity induced the upregulation of intracellular lipid intermediates due to an increased fatty acid uptake that, in turn, alter insulin signaling via the PKC reaction resulting in decreased glucose transport and insulin resistance.

GENETIC LINKS BETWEEN OBESITY AND TYPE 2 DIABETES

It appears that in both humans and animals, monogenic obesity is a rare phenomenon, and genes related to this type of obesity are not involved in etiology of polygenic obesity. By using the approach of genome-wide linkage analysis, several laboratories identified a good number of quantitative trait loci (QTL) related to obesity and diabetes abnormalities such as plasma insulin/glucose levels, fat mass, body weight, etc. [108]. Nevertheless, until now only a limited number of responsible gene variants have been discovered.

Research in this area has been performed mostly on animal models such as the New Zealand obese (NZO) mouse that exhibits the characteristics of morbid obesity, insulin resistance, and related abnormalities (i.e., hypertension and hypercholesterolemia) that ultimately lead to the development of T2D, which is accompanied by β-cell destruction, low-circulating insulin concentration, and hyperglycemia [109]. When a QTL is performed on NZO and control mice of different congenic lines, valuable information is obtained relatively to the genetic interactions of obesity and diabetes [110]. Except the NZO, the mice that carry a db/db mutation (background strain C57BLKS) are also characterized by 100% prevalence of diabetes. In contrast, the ob/ob (background strain C57BL/6J) mice do no develop diabetes while blood sugar levels remain normal due to a vast β-cell proliferation and high-circulating insulin levels [111]. Therefore, scientists use these two strains in order to discover diabetes-sensitive and diabetes-resistant gene traits since incorporation of the ob mutation into certain strains results in diabetic lines whereas the db allele does not induce diabetes [111,112]. By using this methodology, scientists discovered two genes that may be related to onset of diabetes: the *Sorcs1* [113] and the Lisch-like [114].

After researchers identified the most important and suggestive QTLs by crossing the NZO and lean strains, they used a variety of methods to discover genes that may be important. Hence, when using a sequencing of candidate genes related to energy balance and those that were identified in a QTL, a number of gene variants with certain functional modifications were characterized such as that of the leptin receptor and the NMU receptor [115,116]. When researchers used previous genome-wide mutagenesis and siRNA experimentation, certain gene orthologs located in one QTL were found to be related with obesity such as the cholesterol transporter gene variant and the Abcg1 variant [117]. When positional cloning and introgression of a QTL into a different background was utilized, the *Tbc1d1* gene from the Nob1 QTL and the *Zfp69* from the Nidd/SJL QTL were identified [118,119].

A disruption of RabGAP *Tbc1d1* resulted in an attenuation of fatness and diabetes symptoms in NZO mice by inducing a metabolic shift from carbohydrate to fat oxidation [120]. When suppression of *Tbc1d1* results in a reduction of RabGTP hydrolysis and, consequently, upregulation of FFA transport and oxidation, which then attenuates glucose transport [121]. The *Zfp69* gene variant may be another possible candidate with diabetogenic potential. The expression of this transcription factor in adipose tissue may be involved in the pathogenesis of T2Ds [121].

Leptin resistance has been implicated in the etiology of NZO obesity [116]. In agreement with this notion, the NZO mice carry a leptin receptor gene variant that is characterized by four amino acid exchanges including two nonconservative substitutions (A720T, T1044I) [116]. This variant allele seems to contribute to a rise of body weight and insulin levels in the NZO mice, and this effect may depend on other alleles of adipose tissue [122]. Therefore, the specific gene variant may contribute to the development of obesity and diabetes.

Defective phosphatidylcholine metabolism has also been implicated in the etiology of T2D of NZO mice based on the lower hepatic activities of two of its key enzymes [123]. Indeed, the QTL Nidd3, which is responsible for hyperglycemia and hypoinsulinemia, carries the inactive R120H gene variant of the phosphatidylcholine transfer protein (regulates hepatic fat metabolism), which may also have a diabetogenic action [124].

Another gene variant that has been associated with obesity and diabetes is that of the ATP-binding cassette transporter G1 (Abcg1) that catalyzes the export of cholesterol from the cells [117]. The Abcg1 is located in an obesity-related QTL on proximal chromosome 17 and, in NZO mice, has been associated with increased triglyceride stores, especially in WAT [117]. In fact, its disruption induces significant decrements in fat cell size, prevents insulin resistance following a high-fat diet, and increases GLUT4 expression and fatty acid transporter FATP1 [117].

One more gene variant that has been implicated in the etiology of obesity and diabetes is that of the neuromedin U receptor 2 (Nmur2$^{V190M/I202M}$), which is involved in the regulation of energy balance and is located on an obesity-related QTL on chromosome 11 [116]. The specific receptor regulates the effects of the anorexigenic neuromedin on meal frequency at the hypothalamic level. The activity of this receptor is substantially suppressed in the NZO mice as compared to their lean counterparts [116]. Therefore, the suppressed signal transduction of the Nmur2$^{V190M/I202M}$ variant may induce an attenuation of the anorexigenic effect of neuromedin U receptor 2 [116].

In summary, based on studies with NZO mice, there are specific gene variants that have been associated with the pathophysiology of obesity and diabetes by altering fat oxidation, fat storage, fat transport, glucose transport, and energy balance. Although not proven yet, these genes may play a significant role in human obesity and diabetes as well.

ENDOCRINE LINKS BETWEEN OBESITY AND DIABETES

Impaired Catecholamine-Induced Lipolysis in the Obese, Insulin-Resistant State: Cause or Consequence

One of the main characteristics of obesity is fat accumulation in adipose tissue in the form of TAG resulting in excessive lipid outflow in the blood compartment. This increased fat overflow in the circulation may result in elevated fat uptake by other nonadipose peripheral tissues such as the liver, the pancreas, and the skeletal muscle, a phenomenon also known as ectopic fat storage. As stated before, this elevated ectopic fat storage in skeletal muscle may lead to accumulation of lipid intermediates such as DAG, ceramides, etc., which can alter insulin signaling, thereby inducing insulin resistance. It has been suggested that this fat accumulation in both adipose and nonadipose tissues may be attributed to a defective catecholamine-induced lipolysis. The purpose of this section does not include the detailed description of the lipolytic pathway in adipose tissue and skeletal muscle. Therefore, only a brief outline of the lipolytic pathway will be provided. The main focus of this section is to question whether possible disturbances in catecholamine-induced lipolysis in these tissues may be the cause or the result of the obese, insulin-resistant state.

Adipose tissue lipolysis is mainly regulated by catecholamines and insulin, although there may be other potent lipolytic agents such as the natriuretic peptides (NP) acting through a different mechanism especially when β-adrenergic receptors are not functional [125]. After catecholamines bind to β-adrenergic receptors, the latter are coupled with the stimulatory unit of G proteins (Gs) to activate adenylate cyclase (AC), which then will produce cyclic adenosine monophosphate (cAMP). cAMP will then activate protein kinase A (PKA), which will then phosphorylate the hormone-sensitive lipase (HSL) and perilipins. On the other hand, if an agent (e.g., insulin, NPY, and prostaglandins) binds to α2-adrenergic receptors, then the latter will be coupled to the inhibitory unit of G proteins (Gi) that will ultimately inactivate AC and suppress cAMP production, PKA stimulation, and HSL and perilipin phosphorylation. Following its phosphorylation, HSL is translocated to the lipid droplet in the fat cell, while perilipin phosphorylation facilitates HSL action (its access on the lipid droplet surface) to initiate lipolysis by hydrolyzing the lipid core. Docking of fatty acid–binding protein (FABP4) to HSL enhances the exit of the nonesterified fatty acid (NEFA) from the fat cell (following their release from the lipid core due to the action of HSL). HSL docking on the lipid outer surface may be facilitated by the interaction of the lipase with lipotransin. While HSL may be the major lipase during catecholamine-induced lipolysis, another lipase, the adipose triglyceride lipase (ATGL), demonstrates a high substrate affinity for TAG hydrolysis and appears to be the main regulator of basal lipolysis. ATGL's activation by phosphorylation is independent of PKA action. ATGL and HSL hydrolyze 95% of fat cells' TAG. The remaining monoacylglycerol (MAG) is hydrolyzed by the monoacylglycerol lipase (MGL) into one FFA and one glycerol molecule. The lipolytic cascade is concluded with NEFA and glycerol efflux from the fat cell. Fatty acids exit by passive diffusion by several plasma membrane transporters such as fatty acid translocase (FAT/CD36), $FABP_{pm}$, and caveolin and/or by an unidentified ATP-dependent pump. Glycerol exits mainly through the aquaporin-7 (AQP7) channel. The physiological significance of other hormones (growth hormone, TNF-α, etc.) in the upregulation of the lipolytic cascade in humans remains relatively unclear. In contrast, the antilipolytic role of insulin is well established. Insulin, as the main antilipolytic agent, may increase cAMP degradation, suppress AC activation, deactivate β-adrenergic receptors, and dephosphorylate HSL. An increased adipose tissue blood flow may be crucial for fatty acid removal following their release. It appears that, due to differences at the β-adrenergic receptor and postreceptor level, catecholamine-induced lipolysis is greater in visceral fat as compared to subcutaneous fat. On the other hand, insulin exerts a more intense antilipolytic action in subcutaneous fat cells as compared to visceral fat cells due to discrepancies at insulin receptor and postreceptor level.

In obesity, numerous research groups have reported a blunted catecholamine-induced lipolysis in SAT [126–129]. This phenomenon may be either a primary defect predisposing to elevated fat storage in adipose tissue or a consequence of the obese state. This defective response is mainly seen in β2-adrenergic receptors as a result of their reduced number and/or function [130]. Others have indicated that α2-adrenergic receptors may also contribute to this blunted lipolytic response, especially in the abdominal subcutaneous tissue [131]. Several reports also implicate the reduced HSL expression and/or activity in this disturbed basal and exercise-induced lipolytic response in obese humans and animals [132–135]. Some investigators have proposed that catecholamine resistance may also be induced by ATGL deficiency [136]. Nevertheless, ATGL may not be the main contributor for this blunted lipolytic response since HSL is the principal mediator of catecholamine-induced lipolysis in adipose tissue in the obese state. Another factor that might contribute to blunted lipolysis is HSL's and other lipases' access to lipid droplets (substrate) due to a defective lipase translocation [137] as a result of reduced activation and/or expression of perilipins [138]. However, it is not clear whether perilipins' expression and translocation is defective in human adipose tissue of obese adults as compared to their lean counterparts [139,140]. More work is needed in this area. Data from AQP7-deficient animals suggest that in the obese there may be a disturbed glycerol outflow from adipose tissue due to a reduced expression of this catecholamine-regulated protein that contributes to glycerol efflux [141,142]. If glycerol outflow from adipose tissue is inhibited, glycerol concentration increases in the cytoplasm of the adipocytes, thereby elevating glycerol kinase activity that ultimately upregulates G3P levels and triglyceride synthesis [143,144]. Factors such as adipose blood flow [145] and impaired adrenergic stimulation [146] may also promote insulin resistance in the obese.

The regulation of skeletal muscle lipolysis differs from that in adipose tissue. In muscle, catecholamines exert their action only through the β2-adrenergic receptors (via PKA activation), while other lipolytic hormones (such as the ANP) have no effect [147]. Triglyceride hydrolysis is performed by an HSL expressed in human skeletal muscle fibers. The factors regulating HSL activity in skeletal muscle are less clear compared to adipose tissue. For example, muscle contraction may also activate HSL in a synergistic manner with catecholamines [147]. However, the effects of muscle contraction and of catecholamines are mediated by distinct signaling pathways [148]. During muscle contraction, calcium may activate PKC, which, in turn, phosphorylates and activates HSL [149]. During exercise, catecholamines seem to be the main regulators of HSL activity in skeletal muscle [150]. Furthermore, increased glucose availability in skeletal muscle fibers appears to downregulate HSL activity [151]. ATGL may also contribute to TAG hydrolysis, at least in animal models [137]. It appears that skeletal muscle lipolysis is less affected by insulin than that in adipose tissue in both lean and obese subjects [152]. Hyperglycemia, on the other hand, may be a more potent suppressor of skeletal muscle lipolysis than insulin, especially in diabetics [153]. To a lesser extent, perilipins are also involved in skeletal muscle lipolysis [154]. However, their origin is still questionable. Nevertheless, adipose differentiation–related protein (ADRP) may be more important than perilipins for HSL interaction with lipid droplets in skeletal muscle [155]. Glycerol efflux from skeletal muscle is probably mediated by AQP7 [147].

The elevated intramuscular triglycerides (ITG) observed in the obese have been associated with skeletal muscle insulin resistance and reflect an impaired capacity to utilize fat as an energy substrate in the mitochondria [80]. Reduced skeletal muscle lipolysis may also affect insulin signaling and function [156]. However, it remains unclear whether skeletal muscle lipolysis is impaired in humans. In fact, glycerol release from muscle appears similar in obese and lean individuals during fasting [157]. On the other hand, others have reported a reduced glycerol release in the interstitial space from skeletal muscle in obese as compared to their lean counterparts following infusion of a β2 agonist suggesting a blunted lipolysis in response to catecholamine stimulation [158]. This finding may be attributed to either differences in muscle fiber composition of the examined muscles or discrepancies in the β-adrenergic receptor density between lean and obese subjects. It is not known, however, whether this reduced lipolytic response is related to an impaired expression and/or activation of HSL or ATGL (or both) in the obese. In animals, HSL and not ATGL deficiency has been associated with elevated DAG skeletal muscle concentration and insulin resistance [134]. Furthermore, the obese may demonstrate a blunted skeletal muscle blood flow in response to β-adrenergic stimulation as compared to the lean resulting in adequate nutrient supply of the myocytes, which, in turn, may interfere with fat metabolism in muscle tissue [158].

One has to ask whether this blunted catecholamine-induced lipolysis in the obese represents a primary cause predisposing to insulin resistance or a consequence of the obese, insulin-resistant state. The fact that impaired lipolysis (mainly in adipose tissue) is present in childhood obesity [159], is not reversed following weight loss [160], is also evident in first-degree relatives of obese humans [161], and is related to polymorphisms of genes encoding important proteins involved in the lipolytic cascade (adrenergic receptors, HSL, perilipins, etc.) [162] indicates that it is an early adaptation in obesity that contributes to increased fat storage. Therefore, it is possible that early genetic defects induce a catecholamine resistance of the lipolytic pathway that predisposes to excessive fat storage and obesity. On the other hand, one would also ask if there is evidence that this lipolytic resistance to catecholamine stimulation is a consequence of obesity that could worsen insulin resistance. If that was the case, FFA concentration in the circulation should always be higher in the obese compared to the lean. However, such a finding is not always observed when the obese are compared to the lean [129,158]. In fact, fasting glycerol outflow from adipose tissue may be even less in the obese probably due to the presence of hyperinsulinemia [163,164]. One could argue that hyperinsulinemia may be the cause of this blunted lipolytic response. However, when hyperinsulinemia was prevented by a pancreatic hormonal clamp, a blunted lipolysis was still present [128].

In any case, a blunted lipolysis may an important factor in the pathogenesis of obesity and T2D. Future pharmaceutical interventions may target various proteins of the lipolytic cascade in order to offset the deleterious effects of its downregulation. Since lipolysis affects FFA concentration in the circulation, its manipulation by various agents (i.e., drugs) may be considered for the treatment of T2D and other pathological conditions characterized by reduced fat storage such as cachexia and lipodystrophy [147]. In obesity, however, lipase activation may aid against obesity. Exercise helps to hydrolyze stored triglycerides from adipose tissue and oxidize them in skeletal muscle. However, may obese individuals demonstrate an exercise resistance suggesting that their adipose may not be responsive to an exercise stimulus? More research is needed in this area in order to understand the mechanisms regulating adipose tissue lipolysis under various conditions.

Impaired Free Fatty Acid Utilization in Skeletal Muscle

Besides an impaired skeletal muscle lipolysis, obese adults may exhibit a reduced potential for FFA utilization by their skeletal muscles [165], which, in turn, may contribute to the pathogenesis of obesity since a reduced skeletal muscle oxidative potential impairs resting metabolic rate [166]. In fact, obese adults have been reported to demonstrate a reduced uptake and utilization (oxidation) of FFAs by their skeletal muscles and increased glucose uptake and oxidation following β-adrenergic stimulation [167]. Similar results have been obtained by studies using muscle strips from obese and morbidly obese individuals [106,168]. Interestingly, this impaired capacity for FFA handling was not reversed by a weight loss [160]. Therefore, it is not certain whether this reduced potential of skeletal muscle for FFA oxidation contributes to the development of obesity. However, a reduced skeletal muscle fat oxidation may be classified as a risk factor for developing obesity since individuals with high resting respiratory quotient (RQ) have significantly more possibilities to gain weight compared to those with a low RQ [166,169]. This impaired capacity of skeletal muscle to utilize fatty acids may also be attributed to the reduced muscle mass of the obese thereby increasing even further their potential to store energy. This phenomenon is usually observed in sedentary obese individuals who demonstrate reduced muscle capillary bed and energy substrate delivery to muscle resulting in reduced muscle's oxidative potential. The combination of reduced energy expenditure by skeletal muscle and increased energy delivery through diet contributes to the development of obesity.

Reduced fat uptake utilization by skeletal muscle is evident during insulin-resistant, obese, prediabetic, and diabetic states [170,171]. Stable isotope studies in humans have also shown that fat uptake and oxidation in skeletal muscle of obese T2D are reduced compared to that of healthy controls during either a postabsorptive state or β-adrenergic stimulation [172]. There is evidence that in T2D FFAs delivered to skeletal muscle do not enter the oxidation pathways but rather they are likely incorporated into muscle's TAG pool [172,173]. Moreover, obese and obese T2D individuals demonstrate a reduced suppression of FFA uptake and increase fat oxidation in skeletal muscle following insulin stimulation during fasting [174]. In contrast, during fasting, healthy controls switch from fat oxidation to an increased glucose uptake and oxidation [174]. Similarly, a reduced fat oxidation in the obese T2D has been observed during mild cardiovascular exercise [170]. In light of this evidence, it has been proposed that in metabolic inflexible states such as insulin resistance, skeletal muscle may lose its ability to switch between energy substrates (i.e., fat and carbohydrate) resulting in fat accumulation in muscle [174].

This reduced capacity of skeletal muscle to handle fat in obesity and T2D may be attributed to several factors. A reduced blood–muscle concentration gradient has been implicated to the reduced fatty acid uptake by skeletal muscle during fasting and following β-adrenergic stimulation [175]. This may be attributed, at least partly, to a reduced protein content of fatty acid transporters such as fatty acid binding protein (FABPc) in skeletal muscle of individuals with T2D compared to healthy lean controls [171]. A mutation in the gene of another fatty acid carrier protein, the fatty acid translocase (FAT/CD36), has been correlated with hypertriglyceridemia and a defective fat metabolism in skeletal muscle and adipose tissue [176]. The fact that thiazolidinedione (TZD) treatment and an upregulated expression of FAT/CD36 enhanced protein-mediated transport of FFAs in human skeletal muscle provides further support for the important role of fatty acid transport in the impaired skeletal muscle fat oxidation of obese and T2D individuals [177]. However, other reports suggest FFA transport may not contribute to the reduced fat oxidation in skeletal muscle [171,178]. More work is needed in order to determine whether an impaired fatty acid transport across the skeletal muscle fiber plasma membrane contributes to reduced fat oxidation.

Mitochondrial transport of long-chain fatty acids through the carnitine palmitoyltransferase 1 (CPT1) has also been implicated in the etiology of reduced fat oxidation in skeletal muscle of obese and T2D individuals. A rise of malonyl-CoA content due to an increase of acetyl-CoA carboxylase (ACC) activity or an attenuation of malonyl-CoA decarboxylase activity may result in the inhibition of CPT1 and a reduction of fat oxidation. There are several reports suggesting that this assumption may be true. First, obesity and insulin resistance are accompanied by a rise in intramuscular malonyl-CoA content in rodents [179]. Second, a fat oxidation enhancement following lifestyle interventions is accompanied by a reduced ACC mRNA expression indicating that a reduced fatty acid mitochondrial transport may contribute to the reduced fat oxidation in skeletal muscle [180,181]. Third, CPT1 activity is related with FFA uptake in obese adults [167]. Another interesting idea suggests that the increased intramyocellular glucose availability (due to the mass action effect) may inhibit fat oxidation [182]. In fact, glucose uptake and oxidation in skeletal muscle of obese, insulin-resistant, and T2D states is upregulated during fasting and following β-adrenergic stimulation compared to healthy lean controls [105,160,183]. Moreover, hyperglycemia and hyperinsulinemia increase intramuscular malonyl-CoA content, inhibit CPT1 activity, and promote a lower long-chain fatty acid oxidation (and an increased long-chain fatty acid storage) [184] probably due to a defect in CPT1 and mitochondrial content [168] suggesting a possible substrate competition in skeletal muscle.

Obesity and T2D have been associated with a reduced intramyocellular mitochondrial content and size as well as an impaired electron transport chain activity

[185,186]. If one considers the significance of mitochondria in skeletal muscle's fat oxidation potential, we may conclude that an attenuation of electron transport chain activity in mitochondria may represent an integral part of the pathogenesis of insulin resistance in T2D [187]. This reduced mitochondrial content may be linked to a disturbed expression of genes encoding proteins responsible for mitochondrial biogenesis such as the peroxisome proliferator–activated coactivator 1a (PGC-1a) [188,189]. Others believe that the impaired mitochondrial function may be attributed to the accumulation of lipids and lipid peroxides inside the mitochondria thereby damaging this organelle [190].

Other factors that may contribute to a reduced FFA uptake and oxidation in skeletal muscle of the obese and insulin-resistant individuals are impaired catecholamine-mediated lipolysis, the reduced muscle capillarization, and blood flow, as well as the fiber type composition [191,192].

Adipokines

The aforementioned adverse intracellular consequences of energy imbalance and nutrient toxicity in the adipocytes, including ER and mitochondrial (oxidative) stress, also have systemic consequences. Systemic mediators of adipocyte dysfunction include adipokines, FFAs, and inflammatory mediators. Adipokines, including adiponectin, leptin, resistin, ghrelin, and the newly discovered RBP4, are circulating molecules produced by adipocytes that affect energy use and production and appear central to the pathophysiology of obesity and its systemic health effects, including nonalcoholic fatty liver disease, insulin resistance, atherosclerosis, and T2D [193–195]. In addition to their effects on energy use, adipokines influence production of inflammatory mediators. For instance, adiponectin inhibits the synthesis and actions of TNF-α, and in turn, TNF-α negatively affects adiponectin transcription [193]. Leptin increases the synthesis of IL-6 and TNF-α by macrophages and also activates macrophages [193]. Resistin increases TNF-α and IL-6 synthesis, and resistin expression is, in turn, increased by those cytokines [193].

In this inflammatory process, adipokines play multiple roles. Leptin is an adipocyte-derived cytokine, synthesized and released from fat cells in response to changes in body fat. Leptin circulates partially bound to plasma proteins and enters the CNS by diffusion through capillary junctures in the median eminence and by saturable receptor transport in the choroid plexus. In the hypothalamus, leptin binds to receptors that stimulate anorexigenic peptides such as proopiomelanocortin and cocaine- and amphetamine-regulated transcript and inhibit orexigenic peptides, for example, neuropeptide Y and the agouti gene–related protein [196]. Leptin reduces intracellular lipid levels in skeletal muscle, liver, and pancreatic β-cells, thereby improving insulin sensitivity. In muscle, insulin sensitization is achieved through malonyl-CoA inhibition, which increases transport of fatty acids into mitochondria for beta oxidation. These changes are partially mediated by central sympathetic activation of adrenergic receptors [197]. An increase in adipose leptin production has been observed in obese individuals who were not leptin deficient, and this phenomenon introduced the concept of leptin resistance [198]. Apart from mutations in the leptin receptor gene, the molecular basis of leptin resistance has yet to be determined.

A large prospective study—the West of Scotland Coronary Prevention Study (WOSCOPS)—showed, for the first time, that leptin might be an independent risk factor for coronary heart disease [199]. These data suggest that leptin may affect the vascular structure. In fact, in vitro and in vivo assays revealed that leptin has angiogenic activity [200] and contributes to arterial thrombosis through the platelet leptin receptor [201]. It also stimulates production of reactive oxygen species (ROS) as a result of monocyte activation in vitro [202]. Therefore, in an obese subject, leptin may no longer be able to regulate caloric intake and energy balance, but may still exert its angiogenic activity and production of ROS, which affect vessel walls [202].

TNF-α, a multipotential cytokine with several immunologic functions, was initially described as a cause of tumor necrosis in septic animals and associated with cachexia-inducing states, such as cancer and infection [203]. Several mechanisms could account for the effect of TNF-α on obesity-related insulin resistance—increased release of FFA by adipocytes, reduced adiponectin synthesis, and impaired insulin signaling [204]. In vitro and in vivo studies show that TNF-α inhibition of insulin action is, at least in part, antagonized by glitazones, further supporting the role of TNF-α in insulin resistance [205]. Acute ischemia also increases TNF-α levels as has been observed in humans who developed recurrent nonfatal myocardial infarction (MI) or a fatal cardiovascular event in the Cholesterol And Recurrent Events (CARE) trial [206]. TNF-α activates the transcription factor nuclear factor-α, with subsequent inflammatory changes in vascular tissue. These include increased expression of intracellular adhesion molecule (ICAM)-1 and vascular cell adhesion molecule (VCAM)-1 [207,208], which enhances monocyte adhesion to the vessel wall, greater production of MCP-1 and M-CSF from endothelial cells and vascular smooth muscle cells [209,210], and upregulated macrophage expression of inducible nitric oxide (NO) synthase, interleukins, superoxide dismutase, etc. [211,212].

Adiponectin, otherwise termed adipocyte complement–related protein (Acrp 30) because of its homology to complement factor C1q, is almost exclusively expressed in WAT. Adiponectin is present in serum as a trimer, hexamer, or high-molecular-weight isoform [213]. Waki et al. [214] have reported that the high-molecular-weight isoform promotes adenosine monophosphate–activated protein kinase (AMPK) in hepatocytes. In contrast, Tsao et al. [215] have reported that only trimers activate AMPK in muscle. Adiponectin also has antiatherogenic properties, as shown in vitro by its inhibition of monocyte adhesion to endothelial cells, macrophage transformation to foam cells through downregulation of scavenger receptors [216], and endothelial cell activation through reduced production of adhesion molecules and inhibition of TNF-α and transcriptor factor NF-kB [217]. Interleukin (IL-6) and TNF-α are potent inhibitors of adiponectin expression and secretion in human WAT biopsies or cultured adipose cells [218]. Two receptors for adiponectin have been cloned. Adipo R1 and Adipo R2 are expressed predominantly in muscles and liver. Adiponectin-linked insulin sensitization is mediated, at least in part, by activation of AMPK in skeletal muscles and the liver, which increases fatty-acid oxidation and reduces hepatic glucose production [219]. Unlike most adipokines, adiponectin expression and serum concentrations are reduced in obese and insulin-resistant states. In humans, high plasma adiponectin levels are associated with reduced risk of MI in men [220].

In men with T2D, increased adiponectin levels are associated with a moderately decreased risk of coronary heart disease. The association seems to be mediated in part by the effects of adiponectin on high-density lipoprotein (HDL) cholesterol, through parallel increases in both. Although several mechanisms have been hypothesized, it is not yet clear how exactly adiponectin affects HDL cholesterol [221]. In American Indians, who are particularly at risk of obesity and diabetes [222], adiponectin does not correlate with the incidence of coronary heart disease. Moreover, individuals with high adiponectin concentrations are less likely to develop T2D than those with low concentrations [223,224]. Weight loss, caloric restriction, and TZD treatment increase adiponectin plasma levels and gene expression in WAT [223].

IL-6, a pleiotropic circulating cytokine, is reported to have multiple effects ranging from inflammation to host defense and tissue injury. Secreted by many cell types [225] including immune cells, fibroblasts, endothelial cells, skeletal muscle, and adipose tissue, IL-6 circulates as a glycosylated protein. Plasma IL-6 concentrations correlate positively with human obesity and insulin resistance, and high IL-6 levels are predictive of T2D and MI. [226]. Weight loss significantly reduces IL-6 levels in adipose tissue and serum [227]. However, only about 10% of the total IL-6 appears to be produced exclusively by fat cells [228]. Omental fat produces threefold more IL-6 than SAT, and adipocytes isolated from the omental depot also secrete more IL-6 than fat cells from the subcutaneous depot [229]. IL-6 exerts proinflammatory activity in itself and by increasing IL-1 and TNF-α [230]. More recently, IL-6 has been shown to inhibit insulin signal transduction in hepatocytes [231]. This effect has been shown to be related to SOCS-3 (suppressor of cytokine signaling-3), a protein that associates itself with the IR and inhibits its autophosphorylation, the tyrosine phosphorylation of IRS-1, the association of the p85 subunit of PI-3-K (phosphoinositide-3-kinase) to IRS-1, and the subsequent activation of akt. These effects of IL-6 were demonstrated in HepG-2 cells, in vitro, and in mice, in vivo [232]. SOCS-3 might also be the mediator of leptin resistance in the human obesity. IL-6 also stimulates liver production of CRP, which is considered a predictor of atherosclerosis [233]. IL-6 may also influence glucose tolerance by regulation of visfatin. Visfatin, one of the newly discovered adipocytokine in the human visceral fat, exerts insulin-mimetic effects in cultured cells and lowers plasma glucose levels in mice through activation of the insulin receptor [234]. IL-6 has also been related to insulin resistance in patients with high-grade inflammation as a result of cancer [235].

Plasminogen-activating inhibitor (PAI)-1, synthesized in the liver and in adipose tissue, regulates thrombus formation by inhibiting the activity of tissue-type plasminogen activator, an anticlotting factor. PAI-1 serum concentrations increase with visceral adiposity and decline with caloric restriction, exercise, weight loss, and metformin treatment [236]. Omental tissue explants secrete significantly more PAI-1 than subcutaneous tissue from the same subject [237]. PAI-1 concentrations, which are regulated by the transcription factor nuclear factor-α, are abnormally high in hyperglycemia, obesity, and hypertriglyceridemia [238], because of the increased PAI-1 gene expression [239]. PAI-1 inhibits fibrin clot breakdown, thereby favoring thrombus formation upon ruptured atherosclerotic plaques [240]. In humans, circulating PAI-1 levels correlate with atherosclerotic events and mortality, and some studies suggest that PAI-1 is an independent risk factor for coronary artery disease [241].

Angiotensinogen (AGE) is a precursor of angiotensin II (AngII), highly correlated with elevated blood pressure, and cardiovascular risk is mainly produced by the liver, but adipose tissue is the major extrahepatic source of AGE and could raise circulating levels in obese individuals. Increased AGE production could also contribute to enhanced adipose mass because AngII is believed to act locally as a trophic factor for new adipose cell formation [242]. AGE stimulates ICAM-1, VCAM-1, MCP-1, and M-CSF expression in vessel wall cells [243]. AngII also reduces NO bioavailability [244] with loss of vasodilator capacity and with increased platelet adhesion to the vessel wall.

The most recent adipokine to emerge as a contributor to obesity-induced insulin resistance is RBP4. RBP4 levels have been shown to be elevated in several groups of insulin-resistant subjects [24,245]. It has been suggested that increased serum RBP4 levels might contribute to insulin resistance by impairing insulin-stimulated glucose uptake in muscles and elevating hepatic glucose production, although the mechanism is not fully clear [246].

It is well established that in humans, endothelial dysfunction is indicative of the preclinical stages of atherosclerosis and is prognostic of future cardiovascular events [247]. High concentrations of proinflammatory adipokines may contribute to development of endothelial dysfunction, insulin resistance, and T2D. At this stage of disease, the role of resistin is particularly interesting. In vitro studies show resistin "activates" the endothelial cell, which, when incubated with recombinant human resistin, releases more endothelin-1 and VCAM-1 [248]. The physiological role of resistin is not yet clarified, and its role in obesity and insulin resistance and/or diabetes is controversial. In humans, resistin is primarily produced in peripheral blood monocytes and its levels correlate with IL-6 concentrations [249], and this is why its inflammatory role has been raised. Finally, resistin also induces proliferation of smooth muscle cells [250].

In human adipose tissue, aromatase activity is expressed mainly in mesenchymal cells with an undifferentiated preadipocyte phenotype [251]. P450 aromatase, a heme protein product of the *CYP19* gene, converts androstenedione to estrone. Estrogen production in fat rises with body weight and aging [252]. Adipose tissue–derived estrogens drive fat to subcutaneous and breast tissues, whereas androgens promote central or visceral fat accumulation [253,254].

11β-hydroxysteroid dehydrogenases (11β-HSDs) catalyze interconversion of active cortisol and inert cortisone. Two isoenzymes have been discovered, each with unique properties and powerful biological roles. 11β-HSD1 regenerates metabolically active cortisol from cortisone in humans and is increased in adipose tissue from obese subjects. 11β-HSD2 potently inactivates cortisol, protecting key tissues [255]. 11β-HSD1 is located at the ER. Several observations have associated adipose 11β-HSD1 activity with obesity, insulin resistance, and other features of the metabolic syndrome in different groups of obese men and women [256]. However, no difference in 11β-HSD1 activity was detected between obese T2D patients and their obese controls, suggesting that 11β-HSD1 dysregulation probably associates more closely with obesity than with the diabetic phenotype [257].

The fact that obesity, a major risk factor for T2D, and diabetes itself [258,259] are inflammatory conditions led to investigations exploring whether inflammatory mediators predict the development of T2D in populations at risk. Several such studies have confirmed that the presence of inflammation predicts the development of T2D. The first of these studies by Schmidt et al. [260] showed that the presence of inflammatory mediators predicted the future occurrence of T2D in adults and was part of the larger Atherosclerosis Risk in Communities (ARIC) study. Another publication from the same study has shown that elevated plasma concentrations of sialic acid, orosomucoid, IL-6, and CRP predict T2D [261]. Inflammation scores based on these inflammatory markers, along with the total leukocyte count and plasma fibrinogen concentration, have been developed to predict the development of T2D and have been rather indicative. There are at least three other prospective studies confirming the fact that an increase in inflammatory indices at baseline predicts T2D and insulin resistance [262–265]. Similarly, there is also a correlation between fasting insulin concentrations and CRP concentrations in plasma [266–268], indicating that insulin resistance and inflammatory processes are related and that in association with the other facts already discussed there might be a causal link. A significant correlation between the BMI and elevated plasma TNF-α concentrations has also been observed. TNF receptor concentration has also been observed in obese patients [269]. Further work in the area of obesity has confirmed that obesity is a state of chronic inflammation, as indicated by increased plasma concentrations of CRP [266], IL-6 [228], and plasminogen activator inhibitor-1 (PAI-1) [270]. On the other hand, plasma adiponectin concentration has an inverse relationship with adiposity (waist:hip ratio), insulin resistance, diastolic pressure, triglyceride concentration, and TNF-α receptor concentration [271]. Leptin is also elevated in the human obese, has proaggregatory effect on platelets, and might also regulate immune function through a stimulation of responses to inflammatory challenge. The definitive role of leptin in this context in the human has yet to be proved. Data on the association of depression, adiposity, and inflammatory mediators have been strongly suggesting that depression stimulates weight accumulation. This, in turn, activates an inflammatory response through an expanded adipose tissue release of IL-6 and leptin-induced IL-6 release by leukocytes [272]. Leptin also induces oxidative stress and inflammation in endothelial cells [273].

From most of the data available, it seems that TNF-α plays the key role linking inflammation, insulin resistance, obesity, and T2D by inhibiting the autophosphorylation of tyrosine residues of the insulin receptor and by inducing serine phosphorylation of IRS-1, which, in turn, causes serine phosphorylation of the IR in adipocytes and inhibits tyrosine phosphorylation [274]. Moreover, TNF-α in human aortic endothelial cells not only suppresses tyrosine phosphorylation, but it also suppresses the expression of the IR itself [275].

Novel data have now appeared showing that the concomitant presence of promoter polymorphisms of TNF-α (G-308A) and IL-6 (C-124G) in obese subjects with IGT carries twice the risk of conversion to T2D when compared with other genotypes. A G-308A mutation of the TNF-α promoter is associated with increased plasma TNF-α concentrations and a 1.8 higher risk of developing diabetes compared to noncarriers. A C-124G mutation of the IL-6 promoter increases the risk for insulin resistance [276]. Eckel et al. in a recent consensus statement [277] rank the increased production of adipokines/cytokines, including TNF-α, resistin, and RBP4, that contribute to insulin resistance as well as reduced levels of adiponectin [278] among the three most distinct mechanisms that link obesity to insulin resistance and predisposition to T2D.

GLUCOCORTICOIDS

Augmented glucocorticoids may induce insulin resistance and T2D by opposing the antigluconeogenic action of insulin in the hepatic tissue [255]. Although blood glucocorticoid concentration is almost physiological in the obese, the adipose tissue may increase cortisol production by cortisone to cortisol through the action of 11β-HSD type 1 (11β-HSD1) [279]. When 11β-HSD1 is overexpressed, transgenic animals develop visceral insulin resistance, obesity, and T2D due to a rise in glucocorticoids uptake by the liver via the portal vein [280]. Moreover, increased 11β-HSD1 has been detected in the adipose tissue of both humans and animals [281]. Furthermore, glucocorticoid inhibition in the liver attenuates hepatic glucose production and enhances glucose regulation in obese, insulin-resistant animals [282]. These increased glucocorticoid levels are observed in individuals with "apple-shaped" fat distribution as compared to individuals with "pear-shaped" fat distribution [283]. These findings led researchers to suggest that adipose tissue–derived cortisol reaches liver through portal vein circulation and contributes to hepatic insulin resistance [284].

CELL-INTRINSIC MECHANISMS LINKING OBESITY TO DIABETES

Ectopic Fat Storage

When the FFAs and other lipids are chronically elevated in the circulation (as it happens in the obesity), they may lead to ectopic fat storage as TAGs accumulate and store in liver and skeletal muscle [285]. Ectopic fat storage may contribute to the development of insulin resistance [34,286] by facilitating the generation of FFA-derived molecules that participate in intracellular signaling pathway or by triggering the production of ROS, which may cause ER stress and/or mitochondrial dysregulation [156,287]. The molecules activating these pathways are produced during the extensive TAG turnover [288].

The clinical manifestations of obesity are not only associated with the mechanisms by which fat is stored (i.e., adipocyte proliferation vs. adipocyte hypertrophy) but also where fat is stored. Visceral adipose tissue (VAT) may be more metabolically active than SAT, and these depots differ in processes involving lipolysis/lipogenesis, expression of adipocyte receptors, and differ in the secretion of adipokines/cytokines, enzymes, hormones, immune molecules, proteins, and other factors [289]. Derangements in adipose tissue endocrine and immune processes contribute to metabolic diseases.

The various fat depots have unique characteristics. These range from smaller fat depots that track with visceral fat (VAT) such as pericardial [290] and buccal [291] to larger fat depots like the superficial and deep abdominal superficial fat [292,293]. Intra-abdominal fat includes omental and mesenteric (visceral) depots, both of which drain into the portal vein, along with perinephric fat, which drains into the systemic circulation. Subcutaneous lower body fat includes gluteal and leg depots, which may have differing characteristics [294], and adipose tissue in between the major muscle groups (marbling) [295]. Upper body sc fat includes superficial and deep truncal depots noted previously, upper extremity fat, and breast adipose tissue in women. For practical reasons, we characterize human body fat compartments as lower body fat, upper body sc fat, and intra-abdominal/visceral fat. A predominantly upper body fat distribution, commonly associated with increased visceral fat, has been shown to be associated with an abnormal metabolic profile over a wide range of body mass indices [296,297]. Upper body/visceral obesity increases the risk for dyslipidemia [297], hypertension [298,299], T2D [300,301], sleep apnea [302], etc., whether increasing amounts of lower body fat are usually independently associated with a reduced risk of metabolic complication [303]. Among upper body adipose tissue, visceral fat mass (VAT) is more strongly associated with an abnormal metabolic profile than upper body sc fat [304–306]. Enlarged abdominal or visceral adipocytes seen in upper body obesity are resistant to the antilipolytic insulin action. Weight loss with diet and exercise, which reduces the size of the fat cells, improves insulin regulation of lipolysis [307], whereas surgical removal of abdominal sc fat with liposuction, which does not decrease fat cell size, does not [308]. On the other hand, surgical removal of omental fat during bariatric surgery was associated with greater improvement in fasting glucose levels and insulin concentrations along with a significantly greater decrease in BMI compared to those who did not undergo resection of the omentum [309].

Fat depots other than VAT have pathogenic potential [310,311]. Pericardial, subcutaneous abdominal, perimuscular, perivascular, orbital, and paraosseal fat depots also have lipolytic and inflammatory activities [289]. Pericardial and perivascular adiposopathy may have direct pathogenetic effects on the myocardium, coronary arteries, and peripheral vessels through a dysregulated local secretion of vasoactive and inflammatory factors that may contribute to atheroma instability and other cardiovascular pathophysiology [312–315]. Pericardial adiposity has been found to be strongly associated with coronary atherosclerosis in African Americans with T2DM, which may contribute to ethnic disparities in atherosclerosis susceptibility [316]. Even if we believe that atherosclerosis is exclusively a lipid-mediated process of the endothelium, pericardial and perivascular adipose tissue may also directly contribute to the inflammatory atherogenic model [312,313], which is supported by the strong association between pericardial adipose tissue and coronary artery calcification [317].

The reason ectopic fat is present in obesity is that during positive caloric balance, adipocytes are unable to store excess energy, mostly in the form of triglycerides, and so circulating FFAs are increased and are accumulating in nonadipose tissue organs, such as the liver, muscle, pancreas, and blood vessels [318] leading to abnormalities of glucose and lipid metabolism [319] and high blood pressure [320]. The delivery of excess FFA to the liver from systemic and/or VAT lipolysis will prevent the normal insulin-mediated suppression of glucose output by the liver. There is some controversy as to whether the effects of elevated FFA are on hepatic gluconeogenesis or a combination of gluconeogenesis and glycogenolysis. It is proposed that FFAs influence glucose output by creating surpluses of factors such as acetyl-CoA, reduced nicotinamide adenine dinucleotide, ATP, and citrate, perhaps with intrahepatic triglyceride as the intermediate step. Elevated FFAs also stimulate VLDL-triglyceride production in the face of hyperinsulinemia [321], and given the fact that portal FFAs are quite substantially increased during hyperinsulinemia in visceral obesity, this could be an especially important effect of visceral fat [322].

The majority of circulating FFAs actually originate from SAT, because SAT is the largest fat depot, constituting ~80% or more of total body fat. Even the majority of FFAs in the portal system may originate from SAT [323,324]. So while VAT is generally considered the most pathological fat depot [325,326], SAT fat storage is limited or impaired during positive caloric balance and if SAT net FFA release is increased into the circulation, then this SAT dysfunction may adversely affect non-hepatic organs, resulting in lipotoxicity to muscle (causing insulin resistance) and the pancreas (possibly reducing insulin secretion) [327,328].

If organs such as the liver are able to overcome lipotoxicity through inherent predisposition or through the use of therapeutic agents such as peroxisome proliferator–activated receptor (PPAR) gamma agonists [328], then the onset or worsening of metabolic disease may be eliminated. On the other hand, if adiposity occurs without intraorgan (e.g., intrahepatic) fatty infiltration, then the onset or worsening of metabolic disease may be averted [329].

In conclusion, the characteristics of adipose tissue are more important than the amount of body fat in determining the risk of obesity-related metabolic disease; insulin resistance is associated with increased fat-cell size and increased adipose tissue lipolytic activity, and the accumulation of ectopic fat in other organs, particularly the liver, might be a marker of adipose tissue pathology [329].

Oxidative Stress

Oxidative stress represents an imbalance between the generation of very reactive oxygen and nitrogen molecular reactive species (RONS) and the antioxidant defense reserves of the body or individual tissues [330]. Oxidative stress manifestations have been associated with fat accumulation in both humans and animals [288,331]. The evidence of oxidative stress implication in the pathophysiology of insulin resistance came from studies that showed an attenuation or reversal of oxidative stress when insulin resistance is improved in both humans and animals [287,332,333]. Most evidence indicates that oxidative stress is a consequence of insulin resistance–induced hyperglycemia and not a cause in T2D [288,334]. Moreover, the time course of hyperglycemia and insulin resistance onset is different (insulin resistance appears before chronic hyperglycemia) in the prediabetic phase, suggesting that RONS generation should be attributed to hyperglycemia and not insulin resistance [335,336]. The obesity-related rise in the circulating FFA is another contributing factor to the elevation of RONS generation probably due to augmented β-oxidation and mitochondrial uncoupling [337,338]. In fact, FFA infusion elevates oxidative stress and insulin resistance, an effect that is neutralized by antioxidant infusion [339,340]. Based on in vitro experiments, RNOS seem to turn on various serine/threonine kinases (p38 MAPK, JNK, and IKKβ) [325,341–343] that modify the activation of molecules participating in the insulin signaling pathway (i.e., the insulin receptor and the IRS proteins) that ultimately result in the degree of tyrosine phosphorylation through an elevation of serine phosphorylation in IRS-1 and IRS-2 [334,344].

Mitochondrial Dysfunction

Advanced insulin resistance has been linked to marked elevation in triacylglycerol concentration in both skeletal muscle and hepatic tissues probably due to ectopic fat accumulation [345]. As mentioned before, ectopic fat accumulation is associated with impairment in mitochondrial function manifested as reduced mitochondrial oxidative activity and ATP production [156]. In fact, Petersen et al. [187] reported that young insulin-resistant offspring of parents with T2D not only exhibit a predisposition to develop T2D in the later year of their lives, but they also demonstrate a marked reduction in their mitochondrial activity and an accumulation of intramuscular lipid. These observations led researchers to examine whether insulin resistance decreases mitochondrial biogenesis. Hence, studies reported that obese, insulin-resistant or diabetic subjects tend to accumulate more intramuscular fat caused by an impairment in mitochondrial biogenesis probably due to an inhibition in the expression of genes involved in the regulation of mitochondrial biogenesis such as those of PPARγ coactivators 1α and 1β (PGC-1α and PGC-1β) [188,189,346,347]. When PGC-1α expression was restored, mitochondrial function and insulin sensitivity were improved in animal and human models [348,349]. Collectively, these observations suggest that the impaired mitochondrial function may induce insulin resistance. Obesity-related mitochondrial dysfunction results in the accumulation of intracellular lipid (such as fatty acyl-CoA and DAG) and ROS accumulation, which, in turn, may disturb insulin signaling in muscle and liver. However, increased ROS generation requires functional mitochondria. How is then possible to have increased ROS production by dysfunctional mitochondria? It is possible that a rise in ROS generation precedes mitochondrial dysfunction, at an earlier stage of insulin resistance development. These ROS may promote a later mitochondrial dysfunction that leads to intracellular fat accumulation, which then impairs insulin signaling causing insulin resistance.

Endoplasmic Reticulum Stress as an Origin of Inflammation

Insulin resistance has also been associated with ER stress [350–353]. It appears that obesity stresses ER, thereby activating JNK, which, in turn, disturbs insulin intracellular signaling [351]. Studies with transgenic animals overexpressing ER chaperones or with knockdown of ER chaperones further support this hypothesis since in the former obesity-induced T2D was prevented while in the later T2D was developed [350,353]. Moreover, when chemical chaperones were used, obesity-related ER stress was reversed, and insulin sensitivity was restored in experimental animals [352]. It is possible that accumulated fat instigates ER stress simply by inducing sheer mechanical stress and/or disturbance in energy substrate utilization that ultimately lead to deterioration of cellular structure [351,354]. ER stress may also induce a rise in ROS generation, which then, as said before, may induce insulin resistance [355].

Neural Mechanisms

How important is the brain for the regulation of carbohydrate and fat homeostasis? There are reports suggesting that the brain accepts signals from the periphery regarding fatness level. More specifically, signaling to the brain regarding adiposity is mediated by hormones such as leptin and insulin whose levels in the circulation depend on body's fat mass. The brain integrates and processes the feedback provided by these hormones and by energy substrate levels such as the circulating glucose and FFA levels [356–358]. Following the reception of these signals, the brain intervenes by sending its own signals to the periphery in order to adjust feeding responses and energy substrate metabolism aiming to maintain homeostasis of energy fuels. The nervous system uses hormones such as insulin and leptin to control carbohydrate metabolism. In fact, leptin administration to the brain seems to normalize insulin resistance that leptin-deficient animals demonstrate [359,360]. In addition, when insulin receptors at the hypothalamus are disturbed, the animals develop hepatic insulin resistance and impaired glucose metabolism [361]. It appears that although insulin regulates carbohydrate metabolism via both central and peripheral receptors [362], the former may be more critical for insulin-dependent glucose regulation [363].

Studies reporting an enhanced insulin sensitivity following central infusion of oleic acid and an inhibitor of CPT1 in animals suggest that circulating metabolic intermediates such as FFAs may mediate insulin's effects at brain level [356,364]. It has been proposed that CPT1 inhibition in the brain triggers brain stem neurons that regulate parasympathetic input and increase insulin sensitivity via fibers innervating the hepatic tissue [365].

Hyperglycemia and insulin resistance may also result from a disruption of the mechanism regulating the circadian rhythms in the hypothalamus [366]. Food intake irregularities caused by changes in normal daily habits may alter hormonal peptides involved in appetite regulations (i.e., leptin), which then will induce central adaptations that could lead to insulin sensitivity deregulation [367].

COMMON APPROACHES TO TREAT INSULIN RESISTANCE AND OBESITY

BEHAVIORAL APPROACHES

Diabetes is a metabolic disorder related to the obesity pandemic. T2D is expected to reach 366 million cases worldwide by the year 2030 [368]. It must also be considered here that 20%–50% of diabetics are undiagnosed [369]. The financial burden of T2D for the health-care system is extremely high since it has been estimated that diabetes health-care cost for the year 2007 reached the amount of 116 billion dollars [370]. Scientific reports indicate that physical inactivity and obesity are independent modifiable risk factors for the development of insulin resistance and T2D [371,372]. Based on these reports, lifestyle interventions such as behavioral approaches including physical activity and nutritional strategies have been advanced as therapeutic means for humans at high risk for developing T2D. The basic aim of these strategies is to decrease the incidence of obesity and T2D as well as to reduce cardiovascular morbidity and mortality. However, adherence and compliance of participants in these behavioral interventions remains problematic. In the following paragraphs of this chapter, the reader will have the opportunity to be introduced to various behavioral approaches used to prevent or fight obesity, insulin resistance, and T2D with emphasis on exercise and nutrition.

Exercise

One of the main reasons for the obesity pandemic in our world is habitual physical inactivity and food abundance, especially in the industrialized countries, that resulted in a disturbance of the feast-famine cycles that are considered necessary for the preservation of metabolic genotype and function according to the "thrifty genes" theory [373]. Therefore, the modern man can convert very easily energy into adipose tissue TAG, but he cannot convert stored fat to energy as easily as his ancestors due to the lack of movement for survival since periods of famine are scarce in modern times. Consequently, stored fat is chronically elevated, and the original metabolic genotype is converted to more "thrifty" genotype. Obesity due to physical inactivity and overfeeding results in elevated mortality risk, insulin resistance, and T2D via mechanisms already analyzed in previous paragraphs of this chapter. Physical activity and/or exercise training interventions are considered as the most important nonpharmacological treatments for the prevention and care of obesity, insulin resistance, and T2D [374]. A minimum of 150 min/week of mild exercise that is progressively increased to 150 min/week may induce significant health benefits if performed 3–5 days/week according to previous guidelines of the American Heart Association [375]. In fact, systematic physical activity was able to reduce mortality risk from cardiovascular causes by 24% [376]. The purpose of this paragraph is to offer some more analytical description of exercise guidelines for the prevention and/ or treatment of obesity, insulin resistance, and diabetes. In this perspective, optimal exercise should aid in maximizing health benefits (i.e., enhance glycemic control, blood rheology, and endothelial function; reduce low-grade inflammation and oxidative stress, and coronary atherosclerosis; improve vascular remodeling, angiogenesis, and arteriogenesis) and improving cardiovascular conditioning and body composition. For this purpose, various exercise training modalities have been utilized and examined. In addition, exercise training program variables such as intensity and frequency of training as well as duration of the program are key elements for an optimal exercise intervention.

In fact, cardiovascular exercise alone or in combination with energy intake restriction results in fat loss (~10 and 3 kg, respectively) in obese adults [377]. In general, visceral fat loss is greater when cardiovascular exercise is combined with restriction energy intake protocols [378]. This observation is important since visceral adiposity is associated with increased risk of insulin resistance [379]. However, reduced energy intake may result in a decline of habitual physical activity, and this should be taken into consideration in clinical interventions [380]. Exercise training may elicit a lower fat loss in females with lower fat mass at baseline [381]. Fat loss that is obtained through cardiovascular-type exercise is usually accompanied by other positive health adaptations [382]. When resistance exercise is integrated in a general exercise prescription, skeletal muscle loss induced by energy intake restriction is prevented [383].

In regard to the metabolic syndrome (cardiovascular symptoms, dyslipidemia, hypertension, insulin resistance, central obesity), precursor of T2D, regular exercise may improve lipid profile (although its effects may be affected by lipid-lowering medications) [384–386], improve glycemic control and insulin sensitivity [387,388], decreases body weight, central adiposity, and total fat mass [385,387–389], and elevates cardiovascular fitness [385,386,388–390].

Regarding diabetes treatment, systematic exercise may reduce glycosylated hemoglobin (HbA1c) by as much as 0.8% and improve glycemic control following >12 weeks of cardiovascular and resistance exercise training [391,392]. Reduction of HbA1c is associated with a marked decrease in risk for developing micro- and macrovascular complications and lowered mortality rate of diabetics [393,394]. Exercise training improves functional performance, increases fat loss, reduces fasting blood lipids, improves hypertension, and enhances β-cell pancreatic function and skeletal muscle's oxidative capacity and mitochondrial function [395–400]. In regard to diabetes treatment with exercise training, health professionals should be aware that female diabetics as well as diabetics with higher baseline HbA1c and fasting blood glucose levels demonstrate better adaptations compared to male diabetics and diabetics with lower HbA1c and glycemic levels [396,401]. VAT reductions may be responsible for the improvement in glycemic control in diabetics with exercise training [402,403].

It appears that the clinical effectiveness of exercise training interventions is dependent upon training program variables, that is, exercise mode, training intensity, duration, and frequency. Regarding duration, the most effective exercise training programs are those that introduce long-term participation in the form of either habitual physical activity or supervised training [376]. Training programs of long duration seem to be the most effective for enhancing health and performance [381,404–407]. Most experts suggest that exercise or physical activity should become part of the daily life of the patients [374]. Therefore, long-duration exercise training intervention for optimal health and performance gains in diabetics [374,406].

Regarding the exercise mode, cardiovascular exercise was traditionally the main choice of exercise specialists for the obese, T2D patient. Based on cumulative evidence produced during the last two decades, resistance exercise has been included in the clinical guidelines of various agencies for the prevention and treatment of T2D [375]. Resistance exercise training in addition to cardiovascular exercise may induce increased energy expenditure, but it does not produce a greater fat loss in the obese [408–410]. Nevertheless, the addition of resistance exercise training to cardiovascular exercise prevents or attenuates losses of skeletal muscle tissue, thereby preventing the decline of the resting metabolic rate that is associated with reduced food consumption in the obese [411,412]. Hence, resistance exercise training interventions contribute to a long-term maintenance of weight loss. The combination of cardiovascular exercise and resistance training interventions is more effective in enhancing insulin sensitivity (by 77%) [413], reducing circulating levels of HbA1c (by 0.8%) [396], increasing blood glucose disposal due to an increase in skeletal muscle mass [414,415], and augmenting the functional performance (VO_{2peak}) of obese adults with T2D [416–418]. Two very recent review reports suggested that when resistance training is combined with cardiovascular exercise training, it produces significant clinical effects on metabolic syndrome risk factors, glycemic control, and arterial blood pressure and it should be incorporated in the exercise management plan of patients with T2D [419–421].

Regarding exercise intensity, clinical authorities propose a range of 40%–85% of VO_{2peak} for obese, insulin-resistant or diabetic individuals [375]. However, there is a need to define a narrower range of exercise intensity based on the fitness level and clinical status of the individual. Although, traditionally, fat loss has been associated with low-intensity cardiovascular exercise [422], numerous investigations suggested that there are no differences between low- and high-intensity exercise training interventions in respect to adipose tissue loss (when these interventions are of comparable energy expenditure level) [423–425], while one study reported a greater fat loss with high-intensity exercise [426]. In general, although exercise intensity is considered as the most critical variable of an exercise intervention effectiveness for obese, insulin-resistant individuals due its inverse relationship with glycogen utilization rate [427,428], recent evidence indicates that the enhancement of glycemic control as well as the improvement of oxidative capacity and lean body mass by an exercise intervention is independent of exercise intensity [427]. However, low-intensity exercise training has been shown to be more effective in improving insulin sensitivity than a high-intensity training protocol [429]. Nevertheless, high-intensity exercise training programs are associated with a lower compliance rate (higher dropout rates) by previously inactive participants compared to low-intensity interventions, making the former less suitable for the initial phase of an exercise intervention for individuals with metabolic syndrome [430]. In contrast, high-intensity continuous exercise may be more effective in increasing functional performance (VO_{2peak}) than low-intensity exercise interventions [431,432]. Collectively, although exercise intensity level has been debated by clinicians, it seems that low-intensity continuous cardiovascular exercise may be more effective in improving glycemic control and insulin sensitivity and less effective in increasing functional performance in obese, insulin-resistant individuals. More studies are needed in order to identify the proper exercise intensity range for this cohort of patients.

Recently, high-intensity interval training (HIIT) has received considerable attention for its effects on obese individuals with metabolic syndrome symptoms. Compared to continuous exercise training protocols, HIIT utilizes repetitive exercise intervals of brief duration (1–4 min) performed at a high intensity (75–100 VO_{2peak}) alternated with intervals of active rest of the same duration (1–4 min) but of lower intensity (40%–60% VO_{2peak}). HIIT induced an equal fat loss [433] but a greater improvement of insulin sensitivity [390] and functional performance [434–436] when compared to a more traditional low-intensity continuous exercise protocol in patients with metabolic syndrome symptoms. However, there is no evidence regarding the effectiveness of HIIT on glycemic control. Considering the difficulty associated with high-intensity training and the limited data on HIIT, health professionals should be skeptical regarding its application on obese, insulin-resistant individuals.

Regarding the duration of the exercise bouts, clinical guidelines recommend at least 40 min of exercise per training period up to total 60 min (or even more for the obese) per session [374,375]. In general, there is lack of available research evidence regarding exercise duration per session for obese, insulin-resistant individuals, especially in respect to fat loss, glycemic control, and insulin sensitivity. Nevertheless, despite the lack of available data, it seems that greater exercise duration may be more beneficial for glycemic control and mitochondrial biogenesis [437] but not for insulin sensitivity [429] compared to protocols of lower duration per exercise bout. In patients with cardiovascular disease, 40 and 60 min exercise sessions produced similar results in respect to improvement of functional performance during a 7 week training intervention [438]. This finding suggests that these patients may acquire the same results with exercise sessions of smaller volume.

In respect to training frequency, clinical guidelines for obese, insulin-resistant individuals recommend three to five training sessions/week [374,375]. As with exercise durations, training frequency has received limited research attention. In one study, a frequency of five sessions/week was more effective in respect to fat loss magnitude compared to low-frequency regimen of three sessions/week [439]. In patients with cardiovascular disease, two [440,441] but not six [442] training sessions/week were more effective in improving performance indicating that a training frequency of more than two sessions/week may not be necessary for optimal performance adaptations in this cohort of patients. Nevertheless, diabetic patients may need to train more frequently (i.e., three times/week) since training effects on insulin sensitivity enhancement last for only 48 h [443]. More studies are needed in order to explore the effects of training frequency on glycemic control in diabetic patients.

Nutrition

T2D represents a complex metabolic disease that is induced mainly by a combination of lifestyle factors (i.e., obesity and inactivity) and a genetic predisposition [444]. T2D develops over a long-term time period and is preceded by an initial phase characterized by IGT and fasting hyperglycemia [445]. Therefore, the management plan of T2D and insulin resistance includes reduction of body weight and fat as well as an increase of physical activity. Nutrition therapy is an important part of diabetes treatment plan because it can reduce the incidence of potential complications associated with hypertension and poor lipid or glycemic control [446].

Weight loss is recommended for the treatment of T2D and insulin resistance because it improves glycemic control, reduces hypertension, and affects positively the patients' lipid blood profile. However, in the later stages of T2D, as insulin deficiency becomes more prominent than insulin resistance, weight loss may be less effective in respect to glycemic control [447]. At this advanced stage, antidiabetes medications should be combined with optimal nutrition therapy to prevent gain of body weight [447]. Most nutritional interventions for diabetics examined so far were successful in reducing body weight and HbA1c as well as in improving blood's lipid profile and in reducing arterial blood pressure following at least 12 months of treatment [447–453]. Long-term studies using weight loss medications were also successful in reducing weight (4–8.5 kg) and HbA1c (by 0.3%–1.1%) as well as in reducing blood pressure and in improving blood lipid profile [450,451,454–458]. Results from the Look AHEAD clinical trial show that nutrition therapy including meal replacements or structured food protocols along with counseling session and physical activity (175 min/week) result in significant weight loss (~8%), marked elevation in stamina (21%), and a marked improvement in glycemic control (0.6%) in diabetic patients following 12 months of intervention [459]. Other studies showed that the content of carbohydrate of monounsaturated fatty acids (high or low) may or may not be critical for long-term weight loss protocols in diabetics [460–462]. Furthermore, meal replacements and self-selected meals have been shown to be equally effective in reducing body weight in patients with T2D [463]. Regarding energy restriction protocols, experts believe that it is better to err on the side of hypocaloric nutrition rather than on that of overfeeding in the obese, insulin-resistant patient [464]. Despite the fact that the optimal duration of hypocaloric feeding has yet to be defined, it may actually induce some improved health effects in the obese diabetics [464]. Although weight loss is considered critical for patients with T2D, it is uncertain if it alone can enhance glycemic control (reduce HbA1c). The American Dietetic Association suggests that lifestyle interventions such as exercise and nutrition therapy may allow a weight loss of 5%–10% [447].

A very important issue in nutrition therapy for diabetics is the food composition, especially in respect to macronutrients. Carbohydrate consumption determines postprandial glucose levels in blood and hence glycemic control. Therefore, diabetics must regulate carbohydrate intake in their meals. A critical matter for an effective glycemic control for diabetics is the consistency of carbohydrate intake (source and amount) each day [465], and this may also apply to patients receiving insulin treatment [466]. In general, previous studies defend the adjustment of insulin administration relatively to programmed carbohydrate intake since this scheme improves glycemic control [467,468].

However, findings on carbohydrate composition (percentage) in meals are contradictory and inconclusive with some earlier studies suggesting that a lower percentage may be more effective for maintaining glycemic control [465,469] while others supported that a higher percentage would be more beneficial [470]. New evidence suggests that a low-fat vegan diet may be more effective in improving glycemic control than a more conventional diabetes diet [471]. Nevertheless, according to more recent studies, the percentage of carbohydrate in diet may not be a critical factor [460,461]. In contrast, two recent meta-analyses reported that in T2D patients, low-carbohydrate diets (<45%) are more effective in improving glycemic control (one of them) and blood lipid profile than higher-carbohydrate diets (45%–70%) [472,473]. In conclusion, day-to-day carbohydrate intake should be consistent in order to improve glycemic control. Very-low-carbohydrate diets may jeopardize the optimal intake of other important nutrients such as vitamins, minerals, and fiber. Patients receiving insulin should adjust its administration relatively to standard programmed meal for a better glycemic control. In respect to sucrose intake, intakes of 10%–35% appear safe in respect to glycemic control if replaced by isocaloric quantities of starch [447]. Nonnutritive sweeteners may not affect glycemic control, although some of these products may contain carbohydrates that should be considered [447]. Regarding glycemic index, evidence is conflicting relatively to the effects of low- and high-glycemic index foods on HbA1c levels [447]. Fiber consumption of 45–50 g may actually improve glycemic control in patients with T2D, while intakes less than 24 g daily may not affect glycemic control [474,475]. The American Dietetic Association recommends a fiber intake of 25–30 g/day from food and 7–13 g/day from soluble sources for patients with T2D [447]. These intake levels may provide cardioprotective benefits [476].

Protein intake may prevent lean body mass losses during energy restriction protocols and contribute to the regulation of hyperglycemia and body mass. Protein intake should range between 15% and 20% of total daily energy intake if diabetics demonstrate a physiological kidney function [477–480]. Despite the fact that protein ingestion may affect insulin secretion acutely, chronic protein intake at regular daily levels may not affect circulating glucose and lipid levels as well insulin responses [481,482]. A protein intake of 1 g/kg/day may be required for diabetics with nephropathy because at this intake level protein ingestion may improve albuminuria [483]. In diabetics with end-stage renal disease, modifications in protein and energy intakes may help in the management of hypoalbuminemia and prevent malnutrition [484].

Regarding fat intake for obese diabetics, there are no clear guidelines. Neither total fat nor total carbohydrate intake seems to affect the development of T2D [485]. In fact, a higher intake of polyunsaturated fat and long-chain n-3 fatty acids may actually be beneficial for this cohort of patients, whereas an increased intake of saturated fat and trans fat may affect negatively carbohydrate metabolism [485]. Moreover, increased replacing saturated fat and trans fat with non-hydrogenated polyunsaturated fat may actually decrease the risk for developing T2D [485].

IMPROVING INSULIN SENSITIVITY IN OBESITY WITH PHARMACOLOGICAL AGENTS

Pharmacological treatment of obesity should aim not only at weight loss but particularly at a loss of fat mass, changes on the distribution of fat even without weight loss, and/or direct effects on adipose tissue dysfunction. Adipose tissue dysfunction depends on the quantity of adipose tissue and its distribution mainly visceral fat. Decreasing the amount of VAT may be accomplished through the following mechanisms: weight loss per se, loss of fat mass with an increase in fat-free mass such as seen with exercise, or by inducing a shift in fat distribution from visceral to subcutaneous compartments. Apart of reducing calories intake, even changing the dietary content without altering the caloric content may also have a beneficial effect on adipose tissue function. Such an example is the substitution of glucose by fructose on an isocaloric diet. Fructose rather than glucose intake was associated with an increase in VAT in humans altering the visceral and perivascular adipose tissue dysfunction in rats [486].

Diet-induced weight loss is an effective strategy for improving adipose tissue function, but at least 10% weight loss is needed to improve plasma concentrations of adiponectin and inflammatory markers such as CRP [487]. Besides the amount of

weight loss, the duration of the weight loss period might also influence plasma adiponectin levels with adiponectin levels increasing during the weight loss maintenance
period after a weight loss of 11%–12% in 8 weeks [488].

Available Medications for Weight Loss

Orlistat

Orlistat is a lipase inhibitor that decreases intestinal fat absorption after meals. In
a recent meta-analysis of 16 studies including 10,631 patients with a follow-up of
1–4 years, orlistat reduced weight by 2.9 kg and increased absolute percentages of
participants achieving 5% and 10% weight loss thresholds by 21% and 12%, respectively [489]. Weight loss by orlistat was not associated with a change in plasma leptin
and adiponectin concentrations, although resistin levels decreased by 36% after
6 months of treatment [490], but a decrease in the incidence of diabetes type 2 from
9% to 6.2% was observed [491]. When orlistat was combined with a hypocaloric diet
with a 600 kcal restriction, bodyweight decreased by 14%–24%, percentage body
fat decreased by 21%, and plasma concentrations of leptin, CRP, IL-6, TNF-α, and
resistin decreased while adiponectin increased, indicating an improvement in adipose
tissue function [492].

Sibutramine

Sibutramine is a highly selective inhibitor for the reuptake of norepinephrine and
serotonin at nerve endings. Originally developed as an antidepressant, sibutramine has effects on energy intake and, to a lesser extent, on energy expenditure. In a meta-analysis of placebo-controlled randomized trials, sibutramine
decreased bodyweight by 4.2 kg [489]. Compared with placebo, sibutramine
however increased systolic blood pressure by 1.7 mm Hg and pulse rate by 4.5
beats/min. Other common side effects included dry mouth, insomnia, and nausea
in 7%–20%.

Sibutramine-induced weight loss seems to have a greater effect on the release of
adipokines and a greater increase in adiponectin levels than caloric restriction [493].
This effect on adipose tissue function seems to be independent of sole weight loss
probably because sibutramine has an effect on the catecholamine-induced lipolysis
in the VAT and a preferential loss of VAT than in SAT [494].

Recently it has been reported that the use of sibutramine is associated with
an increased risk for nonfatal MI and stroke in patients at high cardiovascular
risk [495], and, thus, sibutramine has therefore been withdrawn from the market
since October 2010.

Cannabinoid-1 Receptor Antagonists

The cannabinoid-1 (CB1) receptor is widely dispersed throughout the body with high
concentration in areas of the brain related to feeding and is also present on adipocytes [496,497]. Rimonabant is a selective CB1 receptor blocker that has been investigated in wide-scale clinical trials. Weight loss by rimonabant is achieved both by
its central effects on satiety as well as its effects on the peripheral endocannabinoid
system in the gut, leading to nausea and diarrhea [498]. In a recent meta-analysis of

placebo-controlled trials, evaluating the clinical effects of rimonabant, it appeared that the mean weight loss was 4.7 kg more than in the placebo group [489]. Furthermore, rimonabant significantly reduced waist circumference, lowered blood pressure, lowered triglyceride levels, and increased HDL cholesterol plasma concentrations.

In patients with T2D, treatment with rimonabant at the highest dose (20 mg) decreased CRP (−26%) and leptin (−2%) levels [499]. In overweight or obese patients with untreated dyslipidemia, rimonabant decreased leptin levels to a greater extent than in patients with diabetes (23%) and significantly increased adiponectin levels by 37% [500]. Rimonabant was withdrawn from the market in 2008 due to adverse effects including an increased incidence of psychiatric disorders (depression, suicidal ideation, anxiety, and aggression). Other CB1 receptor antagonists are still under investigation.

New pharmacological agents are under investigation targeting the central nervous system in order to stimulate endogenous catabolic signals or inhibit anabolic signals. Examples of the former approach include methods to enhance central leptin signaling through intranasal leptin delivery, use of superpotent leptin-receptor agonists, and mechanisms to increase leptin sensitivity by techniques to augment signaling by neurochemical mediators of leptin action that lie downstream of at least some levels of obesity-associated leptin resistance. Strategies to inhibit anabolic molecules, such as neuropeptide Y, melanin-concentrating hormone, ghrelin, and endocannabinoids, are also under development. Modulation of gastrointestinal satiation and hunger signals is being investigated. As we are getting more insights into the mechanisms governing body weight and with the better understanding of the mechanisms underlying the weight loss with bariatric surgery, new and better antiobesity medications may be developed to be used with diet and exercise to facilitate substantial weight loss [501].

Other Nonbehavioral Treatments

Bariatric Surgery

Bariatric surgery is increasingly used as a strategy to reduce body weight and thereby ameliorate risk factors for cardiovascular disease. On average, patients lose 14%–25% weight after bariatric surgery [502]. Patients who underwent gastric bypass surgery showed a significant decline in all-cause mortality as well as coronary artery disease, diabetes, and cancer during 7.1 year follow-up [503]. Patients with recently diagnosed T2D showed greater weight loss after gastric banding compared to conventional therapy (lifestyle advice) as well as a greater chance of remission of T2D [504]. This effect of bariatric surgery on diabetes is probably due to a reduction in body fat mass and, in the case of gastric bypass surgery, changes in gut hormone production such as glucagon-like peptide-1 (GLP-1), gastric inhibitory polypeptide (GIP), and ghrelin [505].

Adiponectin levels have been referred to increase after bariatric surgery in several small-scale studies mainly because of an increase in high-molecular-weight adiponectin [506–508]. After bariatric surgery, plasma concentrations of macrophage inhibitory factor (MIF), PAI-1, RBP-4, MCP-1, and IL-18 are decreased, indicating positive effects on adipose tissue function [509–511].

CONCLUSIONS

Most patients with T2D are obese, and the global epidemic of obesity largely explains the dramatic increase in the incidence and prevalence of T2D over the past 20 years. Recent research investigation has identified "links" between obesity and T2D involving inflammation, cytokines, insulin resistance, disrupted fatty acid metabolism, and cellular processes such as mitochondrial dysfunction and ER stress. The interplay among these mechanisms is very complex with the relative contribution of each process still unclear. Further genetic studies may elucidate additional common pathophysiological pathways linking obesity and diabetes. Identifying the links may lead to future treatment strategies of the diseases.

REFERENCES

1. WHO. Obesity and overweight fact sheet N°311. Updated February 2011.
2. Flegal, K.M., Carroll, M.D., Ogden, C.L., Curtin, L.R. 2010. Prevalence and trends in obesity among US adults, 1999–2008. 2010. *JAMA* 303:235–241.
3. Flegal, K.M., Carroll, M.D., Kuczmarski, R.J., Johnson, C.L. 1998. Overweight and obesity in the United States: Prevalence and trends, 1960–1994. *Int J Obes Rel Metab Disord* 22(1):39–47.
4. Flegal, K.M., Graubard, B., Williamson, D., Gail, M. 2010. Sources of differences in estimates of obesity-associated deaths from first National Health and Nutrition Examination Survey (NHANES I) hazard ratios. *Am J Clin Nutr* 91:519–527.
5. Ogden, C.L., Carroll, M.D., Curtin, L.R., Lamb, M.M., Flegal, K.M. 2010. Prevalence of high body mass index in US children and adolescents, 2007–2008. *JAMA* 303:242–249.
6. Eaton, D.K., Kann, L., Kinchen, S. et al. 2010. Youth risk behavior surveillance—United States, 2009. *MMWR Surveill Summ* 59:1–142.
7. Flegal, K.M., Ogden, C.L., Yanovski, J. et al. 2010. High adiposity and high body mass index–for-age in US children and adolescents overall and by race-ethnic group. *Am J Clin Nutr* 91:1020–1026.
8. Biggs, M., Mukamal, K., Luchsinger, J. et al. 2010. Association between adiposity in midlife and older age and risk of diabetes in older adults. *JAMA* 303:2504–2512.
9. The, N., Suchindran, C., North, K., Popkin, B., Gordon-Larsen, P. 2010. The association of adolescent obesity with risk of severe obesity in adulthood. *JAMA* 304:2042–2047.
10. Yanovski, S., Yanovski, J. 2011. Obesity prevalence in the United States—Up, down, or sideways? *N Engl J Med* 364:11.
11. The Emerging Risk Factor Collaboration. 2011. Separate and combined associations of body-mass index and abdominal adiposity with cardiovascular disease: Collaborative analysis of 58 prospective studies. *Lancet* 377:1085–1095.
12. Montague, C.T., O'Rahilly, S. 2000. The perils of portliness: Causes and consequences of visceral adiposity. *Diabetes* 49:883–893.
13. Bahceci, M., Gokalp, D., Bahceci, S., Tuzcu, A., Atmaca, S., Arikan, S. 2007. The correlation between adiposity and adiponectin, tumor necrosis factor alpha, interleukin-6 and high sensitivity C-reactive protein levels. Is adipocyte size associated with inflammation in adults? *J Endocrinol Invest* 30:210–214.
14. Goossens, G.H. 2008. The role of adipose tissue dysfunction in the pathogenesis of obesity-related insulin resistance. *Physiol Behav* 94:206–218.
15. Corpeleijn, E., Saris, W.H., Blaak, E.E. 2009. Metabolic flexibility in the development of insulin resistance and type 2 diabetes: Effects of lifestyle. *Obes Rev* 10:178–193.

16. Bickerton, A.S., Roberts, R., Fielding, B.A. et al. 2007. Preferential uptake of dietary fatty acids in adipose tissue and muscle in the postprandial period. *Diabetes* 56:168–176.

17. Stephens, M., Ludgate, M., Rees, A. 2011. Brown fat and obesity: The next big thing? *Clin Endocrinol* 74(6):661–670.

18. Hansen, J.B., Kristiansen, K. 2006. Regulatory circuits controlling white versus brown adipocyte differentiation. *Biochem J* 398:153–168.

19. Cypess, A.M., Lehman, S., Williams, G. et al. 2009. Identification and importance of brown adipose tissue in adult humans. *N Engl J Med* 360:1509–1517.

20. Van Baarlen, P., Troost, F.J., van Hemert, S. et al. 2009. Differential NF-kappaB pathways induction by *Lactobacillus plantarum* in the duodenum of healthy humans correlating with immune tolerance. *Proc Natl Acad Sci USA* 106:2371–2376.

21. Bäckhed, F., Ding, H., Wang, T. et al. 2004. The gut microbiota as an environmental factor that regulates fat storage. *Proc Natl Acad Sci USA* 101:15718–15723.

22. Rube, H., Lehrke, M., Parhofer, K.G., Broedi, U.C. 2008. Adipokines and insulin resistance. *Mol Med* 14:741–751.

23. Antuna-Puente, B., Feve, B., Fellahi, S., Bastard, J.P. 2008. Adipokines: The missing link between insulin resistance and obesity. *Diabetes Metab* 34:2–11.

24. Graham, T.E., Yang, Q., Bluher, M. et al. 2006. Retinol-binding protein 4 and insulin resistance in lean, obese, and diabetic subjects. *N Engl J Med* 354:2552–2563.

25. Sul, H.S. 2005. Resistin/ADSF/FIZZ3 in obesity and diabetes. 2004. *Trends Endocrinol Metab* 15:247–249.

26. Kadowaki, T., Yamauchi, T. 2005. Adiponectin and adiponectin receptors. *Endocrinol Rev* 26:439–451.

27. Bays, H. 2011. Adiposopathy: Is "sick fat" a cardiovascular disease? *J Am Coll Cardiol* 57(25):2461–2473.

28. Ravussin, E., Smith, S.R. 2002. Increased fat intake, impaired fat oxidation, and failure of fat cell proliferation result in ectopic fat storage, insulin resistance, and type 2 diabetes mellitus. *Ann N Y Acad Sci* 967:363–378.

29. Thorleifsson, G., Walters, G.B., Gudbjartsson, D.F. et al. 2009. Genome-wide association yields new sequence variants at seven loci that associate with measures of obesity. *Nat Gen* 41:18–24.

30. Mitrakou, A., Kelley, D., Veneman, T., Pangburn, T., Reilly, J., Gerich, J. 1992. Role of reduced suppression of hepatic glucose output and diminished early insulin release in impaired glucose tolerance. *N Engl J Med* 326:22–29.

31. Mitrakou, A., Kelley, D., Veneman, T. et al. 1990. Contribution of abnormal muscle and liver glucose metabolism to postprandial hyperglycemia in non-insulin dependent diabetes mellitus. *Diabetes* 39:1381–1390.

32. Pimenta, W., Mitrakou, A., Jensen, T., Yki-Jarvinen, H., Daily, G., Gerich, J. 1996. Insulin secretion and insulin sensitivity in people with impaired glucose tolerance. *Diabetes Med* 13(9 Suppl. 6):S33–S36.

33. Kahn, S.E. 2003. The relative contributions of insulin resistance and beta-cell dysfunction to the pathophysiology of type 2 diabetes. *Diabetologia* 46:3–19.

34. McGarry, J.D. 2002. Banting lecture 2001: Dysregulation of fatty acid metabolism in the etiology of type 2 diabetes. *Diabetes* 51:7–18.

35. Boden, G. 2006. Obesity, insulin resistance, type 2 diabetes and free fatty acids. *Expert Rev Endocrinol Metab* 1:499–505.

36. Groop, L.C., Bonadonna, R.C., Del Prato, S. et al. 1989. Glucose and FFA metabolism in non-insulin dependent diabetes mellitus. Evidence for multiple sites of insulin resistance. *J Clin Invest* 84:205–215.

37. Randle, P.J., Garland, P.B., Hales, C.N., Newsholme, E.A. 1963. The glucose fatty-acid cycle. Its role in insulin sensitivity and the metabolic disturbances of diabetes mellitus. *Lancet* 1:785–789.

38. Ferrannini, E., Balkau, B. 2002. Insulin: In search of a syndrome. *Diabetes Med* 19:724–729.
39. Turner, R.C., Holman, R.R., Matthews, D. et al. 1979. Insulin deficiency and insulin resistance interaction in diabetes: Estimation of their relative contribution by feedback analysis from basal plasma insulin and glucose concentrations. *Metabolism* 28:1086–1096.
40. Bagdade, J.D., Bierman, E.L., Porte, D. Jr. 1967. The significance of basal insulin levels in the evaluation of the insulin response to glucose in diabetic and nondiabetic subjects. *J Clin Invest* 46:1549–1557.
41. Polonsky, K.S., Given, B.D., Hirsch, L. et al. 1988. Quantitative study of insulin secretion and clearance in normal and obese subjects. *J Clin Invest* 81:435–441.
42. Kloppel, G., Lohr, M., Habich, K., Oberholzer, M., Heitz, P.U. 1985. Islet pathology and the pathogenesis of type 1 and type 2 diabetes mellitus revisited. *Surv Synth Pathol Res* 4:110–125.
43. Butler, A.E., Janson, J., Bonner-Weir, S., Ritzel, R., Rizza, R.A., Butler, P.C. 2003. β-Cell deficit and increased β-cell apoptosis in humans with type 2 diabetes. *Diabetes* 52:102–110.
44. Kahn, S.E., Hull, R.L., Utzschneider, K.M. 2006. Mechanisms linking obesity to insulin resistance and type 2 diabetes. *Nature* 444:840–846.
45. Goodpaster, B.H., Kelley, D.E., Wing, R.R. et al. 1999. Effects of weight loss on regional fat distribution and insulin sensitivity in obesity. *Diabetes* 48:839–847.
46. Rampersaud, E., Damcott, C.M., Fu, M. et al. 2007. Identification of novel candidate genes for type 2 diabetes from a genome-wide association scan in the Old Order Amish: Evidence for replication from diabetes related quantitative traits and from independent populations. *Diabetes* 56:3053–3062.
47. Hayes, M.G., Pluzhnikov, A., Miyake, K. et al. 2007. Identification of type 2 diabetes genes in Mexican Americans through genome-wide association studies. *Diabetes* 56:3033–3044.
48. Zeyda, M., Stulnig, T.M. 2009. Obesity, inflammation, and insulin resistance: A mini-review. *Gerontology* 55:379–386.
49. Hotamisligil, G.S., Shargill, N.S., Spiegelman, B.M. 1993. Adipose expression of tumor necrosis factor-α: Direct role in obesity-linked insulin resistance. *Science* 259:87–91.
50. Wu, D., Ren, Z., Pae, M. et al. 2007. Aging up-regulates expression of inflammatory mediators in mouse adipose tissue. *J Immunol* 179:4829–4839.
51. Ohman, M.K., Shen, Y., Obimba, C.I. et al. 2008. Visceral adipose tissue inflammation accelerates atherosclerosis in apolipoprotein E deficient mice. *Circulation* 117:798–805.
52. Fain, J.N. 2006. Release of interleukins and other inflammatory cytokines by human adipose tissue is enhanced in obesity and primarily due to the nonfat cells. *Vitam Horm* 74:443–477.
53. Weisberg, S.P., McCann, D., Desai, M., Rosenbaum, M., Leibel, R.L., Ferrante, A.W. Jr. 2003. Obesity is associated with macrophage accumulation in adipose tissue. *J Clin Invest* 112:1796–1808.
54. Zeyda, M., Farmer, D., Todoric, J. et al. 2007. Human adipose tissue macrophages are of an anti-inflammatory phenotype but capable of excessive pro-inflammatory mediator production. *Int J Obes (Lond)* 31:1420–1428.
55. Cinti, S., Mitchell, G., Barbatelli, G. et al. 2005. Adipocyte death defines macrophage localization and function in adipose tissue of obese mice and humans. *J Lipid Res* 46:2347–2355.
56. Huber, J., Kiefer, F.W., Zeyda, M. et al. 2008. CC chemokine and CC chemokine receptor profiles in visceral and subcutaneous adipose tissue are altered in human obesity. *J Clin Endocrinol Metab* 93:3215–3221.

57. Kanda, H., Tateya, S., Tamori, Y. et al. 2006. MCP-1 contributes to macrophage infiltration into adipose tissue, insulin resistance, and hepatic steatosis in obesity. *J Clin Invest* 116:1494–1505.

58. Weisberg, S.P., Hunter, D., Huber, R. et al. 2006. CCR2 modulates inflammatory and metabolic effects of high-fat feeding. *J Clin Invest* 116:115–124.

59. Lumeng, C.N., Deyoung, S.M., Bodzin, J.L., Saltiel, A.R. 2007. Increased inflammatory properties of adipose tissue macrophages recruited during diet-induced obesity. *Diabetes* 56:16–23.

60. Zeyda, M., Stulnig, T.M. 2007. Adipose tissue macrophages. *Immunol Lett* 112:61–67.

61. Lumeng, C.N., Bodzin, J.L., Saltiel, A.R. 2007. Obesity induces a phenotypic switch in adipose tissue macrophage polarization. *J Clin Invest* 117:175–184.

62. Clement, K., Viguerie, N., Poitou, C. et al. 2004. Weight loss regulates inflammation-related genes in white adipose tissue of obese subjects. *FASEB J* 18:1657–1669.

63. Friedman, J.M., Halaas, J.L. 1998. Leptin and the regulation of body weight in mammals. *Nature* 395:763–770.

64. Kiefer, F.W., Zeyda, M., Todoric, J. et al. 2008. Osteopontin expression in human and murine obesity: Extensive local up-regulation in adipose tissue but minimal systemic alterations. *Endocrinology* 149:1350–1357.

65. Uysal, K.T., Wiesbrock, S.M., Marino, M.W., Hotamisligil, G.S. 1997. Protection from obesity-induced insulin resistance in mice lacking TNF-α function. *Nature* 389:610–614.

66. Shi, H., Tzameli, I., Bjorbaek, C., Flier, J.S. 2004. Suppressor of cytokine signaling 3 is a physiological regulator of adipocyte insulin signaling. *J Biol Chem* 279:34733–34740.

67. Jager, J., Gremeaux, T., Cormont, M., Le Marchand-Brustel, Y., Tanti, J.F. 2007. Interleukin-1β-induced insulin resistance in adipocytes through down-regulation of insulin receptor substrate-1 expression. *Endocrinology* 148:241–251.

68. Arkan, M.C., Hevener, A.L., Greten, F.R. et al. 2005. IKK-β links inflammation to obesity-induced insulin resistance. *Nat Med* 11:191–198.

69. De Taeye, B.M., Novitskaya, T., McGuinness, O.P. et al. 2007. Macrophage TNF-α contributes to insulin resistance and hepatic steatosis in diet-induced obesity. *Am J Physiol* 293:E713–E725.

70. Zhou, Q., Leeman, S.E., Amar, S. 2009. Signaling mechanisms involved in altered function of macrophages from diet-induced obese mice affect immune responses. *Proc Natl Acad Sci USA* 106(26):10740–10745.

71. Shi, H., Kokoeva, M.V., Inouye, K., Tzameli, I., Yin, H., Flier, J.S. 2006. TLR4 links innate immunity and fatty acid-induced insulin resistance. *J Clin Invest* 116:3015–3025.

72. Kim, E.Y., Kim, B.C. 2011. Lipopolysaccharide inhibits transforming growth factor-beta1-stimulated Smad6 expression by inducing phosphorylation of the linker region of Smad3 through a TLR4-IRAK1-ERK1/2 pathway. *FEBS Lett* 585(5):779–785.

73. McAvoy, E.F., McDonald, B., Parsons, S.A., Wong, C.H., Landmann, R., Kubes, P. 2011. The role of CD14 in neutrophil recruitment within the liver microcirculation during endotoxemia. *J Immunol* 186(4):2592–2601.

74. Hernández Vallejo, S.J., Alqub, M., Luquet, S. et al. 2009. Short-term adaptation of postprandial lipoprotein secretion and intestinal gene expression to a high-fat diet. *Am J Physiol Gastrointest Liver Physiol* 296(4):G782–G792.

75. Cani, P.D., Amar, J., Iglesias, M.A. et al. 2007. Metabolic endotoxemia initiates obesity and insulin resistance. *Diabetes* 56:1761–1772.

76. Erridge, C., Attina, T., Spickett, C.M., Webb, D.J. 2007. A high-fat meal induces low-grade endotoxemia: Evidence of a novel mechanism of postprandial inflammation. *Am J Clin Nutr* 86:1286–1292.

77. Perseghin, G., Ghosh, S., Gerow, K., Shulman, G.I. 1997. Metabolic defects in lean nondiabetic offspring of NIDDM parents: A cross-sectional study. *Diabetes* 46:1001–1009.

78. Krssak, M., Falk Petersen, K., Dresner, A. et al. 1999. Intramyocellular lipid concentrations are correlated with insulin sensitivity in humans: A 1H NMR spectroscopy study.
Diabetologia 42:113–116.

79. Perseghin, G., Scifo, P., De Cobelli, F. et al. 1999. Intramyocellular triglyceride content
is a determinant of in vivo insulin resistance in humans: A 1H-13C nuclear magnetic
resonance spectroscopy assessment in offspring of type 2 diabetic parents. *Diabetes*
48:1600–1606.

80. Pan, D.A., Lillioja, S., Kriketos, A.D. et al. 1997. Skeletal muscle triglyceride levels are
inversely related to insulin action. *Diabetes* 46:983–988.

81. Shulman, G.I., Rothman, D.L., Jue, T., Stein, P., DeFronzo, R.A., Shulman, R.G. 1990.
Quantitation of muscle glycogen synthesis in normal subjects and subjects with non-
insulin-dependent diabetes by 13C nuclear magnetic resonance spectroscopy. *N Engl J
Med* 322:223–228.

82. Rothman, D.L., Shulman, R.G., Shulman, G.I. 1992. ^{1}P nuclear magnetic resonance
measurements of muscle glucose-6-phosphate. Evidence for reduced insulin-dependent
muscle glucose transport or phosphorylation activity in non-insulin-dependent diabetes
mellitus. *J Clin Invest* 89:1069–1075.

83. Roden, M., Price, T.B., Perseghin, G. et al. 1996. Mechanism of free fatty acid-induced
insulin resistance in humans. *J Clin Invest* 97:2859–2865.

84. Dresner, A., Laurent, D., Marcucci, M. et al. 1999. Effects of free fatty acids on glucose
transport and IRS-1-associated phosphatidylinositol 3-kinase activity. *J Clin Invest*
103:253–259.

85. Garvey, W.T., Maianu, L., Zhu, J.H., Brechtel-Hook, G., Wallace, P., Baron, A.D. 1998.
Evidence for defects in the trafficking and translocation of GLUT4 glucose transporters
in skeletal muscle as a cause of human insulin resistance. *J Clin Invest* 101:2377–2386.

86. Choi, C.S., Savage, D.B., Abu-Elheiga, L. et al. 2007. Continuous fat oxidation in acetyl-
CoA carboxylase 2 knockout mice increases total energy expenditure, reduces fat mass,
and improves insulin sensitivity. *Proc Natl Acad Sci USA* 104:16480–16485.

87. Hoehn, K.L., Turner, N., Swarbrick, M.M. et al. 2010. Acute or chronic upregulation of
mitochondrial fatty acid oxidation has no net effect on whole-body energy expenditure
or adiposity. *Cell Metab* 11:70–76.

88. Kim, J.Y., van de Wall, E., Laplante, M. et al. 2007. Obesity-associated improvements
in metabolic profile through expansion of adipose tissue. *J Clin Invest* 117:2621–2637.

89. Krssak, M., Petersen, K.F., Bergeron, R. et al. 2000. Intramuscular glycogen and intramyocellular lipid utilization during prolonged exercise and recovery in man: A ^{13}C and
^{1}H nuclear magnetic resonance spectroscopy study. *J Clin Endocrinol Metab* 85:748–754.

90. Schenk, S., Horowitz, J.F. 2007. Acute exercise increases triglyceride synthesis in skeletal
muscle and prevents fatty acid-induced insulin resistance. *J Clin Invest* 117:1690–1698.

91. Samuel, V.T., Petersen, K.F., Shulman, G.I. 2010. Lipid-induced insulin resistance:
Unravelling the mechanism. *Lancet* 375(9733):2267–2277.

92. Morino, K., Petersen, K.F., Dufour, S. et al. 2005. Reduced mitochondrial density and
increased IRS-1 serine phosphorylation in muscle of insulin-resistant offspring of type 2
diabetic parents. *J Clin Invest* 115:3587–3593.

93. Azevedo, J.L. Jr., Carey, J.O., Pories, W.J., Morris, P.G., Dohm, G.L. 1995. Hypoxia stimulates glucose transport in insulin-resistant human skeletal muscle. *Diabetes* 44:695–698.

94. Dolan, P.L., Tapscott, E.B., Dorton, P.J., Dohm, G.L. 1993. Contractile activity restores
insulin responsiveness in skeletal muscle of obese Zucker rats. *Biochem J* 289:423–426.

95. Goodyear, L.J., Giorgino, F., Sherman, L.A., Carey, J., Smith, R.J., Dohm, G.L. 1995.
Insulin receptor phosphorylation, insulin receptor substrate-1 phosphorylation, and
phosphatidylinositol 3-kinase activity are decreased in intact skeletal muscle strips from
obese subjects. *J Clin Invest* 95:2195–2204.

96. Itani, S.I., Zhou, Q., Pories, W.J., MacDonald, K.G., Dohm, G.L. 2000. Involvement of protein kinase C in human skeletal muscle insulin resistance and obesity. *Diabetes* 49:1353–1358.

97. Bossenmaier, B., Mosthaf, L., Mischak, H., Ullrich, A., Haring, H.U. 1997. Protein kinase C isoforms beta 1 and beta 2 inhibit the tyrosine kinase activity of the insulin receptor. *Diabetologia* 40:863–866.

98. Cortright, R.N., Azevedo, J.L. Jr., Zhou, Q. et al. 2000. Protein kinase C modulates insulin action in human skeletal muscle. *Am J Physiol* 278:E553–E562.

99. Griffin, M.E., Marcucci, M.J., Cline, G.W. et al. 1999. Free fatty acid-induced insulin resistance is associated with activation of protein kinase C theta and alterations in the insulin signaling cascade. *Diabetes* 48:1270–1274.

100. Itani, S.I., Ruderman, N.B., Schmieder, F., Boden, G. 2002. Lipid-induced insulin resistance in human muscle is associated with changes in diacylglycerol, protein kinase C, and IkappaBalpha. *Diabetes* 51:2005–2011.

101. Schmitz-Peiffer, C. 2002. Protein kinase C and lipid-induced insulin resistance in skeletal muscle. *Ann N Y Acad Sci* 967:146–157.

102. Cooney, G.J., Thompson, A.L., Furler, S.M., Ye, J., Kraegen, E.W. 2002. Muscle long-chain acyl CoA esters and insulin resistance. *Ann N Y Acad Sci* 967:196–207.

103. Chavez, J.A., Knotts, T.A., Wang, L.P. et al. 2003. A role for ceramide, but not diacylglycerol, in the antagonism of insulin signal transduction by saturated fatty acids. *J Biol Chem* 278:10297–10303.

104. Kawakami, T., Kawakami, Y., Kitaura, J. 2002. Protein kinase C beta (PKC beta): Normal functions and diseases. *J Biochem (Tokyo)* 132:677–682.

105. Kelley, D.E., Goodpaster, B.H., Wing, R.R., Simoneau, J.A. 1999. Skeletal muscle fatty acid metabolism in association with insulin resistance, obesity, and weight loss. *Am J Physiol* 277:E1130–E1141.

106. Hulver, M.W., Berggren, J.R., Cortright, R.N. et al. 2003. Skeletal muscle lipid metabolism with obesity. *Am J Physiol* 284:E741–E747.

107. MacLean, P.S., Bower, J.F., Vadlamudi, S., Green, T., Barakat, H.A. 2000. Lipoprotein subpopulation distributions in lean, obese, and type 2 diabetic women: A comparison of African and white Americans. *Obes Res* 8:62–70.

108. Schmidt, C., Gonzaludo, N.P., Strunk, S. et al. 2008. A metaanalysis of QTL for diabetes related traits in rodents. *Physiol Genomics* 34:42–53.

109. Leiter, E.H., Reifsnyder, P.C., Flurkey, K., Partke, H.J., Junger, E., Herberg, L. 1998. NIDDM genes in mice. Deleterious synergism by both parental genomes contributes to diabetic thresholds. *Diabetes* 47:1287–1295.

110. Reifsnyder, P.C., Leiter, E.H. 2002. Deconstructing and reconstructing obesity-induced diabetes (diabesity) in mice. *Diabetes* 51:825–832.

111. Coleman, D.L. 1978. Obese and diabetes: Two mutant genes causing diabetes-obesity syndromes in mice. *Diabetologia* 14:141–148.

112. Stoehr, J.P., Nadler, S.T., Schueler, K.L. et al. 2000. Genetic obesity unmasks non-linear interactions between murine type 2 diabetes susceptibility loci. *Diabetes* 49:1946–1954.

113. Clee, S.M., Yandell, B.S., Schueler, K.M. et al. 2006. Positional cloning of *Sorcs1*, a type 2 diabetes quantitative trait locus. *Nat Genet* 38:688–693.

114. Dokmanovic-Chouinard, M., Chung, W.K., Chevre, J.C. et al. 2008. Positional cloning of "Lisch-Like", a candidate modifier of susceptibility to type 2 diabetes in mice. *PLoS Genet* 4:e1000137.

115. Igel, M., Becker, W., Herberg, L., Joost, H.G. 1997. Hyperleptinemia, leptin resistance and polymorphic leptin receptor in the New Zealand Obese (NZO) mouse. *Endocrinology* 138:4234–4239.

116. Schmolz, K., Pyrski, M., Bufe, B. et al. 2007. Regulation of feeding behavior in normal and obese mice by neuromedin-U: A variant of the neuromedin-U receptor 2 contributes to hyperphagia in the New-Zealand obese mouse. *Obes Metab* 3:28–37.

117. Buchmann, J., Meyer, C., Neschen, S. et al. 2007. Ablation of the cholesterol transporter adenosine triphosphate-binding cassette transporter G1 reduces adipose cell size and protects against diet-induced obesity. *Endocrinology* 148:1561–1573.

118. Scherneck, S., Nestler, M., Vogel, H. et al. 2009. Positional cloning of zinc finger domain transcription factor *Zfp69*, a candidate gene for obesity-associated diabetes contributed by mouse locus Nidd/SJL. *PLoS Genet* 5:e1000541.

119. Vogel, H., Nestler, M., Ruschendorf, F. et al. 2009. Characterization of Nob3, a major quantitative trait locus for obesity and hyperglycemia on mouse chromosome 1. *Physiol Genomics* 38:226–232.

120. Chadt, A., Leicht, K., Deshmukh, A. et al. 2008. *Tbc1d1* mutation in lean mouse strain confers leanness and protects from diet-induced obesity. *Nat Genet* 40:1354–1359.

121. Joost, H.G. 2010. The genetic basis of obesity and type 2 diabetes: Lessons from the New Zealand obese mouse, a polygenic model of the metabolic syndrome. *Results Probl Cell Differ* 52:1–11.

122. Kluge, R., Giesen, K., Bahrenberg, G., Plum, L., Ortlepp, J.R., Joost, H.G. 2000. Two quantitative trait loci for obesity and insulin resistance (Nob1, Nob2) and their interaction with the leptin receptor locus (Lepr$^{A720T/T1044I}$) in New Zealand obese (NZO) mice. *Diabetologia* 43:1565–1573.

123. Pan, H.J., Reifsnyder, P., Vance, D.E., Xiao, Q., Leiter, E.H. 2005. Pharmacogenetic analysis of rosiglitazone-induced hepatosteatosis in new mouse models of type 2 diabetes. *Diabetes* 54:1854–1862.

124. Pan, H.J., Agate, D.S., King, B.L. et al. 2006. A polymorphism in New Zealand inbred mouse strains that inactivates phosphatidylcholine transfer protein. *FEBS Lett* 580:5953–5958.

125. Lafontan, M., Langin L. 2009. Lipolysis and lipid mobilization in human adipose tissue. *Prog Lipid Res* 48:275–297.

126. Blaak, E.E., Van Baak, M.A., Kemerink, G.J., Pakbiers, M.T., Heidendal, G.A., Saris, W.H. 1994. Beta-adrenergic stimulation of energy expenditure and forearm skeletal muscle metabolism in lean and obese men. *Am J Physiol* 267:E306–E315.

127. Webber, J., Taylor, J., Greathead, H., Dawson, J., Buttery, P.J., Macdonald, I.A. 1994. A comparison of the thermogenic, metabolic and haemodynamic responses to infused adrenaline in lean and obese subjects. *Int J Obes Relat Metab Disord* 18:717–724.

128. Horowitz, J.F., Klein, S. 2000. Whole body and abdominal lipolytic sensitivity to epinephrine is suppressed in upper body obese women. *Am J Physiol Endocrinol Metab* 278:E1144–E1152.

129. Schiffelers, S.L., Akkermans, J.A., Saris, W.H., Blaak, E.E. 2003. Lipolytic and nutritive blood flow response to beta-adrenoceptor stimulation in situ in subcutaneous abdominal adipose tissue in obese men. *Int J Obes Relat Metab Disord* 27:227–231.

130. Reynisdottir, S., Wahrenberg, H., Carlstrom, K., Rossner, S., Arner, P. 1994. Catecholamine resistance in fat cells of women with upper-body obesity due to decreased expression of beta 2-adrenoceptors. *Diabetologia* 37:428–435.

131. Stich, V., De Glisezinski, I., Crampes, F. et al. 2000. Activation of alpha(2)-adrenergic receptors impairs exercise-induced lipolysis in SCAT of obese subjects. *Am J Physiol Regul Integr Comp Physiol* 279:R499–R504.

132. Lofgren, P., Hoffstedt, J., Ryden, M. et al. 2002. Major gender differences in the lipolytic capacity of abdominal subcutaneous fat cells in obesity observed before and after long-term weight reduction. *J Clin Endocrinol Metab* 87:764–771.

133. Ray, H., Beylot, M., Arner, P. et al. 2003. The presence of a catalytically inactive form of hormone-sensitive lipase is associated with decreased lipolysis in abdominal subcutaneous adipose tissue of obese subjects. *Diabetes* 52:1417–1422.

134. Mulder, H., Sorhede-Winzell, M., Contreras, J.A. et al. 2003. Hormone-sensitive lipase null mice exhibit signs of impaired insulin sensitivity whereas insulin secretion is intact. *J Biol Chem* 278:36380–36388.

135. Chatzinikolaou, A., Fatouros, I., Petridou, A. et al. 2008. Adipose tissue lipolysis is upregulated in lean and obese men during acute resistance exercise. *Diabetes Care* 31:1397–1399.

136. Haemmerle, G., Lass, A., Zimmermann, R. et al. 2006. Defective lipolysis and altered energy metabolism in mice lacking adipose triglyceride lipase. *Science* 312:734–737.

137. Sztalryd, C., Xu, G., Dorward, H. et al. 2003. Perilipin A is essential for the translocation of hormone-sensitive lipase during lipolytic activation. *J Cell Biol* 161:1093–1103.

138. Tansey, J.T., Sztalryd, C., Gruia-Gray, J. et al. 2001. Perilipin ablation results in a lean mouse with aberrant adipocyte lipolysis, enhanced leptin production, and resistance to diet-induced obesity. *Proc Natl Acad Sci USA* 98:6494–6499.

139. Kern, P.A., Di Gregorio, G., Lu, T., Rassouli, N., Ranganathan, G. 2004. Perilipin expression in human adipose tissue is elevated with obesity. *J Clin Endocrinol Metab* 89:1352–1358.

140. Wang, Y., Sullivan, S., Trujillo, M. 2003. Perilipin expression in human adipose tissues: Effects of severe obesity, gender, and depot. *Obes Res* 11:930–936.

141. Fasshauer, M., Klein, J., Lossner, U., Klier, M., Kralisch, S., Paschke, R. 2003. Suppression of aquaporin adipose gene expression by isoproterenol, TNFalpha, and dexamethasone. *Horm Metab Res* 35:222–227.

142. Marrades, M.P., Milagro, F.I., Martinez, J.A., Moreno-Aliaga, M.J. 2006. Differential expression of aquaporin 7 in adipose tissue of lean and obese high fat consumers. *Biochem Biophys Res Commun* 339:785–789.

143. Yeh, J.I., Charrier, V., Paulo, J. et al. 2004. Structures of enterococcal glycerol kinase in the absence and presence of glycerol: Correlation of conformation to substrate binding and a mechanism of activation by phosphorylation. *Biochemistry* 43:362–373.

144. Hara-Chikuma, M., Sohara, E., Rai, T. et al. 2005. Progressive adipocyte hypertrophy in aquaporin-7-deficient mice: Adipocyte glycerol permeability as a novel regulator of fat accumulation. *J Biol Chem* 280:15493–15496.

145. Summers, L.K., Samra, J.S., Humphreys, S.M., Morris, R.J., Frayn, K.N. 1996. Subcutaneous abdominal adipose tissue blood flow: Variation within and between subjects and relationship to obesity. *Clin Sci (Lond)* 91:679–683.

146. Blaak, E.E., van Baak, M.A., Kemerink, G.J., Pakbiers, M.T., Heidendal, G.A., Saris, W.H. 1995. Beta-adrenergic stimulation and abdominal subcutaneous fat blood flow in lean, obese, and reduced-obese subjects. *Metabolism* 44:183–187.

147. Jocken, J.W.E., Blaak, E.E. 2008. Catecholamine-induced lipolysis in adipose tissue and skeletal muscle in obesity. *Physiol Behav* 94:219–230.

148. Langfort, J., Ploug, T., Ihlemann, J. et al. 2003. Additivity of adrenaline and contractions on hormone-sensitive lipase, but not on glycogen phosphorylase, in rat muscle. *Acta Physiol Scand* 178:51–60.

149. Barbe, P., Millet, L., Galitzky, J., Lafontan, M., Berlan, M. 1996. In situ assessment of the role of the beta 1-, beta 2- and beta 3-adrenoceptors in the control of lipolysis and nutritive blood flow in human subcutaneous adipose tissue. *Br J Pharmacol* 117:907–913.

150. Kjaer, M., Howlett, K., Langfort, J. et al. 2000. Adrenaline and glycogenolysis in skeletal muscle during exercise: A study in adrenalectomised humans. *J Physiol* 528(Pt 2):371–378.

151. Watt, M.J., Krustrup, P., Secher, N.H., Saltin, B., Pedersen, B.K., Febbraio, M.A. 2004. Glucose ingestion blunts hormone-sensitive lipase activity in contracting human skeletal muscle. *Am J Physiol Endocrinol Metab* 286:E144–E150.

152. Wicklmayr, M., Dietze, G., Rett, K., Mehnert, H. 1985. Evidence for a substrate regulation of triglyceride lipolysis in human skeletal muscle. *Horm Metab Res* 17:471–475.

153. Qvisth, V., Hagstrom-Toft, E., Enoksson, S., Sherwin, R.S., Sjoberg, S., Bolinder, J. 2004. Combined hyperinsulinemia and hyperglycemia, but not hyperinsulinemia alone, suppress human skeletal muscle lipolytic activity in vivo. *J Clin Endocrinol Metab* 89:4693–4700.

154. Hagstrom-Toft, E., Qvisth, V., Nennesmo, I. et al. 2002. Marked heterogeneity of human skeletal muscle lipolysis at rest. *Diabetes* 51:3376–3383.

155. Yamaguchi, T., Omatsu, N., Matsushita, S., Osumi, T. 2004. CGI-58 interacts with per-ilipin and is localized to lipid droplets. Possible involvement of CGI-58 mislocalization in Chanarin–Dorfman syndrome. *J Biol Chem* 279:30490–30497.

156. Petersen, K.F., Shulman, G.I. 2006. Etiology of insulin resistance. *Am J Med* 119:S10–S16.

157. Bolinder, J., Kerckhoffs, D.A., Moberg, E., Hagstrom-Toft, E., Arner, P. 2000. Rates of skeletal muscle and adipose tissue glycerol release in nonobese and obese subjects. *Diabetes* 49:797–802.

158. Blaak, E.E., Schiffelers, S.L., Saris, W.H., Mensink, M., Kooi, M.E. 2004. Impaired betaadrenergically mediated lipolysis in skeletal muscle of obese subjects. *Diabetologia* 47:1462–1468.

159. Enoksson, S., Talbot, M., Rife, F., Tamborlane, W.V., Sherwin, R.S., Caprio, S. 2000. Impaired in vivo stimulation of lipolysis in adipose tissue by selective beta2-adrenergic agonist in obese adolescent girls. *Diabetes* 49:2149–2153.

160. Blaak, E.E., Van Baak, M.A., Kemerink, G.J., Pakbiers, M.T., Heidendal, G.A., Saris, W.H. 1994. Beta-adrenergic stimulation of skeletal muscle metabolism in relation to weight reduction in obese men. *Am J Physiol* 267:E316–E322.

161. Hellstrom, L., Langin, D., Reynisdottir, S., Dauzats, M., Arner, P. 1996. Adipocyte lipol-ysis in normal weight subjects with obesity among first-degree relatives. *Diabetologia* 39:921–928.

162. Jocken, J.W., Blaak, E.E., Schiffelers, S., Arner, P., van Baak, M.A., Saris, W.H. 2006. Association of a beta-2 adrenoceptor (ADRB2) gene variant with a blunted in vivo lipolysis and fat oxidation. *Int J Obes (Lond)* 31:813–819.

163. Jocken, J.W., Goossens, G.H., van Hees, A.M. et al. 2008. Effect of beta-adrenergic stimulation on whole-body and abdominal subcutaneous adipose tissue lipolysis in lean and obese men. *Diabetologia* 51:320–327.

164. Campbell, P.J., Carlson, M.G., Nurjhan, N. 1994. Fat metabolism in human obesity. *Am J Physiol* 266:E600–E605.

165. Blaak, E.E. 2004. Basic disturbances in skeletal muscle fatty acid metabolism in obesity and type 2 diabetes mellitus. *Proc Nutr Soc* 63:323–330.

166. Zurlo, F., Lillioja, S., Esposito-Del Puente, A. et al. 1990. Low ratio of fat to carbohydrate oxidation as predictor of weight gain: Study of 24-h RQ. *Am J Physiol* 259:E650–E657.

167. Colberg, S.R., Simoneau, J.A., Thaete, F.L., Kelley, D.E. 1995. Skeletal muscle utilization of free fatty acids in women with visceral obesity. *J Clin Invest* 95:1846–1853.

168. Kim, J.Y., Hickner, R.C., Cortright, R.L., Dohm, G.L., Houmard, J.A. 2000. Lipid oxidation is reduced in obese human skeletal muscle. *Am J Physiol Endocrinol Metab* 279:E1039–E1044.

169. Astrup, A., Buemann, B., Christensen, N.J., Toubro, S. 1994. Failure to increase lipid oxidation in response to increasing dietary fat content in formerly obese women. *Am J Physiol* 266:E592–E599.

170. Mensink, M., Blaak, E.E., van Baak, M.A. et al. 2001. Plasma free fatty acid uptake and oxidation are already diminished in subjects at high risk for developing type 2 diabetes. *Diabetes* 50:2548–2554.

171. Blaak, E.E., Wagenmakers, A.J., Glatz, J.F. et al. 2000. Utilization and fatty acid-binding protein content are diminished in type 2 diabetic muscle. *Am J Physiol Endocrinol Metab* 279:E146–E154.

172. Blaak, E.E., Wagenmakers, A.J. 2002. The fate of [U-(13)C]palmitate extracted by skeletal muscle in subjects with type 2 diabetes and control subjects. *Diabetes* 51:784–789.

173. Kelley, D.E., Simoneau, J.A. 1994. Impaired free fatty acid utilization by skeletal muscle in non-insulin-dependent diabetes mellitus. *J Clin Invest* 94:2349–2356.

174. Kelley, D.E., Mandarino, L.J. 2000. Fuel selection in human skeletal muscle in insulin resistance: A reexamination. *Diabetes* 49:677–683.

175. van der Vusse, G.J., van Bilsen, M., Glatz, J.F. et al. 2002. Critical steps in cellular fatty acid uptake and utilization. *Mol Cel Biochem* 239:9–15.

176. Coburn, C.T., Knapp, F.F. Jr., Febbraio, M. et al. 2000. Defective uptake and utilization of long chain fatty acids in muscle and adipose tissues of CD36 knockout mice. *J Biol Chem* 275:32523–32529.

177. Wilmsen, H.M., Ciaraldi, T.P., Carter, L. et al. 2003. Thiazolidinediones upregulate impaired fatty acid uptake in skeletal muscle of type 2 diabetic subjects. *Am J Physiol Endocrinol Metab* 285:E354–E362.

178. Gaster, M., Rustan, A.C., Aas, V., Beck-Nielsen, H. 2004. Reduced lipid oxidation in skeletal muscle from type 2 diabetic subjects may be of genetic origin: Evidence from cultured myotubes. *Diabetes* 53:542–548.

179. Saha, A.K., Vavvas, D., Kurowski, T.G. et al. 1997. Malonyl-CoA regulation in skeletal muscle: Its link to cell citrate and the glucose-fatty acid cycle. *Am J Physiol* 272:E641–E648.

180. Schrauwen, P., van Aggel-Leijssen, D.P., Hul, G. et al. 2002. The effect of a 3-month low-intensity endurance training program on fat oxidation and acetyl-CoA carboxylase-2 expression. *Diabetes* 51:2220–2226.

181. Mensink, M., Blaak, E.E., Vidal, H. et al. 2003. Lifestyle changes and lipid metabolism gene expression and protein content in skeletal muscle of subjects with impaired glucose tolerance. *Diabetologia* 46:1082–1089.

182. Sidossis, L.S., Wolfe, R.R. 1996. Glucose and insulin-induced inhibition of fatty acid oxidation: The glucose-fatty acid cycle reversed. *Am J Physiol* 270:E733–E738.

183. Mandarino, L.J., Consoli, A., Jain, A., Kelley, D.E. 1996. Interaction of carbohydrate and fat fuels in human skeletal muscle: Impact of obesity and NIDDM. *Am J Physiol* 270:E463–E470.

184. Rasmussen, B.B., Holmback, U.C., Volpi, E. et al. 2002. Malonyl coenzyme A and the regulation of functional carnitine palmitoyltransferase-1 activity and fat oxidation in human skeletal muscle. *J Clin Invest* 110:1687–1693.

185. Kelley, D.E., He, J., Menshikova, E.V., Ritov, V.B. 2002. Dysfunction of mitochondria in human skeletal muscle in type 2 diabetes. *Diabetes* 51:2944–2950.

186. Ritov, V.B., Menshikova, E.V., He, J. et al. 2005. Deficiency of subsarcolemmal mitochondria in obesity and type 2 diabetes. *Diabetes* 54:8–14.

187. Petersen, K.F., Dufour, S., Befroy, D. et al. 2004. Impaired mitochondrial activity in the insulin-resistant offspring of patients with type 2 diabetes. *N Engl J Med* 350:664–671.

188. Mootha, V.K., Lindgren, C.M., Eriksson, K.F. et al. 2003. PGC-1alpha-responsive genes involved in oxidative phosphorylation are coordinately downregulated in human diabetes. *Nat Genet* 34:267–273.

189. Patti, M.E., Butte, A.J., Crunkhorn, S. et al. 2003. Coordinated reduction of genes of oxidative metabolism in humans with insulin resistance and diabetes: Potential role of PGC1 and NRF1. *Proc Natl Acad Sci USA* 100:8466–8471.

190. Schrauwen, P., Hesselink, M.K. 2004. Oxidative capacity, lipotoxicity, and mitochondrial damage in type 2 diabetes. *Diabetes* 53:1412–1417.

191. Blaak, E.E. 2005. Metabolic fluxes in skeletal muscle in relation to obesity and insulin resistance. *Best Pract Res Clin Endocrinol Metab* 19(3):391–403.
192. Schiffelers, S.L., Saris, W.H., van Baak, M.A. 2001. The effect of an increased free fatty acid concentration on thermogenesis and substrate oxidation in obese and lean men. *Int J Obes Relat Metab Disord* 25:33–38.
193. Tilg, H., Moschen, A.R. 2006. Adipocytokines: Mediators linking adipose tissue, inflammation and immunity. *Nat Rev Immunol* 6:772–783.
194. Arita, Y., Kihara, S., Ouchi, N. 1999. Paradoxical decrease of an adipose-specific protein, adiponectin, in obesity. *Biochem Biophys Res Commun* 257:79–83.
195. Hotta, K., Funahashi, T., Arita, Y. et al. 2000. Plasma concentrations of a novel, adipose-specific protein, adiponectin, in type 2 diabetic patients. *Arterioscler Thromb Vasc Biol* 20:1595–1599.
196. Ahima, R.S., Saper, C.B., Flier, J.S., Elmquist, J.K. 2000. Leptin regulation of neuroendocrine systems. *Front Neuroendocrinol* 21:263–307.
197. Minokoshi, Y., Kim, Y.B. 2002. Leptin stimulates fatty-acid oxidation by activating AMP-activated protein kinase. *Nature* 415:339–343.
198. Wang, Z., Zhou, Y.T., Kakuma, T. et al. 2000. Leptin resistance of adipocytes in obesity: Role of suppressors of cytokine signaling. *Biochem Biophys Res Commun* 277:20–26.
199. Wallace, A.M., McMahon, A.D., Packard, C.J. et al. 2001. Plasma leptin and the risk of cardiovascular disease in the West of Scotland Coronary Prevention Study (WOSCOPS). *Circulation* 104:3052–3056.
200. Sierra-Honigmann, M.R., Nath, A.K., Murakami, C. et al. 1998. Biological action of leptin as an angiogenic factor. *Science* 281:1683–1686.
201. Bodary, P.F., Westrick, R.J., Wickenheiser, K.J., Shen, Y., Eitzman, D.T. 2002. Effect of leptin on arterial thrombosis following vascular injury in mice. *JAMA* 287:1706–1709.
202. Xu, F.P., Chen, M.S., Wang, Y.Z. et al. 2004. Leptin induces hypertrophy via endothelin-1-reactive oxygen species pathway in cultured neonatal rat cardiomyocytes. *Circulation* 110:1269–1275.
203. Coppack, S.W. 2001. Pro-inflammatory cytokines and adipose tissue. *Proc Nutr Soc* 60:349–356.
204. Ruan, H., Miles, P.D., Ladd, C.M. et al. 2002. Profiling gene transcription in vivo reveals adipose tissue as an immediate target of tumor necrosis factor-alpha: Implications for insulin resistance. *Diabetes* 51:3176–3188.
205. Boyle, P.J. 2004. What are the effects of peroxisome proliferator activated receptor agonists on adiponectin, tumor necrosis factor alpha, and other cytokines in insulin resistance? *Clin Cardiol* 27:1111–1116.
206. Pai, J.K., Pischon, T., Ma, J. et al. 2004. Inflammatory markers and the risk of coronary heart disease in men and women. *N Engl J Med* 351:2599–2610.
207. Landry, D.B., Couper, L.L., Bryant, S.R., Lindner, V. 1997. Activation of the NF-B and I B system in smooth muscle cells after rat arterial injury. Induction of vascular cell adhesion molecule-1 and monocyte chemoattractant protein-1. *Am J Pathol* 151:1085–1095.
208. Iademarco, M.F., McQuillan, J.J., Dean, D.C. 1993. Vascular cell adhesion molecule 1: Contrasting transcriptional control mechanisms in muscle and endothelium. *Proc Natl Acad Sci USA* 90:3943–3947.
209. Eck, S.L., Perkins, N.D., Carr, D.P., Nabel, G.J. 1993. Inhibition of phorbol ester-induced cellular adhesion by competitive binding of NF-B in vivo. *Mol Cell Biol* 13:6530–6536.
210. Clesham, G.J., Adam, P.J., Proudfoot, D., Flynn, P.D., Efstathiou, S., Weissberg, P.L. 1998. High adenoviral loads stimulate NF-κB-dependent gene expression in human vascular smooth muscle cells. *Gene Ther* 5:174–180.
211. Xie, Q.W., Kashiwabara, Y., Nathan, C. 1994. Role of transcription factor NF-κB/Rel in induction of nitric oxide synthase. *J Biol Chem* 269:4705–4708.

212. Goto, M., Katayama, K.I., Shirakawa, F., Tanaka, I. 1999. Involvement of NF-κB p50/p65 heterodimer in activation of the human prointerleukin-1β gene at two subregions of the upstream enhancer element. *Cytokine* 11:16–28.

213. Ouchi, N., Kihara, S., Funahashi, T., Matsuzawa, Y., Walsh, K. 2003. Obesity, adiponectin and vascular inflammatory disease. *Curr Opin Lipid* 14:561–566.

214. Waki, H., Yamauchi, T., Kamon, J. et al. 2003. Impaired multimerization of human adiponectin mutants associated with diabetes: Molecular structure and multimer formation of adiponectin. *J Biol Chem* 278:40352–40363.

215. Tsao, T.S., Tomas, E., Murrey, H.E. et al. 2003. Role of disulfide bonds in Acrp30/adiponectin structure and signaling specificity: Different oligomers activate different signal transduction pathways. *J Biol Chem* 278:50810–50817.

216. Ouchi, N., Kihara, S., Arita, Y. et al. 1999. Novel modulator for endothelial adhesion molecules: Adipocyte-derived plasma protein adiponectin. *Circulation* 100:2473–2476.

217. Tan, K.C., Xu, A., Chow, W.S. et al. 2004. Hypoadiponectinemia is associated with impaired endothelium-dependent vasodilation. *J Clin Endocrinol Metab* 89:765–769.

218. Bruun, J.M., Lihn, A.S., Verdich, C. et al. 2003. Regulation of adiponectin by adipose tissue-derived cytokines: In vivo and in vitro investigations in humans. *Am J Physiol Endocrinol Metab* 285:E527–E533.

219. Yamauchi, T., Kamon, J., Minokoshi, Y. et al. 2002. Adiponectin stimulates glucose utilization and fatty-acid oxidation by activating AMP-activated protein kinase. *Nat Med* 8:1288–1295.

220. Pischon, T., Girman, C.J., Hotamisligil, G.S., Rifai, N., Hu, F.B., Rimm, E.B. 2004. Plasma adiponectin levels and risk of myocardial infarction in men. *JAMA* 291:1730–1737.

221. Schulze, M.B., Shai, I., Rimm, E.B., Li, T., Rifai, N., Hu, F.B. 2005. Adiponectin and future coronary heart disease events among men with type 2 diabetes. *Diabetes* 54:534–539.

222. Howard, B.V., Lee, E.T., Cowan, L.D. et al. 1999. Rising tide of cardiovascular disease in American Indians: The Strong Heart Study. *Circulation* 11:2389–2395.

223. Lindsay, R.S., Funahashi, T., Hanson, R.L. et al. 2002. Adiponectin and development of type 2 diabetes in the Pima Indian population. *Lancet* 360:57–58.

224. Spranger, J., Kroke, A., Mohlig, M. et al. 2003. Adiponectin and protection against type 2 diabetes mellitus. *Lancet* 361:226–228.

225. Mohamed-Ali, V., Pinkney, J.K. 1998. Adipose tissue as an endocrine and paracrine organ. *Int J Obes Relat Metab Disord* 22:1145–1158.

226. Bastard, J.P., Jardel, C., Bruckert, E. et al. 2000. Elevated levels of interleukin 6 are reduced in serum and subcutaneous adipose tissue of obese women after weight loss. *J Clin Endocrinol Metab* 85:3338–3342.

227. Esposito, K., Pontillo, A., Di Palo, C., Giugliano, G., Masella, M., Marfella, R., Giugliano, D. 2003. Effect of weight loss and lifestyle changes on vascular inflammatory markers in obese women: A randomized trial. *JAMA* 289:1799–1804.

228. Mohamed-Ali, V., Goodrick, S., Rawesh, A. et al. 1997. Subcutaneous adipose tissue releases interleukin-6, but not tumor necrosis factor-alpha, in vivo. *J Clin Endocrinol Metab* 82:4196–4200.

229. Fried, S.K., Bunkin, D.A., Greenberg, A.S. 1998. Omental and subcutaneous adipose tissues of obese subjects release interleukin-6: Depot difference and regulation by glucocorticoid. *J Clin Endocrinol Metab* 83:847–850.

230. Yudkin, J.S., Kumari, M., Humphries, S.E., Mohamed-Ali, V. 2000. Inflammation, obesity, stress and coronary heart disease: Is interleukin-6 the link? *Atherosclerosis* 148:209–214.

231. Senn, J.J., Klover, P.J., Nowak, I.A., Mooney, R.A. 2002. Interleukin-6 induces cellular insulin resistance in hepatocytes. *Diabetes* 51:3391–3399.

232. Senn, J.J., Klover, P.J., Nowak, I.A. et al. 2003. Suppressor of cytokine signaling-3 (SOCS-3), a potential mediator of interleukin-6-dependent insulin resistance in hepatocytes. *J Biol Chem* 278:13740–13746.

233. Ridker, P.M., Rifai, N., Rose, L., Buring, J.E., Cook, N.R. 2002. Comparison of C-reactive protein and low-density lipoprotein cholesterol levels in the prediction of first cardiovascular events. *N Engl J Med* 347:1557–1565.

234. Fukuhara, A., Matsuda, M., Nishizawa, M. et al. 2005. Visfatin: A protein secreted by visceral fat that mimics the effects of insulin. *Science* 307:426–430.

235. Makino, T., Noguchi, Y., Yoshikawa, T., Doi, C., Nomura, K. 1998. Circulating interleukin 6 concentrations and insulin resistance in patients with cancer. *Br J Surg* 85:1658–1662.

236. Alessi, M.C., Peiretti, F., Morange, P., Henry, M., Nalbone, G., Juhan-Vague, I. 1997. Production of plasminogen activator inhibitor by human adipose tissue: Possible link between visceral fat accumulation and vascular disease. *Diabetes* 46:860–867.

237. Bastelica, D., Morange, P., Berthet, B. et al. 2002. Stromal cells are the main plasminogen activator inhibitor-1-producing cells in human fat: Evidence of differences between visceral and subcutaneous deposits. *Arterioscler Thromb Vasc Biol* 22:173–178.

238. Stentz, F.B., Umpierrez, G.E., Cuervo, R., Kitabchi, A.E. 2004. Proinflammatory cytokines, markers of cardiovascular risks, oxidative stress, and lipid peroxidation in patients with hyperglycemic crises. *Diabetes* 53:2079–2086.

239. Gabriely, I., Yang, X.M., Cases, J.A., Ma, X.H., Rossetti, L., Barzilai, N. 2002. Hyperglycemia induces *PAI-1* gene expression in adipose tissue by activation of the hexosamine biosynthetic pathway. *Atherosclerosis* 160:115–122.

240. Sobel, B.E. 1999. Increased plasminogen activator inhibitor-1 and vasculopathy: A reconcilable paradox. *Circulation* 99:2496–2498.

241. Thogersen, A.M., Jansson, J.H., Boman, K. et al. 1998. High plasminogen activator inhibitor and tissue plasminogen activator levels in plasma precede a first acute myocardial infarction in both men and women: Evidence for the fibrinolytic system as an independent primary risk factor. *Circulation* 98:2241–2247.

242. Ailhaud, G., Fukamizu, A., Massiera, F., Negrel, R., Saint-Marc, P., Teboul, M. 2000. Angiotensinogen, angiotensin II and adipose tissue development. *Int J Obes Relat Metab Disord* 24:S33–S35.

243. Tham, D.M., Martin-McNulty, B., Wang, Y.X. et al. 2002. Angiotensin II is associated with activation of NF-B-mediated genes and downregulation of PPARs. *Physiol Genomics* 11:21–30.

244. Cai, H., Li, Z., Dikalov, S. et al. 2002. NAD (P) H oxidase-derived hydrogen peroxide mediates endothelial nitric oxide production in response to angiotensin II. *J Biol Chem* 277:48311–48317.

245. Gavi, S., Stuart, L.M., Kelly, P. et al. 2007. Retinol-binding protein 4 is associated with insulin resistance and body fat distribution in nonobese subjects without type 2 diabetes. *J Clin Endocrinol Metab* 92:1886–1890.

246. Yang, Q., Graham, T.E., Mody, N. et al. 2005. Serum retinol binding protein 4 contributes to insulin resistance in obesity and type 2 diabetes. *Nature* 436:356–362.

247. Widlansky, M.E., Gokce, N., Keaney, J.F. Jr., Vita, J.A. 2003. The clinical implications of endothelial dysfunction. *J Am Coll Cardiol* 42:1149–1160.

248. Verma, S., Li, S.H., Wang, C.H. et al. 2003. Resistin promotes endothelial cell activation: Further evidence of adipokine–endothelial interaction. *Circulation* 108:736–740.

249. Savage, D.B., Sewter, C.P., Klenk, E.S. et al. 2001. Resistin/Fizz3 expression in relation to obesity and peroxisome proliferator-activated receptor action in humans. *Diabetes* 50:2199–2202.

250. Calabro, P., Samudio, I., Willerson, J.T., Yeh, E.T. 2004. Resistin promotes smooth muscle cell proliferation through activation of extracellular signal-regulated kinase 1/2 and phosphatidylinositol 3-kinase pathways. *Circulation* 110:3335–3340.

251. Rubin, G.L., Zhao, Y., Kalus, A.M., Simpson, E.R. 2000. Peroxisome proliferator receptor gamma ligands inhibit estrogen biosynthesis in human breast adipose tissue: Possible implication for breast cancer therapy. *Cancer Res* 60:1604–1608.
252. Hemsell, D.L., Grodin, J.M., Brenner, P.F., Siiteri, P.K., MacDonald, P.C. 1974. Plasma precursors of estrogen: Correlation of the extent of conversion of plasma androstenedione to estrone with age. *J Clin Endocrinol Metab* 38:476–479.
253. Bjorntorp, P. 1996. The regulation of adipose tissue distribution in humans. *Int J Obes Relat Metab Disord* 20:291–302.
254. Jones, M.E., Thorburn, A.W., Britt, K.L. et al. 2000. Aromatase-deficient (ArKO) mice have a phenotype of increased adiposity. *Proc Natl Acad Sci USA* 97:12735–12740.
255. Seckl, J.R. 2004. 11beta-hydroxysteroid dehydrogenases: Changing glucocorticoid action. *Curr Opin Pharmacol* 4:597–602.
256. Wake, D.J., Rask, E., Livingstone, D.E., Soderberg, S., Olsson, T., Walker, B.R. 2003. Local and systemic impact of transcriptional up-regulation of 11β-hydroxysteroid dehydrogenase type 1 in adipose tissue in human obesity. *J Clin Endocrinol Metab* 88:3983–3988.
257. Valsamakis, G., Anwar, A., Tomlinson, J.W. et al. 2004. 11β-hydroxysteroid dehydrogenase type 1 activity in lean and obese males with type 2 diabetes mellitus. *J Clin Endocrinol Metab* 89:4755–4761.
258. Crook, M.A., Tutt, P., Pickup, J.C. 1993. Elevated serum sialic acid concentration in NIDDM and its relationship to blood pressure and retinopathy. *Diabetes Care* 16:57–60.
259. Pickup, J.C., Mattock, M.B., Chusney, G.D., Burt, D. 1997. NIDDM as a disease of the innate immune system: Association of acute-phase reactants and interleukin-6 with metabolic syndrome X. *Diabetologia* 40:1286–1292.
260. Schmidt, M.I., Duncan, B.B., Sharrett, A.R. et al. 1999. Markers of inflammation and prediction of diabetes mellitus in adults (atherosclerosis risk in communities study): A cohort study. *Lancet* 353:1649–1652.
261. Duncan, B.B., Schmidt, M.I., Pankow, J.S. et al. 2003. Low-grade systemic inflammation and the development of type 2 diabetes: The atherosclerosis risk in communities study. *Diabetes* 52:1799–1805.
262. Pradhan, A.D., Manson, J.E., Rifai, N., Buring, J.E., Ridker, P.M. 2001. C-reactive protein, interleukin 6, and risk of developing type 2 diabetes mellitus. *JAMA* 286:327–334.
263. Barzilay, J.I., Abraham, L., Heckbert, S.R. et al. 2001. The relation of markers of inflammation to the development of glucose disorders in the elderly: The Cardiovascular Health Study. *Diabetes* 50:2384–2389.
264. Han, T.S., Sattar, N., Williams, K., Gonzalez-Villapando, C., Lean, M.E., Haffner, S.M. 2002. Prospective study of C-reactive protein in relation to the development of diabetes and metabolic syndrome in the Mexico City Diabetes Study. *Diabetes Care* 25:2016–2021.
265. Pradhan, A.D., Cook, N.R., Buring, J.E., Manson, J.E., Ridker, P.M. 2003. C-reactive protein is independently associated with fasting insulin in nondiabetic women. *Arterioscler Thromb Vasc Biol* 23:650–655.
266. Yudkin, J.S., Stehouwer, C.D., Emeis, J.J., Coppack, S.W. 1999. C-reactive protein in healthy subjects: Associations with obesity, insulin resistance, and endothelial dysfunction: A potential role for cytokines originating from adipose tissue? *Arterioscler Thromb Vasc Biol* 19:972–978.
267. Hak, A.E., Stehouwer, C.D., Bots, M.L. et al. 1999. Associations of C-reactive protein with measures of obesity, insulin resistance, and subclinical atherosclerosis in healthy, middle-aged women. *Arterioscler Thromb Vasc Biol* 19:1986–1991.
268. Lemieux, I., Pascot, A., Prudhomme, D. et al. 2001. Elevated C-reactive protein: Another component of the atherothrombotic profile of abdominal obesity. *Arterioscler Thromb Vasc Biol* 21:961–967.

269. Mantzoros, C.S., Moschos, S., Avramopoulos, I. et al. 1997. Leptin concentrations in relation to body mass index and the tumor necrosis factor-α system in humans. *J Clin Endocrinol Metab* 82:3408–3413.

270. Lundgren, C.H., Brown, S.L., Nordt, T.K., Sobel, B.E., Fujii, S. 1996. Elaboration of type-1 plasminogen activator inhibitor from adipocytes: A potential pathogenetic link between obesity and cardiovascular disease. *Circulation* 93:106–110.

271. Fernandez-Real, J.M., Lopez-Bermejo, A., Casamitjana, R., Ricart, W. 2003. Novel interactions of adiponectin with the endocrine system and inflammatory parameters. *J Clin Endocrinol Metab* 88:2714–2718.

272. Miller, G.E., Freedland, K.E., Carney, R.M., Stetler, C.A., Banks W.A. 2003. Pathways linking depression, adiposity, and inflammatory markers in healthy young adults. *Brain Behav Immun* 17:276–285.

273. Matarese, G., La Cava, A., Sanna, V. et al. 2002. Balancing susceptibility to infection and autoimmunity: A role for leptin? *Trends Immunol* 23:182–187.

274. Hotamisligil, G.S., Budavari, A., Murray, D., Spiegelman, B.M. 1994. Reduced tyrosine kinase activity of the insulin receptor in obesity-diabetes: Central role of tumor necrosis factor-α. *J Clin Invest* 94:1543–1549.

275. Aljada, A., Ghanim, H., Assian, E., Dandona, P. 2002. Tumor necrosis factor-α inhibits insulin-induced increase in endothelial nitric oxide synthase and reduces insulin receptor content and phosphorylation in human aortic endothelial cells. *Metabolism* 51:487–491.

276. Kubaszek, A., Pihlajamaki, J., Komarovski, V. et al. 2003. Promoter polymorphisms of the TNF-α (G-308A) and IL-6 (C-174G) genes predict the conversion from impaired glucose tolerance to type 2 diabetes: The Finnish Diabetes Prevention Study. *Diabetes* 52:1872–1876.

277. Eckel, R., Kahn, S., Ferrannini, E. et al. 2011. Obesity and type 2 diabetes: What can be unified and what needs to be individualized? *J Clin Endocrinol Metab* 96:1654–1663.

278. Deng, Y., Scherer, P.E. 2010. Adipokines as novel biomarkers and regulators of the metabolic syndrome. *Ann N Y Acad Sci* 1212:E1–E19.

279. Hautanen, A., Raikkonen, K., Adlercreutz, H. 1997. Associations between pituitary-adrenocortical function and abdominal obesity, hyperinsulinaemia and dyslipidaemia in normotensive males. *J Intern Med* 241:451–461.

280. Masuzaki, H., Paterson, J., Shinyama, H. et al. 2001. A transgenic model of visceral obesity and the metabolic syndrome. *Science* 294:2166–2170.

281. Paulmyer-Lacroix, O., Boullu, S., Oliver, C., Alessi, M.C., Grino, M. 2002. Expression of the mRNA coding for 11-hydroxysteroid dehydrogenase type 1 in adipose tissue from obese patients: An in situ hybridization study. *J Clin Endocrinol Metab* 87:2701–2705.

282. Jacobson, P.B., von Geldern, T.W., Ohman, L. et al. 2005. Hepatic glucocorticoid receptor antagonism is sufficient to reduce elevated hepatic glucose output and improve glucose control in animal models of type 2 diabetes. *J Pharmacol Exp Ther* 314:191–200.

283. Kabir, M., Catalano, K.J., Ananthnarayan, S. et al. 2005. Molecular evidence supporting the portal theory: A causative link between visceral adiposity and hepatic insulin resistance. *Am J Physiol Endocrinol Metab* 288(2):E454–E461.

284. Bergman, R.N., Kim, S.P., Hsu, I.R. et al. 2007. Abdominal obesity: Role in the pathophysiology of metabolic disease and cardiovascular risk. *Am J Med* 120(Suppl. 1):S3–S8.

285. Qatanani, M., Lazar, M.A. 2007. Mechanisms of obesity-associated insulin resistance: Many choices on the menu. *Genes Dev* 21:1443–1455.

286. Unger, R.H., Orci, L. 2000. Lipotoxic diseases of nonadipose tissues in obesity. *Int J Obes Relat Metab Disord* 24(Suppl. 4):S28–S32.

287. Houstis, N., Rosen, E.D., Lander, E.S. 2006. Reactive oxygen species have a causal role in multiple forms of insulin resistance. *Nature* 440:944–948.

288. Evans, J.L., Goldfine, I.D., Maddux, B.A., Grodsky, G.M. 2002. Oxidative stress and stress-activated signaling pathways: A unifying hypothesis of type 2 diabetes. *Endocrinol Rev* 23:599–622.
289. Bays, H.E., Gonzalez-Campoy, J.M., Bray, G.A. et al. 2008. Pathogenic potential of adipose tissue and metabolic consequences of adipocyte hypertrophy and increased visceral adiposity. *Expert Rev Cardiovasc Ther* 6:343–368.
290. Rosito, G.A., Massaro, J.M., Hoffmann, U. et al. 2008. Pericardial fat, visceral abdominal fat, cardiovascular disease risk factors, and vascular calcification in a community-based sample: A Framingham Heart Study. *Circulation* 117:605–661.
291. Levine, J.A. 1998. Relation between chubby cheeks and visceral fat. *N Engl J Med* 339:1946–1947.
292. Kelley, D.E., Thaete, F.L., Troost, F., Huwe, T., Goodpaster, B.H. 2000. Subdivisions of subcutaneous abdominal adipose tissue and insulin resistance. *Am J Physiol Endocrinol Metab* 278:E941–E948.
293. Smith, S.R., Lovejoy, J.C., Greenway, F. et al. 2001. Contributions of total body fat, abdominal subcutaneous adipose tissue compartments, and visceral adipose tissue to the metabolic complications of obesity. *Metabolism* 50:425–435.
294. Tchoukalova, Y.D., Koutsari, C., Karpyak, M.V., Votruba, S.B., Wendland, E., Jensen, M.D. 2008. Subcutaneous adipocyte size and body fat distribution. *Am J Clin Nutr* 87:56–63.
295. Goodpaster, B.H., Thaete, F.L., Kelley, D.E. 2000. Thigh adipose tissue distribution is associated with insulin resistance in obesity and in type 2 diabetes mellitus. *Am J Clin Nutr* 71:885–892.
296. Björntorp, P. 1991. Metabolic implications of body fat distribution. *Diabetes Care* 14:1132–1143.
297. Kissebah, A.H., Krakower, G.R. 1994. Regional adiposity and morbidity. *Physiol Rev* 74:761–811.
298. Cassano, P.A., Segel, M.R., Vokonas, P.S., Weiss, S.T. 1990. Body fat distribution, blood pressure, and hypertension: A prospective cohort study of men in the normative aging study. *Ann Epidemiol* 1:33–48.
299. Seidell, J.C., Cigolini, M., Deslypere, J., Charzewska, J., Ellsinger, B., Cruz, A. 1991. Body fat distribution in relation to serum lipids and blood pressure in 38-year-old European men: The European fat distribution study. *Atherosclerosis* 86:251–260.
300. Carey, V.J., Walters, E.E., Colditz, G.A. et al. 1997. Body fat distribution and risk of non-insulin-dependent diabetes mellitus in women: The Nurses' Health Study. *Am J Epidemiol* 145:614–619.
301. Chan, J.M., Rimm, E.B., Colditz, G.A., Stampfer, M.J., Willett, W.C. 1994. Obesity, fat distribution, and weight gain as risk factors for clinical diabetes in men. *Diabetes Care* 17:961–969.
302. Schafer, H., Pauleit, D., Sudhop, T., Gouni-Berthold, I., Ewig, S., Berthold, H.K. 2002. Body fat distribution, serum leptin, and cardiovascular risk factors in men with obstructive sleep apnea. *Chest* 122:829–839.
303. Snijder, M.B., Dekker, J.M., Visser, M. et al. 2004. Trunk fat and leg fat have independent and opposite associations with fasting and postload glucose levels: The Hoorn study. *Diabetes Care* 27:372–377.
304. Cefalu, W.T., Wang, Z.Q., Webel, S. et al. 1995. Contribution of visceral fat mass to the insulin resistance of aging. *Metabolism* 44:954–959.
305. Seidell, J.C., Bjorntorp, P., Sjostrom, L., Kvist, H., Sannerstedt, R. 1990. Visceral fat accumulation in men is positively associated with insulin, glucose, and C-peptide levels, but negatively with testosterone levels. *Metabolism* 39:897–901.
306. Kuk, J.L., Katzmarzyk, P.T., Nichaman, M.Z., Church, T.S., Blair, S.N., Ross, R. 2006. Visceral fat is an independent predictor of all-cause mortality in men. *Obesity* 14:336–342.

307. Shadid, S., Jensen, M.D. 2006. Pioglitazone increases non-esterified fatty acid clearance in upper body obesity. *Diabetologia* 49:149–157.

308. Klein, S., Fontana, L., Young, V.L. et al. 2004. Absence of an effect of liposuction on insulin action and risk factors for coronary heart disease. *N Engl J Med* 350:2549–2557.

309. Thörne, A., Lönnqvist, F., Apelman, J., Hellers, G., Arner, P. 2002. A pilot study of long-term effects of a novel obesity treatment: Omentectomy in connection with adjustable gastric banding. *Int J Obes* 26:193–199.

310. Bays, H.E., Fox, K.M., Grandy, S. 2010. Anthropometric measurements and diabetes mellitus: Clues to the "pathogenic" and "protective" potential of adipose tissue. *Metab Syndr Relat Disord* 8:307–315.

311. Schaffler, A., Muller-Ladner, U., Scholmerich, J. et al. 2006. Role of adipose tissue as an inflammatory organ in human diseases *Endocrinol Rev* 27:449–467.

312. Baker, A.R., Silva, N.F., Quinn, D.W. et al. 2006. Human epicardial adipose tissue expresses a pathogenic profile of adipocytokines in patients with cardiovascular disease *Cardiovasc Diabetol* 5:1.

313. Mazurek, T., Zhang, L., Zalewski, A. et al. 2003. Human epicardial adipose tissue is a source of inflammatory mediators *Circulation* 108:2460–2466.

314. Torriani, M., Grinspoon, S. 2005. Racial differences in fat distribution: The importance of intermuscular fat. *Am J Clin Nutr* 81:731–732.

315. Engeli, S. 2005. Is there a pathophysiological role for perivascular adipocytes? *Am J Physiol Heart Circ Physiol* 289:H1794–H1795.

316. Divers, J., Wagenknecht, L.E., Bowden, D.W. et al. 2010. Ethnic differences in the relationship between pericardial adipose tissue and coronary artery calcified plaque: African-American-diabetes heart study. *J Clin Endocrinol Metab* 95:5382–5389.

317. Liu, J., Fox, C.S., Hickson, D. et al. 2010. Pericardial adipose tissue, atherosclerosis, and cardiovascular disease risk factors: The Jackson Heart Study. *Diabetes Care* 33:1635–1639.

318. Bays, H., Mandarino, L., DeFronzo, R.A. 2004. Role of the adipocyte, free fatty acids, and ectopic fat in pathogenesis of type 2 diabetes mellitus: Peroxisomal proliferator-activated receptor agonists provide a rational therapeutic approach. *J Clin Endocrinol Metab* 89:463–478.

319. Yu, Y.H., Ginsberg, H.N. 2005. Adipocyte signaling and lipid homeostasis: Sequelae of insulin-resistant adipose tissue. *Circ Res* 96:1042–1052.

320. Wang, H., Li, H., Hou, Z. et al. 2009. Role of oxidative stress in elevated blood pressure induced by high free fatty acids. *Hypertens Res* 32:152–158.

321. Lewis, G.F., Uffelman, K.D., Szeto, L.W., Weller, B., Steiner, G. 1995. Interaction between free fatty acids and insulin in the acute control of very low density lipoprotein production in humans. *J Clin Invest* 95:158–166.

322. Vogelberg, K.H., Gries, F.A., Moschinski, D. 1980. Hepatic production of VLDL-triglycerides: Dependence of portal substrate and insulin concentration. *Horm Metab Res* 12:688–694.

323. Pasarica, M., Xie, H., Hymel, D. et al. 2009. Lower total adipocyte number, but no evidence for small adipocyte depletion in patients with type 2 diabetes. *Diabetes Care* 32:900–902.

324. Klein, S. 2004. The case of visceral fat: Argument for the defense. *J Clin Invest* 113:1530–1532.

325. Johnson, J.A., Fried, S.K., Pi-Sunyer, F.X. et al. 2001. Impaired insulin action in subcutaneous adipocytes from women with visceral obesity. *Am J Physiol Endocrinol Metab* 280:E40–E49.

326. Jensen, M.D. 2006. Is visceral fat involved in the pathogenesis of the metabolic syndrome? Human model. *Obesity (Silver Spring)* 14(Suppl. 1):S20–S24.

327. Jensen, M.D., Johnson, C.M. 1996. Contribution of leg and splanchnic free fatty acid (FFA) kinetics to postabsorptive FFA flux in men and women. *Metabolism* 45:662–666.

328. Goodpaster, B.H., Thaete, F.L., Simoneau, J.A. et al. 1997. Subcutaneous abdominal fat and thigh muscle composition predict insulin sensitivity independently of visceral fat. *Diabetes* 46:1579–1585.

329. Magkos, F., Fabbrini, E., Mohammed, B.S. et al. 2010. Increased whole-body adiposity without a concomitant increase in liver fat is not associated with augmented metabolic dysfunction. *Obesity (Silver Spring)* 18:1510–1515.

330. Halliwell, B. 1995. Antioxidant characterization: Methodology and mechanism. *Biochem Pharmacol* 49:1341–1348.

331. Rosen, P., Nawroth, P.P., King, G., Moller, W., Tritschler, H.J., Packer, L. 2001. The role of oxidative stress in the onset and progression of diabetes and its complications: A summary of a Congress Series sponsored by UNESCO-MCBN, the American Diabetes Association and the German Diabetes Society. *Diabetes Metab Res Rev* 17:189–212.

332. Furukawa, S., Fujita, T., Shimabukuro, M. et al. 2004. Increased oxidative stress in obesity and its impact on metabolic syndrome. *J Clin Invest* 114:1752–1761.

333. Fridlyand, L.E., Philipson, L.H. 2006. Reactive species and early manifestation of insulin resistance in type 2 diabetes. *Diabetes Obes Metab* 8:136–145.

334. Evans, J.L., Goldfine, I.D., Maddux, B.A., Grodsky, G.M. 2003. Are oxidative stress-activated signaling pathways mediators of insulin resistance and β-cell dysfunction? *Diabetes* 52:1–8.

335. DeFronzo, R.A. 2004. Pathogenesis of type 2 diabetes mellitus. *Med Clin N Am* 88:787–835.

336. Reaven, G.M., Chen, Y.D. 1996. Insulin resistance, its consequences, and coronary heart disease: Must we choose one culprit? *Circulation* 93:1780–1783.

337. Rao, M.S., Reddy, J.K. 2001. Peroxisomal β-oxidation and steatohepatitis. *Semin Liver Dis* 21:43–55.

338. Yamagishi, S.I., Edelstein, D., Du, X.L., Kaneda, Y., Guzman, M., Brownlee, M. 2001. Leptin induces mitochondrial superoxide production and monocyte chemoattractant protein-1 expression in aortic endothelial cells by increasing fatty acid oxidation via protein kinase A. *J Biol Chem* 276:25096–25100.

339. Paolisso, G., Di Maro, G., Pizza, G. et al. 1992. Plasma GSH/GSSG affects glucose homeostasis in healthy subjects and non-insulin-dependent diabetics. *Am J Physiol* 263:E435–E440.

340. Paolisso, G., Gambardella, A., Tagliamonte, M.R. et al. 1996. Does free fatty acid infusion impair insulin action also through an increase in oxidative stress? *J Clin Endocrinol Metab* 81:4244–4248.

341. Maddux, B.A., See, W., Lawrence, J.C. Jr., Goldfine, A.L., Goldfine, I.D., Evans, J.L. 2001. Protection against oxidative stress-induced insulin resistance in rat L6 muscle cells by micromolar concentrations of α-lipoic acid. *Diabetes* 50:404–410.

342. Hirosumi, J., Tuncman, G., Chang, L. et al. 2002. A central role for JNK in obesity and insulin resistance. *Nature* 420:333–336.

343. Yuan, M., Konstantopoulos, N., Lee, J. et al. 2001. Reversal of obesity- and diet-induced insulin resistance with salicylates or targeted disruption of *Ikkβ*. *Science* 293:1673–1677.

344. Birnbaum, M.J. 2001. Turning down insulin signaling. *J Clin Invest* 108:655–659.

345. Petersen, K.F., Befroy, D., Dufour, S. et al. 2003. Mitochondrial dysfunction in the elderly: Possible role in insulin resistance. *Science* 300:1140–1142.

346. St-Pierre, J., Lin, J., Krauss, S. et al. 2003. Bioenergetic analysis of peroxisome proliferator-activated receptor γ coactivators 1α and 1β (PGC-1α and PGC-1β) in muscle cells. *J Biol Chem* 278:26597–26603.

347. Wu, Z., Puigserver, P., Andersson, U. et al. 1999. Mechanisms controlling mitochondrial biogenesis and respiration through the thermogenic coactivator PGC-1. *Cell* 98:115–124.

348. Lagouge, M., Argmann, C., Gerhart-Hines, Z. et al. 2006. Resveratrol improves mitochondrial function and protects against metabolic disease by activating SIRT1 and PGC-1α. *Cell* 127:1109–1122.

349. Mensink, M., Hesselink, M.K., Russell, A.P., Schaart, G., Sels, J.P., Schrauwen, P. 2007. Improved skeletal muscle oxidative enzyme activity and restoration of PGC-1α and PPARβ/δ gene expression upon rosiglitazone treatment in obese patients with type 2 diabetes mellitus. *Int J Obes (Lond)* 31(8):1302–1310.

350. Ozawa, K., Miyazaki, M., Matsuhisa, M. et al. 2005. The endoplasmic reticulum chaperone improves insulin resistance in type 2 diabetes. *Diabetes* 54:657–663.

351. Ozcan, U., Cao, Q., Yilmaz, E. et al. 2004. Endoplasmic reticulum stress links obesity, insulin action, and type 2 diabetes. *Science* 306:457–461.

352. Ozcan, U., Yilmaz, E., Ozcan, L. et al. 2006. Chemical chaperones reduce ER stress and restore glucose homeostasis in a mouse model of type 2 diabetes. *Science* 313:1137–1140.

353. Nakatani, Y., Kaneto, H., Kawamori, D. et al. 2005. Involvement of endoplasmic reticulum stress in insulin resistance and diabetes. *J Biol Chem* 280:847–851.

354. Karaskov, E., Scott, C., Zhang, L., Teodoro, T., Ravazzola, M., Volchuk, A. 2006. Chronic palmitate but not oleate exposure induces endoplasmic reticulum stress, which may contribute to INS-1 pancreatic β-cell apoptosis. *Endocrinology* 147:3398–3407.

355. Haynes, C.M., Titus, E.A., Cooper, A.A. 2004. Degradation of misfolded proteins prevents ER-derived oxidative stress and cell death. *Mol Cell* 15:767–776.

356. Obici, S., Feng, Z., Arduini, A., Conti, R., Rossetti, L. 2003. Inhibition of hypothalamic carnitine palmitoyltransferase-1 decreases food intake and glucose production. *Nat Med* 9:756–761.

357. Pocai, A., Lam, T.K., Obici, S. et al. 2006. Restoration of hypothalamic lipid sensing normalizes energy and glucose homeostasis in overfed rats. *J Clin Invest* 116:1081–1091.

358. Seeley, R.J., Woods, S.C. 2003. Monitoring of stored and available fuel by the CNS: Implications for obesity. *Nat Rev Neurosci* 4:901–909.

359. Pocai, A., Morgan, K., Buettner, C., Gutierrez-Juarez, R., Obici, S., Rossetti, L. 2005. Central leptin acutely reverses diet-induced hepatic insulin resistance. *Diabetes* 54:3182–3189.

360. Asilmaz, E., Cohen, P., Miyazaki, M. et al. 2004. Site and mechanism of leptin action in a rodent form of congenital lipodystrophy. *J Clin Invest* 113:414–424.

361. Obici, S., Zhang, B.B., Karkanias, G., Rossetti, L. 2002. Hypothalamic insulin signaling is required for inhibition of glucose production. *Nat Med* 8:1376–1382.

362. Okamoto, H., Nakae, J., Kitamura, T., Park, B.C., Dragatsis, I., Occili, D. 2004. Transgenic rescue of insulin receptor-deficient mice. *J Clin Invest* 114:214–223.

363. Buettner, C., Patel, R., Muse, E.D. et al. 2005. Severe impairment in liver insulin signaling fails to alter hepatic insulin action in conscious mice. *J Clin Invest* 115:1306–1313.

364. Obici, S., Feng, Z., Morgan, K., Stein, D., Karkanias, G., Rossetti, L. 2002. Central administration of oleic acid inhibits glucose production and food intake. *Diabetes* 51:271–275.

365. Pocai, A., Obici, S., Schwartz, G.J., Rossetti, L. 2005. A brain–liver circuit regulates glucose homeostasis. *Cell Metab* 1:53–61.

366. Turek, F.W., Joshu, C., Kohsaka, A. et al. 2005. Obesity and metabolic syndrome in circadian Clock mutant mice. *Science* 308:1043–1045.

367. Suwazono, Y., Sakata, K., Okubo, Y. et al. 2006. Long-term longitudinal study on the relationship between alternating shift work and the onset of diabetes mellitus in male Japanese workers. *J Occup Environ Med* 48:455–461.

368. Wild, S., Roglic, G., Green, A., Sicree, R., King, H. 2004. Global prevalence of diabetes: Estimates for the year 2000 and projections for 2030. *Diabetes Care* 27(5):1047–1053.
369. Australian Institute of Health and Welfare. 2008. Diabetes: Australian facts. In: *Diabetes Series No. 8. Cat. No. CVD 40*. Canberra, Australia: AIHW.
370. American Diabetes Association. 2008. Economic costs of diabetes in the U.S. in 2007. *Diabetes Care* 31(3):596–615.
371. Laaksonen, D.E., Lindstrom, J., Lakka, T.A. et al. 2005. Physical activity in the prevention of type 2 diabetes: The Finnish Diabetes Prevention Study. *Diabetes* 54(1):158–165.
372. Lindstrom, J., Peltonen, M., Tuomilehto, J., Lindstrom, J., Peltonen, M., Tuomilehto, J. 2005. Lifestyle strategies for weight control: Experience from the Finnish Diabetes Prevention Study. *Proc Nutr Soc* 64(1):81–88.
373. Chakravarthy, M.V., Booth, F.W. 2004. Eating, exercise, and 'thrifty' genotypes: Connecting the dots towards an evolutionary understanding of modern diseases. *J Appl Physiol* 96(1):3–10.
374. Hansen, D., Dendale, P., van Loon, L.J.C., Meeusen, R. 2010. The impact of training modalities on the clinical benefits of exercise intervention in patients with cardiovascular disease risk or type 2 diabetes mellitus. *Sports Med* 40(11):921–940.
375. Fletcher, G.F., Balady, G.J., Amsterdam, E.A. et al. 2001. Exercise standards for testing and training: A statement for healthcare professionals from the American Heart Association. *Circulation* 104(14):1694–1740.
376. Tjonna, A.E., Lund Nilsen, T.I., Slordahl, S.A. et al. 2010. The association of metabolic clustering and physical activity with cardiovascular mortality: The HUNT Study in Norway. *J Epidemiol Community Health* 64(8):690–695.
377. Miller, W.C., Koceja, D.M., Hamilton, E.J. 1997. A meta-analysis of the past 25 years of weight loss research using diet, exercise or diet plus exercise intervention. *Int J Obes Relat Metab Disord* 21(10):941–947.
378. Ross, R., Rissanen, J., Pedwell, H. et al. 1996. Influence of diet and exercise on skeletal muscle and visceral adipose tissue in men. *J Appl Physiol* 81(6):2445–2455.
379. Peiris, A.N., Sothmann, M.S., Hoffmann, R.G. et al. 1989. Adiposity, fat distribution, and cardiovascular risk. *Ann Intern Med* 110(11):867–872.
380. Kempen, K.P., Saris, W.H., Westerterp, K.R. 1995. Energy balance during an 8-wk energy-restricted diet with and without exercise in obese women. *Am J Clin Nutr* 62(4):722–729.
381. Wadden, T.A., Vogt, R.A., Andersen, R.E. et al. 1997. Exercise in the treatment of obesity: Effects of four interventions on body composition, resting energy expenditure, appetite, and mood. *J Consult Clin Psychol* 65(2):269–277.
382. Lumini, J.A., Magalhaes, J., Oliveira, P.J., Ascensao, A. 2008. Beneficial effects of exercise on muscle mitochondrial function in diabetes mellitus. *Sports Med* 38(9):735–750.
383. Ballor, D.L., Poehlman, E.T. 1994. Exercise-training enhances fat free mass preservation during diet-induced weight loss: A meta-analytical finding. *Int J Obes* 18(1):35–40.
384. Roussel, M., Garnier, S., Lemoine, S. et al. 2009. Influence of a walking program on the metabolic risk profile of obese postmenopausal women. *Menopause* 16(3):56–75.
385. Yassine, H.N., Marchetti, C.M., Krishnan, R.K. et al. 2009. Effects of exercise and caloric restriction on insulin resistance and cardiometabolic risk factors in older obese adults: A randomized clinical trial. *J Geront A Biol Sci Med Sci* 64(1):90–95.
386. Green, J.S., Stanforth, P.R., Rankinen, T. et al. 2004. The effects of exercise training on abdominal visceral fat, body composition, and indicators of the metabolic syndrome in postmenopausal women with and without estrogen replacement therapy: The HERITAGE Family Study. *Metabolism* 53(9):1192–1196.
387. Dumortier, M., Brandou, F., Perez-Martin, A. et al. 2003. Low intensity endurance exercise targeted for lipid oxidation improves body composition and insulin sensitivity in patients with the metabolic syndrome. *Diabetes Metab* 29(5):509–518.

388. Watkins, L.L., Sherwood, A., Feinglos, M. et al. 2003. Effects of exercise and weight loss on cardiac risk factors associated with syndrome X. *Arch Intern Med* 163(16):1889–1895.

389. Aloulou, I., Varlet-Marie, E., Mercier, J. et al. 2006. Hemorheologic effects of low intensity endurance training in sedentary patients suffering from the metabolic syndrome. *Clin Hemorheol Microcirc* 35(1–2):333–339.

390. Tjønna, A.E., Lee, S.J., Rognmo, Ø. et al. 2008. Aerobic interval training versus continuous moderate exercise as a treatment for the metabolic syndrome. *Circulation* 118(4):346–354.

391. De Feyter, H.M., Praet, S.F., van den Broek, N.M. et al. 2007. Exercise training improves glycemic control in long-standing insulin-treated type 2 diabetic patients. *Diabetes Care* 30(10):2511–2513.

392. Snowling, N.J., Hopkins, W.G. 2006. Effects of different modes of exercise training on glucose control and risk factors for complications in type 2 diabetic patients. *Diabetes Care* 29(11):2518–2527.

393. UK Prospective Diabetes Study Group. 1998. Intensive blood glucose control with sulphonylureas or insulin compared with conventional treatment and risks of complications in patients with type 2 diabetes (UKPDS 33). *Lancet* 352(9131):837–853.

394. Khaw, K., Wareham, N., Luben, R. et al. 2001. Glycated haemoglobin, diabetes and mortality in men in Norfolk cohort of European Prospective Investigation of Cancer and Nutrition (EPIC-Norfolk). *Br Med J* 322(7277):15–18.

395. Boule, N.G., Kenny, G.P., Haddad, E. et al. 2003. Meta-analysis of the effect of structured exercise training on cardiorespiratory fitness in type 2 diabetes mellitus. *Diabetologia* 46(8):1071–1081.

396. Sigal, R.J., Kenny, G.P., Boule, N.G. et al. 2007. Effects of aerobic training, resistance training, or both on glycemic control in type 2 diabetes. *Ann Intern Med* 147(6):357–369.

397. Praet, S.F., van Rooij, E.S.J., Wijtvliet, A. et al. 2008. Brisk walking compared with an individual medical fitness programme for patients with type 2 diabetes: A randomised controlled trial. *Diabetologia* 51(5):736–746.

398. Dela, F., von Linstow, M.E., Mikines, K.J. et al. 2004. Physical training may enhance b-cell function in type 2 diabetes. *Am J Physiol Endocrinol Metab* 287(5):E1024–E1031.

399. Toledo, G.S., Menshikova, E.V., Ritov, V.B. et al. 2007. Effects of physical activity and weight loss on skeletal muscle mitochondria and relationship with glucose control in type 2 diabetes. *Diabetes* 56(8):2142–2147.

400. Fritz, T., Kramer, D.K., Karlsson, H.K.R. et al. 2006. Low-intensity exercise increases skeletal muscle protein expression of PPARd and UCP3 in type 2 diabetic patients. *Diabetes Metab Res Rev* 22(6):492–498.

401. Tessier, D., Menard, J., Fulop, T. et al. 2000. Effects of aerobic physical exercise in the elderly with type 2 diabetes mellitus. *Arch Geron Geriatr* 31(2):121–132.

402. Giannopoulou, I., Fernhall, B., Carhart, R. et al. 2005. Effects of diet and/or exercise on the adipocytokines and inflammatory cytokine levels of postmenopausal women with type 2 diabetes. *Metabolism* 54(7):866–875.

403. Giannopoulou, I., Ploutz-Snyder, L.L., Carhart, R. et al. 2005. Exercise is required for visceral fat loss in postmenopausal women with type 2 diabetes. *J Clin Endocrinol Metab* 90(3):1511–1518.

404. Lan, C., Chen, S.Y., Chiu, S.F. et al. 2003. Poor functional recovery may indicate restenosis in patients after coronary angioplasty. *Arch Phys Med Rehabil* 84(7):1023–1027.

405. Tokmakidis, S.P., Zois, C.E., Volaklis, K.A. et al. 2004. The effects of a combined strength and aerobic exercise program on glucose control and insulin action in women with type 2 diabetes. *Eur J Appl Physiol* 92(4–5):437–442.

406. Hamm, L.F., Kavanagh, T., Campbell, R.B. 2004. Timeline for peak improvements during 52 weeks of outpatient cardiac rehabilitation. *J Cardiopulm Rehabil* 24(4):374–382.

407. Jeffery, R.W., Wing, R.R., Sherwood, N.E. et al. 2003. Physical activity and weight loss: Does prescribing higher physical activity goals improve outcome? *Am J Clin Nutr* 78(4):684–689.

408. Gielen, S., Schuler, G., Hambrecht, R. 2001. Exercise training in coronary artery disease and coronary vasomotion. *Circulation* 103(1):E1–E6.

409. Donnelly, J.E., Jacobsen, D.J., Jakicic, J.M. et al. 1994. Very low calorie diet with concurrent versus delayed and sequential exercise. *Int J Obes* 18(7):469–475.

410. Marks, B.L., Ward, A., Morris, D.H. et al. 1995. Fat-free mass is maintained in women following a moderate diet and exercise program. *Med Sci Sports Exerc* 27(9):1243–1251.

411. Sweeney, M.E., Hill, J.O., Heller, P.A. et al. 1993. Severe vs moderate energy restriction with and without exercise in the treatment of obesity: Efficiency of weight loss. *Am J Clin Nutr* 57(2):127–134.

412. Bryner, R.W., Ullrich, I.H., Sauers, J. et al. 1999. Effects of resistance vs. aerobic training combined with an 800 calorie liquid diet on lean body mass and resting metabolic rate. *J Am Coll Clin Nutr* 18(2):115–121.

413. Cuff, D.J., Meneilly, G.S., Martin, A. et al. 2003. Effective exercise modality to reduce insulin resistance in women with type 2 diabetes. *Diabetes Care* 26(11):2977–2982.

414. Dunstan, D.W., Daly, R.M., Owen, N. et al. 2002. High-intensity resistance training improves glycemic control in older patients with type 2 diabetes. *DiabetesCare* 25(10):1729–1736.

415. Eriksson, J., Taimela, S., Eriksson, K. et al. 1997. Resistance training in the treatment of non-insulin-dependent diabetes. *Int J Sports Med* 18(4):242–246.

416. Delagardelle, C., Feiereisen, P., Autier, P. et al. 2002. Strength/endurance training versus endurance training in congestive heart failure. *Med Sci Sports Exerc* 34(12):1868–1872.

417. Gayda, M., Choquet, D., Ahmaida, S. 2009. Effects of exercise training modality on skeletal muscle fatigue in men with coronary heart disease. *J Electromyogr Kinesiol* 19(2):e32–e39.

418. Marzolini, S., Oh, P.I., Thomas, S.G. et al. 2008. Aerobic and resistance training in coronary disease: Single versus multiple sets. *Med Sci Sports Exerc* 40(9):1557–1564.

419. Strasser, B., Siebert, U., Schobersberger, W. 2010. Resistance training in the treatment of the metabolic syndrome: A systematic review and meta-analysis of the effect of resistance training on metabolic clustering in patients with abnormal glucose metabolism. *Sports Med* 40(5):397–415.

420. Hills, A.P., Shultz, S.P., Soares, M.J. et al. 2010. Resistance training for obese, type 2 diabetic adults: A review of the evidence. *Obes Rev* 11:740–749.

421. Chudyk, A., Petrella, R.J. 2011. Effects of exercise on cardiovascular risk factors in type 2 diabetes: A meta analysis. *Diabetes Care* 34:1228–1237.

422. Friedlander, A.L., Jacobs, K.A., Fattor, J.A. et al. 2007. Contributions of working muscle to whole body lipid metabolism are altered by exercise training and intensity. *Am J Physiol* 292(4):E107–E112.

423. Ballor, D.L., McCarthy, J.P., Wilterdink, E.J. 1990. Exercise intensity does not affect the composition of diet- and exercise-induced body mass loss. *Am J Clin Nutr* 51(2):142–146.

424. Leutholtz, B.C., Keyser, R.E., Heusner, W.W. et al. 1995. Exercise training and severe caloric restriction: Effect on lean body mass in the obese. *Arch Phys Med Rehabil* 76(1):65–70.

425. van Aggel-Leijssen, D., Saris, W.H.M., Wagenmakers, A.J.M. et al. 2002. Effect of exercise training at different intensities on fat metabolism of obese men. *J Appl Physiol* 92(3):1300–1309.

426. Irving, B.A., Davis, C.K., Brock, D.W. et al. 2008. Effect of exercise training intensity on abdominal visceral fat and body composition. *Med Sci Sports Exerc* 40(11):1863–1872.

427. Hansen, D., Dendale, P., Jonkers, R.A. et al. 2009. Continuous low-to-moderate intensity exercise is equally effective as moderate-to-high intensity exercise training at lowering blood HbA1c content in obese type 2 diabetes patients. *Diabetologia* 52(9):1789–1797.

428. Kang, J., Kelley, D.E., Robertson, R.J. et al. 1999. Substrate utilization and glucose turnover during exercise of varying intensities in individuals with NIDDM. *Med Sci Sports Exerc* 31(1):82–89.

429. Johnson, J.L., Slentz, C.A., Houmard, J.A. et al. 2007. Exercise training amount and intensity effects on metabolic syndrome. *Am J Cardiol* 100(12):1759–1766.

430. Perri, M.G., Anton, S.D., Durning, P.E. et al. 2002. Adherence to exercise prescriptions: Effects of prescribing moderate versus higher levels of intensity and frequency. *Health Psychol* 21(5):452–458.

431. Adachi, H., Koike, A., Obayashi, T. et al. 1996. Does appropriate endurance exercise training improve cardiac function in patients with prior myocardial infarction? *Eur Heart J* 17(10):1511–1521.

432. Jensen, B.E., Fletcher, B.J., Rupp, J.C. et al. 1996. Training level comparison study: Effect of high and low intensity training on ventilatory threshold in men with coronary artery disease. *J Cardiopulm Rehabil* 16(4):227–232.

433. Schjerve, I.E., Tyldum, G.A., Tjonna, A.E. et al. 2008. Both aerobic endurance and strength training programmes improve cardiovascular health in obese adults. *Clin Sci* 115(9):283–293.

434. Warburton, D.E., McKenzie, D.C., Haykowski, M.J. et al. 2005. Effectiveness of high-intensity interval training for the rehabilitation of patients with coronary artery disease. *Am J Cardiol* 95(9):1080–1084.

435. Amundsen, B.H., Rognmo, O., Hatlen-Rebhan, G. et al. 2008. High intensity aerobic exercise improves diastolic function in coronary artery disease. *Scand Cardiovasc J* 42(2):110–117.

436. Wisloff, U., Stoylen, A., Loennechen, J.P. et al. 2007. Superior cardiovascular effect of aerobic interval training versus moderate continuous training in heart failure patients: A randomized study. *Circulation* 115(24):3086–3094.

437. Sriwijitkamol, A., Coletta, D.K., Wajcberg, E. et al. 2007. Effect of acute exercise on AMPK signalling in skeletal muscle of subjects with type 2 diabetes. *Diabetes* 56(3):836–848.

438. Hansen, D., Dendale, P., Berger, J. et al. 2008. Importance of training session duration in the rehabilitation of coronary artery disease patients. *Eur J Cardiovasc Prev Rehabil* 15(4):453–459.

439. Whatley, J.E., Gillespie, W.J., Honig, J. et al. 1994. Does the amount of endurance exercise in combination with weight training and a very-low-energy diet affect resting metabolic rate and body composition? *Am J Clin Nutr* 59(5):1088–1092.

440. Dressendorfer, R.H., Franklin, B.A., Cameron, J.L. et al. 1995. Exercise training frequency in early post-infarction cardiac rehabilitation: Influence on aerobic conditioning. *J Cardiopulm Rehabil* 15(4):269–276.

441. Tygesen, H., Wettervik, C., Wennerblom, B. 2001. Intensive home based exercise training in cardiac rehabilitation increases exercise capacity and heart rate variability. *Int J Cardiol* 79(2–3):175–182.

442. Nieuwland, W., Berkhuysen, M.A., van Veldhuizen, D.J. et al. 2000. Differential effects of high-frequency versus low-frequency exercise training in rehabilitation of patients with coronary artery disease. *J Am Coll Cardiol* 36(1):202–207.

443. Henriksen, E.J. 2002. Exercise effects of muscle insulin signaling and action: Effects of acute exercise and exercise training on insulin resistance. *J Appl Physiol* 93(2):788–796.

444. Bassuk, S.S., Manson, J.E. 2005. Epidemiological evidence for the role of physical activity in reducing risk of type 2 diabetes and cardiovascular disease. *J Appl Physiol* 99:1193–1204.

445. Walker, K.Z., O'Dea, K., Gomez, M., Girgis, S., Colagiuri, R. 2010. Diet and exercise in the prevention of diabetes. *J Hum Nutr Diet* 23:344–352.

446. American Diabetes Association. Nutrition recommendations and interventions for diabetes. 2008. A position statement of the American Diabetes Association. *Diabetes Care* 31(Suppl. 1):S61–S78.

447. Franz, M.Z., Powers, M.A., Leontos, C. et al. 2010. The evidence for medical nutrition therapy for type 1 and type 2 diabetes in adults. *J Am Diet Assoc* 110:1852–1889.

448. Wing, R.R., Koeske, R., Epstein, L.H., Nowalk, M.P., Gooding, W., Becker, D. 1987. Long-term effects of modest weight-loss in type II diabetic patients. *Arch Intern Med* 147:1749–1753.

449. Mertz, J.A., Stern, J.S., Kris-Etherton, P. et al. 2000. A randomized trial of improved weight loss with a prepared meal plan in overweight and obese patients: Impact on cardiovascular risk reduction. *Arch Intern Med* 160:2150–2158.

450. Hanefeld, M., Sachse, G. 2002. The effects of orlistat on body weight and glycaemic control in overweight patients with type 2 diabetes: A randomized, placebo-controlled trial. *Diabetes Obes Metab* 4:415–423.

451. Kelley, D.E., Bray, G.A., Pi-Sunyer, F.X. et al. 2002. Clinical efficacy of orlistat therapy in overweight and obese patients with insulin-treated type 2 diabetes: A 1-year randomized controlled trial. *Diabetes Care* 25:1033–1041.

452. Miles, J.M., Leiter, L., Hollander, P. et al. 2002. Effect of orlistat in overweight and obese patients with type 2 diabetes treated with metformin. *Diabetes Care* 25:1123–1128.

453. Berne, C., for the Orlistat Swedish Type 2 Diabetes Study Group. 2005. A randomized study of orlistat in combination with a weight management programme in obese patients with type 2 diabetes treated with metformin. *Diabet Med* 22:612–618.

454. Paisey, R.B., Frost, J., Harvery, P. et al. 2002. Five-year results of a prospective very-low calorie diet or conventional weight loss programme in type 2 diabetes. *J Hum Nutr Diet* 15:121–127.

455. Dhindsa, P., Scott, A.R., Donnelly, R. 2003. Metabolic and cardiovascular effects of very-low-calorie diet therapy in obese patients with type 2 diabetes in secondary failure: Outcomes after 1 year. *Diabet Med* 20:319–324.

456. Derosa, G., Cicero, A.F., Murdolo, G., Ciccarelli, L., Fogari, R. 2004. Comparison of metabolic effects of orlistat and sibutramine treatment in type 2 diabetic obese patients. *Diabetes Nutr Metab* 17:222–229.

457. Sanchez-Reyes, L., Fanghanel, G., Yamamoto, J., Martinez-Rivas, L., Campos-Franco, E., Berber, A. 2004. Use of sibutramine in overweight adult Hispanic patients with type 2 diabetes mellitus: A 12-month, randomized, double-blind placebo-controlled clinical trial. *Clin Ther* 26:1427–1435.

458. Redmon, J.B., Reck, K.P., Raatz, S.K. et al. 2005. Two-year outcomes of a combination of weight loss therapies for type 2 diabetes. *Diabetes Care* 28:1311–1315.

459. The Look AHEAD Research Group. 2007. Reduction in weight and cardiovascular disease risk factors in individuals with type 2 diabetes: One-year results of the Look AHEAD trial. *Diabetes Care* 30:1374–1383.

460. Brehm, B.J., Lattin, B.L., Summer, S.S. et al. 2009. One-year comparison of a high-monounsaturated fat diet with a high-carbohydrate diet in type 2 diabetes. *Diabetes Care* 32:215–220.

461. Davis, N.J., Tomuta, N., Schechter, C. et al. 2009. Comparative study of the effects of a 1-year dietary intervention of a low-carbohydrate diet versus a low-fat diet on weight and glycemic control in type 2 diabetes. *Diabetes Care* 32:1147–1152.

462. Nielsen, J.V., Joensson, E.A. 2008. Low-carbohydrate diet in type 2 diabetes: Stable improvement of bodyweight and glycemic control during 44 months follow-up. *Nutr Metab (Lond)* 5:14–19.

463. Cheskin, L.J., Mitchell, A.M., Jhaveri, A.M. et al. 2008. Efficacy of a meal replacement versus a standard food-based diet for weight loss in type 2 diabetes. *Diabetes Educ* 3:118–127.

464. Reeds, D.N. 2009. Nutrition support in the obese, diabetic patient: The role of hypocaloric feeding. *Curr Opin Gastroenterol* 25:151–154.

465. Boden, G., Sargrad, K., Homko, C., Mozzoli, M., Stein, T.P. 2005. Effect of a low-carbohydrate diet on appetite, blood glucose levels, and insulin resistance in obese patients with type 2 diabetes. *Ann Intern Med* 142:403–411.

466. DAFNE Study Group. 2202. Training in flexible, intensive insulin management to enable dietary freedom in people with type 1 diabetes: Dose adjustment for normal eating (DAFNE) randomized controlled trial. *Br Med J* 325:746–751.

467. Lowe, J., Linjawi, S., Mensch, M., James, K., Attia, J. 2008. Flexible eating and flexible insulin dosing in patients with diabetes: Results of an intensive self-management course. *Diabetes Res Clin Pract* 80:439–443.

468. Bergenstal, R.M., Johnson, M., Powers, M.A. et al. 2008. Adjust to target in type 2 diabetes: Comparison of a simple algorithm with carbohydrate counting for adjustment of mealtime insulin glulisine. *Diabetes Care* 31:1305–1310.

469. Nielsen, J.V., Jonsson, E., Nilsson, A.K. 2005. Lasting improvement of hyperglycemia and body weight: Low-carbohydrate diet in type 2 diabetes: A brief report. *Upsala J Med Sci* 109:179–184.

470. Komiyama, N., Kaneko, T., Sato, A. et al. 2002. The effect of high carbohydrate diet on glucose tolerance in patients with type 2 diabetes mellitus. *Diabetes Res Clin Pract* 57:163–170.

471. Barnard, N.D., Gloede, L., Cohen, J. et al. 2009. A low-fat vegan diet elicits greater macronutrient changes, but is comparable in adherence and acceptability, compared with a more conventional diabetes diet among individuals with type 2 diabetes. *J Am Diet Assoc* 109:263–272.

472. Kirk, J.K., Graves, D.E., Craven, T.E., Lipkin, E.W., Austin, M., Margolis, K.L. 2008. Restricted-carbohydrate diet in patients with type 2 diabetes: A meta-analysis. *J Am Diet Assoc* 108:91–100.

473. Kodama, S., Saito, K., Tanaka, S. et al. 2009. Influence of fat and carbohydrate proportions on the metabolic profile in patients with type 2 diabetes: A meta-analysis. *Diabetes Care* 32:959–965.

474. Chandalia, M., Garg, A., Lutjohann, D., von Bergmann, K., Grundy, S.M., Brinkley, L.J. 2000. Beneficial effects of high dietary fiber intake in patients with type 2 diabetes mellitus. *N Engl J Med* 342:1392–1398.

475. Giacco, R., Parillo, M., Rivellese, A.A. et al. 2000. Long-term dietary treatment with increased amounts of fiber-rich low-glycemic index natural foods improves blood glucose control and reduces the number of hypoglycemic events in type 1 diabetic patients. *Diabetes Care* 23:1461–1466.

476. Van Horn, L., McCoin, M., Kris-Etherton, P.M. et al. 2008. The evidence for dietary prevention and treatment of cardiovascular disease. *J Am Diet Assoc* 108:287–331.

477. Parker, B., Noakes, M., Luscombe, N., Clifton, P. 2002. Effect of a high-protein diet, high-monounsaturated fat weight loss diet on glycemic control and lipid levels in type 2 diabetes. *Diabetes Care* 25:425–430.

478. Luscombe, N.D., Clifton, P.M., Noakes, M., Parker, B., Wittert, G. 2002. Effects of energy-restricted diets containing increased protein on weight loss, resting energy expenditure, and thermic effect of feeding in type 2 diabetes. *Diabetes Care* 25:652–657.

479. Nuttall, F.Q., Gannon, M.C., Saeed, A., Jordan, K., Hoover, H. 2003. The metabolic response of subjects with type 2 diabetes to a high-protein, weight-maintenance diet. *J Clin Endocrinol Metab* 88:3577–3583.

480. Gannon, M.C., Nuttall, F.Q., Saeed, A., Jordan, K., Hoover, H. 2003. An increase in dietary protein improves the blood glucose response in persons with type 2 diabetes. *Am J Clin Nutr* 78:734–741.

481. Nordt, T.K., Besenthal, I., Eggstein, M., Jakober, B. 1991. Influence of breakfasts with different nutrient contents on glucose, C peptide, insulin, glucagon, triglycerides, and GIP in non-insulin-dependent diabetes. *Am J Clin Nutr* 53:155–160.

482. Gannon, M.C., Nuttall, J.A., Damberg, G., Gupta, V., Nuttall, F.Q. 2001. Effect of protein ingestion on the glucose appearance rate in people with type 2 diabetes. *J Clin Endocrinol Metab* 86:1040–1047.

483. Almeida, J.C., Zelmanovitz, T., Vaz, J.S. et al. 2008. Sources of protein and polyunsaturated fatty acids of the diet and microalbuminuria in type 2 diabetes mellitus. *J Am Coll Nutr* 27:528–537.

484. Pa, Y., Guo, L.L., Jin, H.M. 2008. Low-protein diet for diabetic nephropathy: A meta-analysis of randomized controlled trials. *Am J Clin Nutr* 88:660–666.

485. Hu, F.B., van Dam, R.M., Liu, S. 2001. Diet and risk of type II diabetes: The role of types of fat and carbohydrate. *Diabetologia* 44:807–817.

486. Stanhope, K.L., Schwarz, J.M., Keim, N.L. et al. 2009. Consuming fructose-sweetened, not glucose-sweetened, beverages increases visceral adiposity and lipids and decreases insulin sensitivity in overweight/obese humans. *J Clin Invest* 119:1322–1334.

487. Madsen, E.L., Rissanen, A., Bruun, J.M. et al. 2008. Weight loss larger than 10% is needed for general improvement of levels of circulating adiponectin and markers of inflammation in obese subjects: A 3-year weight loss study. *Eur J Endocrinol* 158:179–187.

488. Christiansen, T., Paulsen, S.K., Bruun, J.M., Ploug, T., Pedersen, S.B., Richelsen, B. 2010. Diet-induced weight loss and exercise alone and in combination enhance the expression of adiponectin receptors in adipose tissue and skeletal muscle, but only diet-induced weight loss enhanced circulating adiponectin. *J Clin Endocrinol Metab* 95:911–919.

489. Rucker, D., Padwal, R., Li, S.K., Curioni, C., Lau, D.C. 2007. Long term pharmacotherapy for obesity and overweight: Updated meta-analysis. *BMJ* 335:1194–1199.

490. Valsamakis, G., McTernan, P.G., Chetty, R. et al. 2004. Modest weight loss and reduction in waist circumference after medical treatment are associated with favorable changes in serum adipocytokines. *Metabolism* 53:430–434.

491. Torgerson, J.S., Hauptman, J., Boldrin, M.N., Sjostrom, L. 2004. XENical in the prevention of diabetes in obese subjects (XENDOS) study: A randomized study of orlistat as an adjunct to lifestyle changes for the prevention of type 2 diabetes in obese patients. *Diabetes Care* 27:155–161.

492. Hsieh, C.J., Wang, P.W., Liu, R.T. et al. 2005. Orlistat for obesity: Benefits beyond weight loss. *Diabetes Res Clin Pract* 67:78–83.

493. Jung, S.H., Park, H.S., Kim, K.S. et al. 2008. Effect of weight loss on some serum cytokines in human obesity: Increase in IL-10 after weight loss. *J Nutr Biochem* 6:371–375.

494. Ramis, J.M., Salinas, R., Garcia-Sanz, J.M., Moreiro, J., Proenza, A.M., Llado, I. 2006. Depot and gender-related differences in the lipolytic pathway of adipose tissue from severely obese patients. *Cell Physiol Biochem* 17:173–180.

495. James, W.P., Caterson, I.D., Coutinho, W. et al. 2010. Effect of sibutramine on cardiovascular outcomes in overweight and obese subjects. *N Engl J Med* 363:905–917.

496. Demuth, D.G., Molleman, A. 2006. Cannabinoid signalling. *Life Sci* 78:549–563.

497. Howlett, A.C., Barth, F., Bonner, T.I. et al. 2002. International Union of Pharmacology. XXVII. Classification of cannabinoid receptors. *Pharmacol Rev* 54:161–202.

498. Izzo, A.A., Camilleri, M. 2008. Emerging role of cannabinoids in gastrointestinal and liver diseases: Basic and clinical aspects. *Gut* 57:1140–1155.

499. Scheen, A.J., Finer, N., Hollander, P., Jensen, M.D., Van Gaal, L.F. 2006. Efficacy and tolerability of rimonabant in overweight or obese patients with type 2 diabetes: A randomised controlled study. *Lancet* 368:1660–1672.

500. Despres, J.P., Golay, A., Sjostrom, L. 2005. Effects of rimonabant on metabolic risk factors in overweight patients with dyslipidemia. *N Engl J Med* 353:2121–2134.

501. Foster-Schubert, K., Cummings, D. 2006. Emerging therapeutic strategies for obesity. *Endocrinol Rev* 27:779–793.

502. Sjostrom, L., Narbro, K., Sjostrom, C.D. et al. 2007. Effects of bariatric surgery on mortality in Swedish obese subjects. *N Engl J Med* 357:741–752.

503. Adams, T.D., Gress, R.E., Smith, S.C. et al. 2007. Long-term mortality after gastric bypass surgery. *N Engl J Med* 357:753–761.

504. Dixon, J.B., O'Brien, P.E., Playfair, J. et al. 2008. Adjustable gastric banding and conventional therapy for type 2 diabetes: A randomized controlled trial. *JAMA* 299:316–323.

505. Westerink, J., Visseren, F.L.J. 2011. Pharmacological and non-pharmacological interventions to influence adipose tissue function. *Cardiovasc Diabetol* 10:13.

506. Diker, D., Vishne, T., Maayan, R. et al. 2006. Impact of gastric banding on plasma adiponectin levels. *Obes Surg* 16:1057–1061.

507. Gomez-Ambrosi, J., Salvador, J., Rotellar, F. et al. 2006. Increased serum amyloid A concentrations in morbid obesity decrease after gastric bypass. *Obes Surg* 16:262–269.

508. Haider, D.G., Schindler, K., Schaller, G., Prager, G., Wolzt, M., Ludvik, B. 2006. Increased plasma visfatin concentrations in morbidly obese subjects are reduced after gastric banding. *J Clin Endocrinol Metab* 91:1578–1581.

509. Haider, D.G., Schindler, K., Prager, G. et al. 2007. Serum retinol-binding protein 4 is reduced after weight loss in morbidly obese subjects. *J Clin Endocrinol Metab* 92:1168–1171.

510. Schernthaner, G.H., Kopp, H.P., Kriwanek, S. et al. 2006. Effect of massive weight loss induced by bariatric surgery on serum levels of interleukin-18 and monocytechemoattractant-protein-1 in morbid obesity. *Obes Surg* 16:709–715.

511. van Dielen, F.M., Buurman, W.A., Hadfoune, M., Nijhuis, J., Greve, J.W. 2004. Macrophage inhibitory factor, plasminogen activator inhibitor-1, other acute phase proteins, and inflammatory mediators normalize as a result of weight loss in morbidly obese subjects treated with gastric restrictive surgery. *J Clin Endocrinol Metab* 89:4062–4068.

14 Obesity and the Metabolic Syndrome

Peter W. Grandjean, PhD, FACSM

CONTENTS

ORIGINS OF THE METABOLIC SYNDROME

The physiological construct that is most widely known today as metabolic syndrome (MetS) was born in clinical practice almost a century ago when a Swedish physician recognized that hypertension, hyperglycemia, and gout commonly occurred together.[1] Several years later, a French physician named Jean Vague recorded the keen observation that cardiovascular and metabolic dysfunctions were associated with an accumulation of upper body fat.[2,3] Dr. Vague is credited with introducing the terms android and gynoid phenotypes to describe upper and lower body fat distribution and to document the greater health risk that appeared with the android pattern. The relationships between obesity, android adiposity, and the presence of hyper-insulinemia, hypertension, and elevated triglycerides gained greater recognition with the modernization of assays to reliably measure insulin, lipids, and other blood constituents.[4–7] Prospective clinical studies, conducted just as obesity rates began to climb in the 1980s, confirmed the greater health risks of abdominal fat that were first observed by Vague. The waist circumference measurement was recognized to be a strong correlate of abdominal fat, and the waist-to-hip ratio was introduced as a surrogate marker of body fat phenotypes.[8–14] Evidence to support the theory that insulin resistance[15,16] and hyperinsulinemia[17,18] were metabolic conditions linking obesity, hypertension, and type 2 diabetes was accumulating.

The "tipping point" for scientific and medical recognition of a syndrome came in 1988 when Dr. Gerald Reaven introduced the term "Syndrome X" to describe the contemporary theory that insulin resistance and compensatory hyperinsulinemia— not necessarily excess adiposity—were the pathological conditions underlying the development of dyslipidemia, hypertension, and heightened cardiovascular disease (CVD) risk. The fact that insulin resistance and the associated comorbidities were observed in lean individuals and not necessarily confined to the obese was central to his concept.[19] Others were hesitant to dismiss the impact of adiposity and cautioned that these CVD risk factors occur together and much more frequently in overweight and obese individuals versus those of normal weight.[20] The rising prevalence of MetS among U.S. adults and children concomitant with the surge in obesity rates over the last three decades strongly suggested that obesity contributes to the clustering of CVD risk factors.[21–25] Moreover, sophisticated techniques for studying fat distribution and the discovery that adipose tissue produces and secretes a number of inter-related bioactive peptides with endocrine, paracrine, and autocrine functions have validated the strong involvement of visceral and ectopic fat in insulin resistance and its multiple clinical manifestations.[26,27] Thus, the scientific and medical communities acknowledged a common clustering of cardiovascular and metabolic risk factors that appear to be intricately related to excess adiposity. As a result, the biological concept most commonly referred to as MetS was established.

MetS is known today by a variety of terms: syndrome X,[19] insulin resistance syndrome,[28] the deadly quartet,[29] the hypertriglyceridemic waist phenotype,[14] cardiometabolic syndrome,[30] and dysmetabolic syndrome.[31] No matter what it is called, it is generally agreed that the clinical characteristics of MetS are a waist circumference reflective of excess abdominal obesity, impaired fasting glucose (IFG), elevated triglyceride concentrations, low high-density lipoprotein (HDL)-cholesterol, and high blood pressure.[32,33] In some cases, microalbuminuria is included among the defining characteristics.[34,35] Recent scientific advances describe more subtle characteristics of dyslipidemia, such as lipoprotein particle sizes and densities, and the contributions of chronic inflammation, oxidative stress, and prothrombotic conditions as part of the syndrome.[36–38]

The various names and definitions that have been proposed for MetS are reflective of the ongoing debate regarding its underlying causes. Indeed, there is little agreement from the empirically based discussions regarding the syndrome's physiological origins, and the primary components are extremely hard to quantify (i.e., insulin resistance and adipose tissue dysfunction). Nevertheless, each clinical definition, with its own set of limitations, has essentially been proposed to help physicians and other health-care providers recognize MetS in the clinical setting.[32,34,35,39–42]

Many physicians remain cautious about diagnosing MetS because of the uncertainty that arises from numerous definitions, constant revisions to the definitions, and a variety of ways in which MetS may present in patients. Those who have adopted MetS as a clinical tool advocate for its usefulness in identifying and addressing lifestyle behaviors that appear to promote the aggregation of CVD risk factors. Skeptics contend that any attempt to diagnose MetS does not assist in treating patients and, thus far, has not been demonstrated to improve upon the identification and treatment of separate risk factors for reducing CVD outcomes.[43-45] Both proponents and skeptics acknowledge that MetS is not recommended as a sole means of estimating absolute CVD or diabetes risk since MetS does not include traditional or emerging risk factors that should be part of a thorough medical evaluation (e.g., low-density lipoprotein [LDL]-cholesterol, smoking, family history of CVD, diet and physical activity behaviors, stress, and depression). Controversy even surrounds the International Classification of Disease code (ICD-9) that is used to obtain medical reimbursement for the condition. Indeed, the title for ICD-9 code 277.7, "Dysmetabolic Syndrome X," combines terminologies and generates its own set of reimbursement questions for the practitioner.[46-48]

The objectives of this chapter are not to solve the debate over the clinical usefulness of diagnosing the syndrome. Nor is it to add to the discussion for a unified definition that might ultimately have tremendous potential to aid in the treatment of cardiometabolic dysfunction. Instead, the aim of this chapter is to highlight and describe clinical strategies for identifying, preventing, and managing cardiometabolic dysfunction—otherwise known as MetS. In order to achieve this objective, a current overview of the multiple definitions of MetS, its epidemiology, and its etiology are introduced first. These topics are followed by empirically informed suggestions for managing the components of MetS in medical practice with an emphasis on primary prevention strategies.

ELUSIVE DEFINITION OF METABOLIC SYNDROME

Clinical definitions are important for determining prevalence in a population and within subgroups in a given population. Definitions are also important for determining the effect and severity of the condition on chronic disease risk and outcomes. This information can then be used to establish public policy, identify effective treatment strategies, direct decisions and resources toward primary prevention programs, and ultimately improve clinical diagnosis and management.[33,49]

In 1998—almost 10 years after Syndrome X and the insulin resistance syndrome were introduced—the American Diabetes Association published a consensus statement that recognized central adiposity, glucose intolerance, hypertension, elevated plasma triglyceride and low HDL-cholesterol concentrations, small dense LDL, and a prothrombotic and antifibrinolytic state as physical characteristics associated with insulin resistance.[50] The statement, however, did not include operational definitions or clinical cut points that might be employed in medical management. Instead, the first diagnostic criteria for MetS were established in the same year by the World Health Organization (WHO).[34] Insulin resistance—as determined by euglycemic clamp procedures, IFG, impaired glucose tolerance (IGT), or previously diagnosed type 2 diabetes mellitus (T2DM)—was the WHO's requisite characteristic for diagnosis.[34] Subsequently, the European Group for the Study of Insulin Resistance (EGIR) maintained the premise that insulin resistance was at the heart of MetS; however, they jettisoned the onerous euglycemic clamp procedures and modified the diagnosis of insulin resistance to measures of fasting insulin. Insulin resistance was determined if insulin concentrations were found to be in the top quartile of a background nondiabetic population.[42] The American Academy of Clinical Endocrinologists (AACE), staying with the theory that insulin resistance was the seminal aspect of MetS, again modified the diagnosis of insulin resistance to further aid the clinician. The AACE allowed that it was acceptable to assume insulin resistance if risk factors for insulin resistance were determined from a patient's health history.[41] Risk factors for insulin resistance included any of the following: a body mass index (BMI) of $\geq 25\,kg/m^2$; waist circumference >40″ for men and >35″ for women; sedentary lifestyle; non-Caucasian; a family history of T2DM, hypertension, or CVD; a personal history of polycystic ovarian syndrome and nonalcoholic fatty-liver disease (NAFLD); or the presence of acanthosis nigricans. Once insulin resistance is established with WHO, EGIR, or AACE procedures, any two of the following abnormalities must also be present to fulfill the diagnostic criteria for MetS: obesity or abdominal adiposity, dyslipidemia, elevated blood pressure,[34,41,42] IFG or IGT,[41,42] or microalbuminuria.[34]

The International Diabetes Federation (IDF) established central obesity—rather than insulin resistance—as necessary for MetS diagnosis.[35] The IDF advocated several cut points for waist circumference to verify central obesity because of ethnic and gender variances in health risk at different levels of visceral adiposity. Similar to the other proposals, the IDF required that centrally obese individuals exhibit two additional characteristics for MetS diagnosis: IFG or T2DM, dyslipidemia, elevated blood pressure, or microalbuminuria. The IDF recognized the use of hypoglycemic agents as an alternative diagnosis for IFG. Likewise, the EGIR and IDF recognized the use of antihyperlipidemic drugs as criteria for dyslipidemia, and all four consensus statements include antihypertensive drug treatment as constituting the presence of elevated blood pressure.

In 2001, the National Cholesterol Education Program–Adult Treatment Panel III (NCEP-ATP III) published a new set of criteria for determining MetS.[51] The NCEP-ATP III approach avoided a required diagnosis for both insulin resistance and central obesity. Instead, all of the diagnostic criteria were given equal importance, and MetS could be determined if any three of five abnormalities were observed: large waist circumference, IFG, elevated triglycerides, elevated blood pressure, or low HDL-cholesterol. The NCEP-ATP III cut points were later modified to be consistent with the ADA findings for IFG and to include drug treatment within the definitions for IFG, dyslipidemia, and hypertension.[52,53] Soon after, the American Heart Association and National Heart, Lung, and Blood Institute (AHA/NHLBI) issued diagnostic criteria very similar to the current NCEP guidelines.[32]

Most recently, a Joint Scientific Statement resulted from an attempt to reconcile the different clinical definitions of MetS. Aspects from the IDF, NCEP-ATP III, and AHA/NHLBI procedures were included to harmonize criteria and facilitate the diagnosis of MetS in medical practice.[33] A major emphasis of this international effort was to encourage physicians and health-care providers to direct more attention to obesity and its related comorbidities. See Table 14.1 to compare the different clinical definitions of MetS and the recently proposed harmonized definition.

TABLE 14.1
Comparison of Definitions for MetS

WHO (1998) {Ref. [34] 761/id}	EGIR (1999) {Ref. [42] 765/id}	NCEP-ATP III (2004) {National Cholesterol Education Program, 2002 603/id} {Grundy, 2004 605/id}	AACE (2002) {Einhorn, 2002 766/id}	AHA/NHLBI {Grundy, 2004 763/id}	IDF (2006) {International Diabetes Federation, 2006 764/id; Alberti, 2006 771/id}
Requisite Characteristic or Condition					
Diagnosed T2DM, IFG, IGT, or insulin resistance[a]	Insulin resistance[a]	None	Risk factors for insulin resistance[b]	None	Central obesity (ethnic cut points)[c]
+Two or more of the following:	+Two or more of the following:	Three out of five of the following:	+Two or more of the following:	Three out of five of the following:	+Two or more of the following:
Characteristic/Measure and Cut Points					
Waist:					
	≥94 cm—men	≥102 cm—men		≥102 cm—men	
	≥80 cm—women	≥88 cm—women		≥88 cm—women	
BMI:					
>30 kg/m²					
Waist/hip ratio:					
>0.90—men					
>0.85—women					

(continued)

TABLE 14.1 (continued)
Comparison of Definitions for MetS

	WHO (1998) {Ref. [34] 761/id}	EGIR (1999) {Ref. [42] 765/id}	NCEP-ATP III (2004) {National Cholesterol Education Program, 2002 603/id} {Grundy, 2004 605/id}	AACE (2002) {Einhorn, 2002 766/id}	AHA/NHLBI {Grundy, 2004 763/id}	IDF (2006) {International Diabetes Federation, 2006 764/id; Alberti, 2006 771/id}
IFG:		110–126 mg/dL (>6.1 < 7.0 mmol/L)	≥110 mg/dL (≥6.1 mmol/L)	110–125 mg/dL (>6.1 < 7.0 mmol/L)	≥100 mg/dL (≥5.6 mmol/L) or drug treatment	≥100 mg/dL (≥5.6 mmol/L) or T2DM
IGT:		140–200 mg/dL (>7.8 < 11.1 mmol/L)		140–200 mg/dL[d] (>7.8 < 11.1 mmol/L)		
Triglyceride:	≥150 mg/dL (≥1.7 mmol/L)	≥177 mg/dL (≥2 mmol/L) or drug treatment	≥150 mg/dL (≥1.7 mmol/L) or drug treatment	≥150 mg/dL (≥1.7 mmol/L)	≥150 mg/dL (≥1.7 mmol/L) or drug treatment[e]	≥150 mg/dL (≥1.7 mmol/L) or drug treatment
HDL–cholesterol:	<35 mg/dL—men (<0.9 mmol/L) <39 mg/dL—women (<1 mmol/L)	<39 mg/dL (<1 mmol/L) or on drug treatment	<40 mg/dL—men (1 mmol/L) <50 mg/dL—women (1.3 mmol/L) or on drug treatment[e]	<40 mg/dL—men (1 mmol/L) <50 mg/dL—women (1.3 mmol/L)	<40 mg/dL—men (1 mmol/L) <50 mg/dL—women (1.3 mmol/L) or on drug treatment[e]	<40 mg/dL—men (1 mmol/L) <50 mg/dL—women (1.3 mmol/L) or on drug treatment

Blood pressure: ≥140/90 mm Hg	≥140/90 mm Hg or on drug treatment	≥130/85 mm Hg or on drug treatment	≥130/85 mm Hg	≥130/85 mm Hg or on drug treatment
Microalbuminuria: ≥20 µg/min or ≥30 albumin/creatinine ratio				Albuminuria: ≥30 albumin/creatinine ratio in nondiabetic

Harmonized Clinical Definitions for MetS (AHA/NHLBI and IDF) [Alberti, 2009 772 /id]

Three out of five of the following:

Characteristic/Measure	Cut Points
Waist	Population and country-specific definitions (see reference {Alberti, 2009 772/id})
IFG	≥100 mg/dL (≥5.6 mmol/L) or drug treatment
Triglyceride	≥150 mg/dL (≥1.7 mmol/L) or drug treatment[e]
HDL-cholesterol	<40 mg/dL—men (1 mmol/L); <50 mg/dL—women (1.3 mmol/L) or on drug treatment[e]
Blood pressure	≥130 systolic and/or 85 mm Hg diastolic or on drug treatment

WHO, World Health Organization; EGIR, European Group for the Study of Insulin Resistance; NCEP-ATP III, National Cholesterol Education–Adult Treatment Panel III; AACE, American Association of Clinical Endocrinologists; AHA/NHLBI, American Heart Association and National Heart, Lung, and Blood Institute; IDF, International Diabetes Federation; T2DM, type 2 diabetes mellitus; NAFLD, nonalcoholic fatty-liver disease.

a Population-specific standards for insulin resistance determined by hyperinsulinemic-euglycemic clamp or $HOMA_{IR}$.

b Risk factors for insulin resistance include BMI > 25 kg/m^2; waist > 40″ men or >35″ women; sedentary lifestyle; non-Caucasian; family history of T2DM, hypertension, or CVD; polycystic ovarian syndrome; gestational diabetes; acanthosis nigricans; and NAFLD.

c Central obesity is defined by population and ethnic-specific cut points for waist circumference {Alberti, 2006 771/id}.

d IFG defined as 2 h glucose concentrations following ingestion of 75 g glucose.

e The use of fibrates or niacin is indicative of elevated triglyceride levels and/or low HDL-cholesterol.

DESCRIBING THE METABOLIC SYNDROME
IN THE UNITED STATES OF AMERICA

Prevalence estimates can vary widely within any population depending on the definition that is used to determine MetS.[33,35,54] The NCEP-ATP III criteria are the most frequently recognized among scientists in the United States to establish prevalence and to determine cardiometabolic risk. Because of its simplicity, the NCEP-ATP III definition is also the most widely utilized in clinical practice. Thus, most of the available prevalence estimates in the U.S. population are derived from the NCEP-ATP III criteria with sparse contribution from other clinical definitions.[55]

According to NCEP-ATP III criteria applied to observations from NHANES III (1988–1994) and NHANES 1999–2000 data, MetS increased from 23% to almost 27% of adult Americans 20 years of age or older.[21] The latter estimate of up to 27% equates to approximately 55 million U.S. adults based on the 2000 census.[21,55] More recently, Ford[23] estimated higher rates of MetS (34.5%–39% of U.S. adults) in a study to compare prevalence using NCEP-ATP III and IDF definitions and a larger sample from NHANES 1999–2000. The estimated prevalence across all demographics was greater using IDF criteria; however, the two methods classified 93% of all participants similarly. Ford and Zhao[24] recently verified their higher MetS estimates in U.S. adults using variations of the most recent harmonious definition. These limited findings suggest that MetS occurs in 20%–40% of our population and is becoming increasingly more prevalent among U.S. adults. The syndrome is lowest in younger individuals and increases with age across all race/ethnicities. MetS is estimated to be 11% in men and 18.0% in women 20–39 years of age. Rates increase to 40% and 46% in men and women older than 60 years of age.[21] The domestic frequency of this condition is similar to what is observed in many countries throughout the world.[56]

MetS prevalence varies among race/ethnic group and gender with a greater prevalence among men in some races and women in others.[21–24] However, MetS currently appears to be growing at a faster rate in women versus men.[21] A 57% higher prevalence of MetS was observed in African American women versus men. Likewise, MetS was 26% greater among Mexican American women as compared to men of the same ethnicity. Non-Hispanic white men and women exhibit similar rates of MetS.[22] MetS was least frequent among African American men and greatest in Mexican American women. Among the larger demographic groups in the United States, MetS is observed with greater frequency among Mexican American men and women followed by non-Hispanic whites and African Americans. Asians exhibit some of the lowest prevalence of MetS,[57] whereas Asian Indians[58] and Native Americans[59] demonstrate some of the highest rates.

Increases in overweight and obesity from the mid-1970s have occurred in both sexes and across all age groups and ethnicities.[25,60,61] The latest estimates are that two-thirds of U.S. adults are overweight (BMI $> 25\,kg/m^2$) and fully one-third are obese (BMI $\geq 30\,kg/m^2$), with the greatest prevalence of overweight and obesity observed in Hispanics and non-Hispanic blacks—the most rapidly growing segments of our population.[25] Obesity raises the risk of morbidity from sleep apnea, respiratory complications, gallbladder disease, osteoarthritis, and endometrial, breast, prostate, and colon cancers.[62] However, major problems with excess body weight—and more specifically excess body fat—are that the condition is associated with a greater incidence of morbidity and mortality due to cardiovascular and metabolic disease.[20,62]

Overweight and obesity greatly influence the prevalence of MetS throughout the population, with MetS observed principally in overweight and obese individuals.[63] Thus, it is no surprise to the clinician that most of the major cardiovascular and metabolic disease risk factors are observed more frequently in overweight and obese individuals and that obesity is associated with more health-averse levels of cardiometabolic disease risk.[20,64] In a cross-sectional analysis of 5440 participants from the 1999 to 2004 NHANES data, 23.5% of normal-weight individuals were found to have two or more cardiometabolic abnormalities compared to 49.7% of overweight adults and 69.3% of obese adults.[65] In a recently published multiethnic study, it was demonstrated that blood pressure was elevated (6–20 mm Hg), fasting glucose and triglyceride concentrations were greater (8–17 and 18–55 mg/dL), HDL-cholesterol was lower (4–14 mg/dL), and there were greater concentrations of small LDL particles (109–173 nmol/L) in the obese versus their normal-weight counterparts.[20] Subclinical measures of underlying atherosclerosis, such as greater carotid artery intimal medial thickness, coronary artery calcium scores, and left ventricular mass, are also observed in the obese despite a significantly higher prevalence of antihypertensive and hypoglycemic medication use.

Clinically measured markers of increased cardiometabolic risk described in the obese are rarely observed independently even in normal-weight individuals,[65] and the clustering of risk factors that describe MetS does not occur by random chance.[66] Moreover, it is unlikely that the growing prevalence of MetS over the last 30 years has occurred independent of the surging obesity rates recorded during the same time frame. Indeed, Park et al.[63] partitioned men by BMI and determined that the odds ratios for MetS were 5.2 in overweight and 67.7 in obese men compared to their normal-weight counterparts. The results were similar in overweight and obese women, with the odds ratios being 5.4 and 34.5 versus women of normal weight. The concurrent growth in obesity, MetS, and T2DM in recent years has led to the term "diabesity."[67–69]

Added to age, ethnicity, and obesity, MetS is more prevalent in those who engage in little or no physical activity[70–73] and individuals exhibiting lower levels of physical fitness.[73,74] In addition, MetS occurs more frequently with greater carbohydrate consumption and reduced fiber intake.[70,72,75,76]

CONTROVERSIES OF MetS IN SCIENCE AND MEDICINE

The primary controversy regarding MetS is whether insulin resistance and obesity are unifying causes for the syndrome.[43,45] It is estimated that only 48% of people with insulin resistance have MetS—owing to the tremendous ability of various physiological processes to compensate for impaired insulin-mediated glucose uptake. On the other hand, only 78% of patients that meet criteria for MetS diagnosis have insulin resistance. This suggests that the etiology of the syndrome and its accompanying manifestations is much more complex than insulin resistance or compensatory hyperinsulinemia.[37,77,78] In regard to obesity, there are between 29% and 35%

of obese individuals who do not qualify as having MetS and between 21% and 30% of normal-weight individuals who would be defined as having MetS.[65] Therefore, although obesity does increase cardiometabolic risk,[64] it does not consistently result in metabolic dysfunction. The accumulation of fat at specific sites, such as excess abdominal or visceral adiposity, remains an attractive determinant for MetS.[26,38,79–81] Visceral fat is strongly associated with the development of insulin resistance and MetS but does not always distinguish those who are insulin resistant from those who are not.[82] Nor does visceral fat always identify those who have MetS from those who, by clinical measures, are metabolically healthy.[82]

Measures of insulin resistance—as elusive as these might be in the clinical setting—and surrogate markers of obesity and fat distribution are reasonable components to include in a model to identify MetS. Certainly, obesity and insulin resistance make independent contributions to increased CVD risk, but they are also related.[26,38,77,79–81] Insulin resistance is considered to be the very essence of the syndrome, while obesity—especially visceral obesity—is its most prevalent clinical culprit. However, both advocates and those that are dubious of MetS as a clinical entity acknowledge that the linking mechanisms remain under investigation and relationships to MetS are not completely understood.

Additional controversies stem from the fact that a common etiology for MetS has not been elucidated. These controversies have direct implications for clinical practice. First, the MetS definitions used for clinical screening are ambiguous. Even when the practitioner remains cognizant of the fact that there is a continuous relationship between disease risk and each of the risk factors, they are left to make clinical judgments using ill-defined thresholds and cut points for identifying heightened risk.[43,45,83] Determining hyperinsulinemia, insulin resistance, or even identifying adiposity and specific adipose tissue depots that insidiously impact health are immediate examples.

Next, there are a number of ways that a patient with heightened cardiometabolic risk might present. For example, there are 16 different combinations of MetS if a practitioner is using the NCEP-ATP III to define the syndrome.[43,45] Several more combinations may result if the clinician follows other definitions. If MetS resulted from a common cause, it would be reasonable to suggest that the heightened future cardiometabolic risk is the same regardless of the combination of risk factors that result. However, there is no research to address this particular issue and it is not known if each of these combinations confers the same risk.[43–45] Moreover, there is little evidence to determine whether any combination of three risk factors (i.e., the threshold for diagnosis of MetS from several definitions) is of greater risk than any two risk factors.[45]

Those that oppose the use of MetS in clinical practice understand the importance of identifying CVD and T2DM risks but are not convinced that diagnosing MetS is more effective for these purposes than traditional practice.[45] MetS screening may omit important health information because traditional CVD risk factors (e.g., family history of heart disease, smoking, or LDL-cholesterol) are part of standard clinical assessment but are not included in the MetS algorithm. As well, the defining characteristics of MetS (e.g., glucose intolerance, elevated plasma triglycerides, low HDL-cholesterol, and high blood pressure) are already part of standard clinical screening. Moreover, it is not known whether a diagnosis of MetS would have better predictive value of future CVD or T2DM than the established prediction tools such as the Framingham Risk Score and Diabetes Risk Score.[43] Those that doubt the usefulness of MetS also point out that the identification of any major cardiometabolic risk factor should prompt the clinician to evaluate for the presence of other risk factors, and all risk factors should be individually and aggressively treated.[43]

Proponents of MetS recognize that several cardiometabolic risk factors commonly present together in patients. Many of the observed risk factors are independently related to CVD and diabetes outcomes[84–87]; however, most do not occur alone. This is particularly true in overweight and obese individuals.[20,63] Advocates of MetS in clinical screening contend that the clustering of risk factors that comprise MetS does not appear by random chance, and the synergistic interaction of these risk factors may confer risk for CHD, MI, stroke, and T2DM that may be greater than otherwise expected.[66,88]

Arguably, one of the most important practical issues for the clinician is how well MetS predicts future CVD or T2DM. Specifically, there is considerable interest in determining if the diagnosis of MetS is better for estimating CVD and T2DM risk than other risk predictors or risk prediction models currently employed in the clinical setting. In addition, clinicians would like to know if the diagnosis of MetS offers greater predictive acuity than the sum of its individual components.

PREDICTING CARDIOMETABOLIC RISK FROM MetS

It is generally accepted that MetS—regardless of the definition employed—predicts a heightened risk for a variety of CVD outcomes and incident T2DM. The scientific literature describing the observational relationship between MetS and chronic disease outcomes is now quite substantial. Therefore, the prognostic significance of MetS with respect to CVD and diabetes may be best summarized by describing overarching results from recent quantitative reviews of the literature.[88–91]

Mottillo et al.[88] determined the efficacy of the initial and revised NCEP-ATP III definitions to predict CVD outcomes in a meta-analysis of 87 studies and 951,083 patients. Overall CVD risk was over 2.3 times greater in those with MetS. The risk for CVD mortality was increased 2.4-fold, and the relative risks for all-cause mortality, MI, and stroke were 1.58, 1.99, and 2.27 in those with versus those without MetS, respectively. Gami et al.[89] conducted a meta-analysis of 37 longitudinal studies comprising 43 cohorts and 172,573 patients in order to characterize the relationship between MetS and CVD events and mortality. A greater risk for CVD events and death was reported among participants with MetS than those without the syndrome (RR = 1.78, CI = 1.58–2.00). The association between MetS and CVD outcomes was stronger in women and in studies that enrolled individuals of lower risk. In a review of prospective studies from 1998 to 2004, Ford[90] determined the combined relative risk for NCEP-defined MetS was 65% greater for CDV mortality and almost 200% greater for diabetes than those without MetS. Although MetS conferred a higher risk of CVD death, it was most effective at predicting future diabetes. In a subsequent quantitative analysis of 16 cohorts and 42,419 participants, Ford et al.[91] compared the effectiveness of different MetS definitions to predict incident diabetes and described MetS as consistently having a strong association with incident diabetes.

Variations in the predictive ability of MetS may be attributed in part to the different populations that were studied, several definitions of MetS to study the risk relationship, and the length of the follow-up periods. In addition, it is likely that variations in prognostic significance are due to characteristics or conditions that vary widely in a population and that are known to contribute to the development of MetS, CVD, and diabetes but are not included in the study assessment. At least some of these characteristics and conditions include established risk factors (e.g., family history of CVD and/or diabetes, age, sex, race/ethnicity, and physical activity, smoking, and diet behaviors) as well as emerging factors (e.g., blood measures of inflammation and thrombosis).

Overall, MetS is more strongly associated with incident diabetes than CVD outcomes. Those with MetS are at least twice as likely to develop CVD and even more likely to develop diabetes within the next decade.[88,92–98] Once CVD or diabetes develops, the presence of MetS contributes to disease progression and severity.[99,100] It remains to be determined whether MetS is better at predicting future CVD or diabetes among apparently healthy low-risk adults or whether it is more effective as a prognostic tool in individuals with known disease and of higher risk.[89,91,100]

Whether the diagnosis of MetS is superior to predict future CVD and diabetes than what might be ascertained by its components[66,99,101] or by standard clinical tests, such as health history questionnaires and risk surveys,[95,102,103] or fasting blood glucose[92,97,104] remains inconclusive and a subject of healthy debate.[43–45,83,105,106]

OBESITY AND THE ETIOLOGY OF INSULIN RESISTANCE AND MetS

Insulin resistance in MetS and T2DM is a disturbance that affects insulin signaling pathways differently. There is evidence that the phosphatidylinositol 3-kinase (PI-3K) pathway, leading to cellular glucose uptake, is inhibited, whereas the mitogen-activated protein kinase (MAPK) pathway, with proinflammatory effects, remains unaffected.[37,107,108] In skeletal muscle, insulin-mediated glucose uptake, which accounts for the disposal of up to 90% of ingested glucose, is attenuated. In the liver, endogenous glucose production and secretion continues unabated due to a weaker PI-3K insulin signal. In adipose tissue, the insulin-mediated suppression of non-esterified fatty acid (NEFA) mobilization and secretion is dampened. The resulting systemic metabolic dysfunction is characterized by compensatory hyperinsulinemia, hyperglycemia, elevated NEFA concentrations, and chronic low-grade inflammation.[37,45,106]

Insulin resistance, relative hyperinsulinemia, and other features of MetS are frequently exhibited in obese individuals into overt T2DM.[68,69,79,109] Likewise, CVD risk factors and clinically defined measures of atherosclerosis are more common and observed at greater intensities in obese versus normal-weight individuals.[20] There is little question that a chronic energy imbalance, often attributed to calorically dense, nutrient-poor diets, poor eating habits, stress, lack of sleep, and inadequate physical activity, contributes to insulin resistance, CVD, and to the accumulation of body weight and body fat.[38] Body fat accrual and fat cell hypertrophy have negative and direct influences on cardiometabolic health. Yet, not all obese individuals develop insulin resistance or MetS. Therefore, obesity is an ill-defined CVD risk factor coinciding with several means of presentation—from otherwise apparently healthy to exhibiting multiple risk factors and/or signs and symptoms of cardiometabolic disease.[45,80]

The differing fat patterns, first observed by Dr. Jean Vague, partially explain the heterogeneous risk profiles associated with obesity. Some fat depots, such as gynoid and subcutaneous adipose tissue, are thought to serve as a "metabolic sink" capable of handling wide variations in energy storage. These fat stores appear to prevent the development of insulin resistance and MetS and are consistent with evidence that some fat tissue is necessary for maintaining a healthy metabolic profile.[26,38,80,81] On the other hand, android fat—and more specifically, visceral fat—is associated with insulin resistance and several pathophysiologies related to the development of cardiovascular and metabolic dysfunction.[38,80,81] Visceral fat, as compared to subcutaneous fat, increases risk for hypertension and stroke, congestive heart failure, MI, and CVD mortality independent of total obesity.[110,111]

An explanation for the metabolic differences between fat depots goes well beyond a mere partitioning of adipose tissue stores. According to a recently introduced theory of "ectopic fat accumulation," adipocyte hypertrophy—resulting from persistent energy storage—diminishes the ability of mature adipocytes to hypertrophy and differentiate. Excess fat begins to accumulate in sites that are not well suited for fat storage such as the liver, skeletal and cardiac muscle, pancreas, and kidneys. The additional fat burden within these tissues is "lipotoxic." That is, ectopic fat induces or greatly contributes to insulin resistance, disturbs glucose and lipid metabolism, and contributes to inflammation and heightened oxidative stress.[112–114] It is thought that visceral fat accumulation may be a form of ectopic fat deposition because visceral fat exhibits insulin resistance and diminished inhibition of NEFA mobilization.[26,38,80] In addition, visceral and ectopic fat exacerbates defective metabolism in tissues throughout the body through altered adipokine synthesis and secretion.[115,116] The disturbed adipokine signaling and regulation that is associated with ectopic fat accumulation adds to insulin resistance, vessel dysfunction, inflammation, dyslipidemia, and hypercoagulability (Figure 14.1).[27,57,68,115–117]

Chronic exposure to elevated NEFA concentrations disrupts normal insulin secretion and causes pancreatic beta cell apoptosis and necrosis.[118] In skeletal muscle, elevated NEFA and intracellular fat accumulation aggravates insulin resistance and contributes to disturbances in several related metabolic pathways.[112,114] In the heart, fat deposition and altered fat metabolism may increase myocardial oxygen requirements, predispose the myocardium to ischemia, and result in impaired contractility and a greater risk for cardiac arrhythmias.[111,119] In blood vessels, persistently elevated NEFA concentrations reduce endothelial nitric oxide production, induce adhesion characteristics, facilitate oxidative damage and inflammation, and result in diminished vascular compliance and reactivity.[27,38,68] In addition, the increased production and conversion of angiotensinogen to angiotensin observed with adipocyte hypertrophy, ectopic fat accumulation, and elevated plasma fatty acids increase vascular tone, exacerbate vascular oxidative stress and inflammation, alter renal hemodynamics and electrolyte management, and is associated with the hypertension observed in MetS.[30] In the liver, oversupply of NEFA facilitates triglyceride

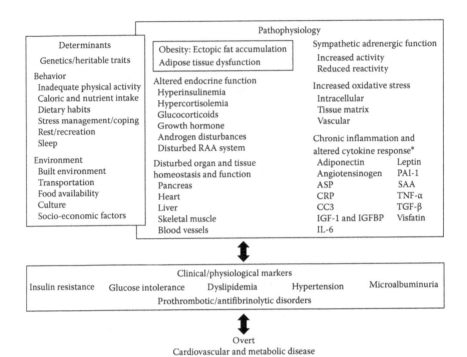

FIGURE 14.1 The pathophysiology of MetS. *, selected adipocytokines; ASP, acylation-stimulating protein; CRP, C-reactive protein; CC3, complement component 3; IGF-1, insulin-like growth factor-1; IGFBP, insulin-like growth factor binding protein; IL-6, interleukin-6; PAI-1, plasminogen activator inhibitor-1; SAA, serum amyloid A; TNF-α, tumor necrosis factor-α; TGF-β, transforming growth factor-β.

synthesis, reduces apolipoprotein B-100 degradation, and enhances the production of triglyceride-rich VLDL. Elevated plasma triglyceride concentrations and triglyceride-rich lipoproteins are observed, owing to increased hepatic production of VLDL and increased intestinal assembly and secretion of triglyceride-rich chylomicrons, and further exacerbated by impaired lipoprotein lipase activities.[38,120,121] The increased actions of hepatic lipase and cholesterol ester transfer protein, observed with insulin resistance and ectopic liver fat, potentiate the transfer of triglyceride from VLDL to HDL and result in the formation of small, dense LDL. Smaller, dense LDL is less likely to be taken up by the normal LDL receptor pathway, more readily penetrates the vascular endothelium, and is more susceptible to oxidative damage. Once in the subendothelial tissue, the modified LDL induces vascular inflammation and contributes to atherosclerotic plaque accumulation and lesion instability.[122,123] Modifications to HDL, resulting from the activities of hepatic lipase and cholesterol ester transfer protein and dysfunctional apolipoprotein metabolism, contribute to greater HDL clearance in the liver. A reduction in HDL quantity and altered HDL composition further impair reverse cholesterol transport and attenuate HDL anti-oxidant potential, thereby adding to dyslipidemia, vascular dysfunction, and atherosclerotic plaque burden.[37,38,114,123]

Even with this cursory overview, it is obvious that the physical manifestations of MetS, although frequently inventoried as independent risk factors or signs/symptoms in the clinic, are intricately related. The clustering of these multiple risk factors in their various combinations is truly a syndrome that likely results from more than one underlying cause. Readers are referred to several excellent reviews for a greater understanding of the cellular and molecular pathophysiology of obesity, insulin resistance, MetS, and related adverse cardiometabolic health outcomes.[26,37,38,80,105,115,116]

SCREENING AND EVALUATION FOR MetS

The inclusion of MetS in clinical practice may encourage the physician to focus on the comorbidities that are frequently associated with obesity and to identify patients at risk of CVD mortality that might otherwise be classified as low risk using traditional risk factors alone (i.e., age, sex, smoking, blood pressure, and cholesterol).[33,124] Physicians that use a MetS inventory in clinical screening suggest that it helps them to consider the underlying causes for risk factor clustering and to address lifestyle behaviors that are known to have a powerful influence on cardiometabolic health (e.g., physical inactivity and poor diet).[105,106,125,126] Identifying patients with MetS may aid the physician in selecting pharmacologic interventions that have greater efficacy and lower side effects in those with the syndrome (i.e., antihypertensive therapy). It may also help physicians recognize the need for more aggressive treatment strategies for risk factor reduction earlier in the treatment regimen (i.e., including the use of antihyperlipidemic therapy).[105,106,126]

Practical approaches for including MetS screening in clinical practice have been proposed and expanded in recent years.[105,126–130] Among these are recommendations to identify and treat MetS in obese patients.[128,131–133] A generally suggested first step in recognizing underlying cardiometabolic dysfunction is to include one of the current MetS definitions into a standard health assessment. The most-recent harmonized definition[33] can serve as a useful means of identifying MetS as the physician considers a patient's family and personal health history and determines the presence of related disorders such as acanthosis nigricans, sleep apnea, fatty liver, lipodystrophies, gallstones, polycystic ovarian syndrome, and microalbuminuria.[126,131,134] An advised "next step" is to calculate the near-term risk for CVD outcomes using an established risk assessment model.[126,127,129] The 10 year Framingham Risk Score[86] is likely the most-often studied and utilized among several assessment models for determining future adverse CVD events.[127,135] The 10 year Framingham model categorizes risk probability as "high" >20%, "moderate" or "intermediate" 10%–20%, and "low" <10%. Blaha et al.[129] further suggest that physicians, utilizing the 10 year Framingham score, consider a more conservative estimate of "moderate risk" (e.g., define moderate or intermediate risk as a 10 year probability of 6%–20% instead of 10%–20%) to account for underestimated CVD risk in those with MetS. This same medical group recently updated their recommendations to add a longer-term estimate of CVD risk[135] that complements the 10 year Framingham score and accounts for the influence of BMI in younger individuals.[126] Others recognize the potential usefulness of measuring C-reactive protein, a marker of chronic inflammation, as part of an overall assessment in those with an intermediate- or high-risk 10 year Framingham score.[127,128,136]

Individuals predisposed to insulin resistance and MetS are those with a family history of T2DM or personal history of IFG or IGT, atherogenic dyslipidemia (elevated triglycerides and low HDL-cholesterol concentrations), elevated C-reactive protein values (>3 mg/dL), microalbuminuria ($\geq$20 μg/min or $\geq$30 albumin/creatinine ratio), or any of the related disorders listed earlier. The information obtained from this health appraisal and estimations of the short- and long-term risk of future cardiovascular events will help the physician to formulate appropriate immediate treatment strategies and long-term management goals for the patient with MetS.

TREATMENT AND MANAGEMENT OF MetS

The primary goal in the clinical management of MetS is to reduce the global risk for cardiovascular and metabolic diseases. Attention should be aimed at reducing the severity and number of traditional risk factors for CVD, such as LDL-cholesterol, high blood pressure, and impaired glucose homeostasis. Aggressive treatment, often including the use of pharmaceutical therapy, is of primary importance for preventing future CVD outcomes in MetS patients with documented or known disease.[126,129,130,134] The current goals and recommendations for managing the components of MetS are described in consensus statements for dyslipidemia, high blood pressure, obesity, diabetes, and physical activity.[49,52,137–140]

LIFESTYLE BEHAVIORS: HEALTHY DIET, PHYSICAL ACTIVITY, AND WEIGHT LOSS

The cornerstone or first-line therapeutic interventions for those with MetS are to engage in regularly practiced physical activity, consume a heart-healthy diet, lose weight, and prevent weight regain after weight loss. All five of the components that define MetS can be mitigated when these lifestyle behaviors are consistently practiced.[141,142] In addition, efforts should be made to quit smoking, improve stress management, and practice individually appropriate behavioral techniques for long-term adherence to healthy lifestyle changes.[134,143] A clinician's guide that describes how to prescribe exercise for most patients and delineates useful strategies for promoting healthy lifestyle changes has recently been published.[144] Strategies for improving patient adherence to lifestyle behavior changes are also available for the physician and health-care practitioner.[143]

Adopting a healthy diet is absolutely critical in treating and managing the components of MetS.[126,128,129,134] A Mediterranean-style diet, composed of wholegrain foods, fruit, vegetables, fish, fiber, and nuts, has demonstrated efficacy in mitigating CVD risk and reducing future CVD events.[145,146] The benefits of a Mediterranean-style diet are due, in part, to the fact that it is low in saturated fats, trans fats, and cholesterol and low in sodium, red meat, simple sugars, and refined grains.[126,129,134,147] In addition, the Mediterranean diet provides nutrients, such as omega-3 fatty acids, polyunsaturated fatty acids, soluble fiber, and carotenoids, all of which are associated with cardiometabolic health.[147] Adopting this type of diet will help those with MetS balance macronutrient intake and avoid succumbing to fad diets. A Mediterranean-style diet is consistent with the NCEP-ATP III recommendations for a dietary fat intake of 25%–35% of total calories.[49] Diets with fat intake exceeding 35% are more likely to include too much saturated fat, contributing to elevated LDL-cholesterol, insulin resistance, and weight gain.[134,148] On the other hand, low-fat, high-carbohydrate diets promote two salient features of atherogenic dyslipidemia, elevated triglycerides, and lower HDL-cholesterol. High-protein diets can increase blood phosphorus levels and may lead to hypercalciuria, acidosis, and insulin resistance, especially in individuals with poor renal function.[130,134,148]

MetS is less prevalent among those consuming moderate amounts of alcohol versus those who report no alcohol use.[141] The incidences of T2DM and coronary artery disease are lower among moderate drinkers as well.[141,149] Although red wine is often associated with the Mediterranean diet, the health benefits of alcohol appear to be unrelated to the type of alcoholic beverage that is consumed.[150] Therefore, patients who are responsible drinkers should be encouraged to continue moderate alcohol use.

Evidenced-based dietary recommendations from the AHA, NCEP-ATP III, and the DASH diet include most of the characteristics described earlier and are widely utilized in clinical practice.[49,137,148] However, it is also important for the clinician to think beyond itemized recommendations for dietary nutrient composition. Patients should be provided with resources to make incremental and lasting behavioral changes in meal planning, food selection, and food preparation. Contingencies for dietary challenges, such as food choices and portion control when dining out, and habits associated with altered eating patterns need to be addressed.[143]

The amount of physical activity recommended for improving and maintaining health in most adults is very attainable. Apparently healthy adults should engage in a minimum of 30 min of moderately intense physical activities on 5 or more days a week. The amount of physical activity can be accumulated throughout the day in sessions lasting as little as 10 min each. The volume of physical activity can be somewhat less when vigorous activity is part of the weekly program. The target is to achieve 450–750 MET·min^{-1} of activity per week (a measure of the accumulated intensity and duration for each activity).[140] All adults are encouraged to resistance train two times per week in order to maintain muscle mass and functional ability. Resistance training is also an effective means of normalizing and maintaining blood glucose control.[151] The health benefits of regularly practiced physical activity, such as improved blood pressure, blood glucose control, lipid measurements, and cardiovascular function, will be enjoyed regardless of weight change or in the absence of noticeable improvements in fitness.[71,73,140,152]

Approximately 150–200 min of moderate-intensity physical activity appears to be effective for preventing weight gain in adults.[139] However, the physical activity needed to achieve weight loss or to enjoy noticeable fitness improvements will be somewhat greater than that recommended for maintaining body weight and achieving health benefits.[139,153] The current body of evidence supports the accumulation of 60–90 min of moderate-intensity physical activity per day for sustained weight loss. Even more physical activity (>250 min/week) may be necessary to prevent weight regain after weight loss targets have been achieved.[139,154] In addition, regularly practiced aerobic and resistance exercise can attenuate the return of cardiometabolic dysfunction in individuals that experience weight regain.[155,156]

The use of intervals, in which periods of low or moderate intense exercise are performed between vigorous periods, appears to have greater efficacy for ameliorating cardiometabolic risk than an equal volume of standard, continuous-intensity exercise. Interval training may also be an excellent means to introduce exercise, to progress exercise for improving fitness, and to enhance weight loss and prevent weight regain.[157,158] All individuals with MetS should undergo risk assessment before beginning an exercise program. It is not necessary for most individuals to undergo an exercise stress test prior to initiating exercise; however, stress testing is recommended for those with known disease or for those who are of high-risk for future CVD events. Individuals with known disease and are of high risk should exercise in a facility that provides medical supervision.[159]

Weight loss is a top priority for obese patients with MetS. The current recommendation is to achieve a 7%–10% reduction in body weight over a 6–12 month period through caloric restriction and increased physical activity. It is generally agreed that this target is best attained through a modest reduction in daily caloric intake (i.e., lower total calories by 500–1000 kcal).[138,139] Achieving a modest weight loss of 7%–10% will positively impact all MetS characteristics.[138,141,160] Daily physical activity will add to the caloric deficit and impart health benefits that may not be achieved through hypocaloric diets alone.[139,140] Weight loss medications may be necessary for those with obesity-related medical conditions or to assist individuals who do not respond to initial weight loss efforts.[133,161] Both drugs currently in use for weight loss, sibutramine and orlistat, have demonstrated short-term benefits for those with MetS.[128] Bariatric surgery for obese patients with MetS appears to have promise as well.[162] The risks associated with weight reduction medications and bariatric surgery may be substantial. As such, physicians and patients considering these interventions should be aware of current guidelines and recommendations.[133,161]

Weight loss achieved by healthy lifestyle behavior may be the most effective means of preventing and treating MetS. Indeed, modest weight reduction, accompanied by regular physical activity, was more effective than pharmacologic intervention for preventing T2DM among those with IGT.[163,164] In addition, weight loss and lifestyle changes were responsible for reducing the incidence of MetS in those previously diagnosed with the syndrome and preventing MetS in a follow-up of individuals without MetS at baseline.[165] Additional health benefits can be realized with greater weight loss and long-term maintenance of the lower body weight.[133,139,142,160] Therefore, individuals who respond well to the initial weight loss goal should be encouraged to continue behaviors conducive to further weight loss or maintenance of their new body weight.

DYSLIPIDEMIA

The primary target for lipid-lowering therapy is LDL-cholesterol even in those with MetS. Current LDL-cholesterol goals range from <70 to <160 mg/dL (<1.8 to <4.1 mmol/L) based on estimates of CVD risk. The target for LDL-cholesterol is <100 mg/dL in patients determined to be at high risk for overt CVD and even lower in very high-risk patients. Less stringent LDL-cholesterol goals of 130 mg/dL for those at intermediate risk and 160 mg/dL for low-risk individuals are recommended.[49]

Statin therapy is frequently used as the first-line treatment for LDL-cholesterol lowering. In standard dosages, statins are capable of reducing LDL-cholesterol by as much as 40% but are limited in their efficacy for lowering triglycerides, increasing HDL-cholesterol, and modifying other aspects of atherogenic dyslipidemia like small dense LDL particles.[53] In addition to lipid-lowering effects, statin treatment may reduce serum uric acid levels,[166] improve renal function,[167] and lower CVD events in patients with MetS and T2DM.[168-170]

Elevated fasting and postprandial triglycerides, low HDL-cholesterol, and small dense LDL particles contribute to the residual CVD risk in MetS after LDL-cholesterol goals have been achieved.[129] This atherogenic dyslipidemia can be approximated in the clinic by calculating non-HDL-cholesterol and measuring triglyceride concentrations. Therefore, non-HDL-cholesterol, which is an aggregate measure of VLDL, chylomicrons, and all triglyceride-rich lipoproteins, is considered the next target for lipid-lowering interventions after LDL-cholesterol goals are met.[49,129] Directly targeting triglyceride concentrations is also of importance in order to avoid acute pancreatitis in those with severe hypertriglyceridemia.[134] Non-HDL-cholesterol goals are generally 30 mg/dL less than those of LDL-cholesterol, and triglyceride concentrations should be reduced to <150 mg/dL or 1.7 mmol/L.[134] HDL-cholesterol, essentially a marker of reverse cholesterol transport, becomes a focus of lipid management after LDL-cholesterol, non-HDL-cholesterol, and triglyceride values have been addressed. There are no clinical targets for raising HDL-cholesterol.[49]

Regular exercise,[171] weight loss,[160] and a variety of dietary elements may be substituted or supplemented to address secondary dyslipidemias. Soluble fiber sources, plant stanol esters, omega-3 fatty acids, and moderate alcohol consumption can boost efforts to address dyslipidemias through lifestyle behaviors.[172]

Fibrates and niacin are effective for lowering triglycerides, increasing HDL-cholesterol, and increasing LDL particle size.[126,128-130,134] As such, these agents are chosen to address atherogenic dyslipidemia—either as first-line therapy when LDL-cholesterol is within normal limits, or in combination with statins. The combination of simvastatin and fenofibrate appears to have an additive and powerful effect on ameliorating all atherogenic characteristics of the lipid/lipoprotein profile.[173,174] Likewise, extended-release niacin improves LDL-cholesterol triglyceride and is very effective at increasing HDL-cholesterol.[175] Niacin also has the added benefit of lowering Lp(a) and fibrinogen levels[176] and, in combination with simvastatin, shows promise in lowering CVD events.[177] Tota-Maharaj et al.[126] published an excellent review of recent clinical trial data supporting the beneficial cardiometabolic effects of antihyperlipidemic medications.

BLOOD PRESSURE

Hypertension therapy should be targeted to reduce blood pressure between 130–135 mm Hg systolic and 80–85 mm Hg diastolic blood pressures or lower in some high-risk patients.[137] Regularly practiced exercise and consistently following the DASH diet are essential elements in any plan to lower blood pressure.[137,178] Obese patients with MetS must also lose body weight for effective blood pressure control.[20,179] Angiotensin-converting enzyme inhibitors (ACEI) and angiotensin receptor blockers (ARB) have gained widespread acceptance as the antihypertensive agents of choice in patients with MetS[126,128–130,134] because these drugs disrupt the altered renin–angiotensin–aldosterone system that often accompanies metabolic dysfunction.[30] In addition to their ability to lower blood pressure, ACEIs and ARBs have demonstrated effectiveness for preventing T2DM,[180] reducing CVD events in T2DM,[181] and attenuating renal function deterioration and microalbuminuria in T2DM patients with nephropathy.[182] However, most of the reduction in CVD risk is attributed to the blood pressure lowering effects of these medications.[126] Thiazide diuretics and beta blockers may be considered for those with MetS but are not generally regarded as first-line antihypertensive agents in patients with MetS because of their negative effects on insulin sensitivity and glucose tolerance.[126,134]

BLOOD GLUCOSE MANAGEMENT

As stated previously, the easiest, most effective and cost-efficient means of addressing all components of MetS, including glucose control, is through lifestyle modification that includes a healthy diet, regular exercise, and weight loss.[133,163–165] Yet, the annual rate at which those with IGT and MetS progress to T2DM may be as high as 19% if left untreated or when patients do not adhere to lifestyle changes.[183] A variety of oral hypoglycemic agents, such as metformin, acarbose, thiazolidinediones, incretin mimetics, and alpha-glucosidase inhibitors, may offer therapeutic options for glycemic control.[126,129,134] These drugs are known to reduce CVD risk in patients with T2DM[130,134]; however, their use is not currently included in clinical recommendations for treating IFG and IGT in patients with MetS because information is lacking regarding the long-term benefits and cost-effectiveness in lowering CVD events.[127,134] As part of an updated approach to the clinical management of MetS, Tota-Maharaj et al.[126] recognized the exciting potential benefits of incretin mimetics in ameliorating glucose abnormalities and dyslipidemia, lowering body weight, and reducing abdominal girth measurements in those with MetS.[184] However, when more aggressive treatment of glucose control in MetS is warranted, metformin currently remains the drug intervention of choice.[164]

ATHEROTHROMBOSIS AND INFLAMMATION

Aspirin is an effective agent for preventing platelet aggregation and reducing the risk for thrombosis. Therefore, low-to-moderate-dose aspirin (75–162 mg/day) is recommended in primary prevention for MetS patients with an intermediate or high 10 year Framingham CVD risk and in older adults without contraindications for gastrointestinal or extracranial bleeding. Omega-3 fatty acids may also be an effective means of lowering atherothrombotic risk and may be considered especially in those with contraindications for aspirin therapy. Niacin appears to have therapeutic value for reducing chronic inflammation and hypercoagulability because of its ability to lower Lp(a) and fibrinogen levels and to reduce the number of small, dense LDL particles.[176,177] Other medications, such as statins, fibrates, ACEIs, and thiazolidinediones, may attenuate chronic systemic inflammation; however, clinical recommendations do not recognize these pharmacologic agents for independently addressing inflammation.[126,129,134]

SUMMARY

Although the increasing rate of obesity is somewhat abating, obesity-related medical expenditures continue to grow. In 2008, medical costs linked to obesity were approximately $147 billion and accounted for up to 9% of all medical costs. This economic toll was almost double the $78.5 billion spent on obesity 10 years before. Unfortunately, the current prevalence of obesity among adults as well as our children and adolescents assures that future generations will be dealing with these health and economic burdens—largely due to cardiometabolic dysfunction—far into the future.[61] Meanwhile, the scientific and medical discussions regarding the primary underlying causes of cardiometabolic dysfunction remain lively. Probably the most debated chronic disease concept over the last 20 years, for clinicians and scientists alike, is the topic of MetS.

The arguments are strong for insulin resistance and chronic hyperinsulinemia being primary factors that precipitate the clinical manifestations of MetS and increase CVD risk. There is also a wealth of data to support the contribution of excess body fat, particularly the presence of ectopic fat to the high prevalence of MetS among overweight and obese individuals. Inflammation, oxidative stress, and predisposition for thrombosis also contribute to the development of MetS. This suggests that the etiology of the syndrome and its accompanying manifestations are not likely to result from a single cause. As a result, definitions for MetS that have been developed with requisite characteristics (i.e., the WHO, EGIR, AACE, and IDF) do not seem to be optimal for diagnosing the syndrome or predicting future CVD or diabetes in individual patients.

A practical approach to diagnosing those with MetS is to incorporate either the NCEP-ATP III[49] or the harmonized definitions[33] into medical evaluations and preventative physical exams.[126] Utilize a 10 year Framingham risk score in order to include traditional CVD risk factors for identifying individuals at intermediate and high risk for future adverse CVD events.[86] In younger individuals, a 30 year risk score may also be helpful for determining strategies to manage cardiometabolic risk factors.[126,135] The diagnosis of MetS can help guide the decision to aggressively treat related health concerns such as blood pressure, dyslipidemia, and elevated blood glucose.

Physicians and other health-care providers should be well versed in recommendations for introducing therapeutic lifestyle changes to their patients. There are several resources available to aid in this regard.[144] Lifestyle modifications for obese individuals with MetS should include weight loss, healthy dieting, and regular physical activity.[127,128,133,134] Behavioral strategies for initiating and maintaining healthy lifestyle choices must be part of this equation.[143] In this regard, the physician should be aware of the surrounding health-care network to support their patients' efforts. Dieticians, health educators, health coaches, and clinical exercise physiologists are well trained for assisting those at increased risk for CVD.

High-risk patients may need pharmacologic interventions to complement lifestyle changes. The most effective medications to ameliorate dyslipidemia and hypertension in those with MetS may be different from the generally prescribed first-line drugs.[126] Appropriate treatment recommendations combined with regularly scheduled follow-up visits to monitor a patient's progress will improve the likelihood that overweight and obese individuals reduce their risk for premature morbidity and mortality due to CVD.

REFERENCES

1. Kylin E. Studien uber das Hypertonie–Hyperglykamie–Hyperurikamiesyndrom. *Zent. fur Innere Medizin.* 1923;44:105–127.
2. Vague J. La differenciation sexuelle, facteur determinant des formes de l' obesite. *Presse Med.* 1947;30:339–340.
3. Vague J. The degree of masculine differentiation of obesities: A factor determining predisposition to diabetes, atherosclerosis, gout and uric acid calculous disease. *Am J Clin Nutr.* 1956;4:20–34.
4. Albrink MJ, Meigs JW. The relationship between serum triglycerides and skinfold thickness in obese subjects. *Ann NY Acad Sci.* 1965;131:673–683.
5. Avogaro P, Crepaldi G, Enzi G, Tiengo A. Associazione di iperlipidemia, diabete mellito e obesita di medio grado. *Acta Diabetol Lat.* 1967;4:36–41.
6. Welborn TA, Breckenridge A, Rubenstein AH, Dollery CT, Fraser TR. Serum-insulin in essential hypertension and in peripheral vascular disease. *Lancet.* 1966;1:1336–1337.
7. Yalow RS, Berson SA. Immunoassay of endogenous insulin in man. *J Clin Invest.* 1960;39:1157–1175.
8. Albrink M, Krauss R, Lindgren F, von der Groben J, Pan S, Wood P. Intercorrelations among high density lipoprotein, obesity, and triglycerides in a normal population. *Lipids.* 1980;15:668–678.
9. Despres J-P, Allard C, Tremblay A, Talbot J, Bouchard C. Evidence for a regional component of body fatness in the association with serum lipids in men and women. *Metabolism.* 1985;34:967–973.
10. Larsson B, Svardsudd K, Welin L, Wilhelmsen L, Bjorntorp P, Tibblin G. Abdominal adipose tissue distribution, obesity, and risk of cardiovascular disease and death: 13.5 years of follow-up of the participants in the study of men born in 1913. *Br Med J.* 1984;288:1401–1404.
11. Lapidus L, Bengtsson C, Larsson B, Pennert K, Rybo E, Sjostrom L. Distribution of adipose tissue and risk of cardiovascular disease and death: A 12 year follow-up of participants in the population study of women in Gothenberg, Sweden. *Br Med J.* 1984;289:1257–1261.
12. Krotkiewski M, Bjorntorp P, Sjostrom L, Smith U. Impact of obesity on metabolism in men and women. Importance of regional adipose tissue distribution. *J Clin Invest.* 1983;72:1150–1162.
13. Despres J-P, Moorjani S, Lupien P, Tremblay A, Nadeau A, Bouchard C. Regional distribution of body fat, plasma lipoproteins, and cardiovascular disease. *Arteriosclerosis.* 1990;10:497–511.
14. Lemieux I, Pascot A, Coulliard C et al. Hypertriglyceridemic waist: A marker of the atherogenic triad (hyperinsulinemia; hyperapolipoprotein B; small, dense LDL) in men? *Circulation.* 2000;102:179–184.
15. DeFronzo RA, Ferrannini E. The pathogenesis of non-insulin-dependent diabetes: An update. *Medicine.* 1982;61:125–140.
16. Ferrannini E, Buzzigoli G, Bonadonna R et al. Insulin resistance in essential hypertension. *N Engl J Med.* 1987;317:350–357.
17. Modan M, Halkin H, Almog S et al. Hyperinsulinemia. A link between hypertension obesity and glucose intolerance. *J Clin Invest.* 1985;75:809–817.
18. Kissebah AH, Vydelingum N, Murray R et al. Relation of body fat distribution to metabolic complications of obesity. *J Clin Endocrinol Metab.* 1982;54:254–260.
19. Reaven GM. Banting lecture 1988. Role of insulin resistance in human disease. *Diabetes.* 1988;37:1595–1607.
20. Burke GL, Bertoni AG, Shea S et al. The impact of obesity on cardiovascular disease risk factors and subclinical vascular disease: The multi-ethnic study of atherosclerosis. *Arch Intern Med.* 2008;168:928–935.

21. Ford ES. Increasing prevalence of the metabolic syndrome among U.S. adults. *Diabetes Care*. 2004;27:2444–2449.
22. Ford ES, Giles WH, Dietz WH. Prevalence of the metabolic syndrome among U.S. adults. Findings from the third National Health and Nutrition Examination Survey. *JAMA*. 2002;287:356–359.
23. Ford ES. Prevalence of the metabolic syndrome defined by the International Diabetes Federation among adults in the U.S. *Diabetes Care*. 2005;28:2745–2749.
24. Ford ES, Zhao G. Prevalence and correlates of metabolic syndrome based on a harmonious definition among adults in the U.S. *J Diabetes*. 2010;3:180–193.
25. Flegal KM, Carroll MD, Ogden CL, Curtin LR. Prevalence and trends in obesity among US adults, 1999–2008. *JAMA*. 2010;303:235–241.
26. Rasouli N, Molavi B, Elbien SC, Kern PA. Ectopic fat accumulation and metabolic syndrome. *Diabetes Obes Metab*. 2007;9:1–10.
27. Koh KK, Han SH, Quon MJ. Inflammatory markers and the metabolic syndrome. Insights from therapeutic interventions. *J Am Coll Cardiol*. 2005;46:1978–1985.
28. DeFronzo RA, Ferrannini E. Insulin resistance. A multifaceted syndrome responsible for NIDDM, obesity, hypertension, dyslipidemia, and atherosclerotic heart disease. *Diabetes Care*. 1991;14:173–194.
29. Kaplan NM. The deadly quartet. Upper-body obesity, glucose intolerance, hypertriglyceridemia, and hypertension. *Arch Intern Med*. 1989;149:1514–1520.
30. Whaley-Connell A, Johnson M, Sowers JR. Aldosterone: Role in the cardiometabolic syndrome and resistant hypertension. *Prog Cardiovasc Dis*. 2010;52:401–409.
31. Groop L, Ortho-Melander M. The dysmetabolic syndrome. *Intern Med*. 2001;250:105–120.
32. Grundy SM, Brewer HB, Cleeman JI, Smith SC, Lenfant C. Definition of metabolic syndrome: Report of the National Heart, Lung, and Blood Institute/American Heart Association conference on scientific issues related to definition. *Circulation*. 2004;109:433–438.
33. Alberti KG, Eckel RH, Grundy SM et al. Harmonizing the metabolic syndrome. A joint interim statement of the International Diabetes Federation Task Force on Epidemiology and Prevention; National Heart, Lung, Blood Institute; American Heart Association; World Heart Federation; International Atherosclerosis Society; and International Association for the Study of Obesity. *Circulation*. 2009;120:1640–1645.
34. Alberti KG, Zimmet PZ. Definition, diagnosis and classification of diabetes mellitus and its complications. Part 1: Diagnosis and classification of diabetes mellitus provisional report of a WHO consultation. *Diabet Med*. 1998;15:539–553.
35. Alberti KG, Zimmet P, Shaw J. Metabolic syndrome—A new worldwide definition. A consensus statement from the International Diabetes Federation. *Diabet Med*. 2006;23:469–480.
36. Bloomgarden ZT. Inflammation, atherosclerosis, and aspects of insulin action. *Diabetes Care*. 2005;28:2312–2319.
37. Miranda PJ, DeFronzo RA, Califf RM, Guyton JR. Metabolic syndrome: Definition, pathophysiology, and mechanisms. *Am Heart J*. 2005;149:33–45.
38. Van Gaal LF, Mertens IL, De Block CE. Mechanisms linking obesity with cardiovascular disease. *Nature*. 2006;444:875–880.
39. National Cholesterol Education Program. Third Report of the Expert Panel on Detection, Evaluation, and Treatment of High Blood Cholesterol in Adults (Adult Treatment Panel II). NIH Publication No. 01–3305. 2001. U.S. Department of Health and Human Services. National Institutes of Health. NHLBI, Bethesda, MD.
40. International Diabetes Federation. The IDF consensus worldwide definition of the metabolic syndrome. 2006. Brussels, Belgium, International Diabetes Federation.
41. Einhorn D, Reaven GM, Cobin RH. American College of Endocrinology position statement on the insulin resistance syndrome. *Endocr Pract*. 2002;9:236–252.

42. Balkau B, Charles MA. Comment on the provisional report from the WHO consultation. European Group for the Study of Insulin Resistance (EGIR). *Diabet Med.* 1999;16:442–443.
43. Kahn R, Buse J, Ferrannini E, Stern M. The metabolic syndrome: Time for a critical appraisal. Joint statement from the American Diabetes Association and the European Association for the Study of Diabetes. *Diabetes Care.* 2005;28:2289–2304.
44. Kahn R. Metabolic syndrome—What is the clinical usefulness? *Lancet.* 2008;371:1892–1893.
45. Reaven GM. The metabolic syndrome: Time to get off the merry-go-round? *J Intern Med.* 2010;269:127–136.
46. Ford ES. Rarer than a blue moon. *Diabetes Care.* 2005;28:1808–1809.
47. Reynolds K, Muntner P, Fonseca V. Metabolic syndrome. Underrated or underdiagnosed? *Diabetes Care.* 2005;28:1831–1832.
48. Boudreau DM, Malone DC, Raebel MA et al. Health care utilization and costs by metabolic syndrome risk factors. *Metab Syndr Relat Disord.* 2009;7:305–314.
49. National Cholesterol Education Program. Third report of the National Cholesterol Education Program (NCEP) expert panel on detection, evaluation and treatment of high cholesterol in adults (Adult Treatment Panel III) final report. *Circulation.* 2002;106:3143–3421.
50. American Diabetes Association. Consensus development conference on insulin resistance. November 5–6, 1977. *Diabetes Care.* 1998;21:310–314.
51. National Cholesterol Education Program. Executive summary of the third report of the National Cholesterol Education Program (NCEP) expert panel on detection, evaluation and treatment of high blood cholesterol in adults (Adult Treatment Panel III). *JAMA.* 2001;285:2486–2497.
52. Genuth S, Alberti KG, Bennett P et al. Follow-up report on the diagnosis of diabetes mellitus. The expert committee on the diagnosis and classification of diabetes mellitus. *Diabetes Care.* 2003;26:3160–3167.
53. Grundy SM, Cleeman JI, Merz NB et al. Implications of recent clinical trials for the National Cholesterol Education Program Adult Treatment Panel III guidelines. *Circulation.* 2004;110:227–239.
54. Dunstan DW, Zimmet PZ, Welborne TA et al. The rising prevalence of diabetes and impaired glucose tolerance. The Australian Diabetes, Obesity and Lifestyle Study. *Diabetes Care.* 2002;25:829–834.
55. Reynolds K, He J. Epidemiology of the metabolic syndrome. *Am J Med Sci.* 2005;330:273–279.
56. Grundy SM. Metabolic syndrome pandemic. *Atheroscler Thromb Vasc Biol.* 2008;28:629–636.
57. Anand SS, Yi Q, Gertein H et al. Relationship of metabolic syndrome and fibrinolytic dysfunction to cardiovascular disease. *Circulation.* 2003;108:420–425.
58. Chandalia M, Abate N, Garg A, Stray-Gundersen J, Grundy SM. Relationship between generalized and upper body obesity to insulin resistance in Asian Indian men. *J Clin Endocrinol Metab.* 2011;84:2329–2335.
59. Resnick HE, Jones K, Ruotolo G et al. Insulin resistance, the metabolic syndrome, and risk of incident cardiovascular disease in nondiabetic American Indians: The Strong Heart Study. *Diabetes Care.* 2003;26:861–867.
60. Flegal KM, Carroll MD, Ogden CL, Johnson CL. Prevalence and trends in obesity among US adults, 1999–2000. *JAMA.* 2002;288:1723–1727.
61. Hedley AA, Ogden CL, Johnson CL, Carroll MD, Curtin LR, Flegal KM. Prevalence of overweight and obesity among US children, adolescents, and adults, 1999–2002. *JAMA.* 2004;291:2847–2850.
62. U.S. Department of Health and Human Services. The Surgeon General's call to action to prevent and decrease obesity. 2001. U.S. Department of Health and Human Services. U.S. Public Health Service. Office of the Surgeon General, Rockville, MD.

63. Park YW, Zhu S, Palaniappan L, Heshka S, Carnethon MR, Heymsfield SB. The metabolic syndrome: Prevalence and associated risk factor findings in the U.S. population from the third National Health and Nutrition Examination Survey, 1988–1994. *Arch Intern Med.* 2003;163:427–436.

64. Arnlov J, Ingelsson E, Sundstrom J, Lind L. Impact of body mass index and the metabolic syndrome on the risk of cardiovascular disease and death in middle-aged men. *Circulation.* 2010;121:230–236.

65. Wildman RP, Munter P, Reynolds K et al. The obese without cardiometabolic risk factor clustering and the normal weight with cardiometabolic risk factor clustering. *Arch Intern Med.* 2008;168:1617–1624.

66. Ninomiya JK, L'Italien G, Criqui MH, Whyte JL, Gamst A, Chen R. Association of the metabolic syndrome with history of myocardial infarction and stroke in the third National Health and Nutrition Examination Survey. *Circulation.* 2004;109:42–46.

67. Zimmet PZ, Alberti KG, Shaw J. Global and societal implications of the diabetes epidemic. *Nature.* 2001;414:782–787.

68. Schmidt MI, Duncan BB. Diabesity: An inflammatory metabolic condition. *Clin Chem Lab Med.* 2003;41:1120–1130.

69. Astrup A, Finer N. Redefining type 2 diabetes: 'Diabesity' or 'obesity dependent diabetes mellitus'? *Obesity Rev.* 2000;1:57–59.

70. Carthenon MR, Loria CM, Hill JO, Sidney S, Savage PJ, Liu K. Risk factors for the metabolic syndrome. *Diabetes Care.* 2004;27:2707–2715.

71. Carroll S, Dudfield M. What is the relationship between exercise and metabolic abnormalities? A review of the metabolic syndrome. *Sports Med.* 2004;34:371–418.

72. Wannamethee SG, Shaper AG, Whincup PH. Modifiable lifestyle factors and the metabolic syndrome in older men: Effects of lifestyle changes. *J Am Geriatric Soc.* 2006;54:1909–1914.

73. Janiszewski PM, Ross R. The utility of physical activity in the management of global cardiometabolic risk. *Obesity.* 2009;17:S3–S14.

74. Gill JR, Malkova D. Physical activity, fitness and cardiovascular disease risk in adults: Interactions with insulin and obesity. *Clin Sci.* 2006;110:409–425.

75. Wirfalt E, Hedblad B, Gullberg B et al. Food patterns and components of the metabolic syndrome in men and women: A cross-sectional study within the Malmo Diet and Cancer cohort. *Am J Epidemiol.* 2001;154:1150–1159.

76. McKeown NM, Meigs JB, Liu S, Saltzman E, Wilson PWF, Jacques PF. Carbohydrate nutrition, insulin resistance, and the prevalence of the metabolic syndrome in the Framingham Offspring cohort. *Diabetes Care.* 2004;27:538–546.

77. McLaughlin T, Allison G, Abbasi F, Lamendola C, Reaven GM. Prevalence of insulin resistance and associated cardiovascular disease risk factors among normal weight, overweight, and obese individuals. *Metabolism.* 2004;53:495–499.

78. Stolar M. Metabolic syndrome: Controversial but useful. *Cleve Clin J Med.* 2007;74:199–208.

79. Despres J-P, Lemieux I, Bergeron J et al. Abdominal obesity and the metabolic syndrome: Contribution to global cardiometabolic risk. *Atheroscler Thromb Vasc Biol.* 2008;28:1039–1049.

80. Despres J-P, Lemieux I. Abdominal obesity and metabolic syndrome. *Nature.* 2006;444:881–887.

81. Despres J-P. Cardiovascular disease under the influence of excess visceral fat. *Crit Pathw Cardiol.* 2007;6:51–59.

82. Stefan N, Kantartzis K, Machann J et al. Identification and characterization of metabolically benign obesity in humans. *Arch Intern Med.* 2008;168:1609–1616.

83. Kim SH, Reaven GM. The metabolic syndrome: One step forward, two steps back. *Diabetes Vasc Dis Res.* 2004;2:68–75.

84. Yusuf S, Hawken S, Ounouu S et al. Effect of potentially modifiable risk factors associated with myocardial infarction in 52 countries (the INTERHEART study): Case-control study. *Lancet.* 2005;366:1640–1649.

85. Vasan RS, Larson MG, Leip EP et al. Impact of high-normal blood pressure on the risk of cardiovascular disease. *N Engl J Med.* 2001;345:1291–1297.

86. Wilson PWF, D'Agostino RB, Levy D, Belanger AM, Silbershatz H, Kannel WB. Prediction of coronary heart disease using risk factor categories. *Circulation.* 1998;97:1837–1847.

87. Wilson PWF, Meigs JB, Sullivan L, Fox CS, Nathan DM, D'Agostino RB. Prediction of incident diabetes mellitus in middle-aged adults. *Arch Intern Med.* 2007;167:1068–1074.

88. Mottillo S, Filion KB, Genest J et al. The metabolic syndrome and cardiovascular risk. *J Am Coll Cardiol.* 2010;56:1113–1132.

89. Gami AS, Witt BJ, Howard DE et al. Metabolic syndrome and risk of incident cardiovascular events and death. *J Am Coll Cardiol.* 2007;49:403–414.

90. Ford ES. Risks for all-cause mortality, cardiovascular disease, and diabetes associated with the metabolic syndrome. *Diabetes Care.* 2005;28:1769–1778.

91. Ford ES, Li C, Sattar N. Metabolic syndrome and incident diabetes. *Diabetes Care.* 2008;31:1898–1904.

92. Wilson PWF, D'Agostino RB, Parise H, Sullivan L, Meigs JB. Metabolic syndrome as a precursor of cardiovascular disease and type 2 diabetes mellitus. *Circulation.* 2005;112:3066–3072.

93. Lakka H-M, Laaksonen DE, Lakka T et al. The metabolic syndrome and total and cardiovascular disease mortality in middle-aged men. *JAMA.* 2002;288:2709–2716.

94. Kurl S, Laukkanen JA, Niskanen L et al. Metabolic syndrome and the risk of stroke in middle-aged men. *Stroke.* 2006;37:806–811.

95. McNeill AM, Rosamond WD, Girman CJ et al. The metabolic syndrome and 11-year risk of incident cardiovascular disease in the atherosclerosis risk in communities study. *Diabetes Care.* 2005;28:385–390.

96. Lorenzo C, Williams K, Hunt KJ, Haffner SM. The National Cholesterol Education Program-Adult Treatment Panel III, International Diabetes Federation, and World Health Organization definitions of the metabolic syndrome as predictors of incident cardiovascular disease and diabetes. *Diabetes Care.* 2007;30:8–13.

97. Sattar N, McConnachie A, Shaper AG et al. Can metabolic syndrome usefully predict cardiovascular disease and diabetes? Outcome data from two prospective studies. *Lancet.* 2008;371:1927–1935.

98. Sattar N, Gaw A, Scherbakova O et al. Metabolic syndrome with and without C-reactive protein as a predictor of coronary heart disease and diabetes in the West of Scotland Coronary Prevention Study. *Circulation.* 2003;108:414–419.

99. Guzder RN, Gatling W, Mullee MA, Byrne CD. Impact of metabolic syndrome criteria on cardiovascular disease risk in people with newly diagnosed type 2 diabetes. *Diabetologia.* 2006;49:49–55.

100. Butler J, Rodondi N, Zhu Y et al. Metabolic syndrome and the risk of cardiovascular disease in older adults. *J Am Coll Cardiol.* 2011;47:1595–1602.

101. Wang J, Ruotsalainen S, Moilanen L, Lepisto P, Laakso M, Kuusisto J. The metabolic syndrome predicts cardiovascular mortality: A 13-year follow-up study in elderly non-diabetic Finns. *Eur Heart J.* 2007;28:857–864.

102. Stern MP, Williams K, Gonzalez-Villalpando C, Hunt KJ, Haffner SM. Does the metabolic syndrome improve identification of individuals at risk of type 2 diabetes and/or cardiovascular disease? *Diabetes Care.* 2004;27:2676–2681.

103. Wannamethee SG, Shaper AG, Lennon L, Morris RW. Metabolic syndrome vs Framingham Risk Score for prediction of coronary heart disease, stroke, and type 2 diabetes. *Arch Intern Med.* 2005;165:2644–2650.

104. Cameron AJ, Magliano DJ, Zimmet PZ et al. The metabolic syndrome as a tool for predicting future diabetes: The AusDiab Study. *J Intern Med.* 2008;264:177–186.

105. Eckel RH, Grundy SM, Zimmet PZ. The metabolic syndrome. *Lancet.* 2005;365:1415–1428.

106. Grundy SM. A constellation of complications: The metabolic syndrome. *Cardiometab Risk Manag.* 2005;7:36–45.

107. Le Roith D, Zick Y. Recent advances in our understanding of insulin action and insulin resistance. *Diabetes Care.* 2001;24:588–597.

108. Cusi K, Maezono K, Osman A et al. Insulin resistance differentially affects the PI-3 kinase- and MAP-kinase-mediated signaling in human muscle. *J Clin Invest.* 2000;105:311–320.

109. DeFronzo RA. Pathogenesis of type 2 diabetes mellitus. *Med Clin N Am.* 2004;88:787–835.

110. Lakka TA, Lakka H-M, Salonen R, Kaplan GA, Salonen JT. Abdominal obesity is associated with accelerated progression of carotid atherosclerosis in men. *Atherosclerosis.* 2001;154:497–504.

111. Kenchaiah S, Evans JC, Levy D et al. Obesity and the risk of heart failure. *N Engl J Med.* 2002;347:305–313.

112. Eckhardt K, Taube A, Eckel J. Obesity-associated insulin resistance in skeletal muscle: Role of lipid accumulation and physical inactivity. *Rev Endocr Metab Disord.* 2011; 12:163–172.

113. Meijer RI, Serne EH, Smulders YM, van Hinsbergh VWM, Yudkin JS, Eringa EC. Perivascular adipose tissue and its role in type 2 diabetes and cardiovascular disease. *Curr Diabetes Rep.* 2011;11:211–217.

114. Aguilera CM, Gil-Campos M, Canete R, Gil A. Alterations in plasma and tissue lipids associated with obesity and metabolic syndrome. *Clin Sci.* 2008;114:183–193.

115. Deng Y, Scherer PE. Adipokines as novel biomarkers and regulators of the metabolic syndrome. *Ann NY Acad Sci.* 2010;1212:E1–E19.

116. Singla P, Bardoloi A, Parkash A. The metabolic effects of obesity: A review. *World J Diabetes.* 2010;1:76–88.

117. Cancello R, Clement K. Is obesity an inflammatory illness? Role of low-grade inflammation and macrophage infiltration in human white adipose tissue. *BJOG.* 2006;113:1141–1147.

118. Giacca A, Xiao C, Oprescu A, Carpentier A, Lewis G. Lipid-induced pancreatic B-cell dysfunction: Focus on in vivo studies. *Am J Physiol Endocrinol Metab.* 2011;300:E255–E262.

119. McGavock JM, Victor RG, Unger RH, Szczepaniak LS. Adiposity of the heart, revisited. *Ann Intern Med.* 2006;144:517–524.

120. Adiels M, Taskinen M-R, Packard CJ et al. Overproduction of VLDL particles is driven by increased liver fat content in man. *Diabetologia.* 2006;49:755–765.

121. Seppala-Lindroos A, Vehkavaara S, Hakkinen A-H et al. Fat accumulation in the liver is associated with defects in insulin suppression of glucose production and serum free fatty acids independent of obesity in normal men. *J Clin Endocrinol Metab.* 2002;87:3023–3028.

122. Kwiterovich PO. Clinical relevance of the biochemical, metabolic, and genetic factors that influence low-density lipoprotein heterogeneity. *Am J Cardiol.* 2002;90:30i–47i.

123. Tomkin GH. Targets for intervention in dyslipidemia in diabetes. *Diabetes Care.* 2008;31:S241–S248.

124. Balkau B, Qiao Q, Tuomilehto J, Borch-Johnsen K, Pyorala K. Does the metabolic syndrome detect further subjects at high risk of cardiovascular death, or is a cardiovascular risk score adequate? *Diabetologia*. 2005;48:abstr 315.

125. James PT, Rigby N, Leach R. The obesity epidemic, metabolic syndrome and future prevention strategies. International Obesity Task Force. *Eur J Cardiovasc Prev Rehabil*. 2004;11:3–8.

126. Tota-Maharaj R, Defilipps AP, Blumenthal RS, Blaha MJ. A practical approach to the metabolic syndrome: Review of current concepts and management. *Curr Opin Clin Cardiol*. 2010;25:502–512.

127. Grundy SM. Metabolic syndrome: Therapeutic considerations. *Hand Exp Pharmacol*. 2005;170:107–133.

128. Liberopoulos EN, Mikhailidis DP, Elisaf MS. Diagnosis and management of the metabolic syndrome in obesity. *Obes Rev*. 2005;6:283–296.

129. Blaha MJ, Bansal S, Rouf R, Golden SH, Blumenthal RS, Defilipps AP. A practical "ABCDE" approach to the metabolic syndrome. *Mayo Clin Proc*. 2008;83:932–943.

130. Wagh A, Stone NJ. Treatment of metabolic syndrome. *Expert Rev Cardiovasc Ther*. 2004;2:213–228.

131. Silk AW, McTigue KM. Reexamining the physical examination for obese patients. *JAMA*. 2011;305:193–194.

132. Reaven GM. Importance of identifying the overweight patient who will benefit the most by losing weight. *Ann Intern Med*. 2003;138:420–423.

133. Lyznicki JM, Young DC, Riggs JA, Davis RM. Obesity: Assessment and management in primary care. *Am Fam Physician*. 2001;63:2185–2196.

134. Grundy SM, Cleeman JI, Daniels SR et al. Diagnosis and management of the metabolic syndrome. An American Heart Association/National Heart, Lung, and Blood Institute Scientific Statement. *Circulation*. 2005;112:2735–2752.

135. Pencina MJ, D'Agostino RB, Larson MG, Massaro JM, Vasan RS. Predicting the 30-year risk of cardiovascular disease: The Framingham Heart Study. *Circulation*. 2009;119:3078–3084.

136. Rutter MK, Meigs JB, Sullivan LM, D'Agostino RB, Wilson PWF. C-reactive protein, the metabolic syndrome, and prediction of cardiovascular events in the Framingham Offspring Study. *Circulation*. 2004;110:380–385.

137. Chobanian AV, Bakris GL, Black HR et al. National Heart, Lung, and Blood Institute Joint National Committee on Prevention, Detection, Evaluation, and Treatment of High Blood Pressure; National High Blood Pressure Education Program Coordinating Committee. The seventh report of the Joint National Committee on Prevention, Detection, Evaluation, and Treatment of High Blood Pressure: The JNC 7 report. *JAMA*. 2003;289:2560–2572.

138. National Institutes of Health. Clinical guidelines on the identification, evaluation, and treatment of overweight and obese adults—The evidence report. National Institutes of Health. *Obes Res*. 1998;6:51S–209S.

139. Donnelly J, Blair S, Jakicic J, Manore M, Rankin J, Smith B. Appropriate physical activity intervention strategies for weight loss and prevention of weight regain for adults. *Med Sci Sports Exerc*. 2009;41:459–471.

140. Haskell WL, Lee I, Pate R et al. Physical activity and public health: Updated recommendation for adults from the American College of Sports Medicine and the American Heart Association. *Med Sci Sports Exerc*. 2007;39:1423–1434.

141. Zhu S, St-Onge MP, Heshka S, Heymsfeild SB. Lifestyle behaviors associated with lower risk of having the metabolic syndrome. *Metabolism*. 2004;53:1503–1511.

142. Ratner R, Goldberg R, Haffner S et al. Impact of intensive lifestyle and metformin therapy on cardiovascular disease risk factors in the diabetes prevention program. *Diabetes Care*. 2005;28:888–894.

143. Fappa E, Yannakoulia M, Pitsavos C, Skoumas I, Valourdou S, Stefanadis C. Lifestyle intervention in the management of metabolic syndrome: Could we improve adherence issues? *Nutrition*. 2008;24:286–291.

144. Capell J, Jonas S, Kaplan-Liss E, Phillips EM, Renna ME. *ACSM's Exercise is Medicine. A Clinician's Guide to Exercise Prescription*. Philadelphia, PA: Wolters Kluwer/Lippincott Williams & Wilkins; 2009.

145. De Lorgeril M, Salen P, Martin J, Monjaud I, Delaye J, Mamelle N. Mediterranean diet, traditional risk factors, and the rate of cardiovascular complications after myocardial infarction: Final report of the Lyon Diet Heart Study. *Circulation*. 1999;99:779–785.

146. Rumawas ME, Meigs JB, Dwyer JT, McKeown NM, Jacques PF. Mediterranean-style dietary pattern, reduced risk of metabolic syndrome traits, and incidence in the Framingham Offspring Cohort. *Am J Clin Nutr*. 2009;90:1608–1614.

147. Bautista MC, Engler MM. The Mediterranean diet. Is it cardioprotective? *Prog Cardiovasc Nurs*. 2005;20:70–76.

148. Krauss RM, Eckel RH, Howard B et al. AHA dietary guidelines: Revision 2000: A statement for healthcare professionals from the Nutrition Committee of the American Heart Association. *Circulation*. 2000;102:2284–2299.

149. Howard AA, Arnsten JH, Gourevitch MN. Effect of alcohol consumption on diabetes mellitus. A systematic review. *Ann Intern Med*. 2004;140:211–219.

150. Djousse L, Arnett DK, Eckfeldt JH, Province MA, Singer MR, Ellison RC. Alcohol consumption and the metabolic syndrome: Does the type of beverage matter? *Obes Res*. 2004;12:1375–1385.

151. Strasser B, Siebert U, Schobersberger W. Resistance training in the treatment of the metabolic syndrome. A systematic review and meta-analysis of the effect of resistance training on metabolic clustering in patients with abnormal glucose metabolism. *Sports Med*. 2010;40:397–415.

152. Kraus WE, Houmard JA, Duscha BD et al. Effects of the amount and intensity of exercise on plasma lipoproteins. *N Eng J Med*. 2002;347:1483–1492.

153. Institute of Medicine. Physical activity. In: Institute of Medicine, ed. *Dietary Reference Intakes for Energy, Carbohydrate, Fiber, Fatty Acids, Cholesterol, Protein and Amino Acids*. Washington, DC: National Academies Press; 2002, pp. 880–935.

154. Wing RR, Phelan S. Long-term weight loss maintenance. *Am J Clin Nutr*. 2005;82:222S–225S.

155. Thomas TR, Warner SO, Dellsperger KC et al. Exercise and metabolic syndrome with weight regain. *J Appl Physiol*. 2010; 109:3–10.

156. Warner SO, Linden MA, Liu Y et al. The effects of resistance training on metabolic health with weight regain. *J Clin Hypertens*. 2010;12:64–72.

157. Tremblay A, Simoneau J-A, Bouchard C. Impact of exercise intensity on body fatness and skeletal muscle metabolism. *Metabolism*. 1994;43:814–818.

158. Tjonna AE, Lee SJ, Rognomo O et al. Aerobic interval training versus continuous moderate exercise as a treatment for the metabolic syndrome. A pilot study. *Circulation*. 2008;118:346–354.

159. American College of Sports Medicine. *ACSM's Guidelines for Exercise Testing and Prescription*. 8th edn. Philadelphia, PA: Lippincott Williams & Wilkins; 2009.

160. Poobalan A, Aucott L, Smith WC et al. Effects of weight loss in overweight/obese individuals and long-term lipid outcomes—A systematic review. *Obes Rev*. 2004;5:43–50.

161. Snow V, Barry P, Fitterman N, Qaseem A, Weiss K. Pharmacological and surgical management of obesity in primary care: A clinical practice guideline from the American College of Physicians. *Ann Intern Med*. 2005;142:525–531.

162. Lee WJ, Huang MT, Wang W, Lin CM, Chen TC, Lai R. Effects of obesity surgery on the metabolic syndrome. *Arch Surg*. 2004;139:1088–1092.

163. Tuomilehto J, Lindstrom J, Eriksson JG et al. Prevention of type 2 diabetes mellitus by changes in lifestyle among subjects with impaired glucose tolerance. *N Engl J Med.* 2001;344:1343–1350.

164. Knowler WC, Barrett-Conner E, Fowler S et al. Reduction in the incidence of type 2 diabetes with lifestyle intervention or metformin. *N Engl J Med.* 2002;346:393–403.

165. Orchard TJ, Temprosa M, Goldberg R et al. The effect of metformin and intensive lifestyle intervention on the metabolic syndrome: The Diabetes Prevention Program randomized trial. *Ann Intern Med.* 2005;142:611–619.

166. Athyros VG, Elisaf M, Papageorgiou AA et al. Effects of statins versus untreated dyslipidemia on serum uric acid levels in patients with coronary heart disease: A subgroup analysis of the GREek atorvastatin and coronary heart disease evaluation (GREACE) study. *Am J Kidney Dis.* 2004;43:589–599.

167. Athyros VG, Mikhailidis DP, Papageorgiou AA et al. Effects of statins versus untreated dyslipidemia on renal function in patients with coronary heart disease: A subgroup analysis of the GREek atorvastatin and coronary heart disease evaluation (GREACE) study. *J Clin Pathol.* 2004;57:728–734.

168. Colhoun HM, Betteridge DJ, Durrington PN et al. Primary prevention of cardiovascular disease with atorvastatin in type 2 diabetes in the Collaborative Atorvastatin Diabetes Study (CARDS): Multicentre randomized placebo-controlled trial. *Lancet.* 2004;364:685–696.

169. Pyorala K, Ballantyne CM, Gumbiner B et al. Reduction of cardiovascular events by simvastatin in non-diabetic coronary heart disease patients with and without the metabolic syndrome: Subgroup analyses of the Scandinavian Simvastatin Survival Study (4S). *Diabetes Care.* 2004;27:1735–1740.

170. Ballantyne CM, Olsson AG, Cook TJ, Mercuri MF, Pedersen TR, Kjekshus J. Influence of low high-density lipoprotein cholesterol and elevated triglyceride on coronary heart disease events and response to simvastatin therapy in 4S. *Circulation.* 2001;104:3046–3051.

171. Durstine JL, Grandjean PW, Davis PG, Ferguson MA, Alderson NL, DuBose KD. Blood lipid and lipoprotein adaptations to exercise: A quantitative analysis. *Sports Med.* 2001;31:1033–1062.

172. Grandjean PW, Crouse SF. Lipid and lipoprotein disorders. In: LeMura LM, von Duvillard SP, eds. *Clinical Exercise Physiology: Application and Physiological Principles.* Philadelphia, PA: Lippincott Williams & Wilkins; 2004, pp. 55–86.

173. Vega GL, Ma PTS, Cater NB. Effects of adding fenofibrate (200 mg/day) to simvastatin (10 mg/dy) in patients with combined hyperlipidemia and metabolic syndrome. *Am J Cardiol.* 2003;91:956–960.

174. Athyros VG, Papageorgiou AA, Athyrou VV, Demitriadis DS, Kontopoulos AG. Atorvastatin and micronized fenofibrate alone and in combination in type 2 diabetes with combined hyperlipidemia. *Diabetes Care.* 2002;25:1198–1202.

175. Plaisance EP, Grandjean PW, Mahurin AJ. Independent and combined effects of aerobic exercise and pharmacological strategies on serum triglyceride concentrations: A qualitative review. *Phys Sportsmed.* 2009;37:1–9.

176. Guyton JR, Blazing MA, Hagar J. Extended release niacin vs. gemfibrozil for the treatment of low levels of high-density lipoprotein cholesterol. *Arch Intern Med.* 2000;160:1177–1184.

177. Brown BG, Zhao XQ, Chait A. Simvastatin and niacin, anti-oxidant vitamins, or the combination for the prevention of coronary disease. *N Engl J Med.* 2001;345:1583–1592.

178. Pescatello LS, Franklin BA, Fagard R, Farquhar WB, Kelley GA, Ray CA. American College of Sports Medicine position stand: Exercise and hypertension. *Med Sci Sports Exerc.* 2004;36:533–553.

179. Reisen E, Abel R, Modan M, Silverberg DS, Eliahou HE, Modan B. Effect of weight loss without salt restriction on the reduction of blood pressure in overweight hypertensive patients. *N Engl J Med.* 1978;298:1–6.

180. Scheen AJ. Renin–angiotensin system inhibition prevents type 2 diabetes mellitus. Part 1. A meta-analysis of randomized clinical trials. *Diabetes Metab.* 2004;30:487–496.

181. The Heart Outcomes Prevention Evaluation Study Investigators. Effects of ramipril on cardiovascular and microvascular outcomes in people with diabetes mellitus: Results of the HOPE study and MICRO-HOPE substudy. *Lancet.* 2000;355:253–259.

182. Brenner BM, Cooper ME, de Zeeuw D et al. Effects of losartan on renal and cardiovascular outcomes in patients with type 2 diabetes and nephropathy. *N Engl J Med.* 2001;345:861–869.

183. Hanefeld M, Karasik A, Koehler C. Metabolic syndrome and its single traits as risk factors for diabetes in people with impaired glucose tolerance: The STOP NIDDM trial. *Diabetes Vasc Dis Res.* 2009;6:32–37.

184. Bhushan R, Elkind-Hirsch KE, Bhushan M. Improved glycemic control and reduction of cardiometabolic risk factors in subjects with type 2 diabetes and metabolic syndrome treated with exanetide in a clinical practice setting. *Diab Technol Ther.* 2009;11:353–359.

15 Obesity and Cancer

Clarence H. Brown, III, MD

CONTENTS

Cancer is a group of diseases that result from uncontrolled growth and spread of genetically altered cells. Cancers are caused by both external factors (tobacco, infectious organisms, radiation, and chemicals) and internal factors (inherited mutations, hormones, immune conditions, and metabolic abnormalities). Interactions among these causative factors are thought to lead to genetic changes that transform normal cells into those that no longer respond to the normal homeostatic mechanisms enjoyed by normal tissue. At least two external factors are controllable, and, were they to be eliminated, a large number of cancers could be prevented. The use of tobacco products and excessive body fat contribute greatly to the incidence of several of the most serious forms of cancer.

For more than half a century, it has been appreciated that a causal relationship between cigarette smoking and lung cancer exists [1]. Of interest, it was German scientists during the 1930s under Adolph Hitler, who were the first to link smoking to lung cancer [2]. Beginning in the mid-twentieth century, investigators began identifying other malignancies that are associated with smoking [3], and medical professionals have become accustomed to advising their patients who smoke to discontinue that particular lifestyle. From those efforts and from a number of government [4] and nongovernmental initiatives, the number of Americans who continue to smoke has significantly decreased [5,6]. Between 1965 and 2004, cigarette smoking among adults aged 18 and older declined by half from 42% to 21%. By 2007, that rate diminished to 20%. Thus, a considerable reduction in the incidence of tobacco-related diseases, including several cancers, has occurred [7].

As numerous efforts to eliminate smoking appear to be effective, that lifestyle factor is declining [7], but unfortunately the other controllable lifestyle factor, being overweight or obese, is doing just the opposite. Many sources have substantiated the fact that there is a frightening rise in the number of Americans, including children, who are obese [8,9]. And, while there has long been an association of obesity with heart disease and other noncancerous medical conditions, only during the past 10–20 years has the etiologic relationship between obesity and cancer been fully appreciated [10,11]. In fact, some authorities feel that obesity and lack of physical activity have or soon will surpass tobacco use as the leading cause of cancer [12,13], not rare cancers, but some of the more common and serious forms of cancer including colon, breast (postmenopausal), endometrial, renal, and esophagus [11]. In addition, some studies have also reported links between obesity and cancers of the gallbladder, ovaries, and pancreas [12].

This chapter will describe what is known about the relationship between obesity and cancer and examine the possible etiologic factors that research has uncovered in this most troubling, yet potentially controllable, situation. Since obesity and a sedentary lifestyle have, for all practical purposes, a cause and effect relationship, much of the reported evidence relating obesity and cancer refers as much to the lack of physical activity as to body weight or body mass index (BMI).

The National Health and Nutrition Examination Survey (NHANES), a program within the Centers for Disease Control and Prevention (CDC), reported that, in the year 2008, approximately 34% of U.S. adults over the age of 20 were overweight and more than one-third (33.8%) were classified as obese [9]. In 2008, 16.9% of children, 2–19 years of age, were overweight, more than triple the number two decades earlier [8]. A startling statistic reported by NHANES is that since 1976 the percentage of adult Americans with BMI values above 30.0 ("obese") has doubled. Studies have shown that being overweight or obese directly relates to both a lack of physical activity and the ingestion of a highly caloric and/or fatty diet.

In 2001, the International Agency for Research on Cancer of the World Health Organization convened a group of experts to evaluate the evidence for the role of physical activity and weight control in cancer prevention. The group concluded that being overweight or obese increases the risk of breast cancer (postmenopausal); cancers of the colon, endometrium, kidney (renal cell), and esophagus (adenocarcinoma); and possibly thyroid cancer. And, by losing weight, one may reduce his or her risk of developing these cancers, but that there is insufficient evidence to definitively conclude that such is the case. These experts determined that physical activity plays a significant role in preventing cancers of the colon and breast. Taken together, they concluded that excess body weight and physical inactivity account for approximately a quarter to one-third of cancers of the colon, breast, endometrium, kidney (renal cell), and esophagus (adenocarcinoma). Thus lack of physical activity and being overweight or obese appear to be the most important lifestyle factors causing these cancers [12].

More than 150 epidemiologic studies of physical activity and cancer risk have been carried out. Several possible biological mechanisms relating physical activity and cancer have been proposed, including changes in androgen, estrogen, and metabolic hormone levels and various growth factors; decreased BMI; and possibly changes in immune function. Excess weight and central adiposity have been implicated in promoting metabolic conditions that relate to carcinogenesis [13,14].

One of the most in-depth studies to estimate the number of obesity-related cancers in the United States was reported in 2008 [10]. Using published meta-analyses and/or large cohort studies, it was estimated that 33,966 new cancers (4% of all cancers) in males and 50,535 (7% of all cancers) in females, diagnosed in 2007, or 6% of all cancers, may be attributable to obesity.

Regarding mortality, if the correlation between obesity and cancer is indeed causal, it was estimated that in 2004, obesity accounted for one in seven (14%) cancer deaths in American men and one in five (20%) cancer deaths in American women, or a total of 17% of all cancer deaths in the United States [11]. More recent data would suggest that as many as one-third of the 562,340 cancer deaths in 2009 were related to overweight or obesity, physical inactivity, and poor nutrition. Reflecting on the relationship between tobacco use and cancer, the American Cancer Society reported that, in 2009, approximately 30% of all cancer deaths in the United States were related to the use of tobacco [15]. If these numbers are factual, then obesity may have passed tobacco use as the number one cause of cancer in the United States.

What follows is a more in-depth narrative of the relationship between being overweight or obese and certain cancers that are causally linked to this lifestyle factor.

BREAST CANCER

There is rather irrefutable evidence that obesity increases the risk of a woman developing breast cancer and depends upon a woman's menopausal status. Premenopausal women who are obese actually have a lower risk of developing breast cancer than nonobese premenopausal women [16–19]. Women who are postmenopausal and obese are those who have an increased risk of developing breast cancer, as much as 1.5 times that of women with healthy weights [16,17,20].

While the evidence is not conclusive, studies suggest that the distribution of the adipose tissue in obese women may have significance. Women with abdominal distribution of fat are at greater risk of developing breast cancer rather than those whose fat is predominantly deposited over the hips, buttocks, and thighs [21,22].

It is believed that the increased risk of breast cancer in obese women is due to their having higher levels of estrogen. While the main source of estrogen is the ovaries, adipose tissue is also a producer of this female hormone and becomes the main source of estrogen in the postmenopausal state. Obese postmenopausal women produce nearly twice the level of estrogen as postmenopausal women with healthy weights [18]; therefore, estrogen-sensitive tissues such as estrogen-responsive breast cancers are more apt to be stimulated to grow.

An additional statistic related to obesity and breast cancer is the observation that death rates for this disease are higher in overweight women. Experts believe this can be attributed to a delay in detecting a palpable tumor mass in the obese breast, thus leading to a later stage of disease at diagnosis [19].

While being overweight does not seem to confer a greater risk of developing the disease in African American women, these women, obese or not, have a greater likelihood of having a more advanced stage of disease at diagnosis [23]. Hispanic women who are overweight have a higher risk of breast cancer, irrespective of menopausal status [24].

COLON CANCER

While there is strong evidence for a relationship between obesity and the risk of developing colon cancer, this has been consistently reported for men [25–28], but not for women [25,28,29].

Just as with breast cancer, the distribution of adipose tissue appears to be a factor in those who are obese and at risk for developing colon cancer. Since men with high BMI are generally obese with an increase in abdominal fat, and women with high BMI are more likely to have their adipose tissue distributed around hips, buttocks, and thighs, the risk of colon cancer appears to relate to abdominal fat [27,28].

The mechanism responsible for the increased risk of colon cancer, especially in obese males, is not determined; however, there is some evidence that high levels of insulin or insulin-related growth factors may enhance adenomatous growth in the colon and thereby lead to the evolution of a cancerous tumor [30].

An additional comparison to breast cancer and obesity is the possible causative factor of estrogen. Unlike for breast cancer and uterine cancer (see the following section), the presence of estrogen appears to be protective for colon cancer in women [31]. However, obese women who also take estrogenic hormone replacement therapy (HRT), regardless of menopausal status, increase their risk of developing colon cancer not dissimilar to the risk seen in obese men [32].

ENDOMETRIAL (UTERINE) CANCER

Obesity accounts for more than a third of all cases of endometrial (uterine) cancers [33], and obese women have nearly a four times greater risk of developing uterine cancer than women with healthy weights, irrespective of menopausal status [34–37].

Evidence suggests that high levels of estrogen and higher than normal levels of insulin in overweight or obese women may account for this increased risk [34–36].

ESOPHAGEAL AND GASTRIC CANCER

There is an increase in esophageal and gastric cancer of a particular histology, specifically adenocarcinoma, and location (distal esophagus and gastric cardia at the esophageal–gastric juncture) in obese individuals [38–42]. Obesity confers a two-times greater risk of developing one of these cancers than for individuals who have healthy weights [38–40].

Since it is known that gastric reflux may lead to the development of Barrett's esophagus, a precancerous condition affecting the distal esophagus, reflux has been postulated to be the mechanism that is responsible for the increased risk of adenocarcinoma of the esophagus. However, the evidence is inconclusive, and a precise mechanism has not been determined [41].

KIDNEY CANCER

Obese women are at increased risk of developing kidney cancer (renal cell carcinoma) [43–47]. This risk may be as high as four times that for women who are not overweight. For men, there does not seem to be this association between obesity and renal cell carcinoma [43]. Like other cancers associated with obesity, the exact mechanism is uncertain, but estrogen exposure certainly has been considered an etiologic factor since the risk is gender related.

PROSTATE CANCER

While the overall risk for obese men developing prostate cancer appears to be no greater, perhaps even slightly less, than for men with healthy weights, obese men appear to be at greater risk of developing the more aggressive forms of prostate cancer [48–51].

The observation that obese men may have lower rates of prostate cancer than thinner men may not reflect an actual lower risk, but a lower rate of early detection through prostate cancer screening. Using data from three U.S. government health surveys, researchers found that among men who underwent prostate cancer screening with a prostate-specific antigen (PSA) blood test, obese men generally had lower PSA levels than thinner men. They were also less likely to have their PSA test followed up with a biopsy to rule out or confirm prostate cancer. Of obese men who had ever had PSA screening, 4.6% had undergone a biopsy, versus 5.8% of normal-weight men [52].

Furthermore, mortality studies have yielded conflicting data, at least one such study suggesting that obese men may in fact have a better prognosis than nonobese men with prostate cancer [53].

OTHER CANCERS

An association between obesity and ovarian cancer has not been delineated [54,55]; however, one study described an increased incidence of this cancer in women who were overweight or obese during adolescence or young adulthood [56].

Obesity as a risk factor for pancreatic cancer has been reported in one study [57], but such an association was not confirmed in other reports [58]. It has been suggested that persons who exhibit physical inactivity are at increased risk of developing pancreatic cancer [59].

Women who are obese are at increased risk of developing cancer of the gallbladder [60,61]. Obesity is associated with a high frequency of gallstones, and the relationship between gallbladder cancer and gallstones is a recognized phenomenon.

PHYSICAL ACTIVITY

While caloric intake is the most important determinant of BMI, not to be overlooked in the variables that contribute to one's BMI is the amount of physical activity that an individual undertakes. Clearly, when there is a high intake of calories accompanied by a sedentary lifestyle, the chance of one becoming overweight or obese is greatly increased. Therefore, one may conclude that those cancers that are associated with obesity as a causative factor might become less common in a population that exhibits regular physical activity.

In fact, with colon cancer, such has been observed. Even with moderate levels of physical activity, the risk of developing colon cancer was reduced by 50% [62,63].

With respect to breast cancer, most studies have looked at the effects of physical activity in postmenopausal women where it has been shown that moderate levels of physical activity (e.g., walking approximately 30 min each day) reduced the risk of developing breast cancer by nearly 20%, the greatest benefit experienced by women who were not overweight, with no benefit seen in obese women [64].

The beneficial effects of increased physical activity as it relates to other cancers with a known association with overweight and obesity are unknown. Virtually no controlled studies to examine this question have been undertaken.

A summary of the foregoing information relating to the causality of obesity and certain cancers and data relating to proposed mechanisms and the relationship of physical activity to the respective cancer is shown in Table 15.1.

TABLE 15.1
Obesity: A Causality Factor for Certain Cancers and Related Data

Cancer	Overweight/ Obesity Related	Population at Risk	Proposed Mechanism of Relationship	Physical Activity Related
Breast	+++++	• Obese postmenopausal • Obese Hispanic women	• Estrogen	++ • Postmenopausal women • Women with healthy weight
Colon	+++++	• Obese men • Obese women on HRT	• Abdominal fat • Insulin • Insulin-related growth factors	+++
Uterine	++++	• Obese pre- and postmenopausal	• Estrogen • Insulin	Not studied
Kidney	+++	• Obese women	• Estrogen	Not studied
Esophageal	++	• Obese men and women • Distal esophagus	• Gastric reflux	Not studied
Gastric	++	• Gastric cardia	• Gastric reflux	Not studied
Gallbladder	++	• Obese women	• Gallstones	Not studied
Ovarian	+	• Obesity during youth or early adulthood	• Unknown	Not studied
Pancreatic	+	• Obese men and women	• Decreased physical inactivity	Not studied
Prostate	+	• Obese men with aggressive form	• Unknown	Not studied

+++++, conclusive evidence; ++++, strong evidence; +++, moderate evidence; ++, inconclusive evidence; +, weak evidence.

DIET

Evidence is rather compelling that dietary patterns and dietary elements are etiologic factors for several types of cancer. As many as 35% of cancer deaths may be related to dietary factors [65]. Research shows that diets low in fat and high in fiber, fruits, vegetables, and grains are associated with reduced risks for certain cancers.

Diets high in fat have been linked to breast, colon, and prostate cancers and possibly to pancreas, ovary, and endometrial cancers [66]. The average U.S. diet is estimated to contain nearly 40% of calories from fat, which is significantly higher than that needed to meet the physiological needs for energy and essential fatty acids. The major sources of fat in the American diet are added fats and oils used as spreads, cooking fats, and salad oils, as well as the fat in meats and whole milk dairy products.

Because dietary fat intake is highly correlated with calorie intake, there is the issue as to whether fat intake or caloric intake is the major dietary factor affecting cancer risk. Several studies have looked at the importance of fat intake versus caloric intake and suggest that both have independent effects. Since dietary fat is the most concentrated source of energy of all the nutrients and supplies (9 cal/g compared to 4 cal/g from either carbohydrate or protein), a reduction in dietary fat intake is accompanied by a decrease in total calorie intake and body weight [67,68].

Evidence suggests that diets high in fiber are associated with a reduced risk for cancer, especially cancer of the colon [69]. This may also be true for cancers of the breast, rectum, oral cavity, pharynx, and stomach [70].

With respect to fruits and vegetables, it has been observed that populations whose diets are rich in fruits and vegetables have a lower risk for cancers of the lung, colon and rectum, breast, oral cavity, esophagus, stomach, pancreas, uterine cervix, and ovary. Fruits, vegetables, and grains contain a number of nutrients, including carotenoids, vitamin A, and vitamin C. For most cancer sites, especially those of the respiratory and digestive tracts, persons with low fruit and vegetable intake had about twice the risk of cancer as those with high intake [71].

The current dietary recommendation is for five servings of fruit and vegetables a day, and Americans fall somewhat short of this goal. Only approximately 20% of the population is achieving this goal with the average daily intake of only three and a half daily servings of fruits and vegetables [72].

In addition to vitamins A and C and the carotenoids, fruits, vegetables, and grains contain other vitamins and minerals associated with a protective effect against cancer.

Vitamin E has inhibited tumors in experimental animals and been linked to reduced risks of oral, stomach, and other cancer in epidemiologic studies. Selenium also may have a protective effect. In a recent randomized large-population trial testing the effectiveness of vitamin/mineral supplementation among persons in high-risk areas of China, those who received daily supplements with a combination of beta-carotene, vitamin E, and selenium for 5 years had a significantly lower cancer death rate [73]. The findings do not automatically translate to Western populations—in that the Chinese population studied was chronically deficient in a number of nutrients—but offer a hopeful sign that certain vitamins and minerals may lower risk of some cancers. However, two other recent large randomized trials of supplements, one testing the effect of supplemental beta-carotene or alpha-tocopherol in the prevention of lung cancer among smokers and the other testing the effect of supplemental beta-carotene and vitamins C and E in the prevention of adenomatous polyps (a precursor lesion for colorectal cancer), suggest that supplemental use of these nutrients does not reduce the risk of either lung or colorectal cancer [74,75]. In the study of the effect of beta-carotene or alpha-tocopherol on lung cancer among smokers, dietary intake of these nutrients from foods was associated with a reduced risk for lung cancer [74]. Some studies suggest that calcium may play a protective role in colon cancer. A 19 year prospective study in men showed the risk for colon cancer was lower in those with the highest calcium intake [76]. In addition to dairy products, certain vegetables are good sources of calcium, notably roots, okra, and dark green leafy vegetables such as collard greens.

REFERENCES

1. White, C. 1990. Research on smoking and lung cancer: A landmark in the history of chronic disease epidemiology. *Yale Journal of Biology and Medicine* 63: 29–46.
2. Proctor, R.N. 1997. The Nazi war on tobacco: Ideology, evidence, and possible cancer consequences. *Bulletin of the History of Medicine* 71: 435–488.
3. U.S. Department of Health and Human Services. 2004. The health consequences of smoking. A Report of the Surgeon General. Atlanta, GA: U.S. Department of Health and Human Services, Centers for Disease Control and Prevention, National Center for Chronic Disease Prevention and Health Promotion, Office on Smoking and Health.
4. U.S. Department of Health and Human Services. 2000. Reducing tobacco use. A Report of the Surgeon General. Atlanta, GA: U.S. Department of Health and Human Services, Public Health Service, Centers for Disease Control and Prevention, National Center for Chronic Disease Prevention and Health Promotion, Office on Smoking and Health.
5. Kotlyar, M. and Hatsukami, D.K. 2002. Managing nicotine addiction. *Journal of Dental Education* 66: 1061–1073.
6. George, T.P. and O'Malley, S.S. 2004. Current pharmacological treatments for nicotine dependence. *Trends in Pharmacological Sciences* 25: 42–48.
7. Jemal, A., Siegel, R., Xu, J. et al. 2010. Cancer statistics, 2010. *CA: A Cancer Journal for Clinicians* 60: 277–300.
8. Ogden, C.L., Carroll, M.D., Curtin, L.R., et al. 2010. Prevalence of high body mass index in US children and adolescents, 2007–2008. *Journal of the American Medical Association* 303(3): 242–249.
9. Flegal, K.M., Carroll, M.D., Ogden, C.L., et al. 2010. Prevalence and trends in obesity among US adults, 1999–2008. *Journal of the American Medical Association* 303(3): 235–241.
10. Polednak, A.P. 2008. Estimating the number of U.S. incident cancers attributable to obesity and the impact on temporal trends in incidence rates for obesity-related cancers. *Cancer Detection and Prevention* 32: 190–199.
11. Calle, E.E. and Thun, M.J. 2004. Obesity and cancer: Review. *Oncogene* 23: 6365–6378.
12. Vainio, H., Kaaks, R., and Bianchini, F. 2002. Weight control and physical activity in cancer prevention: International evaluation of the evidence: Review. *European Journal of Cancer Prevention* 11 (Suppl. 2): 94–100.
13. Friedenreich, C.M. 2001. Physical activity and cancer prevention: From observational to intervention research. *Cancer Epidemiology, Biomarkers and Prevention* 10: 287–301.

14. Friedenreich, C.M. and Orenstein, M.R. 2002. Physical activity and cancer prevention: Etiologic evidence and biological mechanisms. *Journal of Nutrition* 132 (11 Suppl.): 3456–3464.

15. American Cancer Society. Cancer prevention and early detection facts and figures 2008. http://www.cancer.org/Research/CancerFactsFigures/CancerFactsFigures/cancer-facts-figures-2008

16. van den Brandt, P.A., Spiegelman, D., Yuan, S.S. et al. 2000. Pooled analysis of prospective cohort studies on height, weight, and breast cancer risk. *American Journal of Epidemiology* 152: 514–527.

17. Trentham-Dietz, A., Newcomb, P.A., Storer, B.E. et al. 1997. Body size and risk of breast cancer. *American Journal of Epidemiology* 145: 1011–1019.

18. Huang, Z., Hankinson, S.E., Cloditz, G.A. et al. 1997. Dual effects of weight and weight gain on breast cancer risk. *Journal of the American Medical Association* 278: 1407–1411.

19. Cui, Y., Whiteman, M.K., Flaws, J.A. et al. 2002. Body mass and stage of breast cancer at diagnosis. *International Journal of Cancer* 98: 279–283.

20. Yoo, K.Y., Tajima, K., Park, S. et al. 2001. Postmenopausal obesity as a breast cancer risk factor according to estrogen and progesterone receptor status (Japan). *Cancer Letters* 167: 57–63.

21. Friedenreich, C.M. 2001. Review of anthropometric factors and breast cancer risk. *European Journal of Cancer Prevention* 10: 15–32.

22. Kaaks, R., Van Noord, P.A.H., Den Tonkelaar, I. et al. 1998. Breast cancer incidence in relation to height, weight and body-fat distribution in the Dutch "DOM" cohort. *International Journal of Cancer* 76: 647–651.

23. Cui, Y., Whiteman, M.K., Langenberg, P. et al. 2002. Can obesity explain the racial difference in stage of breast cancer at diagnosis between black and white women? *Journal of Women's Health and Gender-Based Medicine* 11: 527–536.

24. Wenten, M., Gilliland, F.D., Baumgartner, K. et al. 2001. Associations of weight, weight change, and body mass with breast cancer risk in Hispanic and non-Hispanic white women. *Annals of Epidemiology* 12: 435–444.

25. Caan, B.J., Coates, A.O., Slattery, M.L. et al. 1998. Body size and the risk of colon cancer in a large case-control study. *International Journal of Obesity and Related Metabolic Disorders* 22: 178–184.

26. Shike, M. 1996. Body weight and colon cancer. *American Journal of Clinical Nutrition* 63 (3 Suppl.): 442–444.

27. Giacosa, A., Franceschi, S., La Vecchia, C. et al. 1999. Energy intake, overweight, physical exercise and colorectal cancer risk. *European Journal of Cancer Prevention* 8(Suppl. 1): S53–S60.

28. Murphy, T.K., Calle, E.E., Rodriguez, C. et al. 2000. Body mass index and colon cancer mortality in a large prospective study. *American Journal of Epidemiology* 152: 847–854.

29. Phillips, R.L. and Snowdon, D.A. 1985. Dietary relationships with fatal colorectal cancer among Seventh-Day Adventists. *Journal of the National Cancer Institute* 74: 307–317.

30. McKeown-Eyssen, G. 1994. Epidemiology of colorectal cancer revisited: Are serum triglycerides and/or plasma glucose associated with risk? *Cancer Epidemiology, Biomarkers and Prevention* 3: 687–695.

31. Writing Group for the Women's Health Initiative Investigators. 2002. Risks and benefits of estrogen plus progestin in healthy postmenopausal women: Principal results from the Women's Health Initiative randomized controlled trial. *Journal of the American Medical Association* 288: 321–333.

32. Slattery, M.L., Ballard-Barbash, R., Edwards, S. et al. 2003. Body mass index and colon cancer: An evaluation of the modifying effects of estrogen (United States). *Cancer Causes and Control* 14: 75–84.

33. Bergstrom, A., Pisani, P.M., Tenet, V. et al. 2001. Overweight as an avoidable cause of cancer in Europe. *International Journal of Cancer* 91: 421–430.

34. Salazar-Martínez, E., Lazcano-Ponce, E.C., Lira-Lira, G.G. et al. 2000. Case-control study of diabetes, obesity, physical activity and risk of endometrial cancer among Mexican women. *Cancer Causes and Control* 11: 707–711.

35. Shoff, S.M. and Newcomb, P.A. 1998. Diabetes, body size, and risk of endometrial cancer. *American Journal of Epidemiology* 148: 234–240.

36. Weiderpass, E., Persson, I., Adami, H.O. et al. 2000. Body size in different periods of life, diabetes mellitus, hypertension, and risk of postmenopausal endometrial cancer (Sweden). *Cancer Causes and Control* 11: 185–192.

37. Goodman, M.T., Hankin, J.H., Wilkens, L.R. et al. 1997. Diet, body size, physical activity, and the risk of endometrial cancer. *Cancer Research* 57: 5077–5085.

38. Brown, L.M., Swanson, C.A., Gridley, G. et al. 1995. Adenocarcinoma of the esophagus: Role of obesity and diet. *Journal of the National Cancer Institute* 87: 104–109.

39. Chow, W.H., Blot, W.J., Vaughan, T.L. et al. 1998. Body mass index and risk of adenocarcinomas of the esophagus and gastric cardia. *Journal of the National Cancer Institute* 90: 150–155.

40. Li, S.D. and Mobarhan, S. 2000. Association between body mass index and adenocarcinoma of the esophagus and gastric cardia. *Nutrition Reviews* 58: 54–56.

41. Lagergren, J., Bergström, R., and Nyrén, O. 1999. Association between body mass and adenocarcinoma of the esophagus and gastric cardia. *Annals of Internal Medicine* 130: 883–890.

42. Ji, B.T., Chow, W.H., Yang, G. et al. 1997. Body mass index and the risk of cancers of the gastric cardia and distal stomach in Shanghai, China. *Cancer Epidemiology, Biomarkers and Prevention* 6: 481–485.

43. Chow, W.H., McLaughlin, J.K., Mandel, J.S. et al. 1996. Obesity and risk of renal cell cancer. *Cancer Epidemiology, Biomarkers and Prevention* 5: 17–21.

44. Yuan, J.M., Castelao, J.E., Gago-Domingues, M. et al. 1998. Hypertension, obesity and their medications in relation to renal cell carcinoma. *British Journal of Cancer* 77: 1508–1513.

45. Lindblad, P., Wolk, A., Bergstrom, R. et al. 1994. The role of obesity and weight fluctuations in the etiology of renal cell cancer: A population-based case-control study. *Cancer Epidemiology, Biomarkers and Prevention* 3: 631–639.

46. Hu, J., Mao, Y., White, K. 2003. Overweight and obesity in adults and risk of renal cell carcinoma in Canada. *Sozial-und Präventivmedizin* 48: 178–185.

47. Bergstrom, A., Hsieh, C.C., Lindblad, P. et al. 2001. Obesity and renal cell cancer—A quantitative review. *British Journal of Cancer* 85: 984–990.

48. Nomura, A.M. 2001. Body size and prostate cancer. *Epidemiologic Reviews* 23: 126–131.

49. Cerhan, J.R., Torer, J.C., Lynch, C.F. et al. 1997. Association of smoking, body mass, and physical activity with risk of prostate cancer in the Iowa 65+ Rural Health Study (United States). *Cancer Causes and Control* 8: 229–238.

50. Putnam, S.D., Cerhan, J.R., Parker, A.S. et al. 2000. Lifestyle and anthropometric risk factors for prostate cancer in a cohort of Iowa men. *Annals of Epidemiology* 10: 361–369.

51. Irani, J., Lefebvre, O., Murat, F. et al. 2003. Obesity in relation to prostate cancer risk: Comparison with a population having benign prostatic hyperplasia. *British Journal of Urology International* 91(6): 482–484.

52. Parekh, N., Lin, Y., DiPaola, R.S. et al. 2010. Obesity and prostate cancer detection: Insights from three national surveys. *American Journal of Medicine* 123: 829–835.

53. Daniell, H.W. 1996. A better prognosis for obese men with prostate cancer. *Journal of Urology* 155: 220–225.

54. Greggi, S., Parazzini, F., Paratore, M.P. et al. 2000. Risk factors for ovarian cancer in central Italy. *Gynecologic Oncology* 79: 50–54.

55. Hartge, P., Schiffman, M.H., Hoover, R. et al. 1989. A case-control study of epithelial ovarian cancer. *American Journal of Obstetrics and Gynecology* 161: 10–16.

56. Engeland, A., Tretli, S., and Bjorge, T. 2003. Height, body mass index, and ovarian cancer: A follow-up of 1.1 million Norwegian women. *Journal of the National Cancer Institute* 95: 1244–1248.

57. Berrington de Gonzalez, A., Sweetland, S., and Spencer, E. 2003. A meta-analysis of obesity and the risk of pancreatic cancer. *British Journal of Cancer* 89: 519–523.

58. Ji, B.T., Hatch, M.C., Chow, W.H. et al. 1996. Anthropometric and reproductive factors and the risk of pancreatic cancer: A case-control study in Shanghai, China. *International Journal of Cancer* 66: 432–437.

59. Michaud, D., Giovannucci, E., Willett, W.C. et al. 2001. Physical activity, obesity, height, and the risk of pancreatic cancer. *Journal of the American Medical Association* 286: 921–929.

60. Lowenfels, A.B., Maisonneuve, P., Boyle, P. et al. 1999. Epidemiology of gallbladder cancer. *Hepato-Gastroenterology* 46: 1529–1532.

61. Moerman, C.J. and Bueno-de-Mesquita, H.B. 1999. The epidemiology of gallbladder cancer: Lifestyle-related risk factors and limited surgical possibilities for prevention. *Hepato-Gastroenterology* 46: 1533–1539.

62. Vainio, H. and Bianchini, F. 2002. *IARC Handbooks of Cancer Prevention* Volume 6: *Weight Control and Physical Activity*. Lyon, France: IARC Press.

63. Martinez, M.E., Giovanucci, E., Speigelman, D. et al. 1997. Leisure-time physical activity, body size and colon cancer in women. Nurses' Health Study Research Group. *Journal of the National Cancer Institute* 89: 948–955.

64. McTiernan, A., Kooperberg, C., White, E. et al. 2003. Recreational physical activity and the risk of breast cancer in postmenopausal women: The Women's Health Initiative Cohort Study. *Journal of the American Medical Association* 290: 1331–1336.

65. Doll, R. and Peto, R. 1981. The causes of cancer: Quantitative estimates of avoidable risks of cancer in the United States today. *Journal of the National Cancer Institute* 66: 1191–1308.

66. U.S. Department of Health and Human Services. 1988. The Surgeon General's Report on Nutrition and Health. DHHS (PHS) Publ. No. 88-50210. Washington, DC: Department of Health and Human Services, Public Health Service.

67. Boyd, N.F., Cousins, M., Lockwood, G. et al. 1990. The feasibility of testing experimentally the dietary fat-breast cancer hypothesis. *British Journal of Cancer* 62: 878–881.

68. Henderson, M.M., Kushi, L.H., Thompson, D.J. et al. 1990. Feasibility of a randomized trial of a low-fat diet for the prevention of breast cancer: Dietary compliance in the Women's Health Trial Vanguard Study. *Preventive Medicine* 19: 115–133.

69. Trock, B., Lanza, E., and Greenwald, P. 1990. Dietary fiber, vegetables and colon cancer: Critical review and meta-analysis of the epidemiologic evidence. *Journal of the National Cancer Institute* 82: 650–661.

70. Lanza, E., Shankar, S., and Trock, B. 1992. Dietary fiber. In *Macronutrients: Investigating their Role in Cancer*, Micozzi, M.S., Moon, T.E., eds. New York: Marcel Dekker, Inc., pp. 293–319.

71. Block, G., Patterson, B., and Subar, A. 1992. Fruit, vegetables, and cancer prevention: A review of the epidemiologic evidence. *Nutrition and Cancer* 18: 1–29.

72. Subar, A.S., Heimendinger, J., and Krebs-Smith, S. 1992. 5-A-Day for better health: A baseline study of American fruit and vegetable consumption. Rockville, MD: NCI, NIH (Executive summary).

73. Blot, W.J., Li, J.Y., Taylor, P.R. et al. 1993. Nutrition intervention trials in Linxian, China: Supplementation with specific vitamin/mineral combinations, cancer incidence, and disease-specific mortality in the general population. *Journal of the National Cancer Institute* 85: 1483–1492.

74. The ATBC Cancer Prevention Study Group. 1994. The effect of vitamin E and beta-carotene on the incidence of lung cancer and other cancers in male smokers. *The New England Journal of Medicine* 330: 1029–1035.

75. Greenberg, E.R., Baron, J.A., Tosteson, T.D. et al. 1994. A clinical trial of antioxidant vitamins to prevent colorectal adenoma. *The New England Journal of Medicine* 331: 141–144.

76. Garland, C., Barrett-Connor, E., Rossof, A.H. et al. 1985. Dietary vitamin D and calcium and risk of colorectal cancer: A 19-year prospective study in men. *Lancet* 1: 307–309.

16 Obesity and Arthritis

Antonios Stavropoulos-Kalinoglou, PhD,
Athanasios Z. Jamurtas, PhD, Yiannis
Koutedakis, PhD, and George D. Kitas, MD, PhD

CONTENTS

INTRODUCTION

The term "arthritis" (from Greek: *arthro-*, joint, and *-itis*, inflammation) was first introduced by Hippocrates (ca. 460 BC to ca. 370 BC) who saw the condition primarily as a metabolic disease, although its main manifestations are in the joints and articular structures. We now know that arthritis may affect any of the structures inside a joint, such as the synovium, bones, cartilage, or supporting tissues. As any inflammatory condition, arthritis gives rise to the five cardinal signs of inflammation as identified by Celsus (30 BC to AD 32) and R.L.K. Virchow (1821–1902): pain (dolor), heat (calor), redness (rubor), swelling (tumor), and, if left untreated, loss of function (functio laesa) [1].

Inflammation is the normal response of the immune system to antigens; it is a complex biological reaction of the vascularized connective tissue that leads to accumulation of fluid and leukocytes in extravascular tissue. Inflammation, fundamentally a protective response, is tightly controlled by the immune system as uncontrolled inflammation can be harmful or even fatal. Life-threatening allergies and common chronic inflammatory and autoimmune diseases are such examples [2]; in general, inflammation can be divided into acute and chronic patterns. Both patterns of inflammation aim to destroy, dilute, or fend off the harmful agents, but also they initiate the process of healing in the damaged tissues.

Acute inflammation is the immediate and early response to an infectious agent; it is of short duration, usually lasting minutes, hours, or even a few days. Transition from acute to chronic inflammation occurs when the former cannot be resolved due to the persistence of the infectious agent or to some interference in the process of healing [2]. Chronic inflammation is of longer duration, and although it may follow acute inflammation, the chronic stage often begins insidiously, as a low grade, initially asymptomatic response. This latter type of chronic inflammation is the cause of some common diseases, including certain types of arthritis.

Several different types of arthritis have been indentified (Table 16.1). They occur either as primary or secondary conditions due to underlying diseases. Even though "inflammation" is inherent in the definition of any type of arthritis, arthritides are often categorized as noninflammatory and inflammatory, mostly due to their pathogenesis. Noninflammatory arthritides are usually products of mechanical misuse or overuse of a joint while the inflammatory equivalents have an autoimmune component. Osteoarthritis (OA) is the most common noninflammatory arthritis with a prevalence of >10% in the general population and increasing with age [3]—*it has been recently shown that low-grade inflammation is involved in its pathogenesis.* The most common high-grade inflammatory arthritis is rheumatoid arthritis (RA) with a prevalence of 0.5%–1% in the westernized countries [4]. The other types of arthritis are more rare, and thus the focus of this chapter will be on OA and RA. The exact causes for both cases are still unknown; what is clear, however, is that genetic and environmental factors contribute to their development.

TABLE 16.1
Different Types of Arthritis

OA
RA
Septic arthritis
Gout and pseudogout
Juvenile idiopathic arthritis
Still's disease
Ankylosing spondylitis
Ehlers–Danlos syndrome (hypermobility)
Psoriatic arthritis
Reactive arthritis

OSTEOARTHRITIS

OA refers to a clinical syndrome of joint pain accompanied by varying degrees of functional limitation and reduced quality of life. It is by far the most common form of arthritis and one of the leading causes of pain and disability worldwide. It can affect any synovial joint, particularly knees, hips, and small hand joints [5]. Symptoms usually include joint pain, tenderness, stiffness, swelling, and reduced function; asymptomatic cases with obvious structural alterations are commonly observed.

Key pathological changes include localized loss of articular (hyaline) cartilage and remodeling of adjacent bone with new bone formation (osteophyte). This combination of tissue loss and new tissue synthesis supports the view of OA as the repair process of synovial joints. A variety of joint traumas may trigger the need to repair, but once initiated, all the joint tissues take part, showing increased cell activity and new tissue production. In general, OA is a slow but efficient repair process that often compensates for the initial trauma, resulting in a structurally altered but symptom-free joint. In some people, however, either because of overwhelming insult or compromised repair potential, the OA process cannot compensate, resulting in continuing tissue damage and eventual presentation with symptomatic OA or "joint failure" [6]. The fact that OA favors certain joints remains unexplained; one hypothesis suggests an evolutionary fault where joints that have most recently altered are biomechanically underdesigned and thus fail more often. The end result of this is partial or complete damage to the joint cartilage that protects the bones; when this protection is lost, bone may be exposed and damaged resulting in significant pain and joint disuse. The latter has been linked to atrophy of regional musculature and ligament laxity [5].

POTENTIAL CAUSES OF OA AND THE ROLE OF OBESITY

OA is a multifactorial condition with no single etiology; there are multiple risk factors that contribute to its development. These are generally divided into three categories: genetic, biomechanical, and constitutional factors [5].

Evidence of a genetic influence comes from a number of sources, including epidemiological studies of family history and family clustering, twin studies, and exploration of rare genetic disorders. Classic twin studies have shown that the influence of genetic factors is between 39% and 65% in radiographic OA of the hand and knee in women, about 60% in OA of the hip, and about 70% in OA of the spine. Taken together, these estimates suggest a heritability of OA of more than 50%, indicating that at least half of the variation in susceptibility to disease can be explained by genetic factors alone. Studies have implicated linkages to OA on chromosomes 2q, 9q, 11q, and 16p, among others. Genes concerned include VDR, AGC1, IGF-1, ER alpha, transforming growth factor beta (TGF beta), CRTM (cartilage matrix protein), CRTL (cartilage link protein), GPR22, and collagens II, IX, and XI. Genes may operate differently in the two sexes, at different body sites, and on different disease features within body sites [7]. Recent studies have also identified genes in the bone morphogenetic pathway (e.g., GDF5), the thyroid regulation pathway (DIO2), and apoptotic pathways as involved in genetic risk of large joint OA. Genome-wide associations have reported structural genes (COL6A4), inflammation-related genes (PTGS2/PLA2G4A), and a locus on chromosome 7q22 (GPR22 and four other genes in the same linkage disequilibrium block) associated with OA [8].

Biomechanical risk factors such as previous joint injury, occupational and recreational usage, reduced muscle strength, joint laxity, or joint malalignment are commonly reported by OA patients. However, their validity as risk factors is not clear. In a recent meta-analysis, previous joint injury was identified as one of the most significant risk factors consistently associated with the development of OA (odds ratio [OR] = 3.86; 95% confidence interval [CI] = 2.61, 5.70) [9]. Results from studies looking at occupational usage are not equivocal. Overall, a protective effect of sitting (<2 h per day) has been reported, whereas excessive kneeling, squatting, climbing steps, standing (>2 h per day), and lifting may associate with OA. Recreational exercise such as walking does not normally associate with OA. Conversely, in athletes and people who exercise excessively or intensively, OA is more common than the general population [9].

Constitutional factors such as bone mineral density, age, gender, and body weight have also been implicated in the development and progression of OA. Bone mineral density has shown a consistent strong association with knee OA [10,11]. Similarly, increasing age associates with a higher incidence of OA [9], most likely due to the length of exposure to joint damaging forces. The effect of age seems to diminish after an age of 80 [12]. Women have higher incidence rates of knee OA [12] and are almost twice as likely as men to develop the condition (OR = 1.84; 95% CI = 1.32, 2.55) [9]. The cause of that is not clear, as estrogens seem to have a protective effect against OA. The fact that women usually live to an older age than men might explain part of the variance. However, the most possible explanation is that women naturally have higher body fat reserves than men. Indeed, obesity is the single strongest and most consistent constitutional risk factor for OA. The association of obesity with OA was first established in 1945 [13], since then numerous studies have verified the significant impact of obesity on the joints and especially the knee [14,15]. Overall, two-thirds of adults with doctor-diagnosed OA are overweight or obese (compared to 53% without OA) [16], while >30% of obese individuals suffer from OA compared to ~15% of nonobese adults [3]. Women with OA have on average a BMI that is about 24% higher than that of women without OA [17]. Similarly, twins with OA are 3–5 kg heavier than their non-OA co-twin. For every kilogram increase in body weight, a twin has 9%, 14%, and 32% increased risk for developing carpometacarpal, tibiofemoral, or patellofemoral osteophytes, respectively, compared to its co-twin [18,19].

OBESITY AND KNEE OA

Knee OA shows the highest associations with obesity. In a study in the 1970s, when obesity was not as frequent as it is today, 83% of females diagnosed with OA of the knee were reported to be obese (compared to 42% in the control group) [20]. In a recent meta-analysis on the same subject [9], the authors found 36 papers discussing the association of obesity with OA. All papers agreed that overweight or obesity is a risk factor for future knee problems. Overall, being overweight is more than twice as likely (OR = 2.18; 95% CI = 1.86, 2.55) to lead to knee OA, while being obese

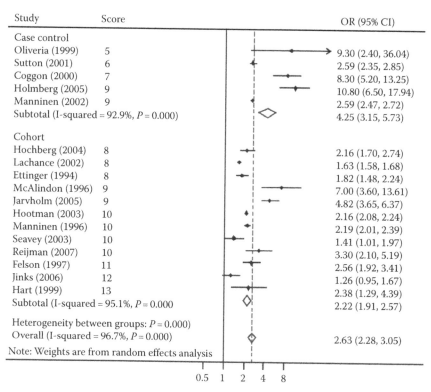

Study	Score		OR (95% CI)
Case control			
Oliveria (1999)	5		9.30 (2.40, 36.04)
Sutton (2001)	6		2.59 (2.35, 2.85)
Coggon (2000)	7		8.30 (5.20, 13.25)
Holmberg (2005)	9		10.80 (6.50, 17.94)
Manninen (2002)	9		2.59 (2.47, 2.72)
Subtotal (I-squared = 92.9%, P = 0.000)			4.25 (3.15, 5.73)
Cohort			
Hochberg (2004)	8		2.16 (1.70, 2.74)
Lachance (2002)	8		1.63 (1.58, 1.68)
Ettinger (1994)	8		1.82 (1.48, 2.24)
McAlindon (1996)	9		7.00 (3.60, 13.61)
Jarvholm (2005)	9		4.82 (3.65, 6.37)
Hootman (2003)	10		2.16 (2.08, 2.24)
Manninen (1996)	10		2.19 (2.01, 2.39)
Seavey (2003)	10		1.41 (1.01, 1.97)
Reijman (2007)	10		3.30 (2.10, 5.19)
Felson (1997)	11		2.56 (1.92, 3.41)
Jinks (2006)	12		1.26 (0.95, 1.67)
Hart (1999)	13		2.38 (1.29, 4.39)
Subtotal (I-squared = 95.1%, P = 0.000			2.22 (1.91, 2.57)
Heterogeneity between groups: P = 0.000)			
Overall (I-squared = 96.7%, P = 0.000)			2.63 (2.28, 3.05)
Note: Weights are from random effects analysis			

0.5   1   2   4   8

FIGURE 16.1 Forest plot of effect of obesity on onset of knee OA. (From Blagojevic, M. et al., *Osteoarthr. Cartil.*, 18, 24, 2010. With permission.)

is 2.63 times as likely (2.28, 3.05) compared to normal weights. Overall, a BMI of more than $25\,kg/m^2$ (i.e., being either overweight or obese) has an almost threefold increase in OA risk (OR = 2.96; 2.56, 3.43). Figure 16.1 shows the variation in OR across studies for obesity.

The associations of obesity with knee OA seem to be independent of age and gender [21]. However, they are affected by degree of obesity [22]. For every 2 units of BMI gain, the risk of knee OA increases by 36% [23] with class III overweight individuals (BMI > $40\,kg/m^2$) having an almost 10-fold relative risk for OA development [24]. Time of exposure (i.e., years of being obese) is also important; people developing obesity at an earlier age have higher risk for OA. However, even small increases in body weight during adulthood increase the risk of developing OA [25]. Interestingly, increasing weight from normal to overweight during adult life may give a slightly higher risk of developing knee OA leading to arthroplasty than being constantly overweight during adult life [26].

From the previous discussion, obesity seems to be a cause rather than a result of OA. And weight loss may significantly reduce the odds for developing OA [27,28]. The importance of prevention of knee OA is further highlighted by the subsequent burden of surgery [29]. An estimated 69% of knee replacements in middle-aged women in the United Kingdom have been attributable to obesity [30].

OBESITY AND HAND OA

The site most commonly affected by OA is the small joints of the hand. In contrast to knee OA, data regarding the association of obesity with hand OA are conflicting. A significant association between obesity and OA of the distal interphalangeal joints has been reported, even though this is more prevalent in men [31]. The New Haven Survey identified obesity as a significant predictor for finger OA especially in women [32], and a longitudinal, prospective study in Sweden also showed an association of obesity with hand OA in people over the age of 70 [33]. Data from prospective studies have shown that obesity is a good predictor for hand OA [34,35] with obese individuals having a greater than fivefold increased risk [34]. In recent years, a 10 year follow-up study by Grotle et al. [36] found a significant association of initial BMI with hand OA (OR = 2.59; 1.08–6.19).

These results are not consistently confirmed. Data from the National Health Examination Survey indicated a significant association of obesity with hand OA, but only following adjustment for age, race, and skinfold thickness; further adjustments for waist circumference and seat breadth eliminated these associations [37]. Similarly, other large cross-sectional studies have failed to show significant associations between obesity and hand OA [38,39]. More recently, this notion was further supported by a review of Doherty et al. [40] who concluded that BMI and waist circumference were not significant predictors of hand OA. Furthermore, Kalichman and Kobyliansky were not able to find any association between BMI or waist circumference with hand OA concluding that obesity is a mechanical rather than a systemic risk factor [41].

OBESITY AND HIP OA

Similarly to hand OA, the association of hip OA with obesity is not consistent. In the National Health and Nutrition Examination Study (NHANES), relative weight was faintly associated with OA of the hips only in white women and nonwhite men [42]. Other studies have reported stronger associations where obesity associates with a two to threefold increased risk for hip OA compared to normal weight [43–45]. Two Swedish case-control studies examined BMI in men and women who had undergone total hip replacement surgery and compared them to the general population. Men with a BMI greater than one standard deviation above the mean had an increased risk for developing hip OA, while those who were obese at the age of 40 had a 2.5-fold increased risk for later surgery of the hip [46]. Likewise, overweight women at the age of 40 had a 2.9 increase in risk for surgery by the age of 50 [47].

In contrast, large longitudinal studies failed to find any associations between obesity and hip OA [48–50]. These studies included more than 7000 participants and were able to control for several potential confounding factors. However, obesity was not a significant predictor of hip OA in either young (20–29 years) [49] or older [48] individuals. On the same line, Grotle et al. [36], in their 10 year follow up study, were unable to uncover any associations of obesity and hip OA (OR = 1.11; 0.41–2.97).

MECHANISMS FOR OBESITY IN THE PATHOGENESIS OF OA

The exact way by which obesity increases the risk for OA is not clear. However, two potential mechanisms are most likely to play a significant role: (1) direct biomechanical factors from the increased load on weight-bearing joints and (2) indirect systemic factors from the inflammatory nature of obesity.

Biomechanical Factors

Increasing body weight has a direct effect on vertical ground reaction forces (GRFs). Simply for standing, obese males exert 53% more GRF, while females 45% [51]. During walking at normal speeds, this difference reaches up to 60% [52]. This has a direct effect on plantar pressures (Figure 16.2) and results in a larger forefoot width while standing and walking [53] commonly causing plantar fasciitis and heel pain [54,55], also present in older adults with OA [56].

Increased GRF may initiate cartilage breakdown or promote joint destruction after the initial incipient lesion most likely due to increased forces on the cartilage [57]. Moreover, obesity is known to increase subchondral bony stiffness; this could further increase the forces applied to the cartilage by making subchondral bone less deformable to increased loads thus transmitting greater forces to the overlying cartilage [58]. It may also reduce joint space within the knee [59].

In theory, increased GRFs initiate muscle synthesis and, in conjunction with the fact that during periods of weight gain both fat and fat-free mass increase, could lead to stronger obese individuals compared to their nonobese counterparts [60]. However, when strength is corrected for body weight, both obese males and females are weaker compared to controls irrespective of age [61]. In adults 60–80 years of age, mean knee strength in obese males and females is 65% and 50% of body weight, respectively, compared to 77% and 62% for their nonobese counterparts [61,62].

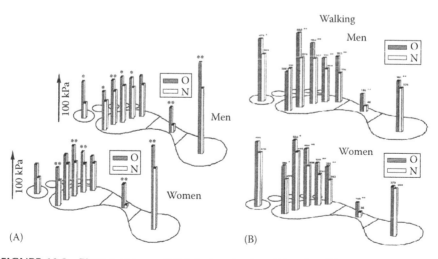

FIGURE 16.2 Plantar pressures (kPa) during standing (A) and walking (B) for obese (O) vs. nonobese (N) men and women. *$P < 0.05$; **$P < 0.01$. (From Hills, A.P. et al., *Int. J. Obes. Relat. Metab. Disord.*, 25, 1674, 2001. With permission.)

This relative muscular weakness is also a significant predictor for falls [63], the leading cause for injury and death in the elderly. Obesity further adds to such risk by affecting balance [64,65]. Indeed, risk of injury increases with BMI; normal-weight individuals have a 15% risk while obese a 48% [66].

This fear is a very likely explanation for some of the observed changes in the gait of obese people. They tend to walk with bilateral abducted forefeet (toes pointing outward) [67]. Most likely this is an adjustment to counteract the imbalance caused by their excess weight and minimize their chances of falling. A wider stance increases the surface area allowing for more sidewise movement. However, this reduces their ability to move effectively and swiftly in a straight line. Moreover, obese people have more rear-foot motion. Touchdown angle, pronation range of motion, and pronation velocity are increased, all of which may result in injury and pain further contributing to the development and progression of OA [67].

Despite the larger mass obese people need to carry when walking, hip and knee torques seem to be unaffected, while ankle torques increase [68]. Specifically, the ankle plantar flexors act eccentrically to control the forward motion of the leg throughout stance, to stabilize body mass, and, at toe-off, to assist in propulsion. The greater mass in obese people requires more ankle plantar flexor torque to perform these tasks [62]. The lack of differences for the knee and hip joint is most likely due to a shortening in stride length observed among obese. BMI associates inversely with stride length and ratio of knee extensor/flexor torque. At high BMIs, flexor torque becomes greater than extensor torque making hamstring muscles, instead of quadriceps, responsible for knee stabilization [68].

Systemic Factors

Low-grade inflammation may be implicated in the pathogenesis of OA. It may contribute to functional limitation, disease progression, and lower pain threshold [62]. OA patients exhibit increased levels of circulating inflammatory markers such as the cytokines interleukin-6 (IL-6) and tumor necrosis factor alpha (TNF-α) and the acute-phase reactant C-reactive protein. High serum levels of these markers predict increased radiographic progression of knee OA as much as 5 years later. Inflammation also associates with OA severity and physical function. Interleukin-1 beta (IL-1β) is present in the joint fluids of patients with OA and is believed to play a role in mediating joint inflammation and cartilage degradation. Diffusion of cytokines from the synovial fluid into the cartilage could contribute to the cartilage matrix loss observed in OA by stimulating chondrocyte catabolic activity and inhibiting anabolic activity [62].

Obesity has been increasingly recognized as a low-grade inflammatory condition, and adipose tissue is not considered merely an energy storage depot but an active endocrine/paracrine organ that secretes a number of bioactive molecules called adipokines [69]. The term "adipokine" refers to bioactive molecules found in the adipocytes; however, these bioactive molecules might be synthesized at other sites and participate in functions unrelated to the adipose tissue [70]. Adipokines have several different functions such as regulation of energy intake and expenditure [71,72]; most of them are also implicated in regulation of inflammation [69] (Table 16.2). As a general rule, increased adiposity associates with heightened production of

TABLE 16.2

Association of Adipokines with Obesity and Inflammation

Adipokine	Effect of Obesity	Effects on Inflammation
Leptin	↑ Plasma concentration	↑ T-cell activation
		↓ Thymocyte apoptosis
		↑ Thymocyte maturation
		↑ Proliferation and apoptosis of naive T cells
		↓ Proliferation of memory T cells
		↓ Apoptosis of B cells
		↑ Peripheral B-cell pool
		↑ Lymphopoiesis
		↑ Monocyte/macrophage proliferation, phagocytosis, and production of IL-1, IL-6, and TNF
		↑ IL-1RA, CD25, CD71
		↑ NOS, LTB4, COX2
		↑ Chemotaxis of neutrophils
		↑ Hydrogen peroxide production
		↓ Apoptosis of dendritic cells
		↑ Maturation of dendritic cells and production of T_H1, T_H2 cytokines, IL-1β, IL-12, IL-6, and TNF
		↑ Survival and cytotoxicity of NK cells
Adiponectin	↓ Plasma concentration	↓ B-cell lymphopoiesis
		↓ T-cell responses
		↓ Phagocytosis
		↓ Endothelial adhesion molecules
		↑ IL-10, IL-1RA, IFNγ
		↓ TNF, NF-κβ, IL-6
		↑ IL-8 (CXCL8) HMW form +LPS
Resistin	↑, ↓, or = Plasma concentration	↑ Endothelial adhesion molecules
		↑ NF-κβ
		↑ IL-1β, IL-12, IL-6, TNF
Visfatin	↑ Plasma concentration	↓ Neutrophil apoptosis
		↑ Chemotaxis
		↑ IL-1RA, IL-1β, IL-8, IL-6, TNF

pro-inflammatory molecules, whereas reduced adiposity associates with decreased concentration of pro-inflammatory and increased concentration of anti-inflammatory molecules; for that reason, obesity is now considered a pro-inflammatory state [73]. Among the various adipokines, leptin seems to be the one with the most potential for affecting OA [74]. Leptin is significantly increased in obesity, and it is known to increase, among others, alkaline phosphatase activity, osteocalcin release, collagen type 1, and TGF beta production within the joint; it also stimulates cell proliferation leading to abnormal osteoblast function [75] stimulating osteophyte formation [76].

In contrast, adiponectin seems to have a protective role against OA [77], although not all workers agree with this observation [78,79].

EFFECTS OF WEIGHT LOSS ON OA

Obesity is the most significant *modifiable* risk factor for the development and progression of OA. Maintaining a healthy body weight may prevent the development of this condition, while reducing the body weight of an OA patient may decelerate its progression by dropping the forces applied on the joints, as well as the systemic inflammatory load. Indeed, in the Framingham cohort, weight loss in mid- and later adult life substantially reduced the risk for symptomatic OA of the knee [27]. Weight change significantly affected the risk for developing OA; a decrease in BMI of 2 units (~5 kg on average) in the 10 years prior to the assessment decreased the chances for OA development by 50% irrespective of initial BMI. In patients with established OA, a meta-analysis of 35 potential trials (with only four meeting their inclusion criteria) suggested that physical disability of overweight and obese patients with knee OA could be significantly improved with a weight loss greater than 5% achieved within a 20 week period, that is, a weekly rate of ~0.25%. Clinical efficacy on pain reduction was present, although not predictable after weight loss [80]. The aforementioned discussions highlight the role of weight reduction as a primary intervention for OA treatment [81]. The two most effective nonpharmacological treatments of increased body weights are diet and exercise.

DIETARY INTERVENTIONS IN OA

The interventions used aimed at caloric intake reductions with concomitant generation of energy deficits of 800–1000 kcal per day, with a minimum intake of 1100 and 1200 kcal for women and men, respectively [82]. Such interventions had an 80% adherence rate, and 50% of the participants achieved the target weight loss of 5% within 20 weeks [83]. Similar results were achieved by other studies [81,84], and this reduction in body weight was associated with a significant improvement of function and disability. Weight-loss via dietary interventions reduced both GRF [85] and inflammatory load (CRP, IL-6, and TNF-α) [86]. However, as with any weight-loss intervention, the greatest challenge is weight-loss maintenance after the end of the intervention. Indeed, the Arthritis, Diet, and Activity Promotion Trial (ADAPT) reported a 33% regain within a year from the end of the intervention [83]. Longer intervention periods, follow-up meetings, education, and individualized plans could improve body-weight maintenance.

EXERCISE INTERVENTIONS IN OA

Until fairly recently, suggesting that a patient with OA could exercise might have seemed impossible due to the increased joint pain and the notion that excessive movement might cause further joint damage. Patients with OA would usually lead a sedentary lifestyle with limited movement. This has a detrimental impact on their aerobic capacity as well as their muscular strength. However, in recent years, exercise has become a valuable tool in the prevention and treatment of OA and is regularly included in treatment guidelines [3,87,88]. Exercise is also a very effective means for reducing body weight *in OA; weight loss of ≥3% is commonly observed especially when combined with diet* [62,89].

One common misconception when discussing exercise is that most people think of heavy, exhaustive drills. However, in patient populations and especially those with musculoskeletal problems, even very light activity over a long period of time can have beneficial effects. Low-intensity aerobic exercise can significantly improve pain and disability [90]. Walking, the most common and readily available form of aerobic exercise, decreases pain (26%) and improves physical function (31%) within a short period of time (8–12 weeks) [91,92]. These improvements, nonetheless, are reversed if the intervention stops [93]. In longer-term interventions or intervention with a long follow-up period, [94,95], the improvements in pain and function are observable for longer. These changes seem to be primarily due to increased strength in the muscles surrounding the joints resulting in greater knee and ankle angular velocities and anterior–posterior propulsive forces leading to faster walking speed [62]. Indeed, patients in the ADAPT study, who combined aerobic and low-resistance exercise training, had significant long-term improvements in their mobility compared to patients performing only aerobic exercise and controls [83]. This indicates that resistance training might also be useful in OA.

Muscle weakness is a significant contributor to pain and disability among OA patients, and resistance training is the best means for stimulating muscle regeneration. In OA patients, strength training is beneficial, but optimum exercise intensity and effect of long-term interventions are still unclear. Low-resistance training is most commonly used. It has been shown to increase knee-extensor strength by 15% within 8 weeks [96]. However, high-resistance training is more effective in that respect (23% improvement) [97] and is known to be safe by causing no additional pain or joint damage even in 80–89 years old participants [96]. Resistance training seems to have a time effect as longer-term interventions (12 weeks) elicit even more pronounced strength gains (28% and 30% gains in knee extensor and flexor strength, respectively) [98]. If this behavior is maintained over a long period of time (18 months in this study [95]), function, pain, and strength significantly improve.

When focusing on weight loss, aerobic exercise is an effective means of reducing body weight, although the combination of both diet and exercise is optimal [62]. These authors found that the exercise only group lost 3.7% of their baseline body weight. The diet only group lost 4.9% while the diet plus exercise group 5.7%. On the same line, preliminary results from the same group show an ~2 kg weight loss for patients doing aerobic exercise vs. 8.5 kg for patients on a diet and exercise regime over a period of 6 months [89]. Resistance training has also the potential of reducing body weight, although this has not been tested in OA patients. Nevertheless, the greatest benefits of resistance training in OA are more likely to be derived from strength increases and improvements in body composition (increased fat-free mass and reduced fat mass) rather than net body weight loss.

RHEUMATOID ARTHRITIS

RA refers to a chronic, progressive, autoimmune, inflammatory condition that affects synovial joints. Common symptoms include joint pain, swelling, and stiffness [99]. As the disease progresses, the majority of the patients develop polyarthritis and experience unexplained flares and remissions. The changes to the synovium (i.e., edema, increased vascularity, and hyperplasia), the primary site of inflammation in RA, are important to the course of the disease [100]. Even though the course of the disease differs between individuals, most RA patients develop destructive arthritis, which can be disabling [101]. Among patients with long-standing disease (i.e., >10 years), only 17% are free from any disability while 16% are completely disabled [102]. More worryingly though, survival rates of RA patients are significantly lower compared to controls [103].

RA associates with reduced life expectancy compared to the general population [104] mainly due to increased prevalence of and worse outcomes from cardiovascular disease (CVD) [105]. The exact cause for this remains unknown; however, genetic predisposition [106–109], classical CVD risk factors [110,111], and the effects of systemic inflammation on the vasculature [112,113] are all thought to contribute. RA also associates with altered body composition. The chronic inflammation of the disease, particularly activation of the nuclear factor kappa-beta (NF-κβ) pathway, triggers metabolic alterations [114] leading to the degradation of lean tissue, especially muscle mass [115]. In combination with inactive lifestyle, this frequently leads to reduced muscle mass in the presence of increased accumulation of body fat and stable or slightly increased body weight [116], a condition known as rheumatoid cachexia [115]. The study of rheumatoid cachexia has received significant scientific attention as it has a detrimental effect on the morbidity and mortality of RA patients [117,118]. Nevertheless, there is still no consensus on the exact methods for identifying such patients, and the prevalence of rheumatoid cachexia, depending on the method used, ranges from as low as 10% [119] up to 67% [120]. However, one observation is common to all such studies: rheumatoid cachexia seems to occur almost exclusively in under-weight and normal-weight individuals; its prevalence decreases as weight increases, and it effectively does not exist in the obese [121,122]. Thus, although both obesity and rheumatoid cachexia are clearly related to body composition, they are different entities and as such require separate attention and study.

The etiology of RA is not clear. It is believed that RA is triggered when an immunogenetically susceptible host is exposed to an antigen. In this manner, an acute inflammatory reaction is initiated. The antigen(s) that triggers the initial inflammatory reaction has not been positively recognized; however, several potential risk factors have been identified. The most consistent genetic association of RA is with the human leukocyte antigen (HLA) alleles [100]. These share a common region of four amino acids located in the antigen-binding cleft of the DR molecule adjacent to the T-cell receptor. This is referred to as "the shared" or "the rheumatoid epitope" [4] and is presumably the specific binding site of the antigen that initiates the inflammation of the joints. Most epidemiological studies suggest an age of disease onset during or after the fifth decade of life [4]. However, no age is immune to RA as even young children suffer from it [99]. Women are affected two to three times more often than men [123], indicating a role for gender and respective hormones. Infectious agents, such as the Epstein–Barr virus, have been suggested as possible initiators of RA; similarly smoking, diet, and ethnicity have been implicated in the pathogenesis of RA [100].

Obesity in RA

It is not clear whether obesity predates or comes as a result of RA; however, the mean BMI reported for RA patients (ranging from 26.5 to 28.2 kg/m²) [116,124,125] is similar to that of the general population (~27 kg/m²) [126]. Prevalence of overweight and obesity in RA appears to be subject to geographic variation. A worldwide study identified 18% of RA patients as obese [127], while a U.K.-based study found a higher prevalence of 31% [128]. However, in both studies, >60% of RA patients exhibited BMI above the desired levels (>25 kg/m², i.e., were overweight or obese). These results are comparable to those of the general population in the United Kingdom, where ~35% are overweight and ~25% obese [129]. Results from other studies lie within this range indicating that overweight and obesity are at least as prevalent among RA patients, as they are in the general population [130,131].

RA pathogenesis: The close association of obesity with the pathogenesis of OA triggered several early studies to test the association of obesity with RA development. In the first studies to investigate this, obesity was found to associate with increased risk for developing RA. Specifically, in a comparison between 349 incident cases of RA and 1457 controls, obesity in females was associated with an OR for RA of 1.4 (95% CI = 1.0–2.0) [132]. Similarly, in a prospective case-control study of 165 pairs including both genders, obesity was associated with almost a fourfold (OR = 3.74; 95% CI = 1.14–12.27) increase in the risk for developing RA; this association was more pronounced in women (OR = 4.96; 95% CI = 1.19–20.71) than men (OR = 1.15; 95% CI = 0.05–24.63) [133], and still some authors consider obesity as a potential contributor to the development of RA [134]. Newer studies, however, consistently suggest that obesity is not a predisposing factor for RA [135–137] apart from the proportion of RA patients who test negative for anti-cyclic citrullinated peptide (anti-CCP) antibodies (OR = 3.45; 95% CI = 1.73–6.87) [138]. Even though the reason for this discrepancy is not usually discussed, it seems that methodological differences and tight standardization for possible confounders in recent studies eliminate the previous positive findings for the association of obesity with RA development [139].

RA progression: In contrast with what is regularly observed for OA, the results on whether obesity increases activity of RA are controversial. Studies in patients with early RA, of up to 3 year duration, surprisingly suggest that obesity (as assessed by the BMI) may protect against joint damage [140–142]. Similarly, changes in body weight over a 1 year period do not correlate with changes in disease activity during the same period [143]. The protective effect of high BMI seems to be present prior to the diagnosis of RA, with overweight or obese RA patients exhibiting less joint damage than their normal weight counterparts at the time of diagnosis [140]. Adiponectin concentrations could provide a potential explanation, as it might induce disease activity in the joint resulting in more active disease in lean (i.e., higher adiponectin levels) and less active in obese (i.e., lower adiponectin levels) patients [144].

In contrast to these observations, studies in unselected (for disease duration) RA patients suggest that obesity associates independently with worse quality of life [145], joint space narrowing in the knees [146], disease activity, and functional disability [147]. These indicate that the potential protective effects of obesity in early RA may be diminished or reversed later on in the course of the disease. Interestingly, all studies suggest a clear association between low BMI and worse disease activity, severity, and quality of life. In this case, it is most likely that significantly reduced BMI is the result rather than the cause of highly active disease over many years [115].

Cardiovascular risk: Obesity is a well-established, independent risk factor for CVD in the general population [148]. It is also considered to be the underlying cause of many other CVD risk factors such as hypertension, dyslipidemia, and insulin resistance [149] and a potent contributor to the inflammatory pathogenesis of atherosclerosis [150]. In RA, however, the results are again conflicting. Obesity independently associates with classical CVD risk factors in RA [110,151]. Obese RA patients are more likely to have such risk factors [128] and a higher 10 year CVD risk event probability [152]. Obesity is also thought to affect the expression of some pro-inflammatory genes that associate with CVD in RA [108]. However, obesity does not seem to predict occurrence of myocardial infarction in RA [153]. Moreover, a BMI of $>30\,kg/m^2$ had lower all-cause mortality; as BMI decreased, mortality increased, and patients with a low BMI ($<20\,kg/m^2$) had the most significantly increased mortality rates [154]. QUEST-RA, a large multinational study, also found no associations between obesity and CVD morbidity [127]. These observations suggest a "reverse epidemiology," that is, paradoxical epidemiological associations between survival outcomes and traditional CVD risk factors such as obesity [155]. In diseases associated with accelerated loss of fat-free mass, such as RA, overnutrition might protect against the significant health consequences of reduced fat-free mass while undernutrition might enhance muscle wasting and through it accelerate mortality [156]. Nonetheless it is still not clear whether this is a true effect or an artifact from interference with other factors such as treatment, smoking, and disease activity [139].

CONSIDERATIONS ABOUT THE STUDY OF OBESITY IN RA

Most of the studies assessing body weight in RA use the WHO *criteria* [157] for overweight and obesity (i.e., overweight: BMI $25\text{--}30\,kg/m^2$; obese: BMI $> 30\,kg/m^2$). Even though *this method of classification* is valid for the general population, it has been proven inaccurate for certain populations with altered body composition. For example, Asian Indians exhibit increased levels of fat [158], while athletes exhibit increased levels of fat-free mass (i.e., predominantly muscle) [159], for a given BMI. Similarly, RA associates with metabolic alterations that lead to reduction in fat-free mass without any obvious change in total body weight; abnormal body composition phenotypes are overrepresented in RA patients, especially in those within the "normal-weight" BMI category [121].

Like Asian Indians, RA patients exhibit reduced fat-free mass for a given BMI, and the general (WHO) BMI cut-off points might not be able to identify RA individuals with increased body fat [116]. This suggests that the definition of obesity in RA requires an "RA-specific" approach such as lowering BMI cutoffs for RA patients by

2 units to 23 and 28 kg/m^2 for overweight and obesity, respectively [116]. The clinical significance and long-term associations of this recent, RA-specific, definition of obesity remains to be proven. However, BMI has the inherent problem that it does not take into account body composition. Thus, in populations with significant body composition alterations, BMI might not be a good measure of obesity altogether, and any adjustments might not rectify this.

CAUSES OF OBESITY AND ITS CONTROL IN RA

As in the general population, energy intake and energy expenditure are the most significant predictors of obesity *in RA* [160]. Specifically, obesity associates with low levels of physical activity, while an underweight state associates with low-energy intake. Inflammation, even though it is suggested to affect body composition in RA, does not appear to associate with it either. Also smoking has a significant impact on body weight of RA patients, with smokers having the lowest BMI, body fat and waist circumference, as well as the lowest prevalence of obesity. In contrast, ex-smokers present with the highest BMI, body fat, and waist circumference, as well as with the highest prevalence of obesity [161]. These findings are similar to those in the general population [162,163] and suggest that lifestyle factors are very important in this context: increasing physical activity is important for obesity control, improving energy intake may prevent an underweight state, and smoking cessation should be accompanied by other lifestyle changes to prevent weight and fat accumulation in patients with RA.

Dietary interventions: Few studies have attempted to reduce body weight by means of diet in RA. In one study, caloric restriction over a period of 12 weeks was used, in combination with a protein-rich diet and low-intensity physical activity. This intervention resulted in modest weight loss (2.7 kg, i.e., ~3.5%), most of which (1.7 kg) was from reduction in fat-free mass [164]. A different study with a similar dietary intervention (i.e., 12 weeks of caloric restriction with protein supplementation) additionally utilized physical activity of moderate intensity. This resulted in a larger body-weight reduction (4.5 kg, i.e., ≥5%) with only minimal loss of fat-free mass (<1 kg) [165]. Both studies were relatively small, and no safe conclusions can be drawn. Nevertheless, their findings are in line with studies investigating ways to reverse rheumatoid cachexia. Marcora et al. [166] investigated the effects of 12 weeks of protein supplementation on lean body mass of RA patients. They suggested that increased protein intake can reverse rheumatoid cachexia and significantly increase lean body mass in RA patients, at least in the short term. However, they were not able to find any changes in body fat.

Exercise interventions: Discussing exercise in RA seems counterintuitive as >70% of RA patients do not perform any type of physical activity. Fear for disease aggravation and an indefensible traditional approach of rheumatology health professionals to recommend exercise restriction may account for the inactive lifestyle of this population [167,168]. It is now established that well-designed physical exercise programs promote prolonged improvements without inducing harmful effects on disease activity and joint damage [169,170]. In general, two approaches have been used in RA, aerobic exercise to improve function and overall fitness and resistance exercise to improve components of rheumatoid cachexia. Very few studies have looked directly at obesity or fat mass. In a 12 week moderate-to-high resistance exercise intervention, lean body mass was increased as a result of the exercise; interestingly, and even though that was not one of the primary objectives of the trial, total body fat was marginally (1.1%) but significantly reduced, while truncal fat also showed a tendency to reduce [171]. These results were further confirmed in a 24 week high-intensity progressive resistance training program; significant increases in lean body mass, reduced fat mass including trunk adiposity, and substantial improvements in muscle strength and physical function were observed [172]. The increases in muscle mass of RA patients following such training are comparable to these observed in the general population [173], indicating that RA patients are not resistant to the anabolic effects of exercise [174].

CONSIDERATIONS FOR WEIGHT-LOSS INTERVENTIONS IN ARTHRITIC POPULATIONS

In this chapter, we have summarized the main associations between obesity and arthritis. Both OA and RA patients can gain significant benefits from weight-loss and optimum body composition. However, any interventions need to be planned with the specific needs of these patients in mind.

Long periods of caloric restriction may result in decreased bone mineral density, increased bone turnover, and fracture rates [175,176]. Similarly, most energy restriction regimens result in a decrease of muscle mass [177], this decrease is proportional to the energy deficit [178], and usually about one-third of the total weight lost via caloric restriction is from muscle mass. Both of these effects of dieting are a very good argument against any such intervention in patients with apparent musculoskeletal conditions. Especially for RA patients, where muscle wasting is very prevalent and clinically significant, dieting needs to be closely monitored *by qualified personnel*. Increasing protein intake during periods of reduced energy intake could protect against losing fat-free mass and developing rheumatoid cachexia. Protein supplementation could also help during periods of high disease activity when protein turnover is increased. In both conditions, the combination of diet with exercise proved to be the optimum strategy. Appropriate exercise, apart from its direct effect on body-weight reduction, can also prevent muscle wasting making it an essential part in any weight-loss regimen.

CONSIDERATIONS FOR EXERCISE PRESCRIPTION IN ARTHRITIC POPULATIONS

Exercise prescription in these two populations is challenging. It is now clear that these patients respond to exercise in the same way and have the same potential for *improvements in physical fitness* as the general population [174]. However, the variation of the disease (i.e., different joints affected, flares) should be taken into account. Most likely, exercise professionals will not be able to apply a given formula for exercise prescription to all OA and RA patients. This highlights the need for individualized exercise prescription. The main differentiations with a normal exercise prescription would be that at the beginning at least, patients would need a long recovery period between exercise sessions; no more than two to three sessions per week should be practiced. For the first few weeks (3–4), the patient should focus on increasing exercise duration at a comfortable intensity. When the desired duration has been achieved, only then intensity should start to be increased. Finally, due to the nature of the disease, putting strain continuously on the same joints should be avoided. A useful technique is to use short (4–5 min) bouts of different types of exercise (walking, cycling, and rowing) in a cyclic fashion so that the patient eventually does two to three sets of these exercises. Overall, the aim should be for the patients to be able to achieve a frequency of three to five times a week, with duration of ~1 h. Intensity should be eventually increased to >65% of aerobic capacity or strength. Also note that several of these people may not have participated in similar exercise programs before, so supervision and encouragement during the first weeks would be necessary. For patients with RA, exercise professionals should allow for variation in the exercise program to accommodate any flares a patient might experience.

However, as with any weight-loss and lifestyle intervention, adherence is very important. Several behavioral strategies have been developed based on social cognitive theory and self-determination theory. Application of these techniques may also improve maintenance of the newly acquired behavior after the intervention has finished. In any case, prevention is always easier than treatment, so the earlier an intervention starts, the more effective it can be.

REFERENCES

1. Stedman TL: *Stedman's Medical Dictionary*. 28th edn. Philadelphia, PA: Lippincott Williams & Wilkins; 2005.
2. Cotran RS, Kumar V, Collins T: *Pathologic Basis of Disease*. 6th edn. Philadelphia, PA: W.B. Saunders Company; 1999.
3. Morbidity and Mortality Weekly Report (MMWR): Prevalence of Doctor-Diagnosed Arthritis and Arthritis-Attributable Activity Limitation - United States, 2007–2009 October 8, 2010/59(39);1261–1265. http://www.cdc.gov/mmwr/preview/mmwrhtml/mm5939a1.htm?s_cid=mm5939a1_w. Accessed: December 12, 2010.
4. Alamanos Y, Drosos AA: Epidemiology of adult rheumatoid arthritis. *Autoimmun Rev* 2005, 4:130–136.
5. National Collaborating Centre for Chronic Conditions (UK): *Osteoarthritis: National Clinical Guideline for Care and Management in Adults*. London, U.K.: Royal College of Physicians; 2008.
6. Nuki G: Osteoarthritis: A problem of joint failure. *Z Rheumatol* 1999, 58:142–147.
7. Spector TD, MacGregor AJ: Risk factors for osteoarthritis: Genetics. *Osteoarthr Cartil* 2004, 12 Suppl A:S39–S44.
8. Valdes AM, Spector TD: The genetic epidemiology of osteoarthritis. *Curr Opin Rheumatol* 2010, 22:139–143.
9. Blagojevic M, Jinks C, Jeffery A, Jordan KP: Risk factors for onset of osteoarthritis of the knee in older adults: A systematic review and meta-analysis. *Osteoarthr Cartil* 2010, 18:24–33.
10. Stewart A, Black AJ: Bone mineral density in osteoarthritis. *Curr Opin Rheumatol* 2000, 12:464–467.
11. Bergink AP, Uitterlinden AG, Van Leeuwen JP, Hofman A, Verhaar JA, Pols HA: Bone mineral density and vertebral fracture history are associated with incident and progressive radiographic knee osteoarthritis in elderly men and women: The Rotterdam Study. *Bone* 2005, 37:446–456.

12. Oliveria SA, Felson DT, Reed JI, Cirillo PA, Walker AM: Incidence of symptomatic hand, hip, and knee osteoarthritis among patients in a health maintenance organization. *Arthritis Rheum* 1995, 38:1134–1141.

13. Fletcher E, Lewis-Fanning E: Chronic rheumatic diseases-part IV: A statistical study of 1,000 cases of chronic rheumatism. *Postgrad Med J* 1945, 21:176–185.

14. Messier SP: Obesity and osteoarthritis: Disease genesis and nonpharmacologic weight management. *Med Clin N Am* 2009, 93:145–159, xi–xii.

15. Messier SP: Obesity and osteoarthritis: Disease genesis and nonpharmacologic weight management. *Rheum Dis Clin N Am* 2008, 34:713–729.

16. Shih M, Hootman JM, Kruger J, Helmick CG: Physical activity in men and women with arthritis: National Health Interview Survey, 2002. *Am J Prev Med* 2006, 30:385–393.

17. Sowers MF, Yosef M, Jamadar D, Jacobson J, Karvonen-Gutierrez C, Jaffe M: BMI vs. body composition and radiographically defined osteoarthritis of the knee in women: A 4-year follow-up study. *Osteoarthr Cartil* 2008, 16:367–372.

18. Cicuttini FM, Spector T, Baker J: Risk factors for osteoarthritis in the tibiofemoral and patellofemoral joints of the knee. *J Rheumatol* 1997, 24:1164–1167.

19. Cicuttini FM, Baker JR, Spector TD: The association of obesity with osteoarthritis of the hand and knee in women: A twin study. *J Rheumatol* 1996, 23:1221–1226.

20. Leach RE, Baumgard S, Broom J: Obesity: Its relationship to osteoarthritis of the knee. *Clin Orthop Relat Res* 1973, 93:271–273.

21. Davis MA, Ettinger WH, Neuhaus JM, Hauck WW: Sex differences in osteoarthritis of the knee: The role of obesity. *Am J Epidemiol* 1988, 127:1019–1030.

22. Davis MA, Ettinger WH, Neuhaus JM: Obesity and osteoarthritis of the knee: Evidence from the National Health and Nutrition Examination Survey (NHANES I). *Semin Arthritis Rheum* 1990, 20:34–41.

23. Lementowski PW, Zelicof SB: Obesity and osteoarthritis. *Am J Orthop (Belle Mead NJ)* 2008, 37:148–151.

24. Coggon D, Reading I, Croft P, McLaren M, Barrett D, Cooper C: Knee osteoarthritis and obesity. *Int J Obes Relat Metab Disord* 2001, 25:622–627.

25. Holmberg S, Thelin A, Thelin N: Knee osteoarthritis and body mass index: A population-based case-control study. *Scand J Rheumatol* 2005, 34:59–64.

26. Manninen P, Riihimaki H, Heliovaara M, Suomalainen O: Weight changes and the risk of knee osteoarthritis requiring arthroplasty. *Ann Rheum Dis* 2004, 63:1434–1437.

27. Felson DT, Zhang Y, Anthony JM, Naimark A, Anderson JJ: Weight loss reduces the risk for symptomatic knee osteoarthritis in women: The Framingham Study. *Ann Intern Med* 1992, 116:535–539.

28. Sutton AJ, Muir KR, Mockett S, Fentem P: A case-control study to investigate the relation between low and moderate levels of physical activity and osteoarthritis of the knee using data collected as part of the Allied Dunbar National Fitness Survey. *Ann Rheum Dis* 2001, 60:756–764.

29. Kulie T, Slattengren A, Redmer J, Counts H, Eglash A, Schrager S: Obesity and women's health: An evidence-based review. *J Am Board Fam Med* 2011, 24:75–85.

30. Liu B, Balkwill A, Banks E, Cooper C, Green J, Beral V: Relationship of height, weight and body mass index to the risk of hip and knee replacements in middle-aged women. *Rheumatology (Oxford)* 2007, 46:861–867.

31. van Saase JL, Vandenbroucke JP, van Romunde LK, Valkenburg HA: Osteoarthritis and obesity in the general population: A relationship calling for an explanation. *J Rheumatol* 1988, 15:1152–1158.

32. Acheson RM, Collart AB: New Haven survey of joint diseases. XVII. Relationship between some systemic characteristics and osteoarthrosis in a general population. *Ann Rheum Dis* 1975, 34:379–387.

33. Bagge E, Bjelle A, Eden S, Svanborg A: Factors associated with radiographic osteoarthritis: Results from the population study 70-year-old people in Goteborg. *J Rheumatol* 1991, 18:1218–1222.

34. Oliveria SA, Felson DT, Cirillo PA, Reed JI, Walker AM: Body weight, body mass index, and incident symptomatic osteoarthritis of the hand, hip, and knee. *Epidemiology* 1999, 10:161–166.

35. Carman WJ, Sowers M, Hawthorne VM, Weissfeld LA: Obesity as a risk factor for osteoarthritis of the hand and wrist: A prospective study. *Am J Epidemiol* 1994, 139:119–129.

36. Grotle M, Hagen KB, Natvig B, Dahl FA, Kvien TK: Obesity and osteoarthritis in knee, hip and/or hand: An epidemiological study in the general population with 10 years follow-up. *BMC Musculoskelet Disord* 2008, 9:132.

37. Davis MA, Neuhaus JM, Ettinger WH, Mueller WH: Body fat distribution and osteoarthritis. *Am J Epidemiol* 1990, 132:701–707.

38. Hochberg MC, Lethbridge-Cejku M, Scott WW, Jr., Plato CC, Tobin JD: Obesity and osteoarthritis of the hands in women. *Osteoarthr Cartil* 1993, 1:129–135.

39. Hochberg MC, Lethbridge-Cejku M, Plato CC, Wigley FM, Tobin JD: Factors associated with osteoarthritis of the hand in males: Data from the Baltimore Longitudinal Study of Aging. *American Journal of Epidemiology* 1991, 134:1121–1127.

40. Doherty M, Spector TD, Serni U: Epidemiology and genetics of hand osteoarthritis. *Osteoarthr Cartil* 2000, 8 Suppl A:S14–S15.

41. Kalichman L, Kobyliansky E: Age, body composition, and reproductive indices as predictors of radiographic hand osteoarthritis in Chuvashian women. *Scand J Rheumatol* 2007, 36:53–57.

42. Hartz AJ, Fischer ME, Bril G et al.: The association of obesity with joint pain and osteoarthritis in the HANES data. *J Chronic Dis* 1986, 39:311–319.

43. Cooper C, Inskip H, Croft P et al.: Individual risk factors for hip osteoarthritis: Obesity, hip injury and physical activity. *Am J Epidemiol* 1998, 147:516–522.

44. Jarvholm B, Lewold S, Malchau H, Vingard E: Age, bodyweight, smoking habits and the risk of severe osteoarthritis in the hip and knee in men. *Eur J Epidemiol* 2005, 20:537–542.

45. Heliovaara M, Makela M, Impivaara O, Knekt P, Aromaa A, Sievers K: Association of overweight, trauma and workload with coxarthrosis: A health survey of 7,217 persons. *Acta Orthop Scand* 1993, 64:513–518.

46. Vingard E: Overweight predisposes to coxarthrosis: Body-mass index studied in 239 males with hip arthroplasty. *Acta Orthop Scand* 1991, 62:106–109.

47. Vingard E, Alfredsson L, Malchau H: Lifestyle factors and hip arthrosis: A case referent study of body mass index, smoking and hormone therapy in 503 Swedish women. *Acta Orthop Scand* 1997, 68:216–220.

48. Reijman M, Pols HA, Bergink AP et al.: Body mass index associated with onset and progression of osteoarthritis of the knee but not of the hip: The Rotterdam Study. *Ann Rheum Dis* 2007, 66:158–162.

49. Gelber AC, Hochberg MC, Mead LA, Wang NY, Wigley FM, Klag MJ: Body mass index in young men and the risk of subsequent knee and hip osteoarthritis. *Am J Med* 1999, 107:542–548.

50. Tepper S, Hochberg MC: Factors associated with hip osteoarthritis: Data from the First National Health and Nutrition Examination Survey (NHANES-I). *Am J Epidemiol* 1993, 137:1081–1088.

51. Gravante G, Russo G, Pomara F, Ridola C: Comparison of ground reaction forces between obese and control young adults during quiet standing on a baropodometric platform. *Clin Biomech (Bristol, Avon)* 2003, 18:780–782.

52. Browning RC, Kram R: Effects of obesity on the biomechanics of walking at different speeds. *Med Sci Sports Exerc* 2007, 39:1632–1641.

53. Hills AP, Hennig EM, McDonald M, Bar-Or O: Plantar pressure differences between obese and non-obese adults: A biomechanical analysis. *Int J Obes Relat Metab Disord* 2001, 25:1674–1679.

54. Irving DB, Cook JL, Young MA, Menz HB: Obesity and pronated foot type may increase the risk of chronic plantar heel pain: A matched case-control study. *BMC Musculoskelet Disord* 2007, 8:41.

55. Riddle DL, Pulisic M, Pidcoe P, Johnson RE: Risk factors for plantar fasciitis: A matched case-control study. *J Bone Jt Surg Am* 2003, 85-A:872–877.

56. Messier SP, Ettinger WH, Doyle TE, James MK, Morgan T, Burns R: Obesity: Effects on gait in an osteoarthritic population. *J Appl Biomech* 1996, 12:161–172.

57. Cicuttini FM, Spector T: Obesity, arthritis, and gout. In *Handbook of Obesity*. 1st edn. Bray GA, Bouchard C, James WPT, Eds. New York: Marcel Dekker; 1998, pp. 741–752.

58. Dequeker J, Goris P, Uytterhoeven R: Osteoporosis and osteoarthritis (osteoarthrosis): Anthropometric distinctions. *JAMA* 1983, 249:1448–1451.

59. Cimen OB, Incel NA, Yapici Y, Apaydin D, Erdogan C: Obesity related measurements and joint space width in patients with knee osteoarthritis. *Ups J Med Sci* 2004, 109:159–164.

60. Sartorio A, Proietti M, Marinone PG, Agosti F, Adorni F, Lafortuna CL: Influence of gender, age and BMI on lower limb muscular power output in a large population of obese men and women. *Int J Obes Relat Metab Disord* 2004, 28:91–98.

61. Miyatake N, Fujii M, Nishikawa H et al.: Clinical evaluation of muscle strength in 20–79-years-old obese Japanese. *Diabetes Res Clin Pract* 2000, 48:15–21.

62. Messier SP: Diet and exercise for obese adults with knee osteoarthritis. *Clin Geriatr Med* 2010, 26:461–477.

63. Rubenstein LZ: Falls in older people: Epidemiology, risk factors and strategies for prevention. *Age Ageing* 2006, 35 Suppl 2:ii37–ii41.

64. Kejonen P, Kauranen K, Vanharanta H: The relationship between anthropometric factors and body-balancing movements in postural balance. *Arch Phys Med Rehabil* 2003, 84:17–22.

65. Jadelis K, Miller ME, Ettinger WH, Jr., Messier SP: Strength, balance, and the modifying effects of obesity and knee pain: Results from the Observational Arthritis Study in Seniors (oasis). *J Am Geriatr Soc* 2001, 49:884–891.

66. Finkelstein EA, Chen H, Prabhu M, Trogdon JG, Corso PS: The relationship between obesity and injuries among U.S. adults. *Am J Health Promot* 2007, 21:460–468.

67. Messier SP, Davies AB, Moore DT, Davis SE, Pack RJ, Kazmar SC: Severe obesity: Effects on foot mechanics during walking. *Foot Ankle Int* 1994, 15:29–34.

68. DeVita P, Hortobagyi T: Obesity is not associated with increased knee joint torque and power during level walking. *J Biomech* 2003, 36:1355–1362.

69. Mohamed-Ali V, Pinkney JH, Coppack SW: Adipose tissue as an endocrine and paracrine organ. *Int J Obes Relat Metab Disord* 1998, 22:1145–1158.

70. Fantuzzi G: Adipose tissue, adipokines, and inflammation. *J Allergy Clin Immunol* 2005, 115:911–919; quiz 920.

71. Houseknecht KL, Baile CA, Matteri RL, Spurlock ME: The biology of leptin: A review. *J Anim Sci* 1998, 76:1405–1420.

72. Chandran M, Phillips SA, Ciaraldi T, Henry RR: Adiponectin: More than just another fat cell hormone? *Diabetes Care* 2003, 26:2442–2450.

73. Ramos EJB, Xu Y, Romanova I et al.: Is obesity an inflammatory disease? *Surgery* 2003, 134:329–335.

74. Dumond H, Presle N, Terlain B et al.: Evidence for a key role of leptin in osteoarthritis. *Arthritis Rheum* 2003, 48:3118–3129.

75. Mutabaruka M-S, Aoulad Aissa M, Delalandre A, Lavigne M, Lajeunesse D: Local leptin production in osteoarthritis subchondral osteoblasts may be responsible for their abnormal phenotypic expression. *Arthritis Res Ther* 2010, 12:R20.

76. Scharstuhl A, Glansbeek HL, van Beuningen HM, Vitters EL, van der Kraan PM, van den Berg WB: Inhibition of endogenous TGF-beta during experimental osteoarthritis prevents osteophyte formation and impairs cartilage repair. *J Immunol* 2002, 169:507–514.

77. Chen TH, Chen L, Hsieh MS, Chang CP, Chou DT, Tsai SH: Evidence for a protective role for adiponectin in osteoarthritis. *Biochim Biophys Acta* 2006, 1762:711–718.

78. Kang EH, Lee YJ, Kim TK et al.: Adiponectin is a potential catabolic mediator in osteoarthritis cartilage. *Arthritis Res Ther* 2010, 12:R231.

79. Griffin TM, Fermor B, Huebner JL et al.: Diet-induced obesity differentially regulates behavioral, biomechanical, and molecular risk factors for osteoarthritis in mice. *Arthritis Res Ther* 2010, 12:R130.

80. Christensen R, Bartels EM, Astrup A, Bliddal H: Effect of weight reduction in obese patients diagnosed with knee osteoarthritis: A systematic review and meta-analysis. *Ann Rheum Dis* 2007, 66:433–439. doi: 10.1136/ard.2006.065904

81. Christensen R, Astrup A, Bliddal H: Weight loss: The treatment of choice for knee osteoarthritis? A randomized trial. *Osteoarthr Cartil* 2005, 13:20–27.

82. Messier SP, Legault C, Mihalko S et al.: The Intensive Diet and Exercise for Arthritis (IDEA) trial: Design and rationale. *BMC Musculoskelet Disord* 2009, 10:93.

83. Messier SP, Loeser RF, Miller GD et al.: Exercise and dietary weight loss in overweight and obese older adults with knee osteoarthritis: The Arthritis, Diet, and Activity Promotion Trial. *Arthritis Rheum* 2004, 50:1501–1510.

84. Miller GD, Nicklas BJ, Davis C, Loeser RF, Lenchik L, Messier SP: Intensive weight loss program improves physical function in older obese adults with knee osteoarthritis. *Obesity (Silver Spring)* 2006, 14:1219–1230.

85. Messier SP, Gutekunst DJ, Davis C, DeVita P: Weight loss reduces knee-joint loads in overweight and obese older adults with knee osteoarthritis. *Arthritis Rheum* 2005, 52:2026–2032.

86. Nicklas BJ, Ambrosius W, Messier SP et al.: Diet-induced weight loss, exercise, and chronic inflammation in older, obese adults: A randomized controlled clinical trial. *Am J Clin Nutr* 2004, 79:544–551.

87. Zhang W, Moskowitz RW, Nuki G et al.: OARSI recommendations for the management of hip and knee osteoarthritis, Part II: OARSI evidence-based, expert consensus guidelines. *Osteoarthr Cartil* 2008, 16:137–162.

88. Richmond J, Hunter D, Irrgang J et al.: Treatment of osteoarthritis of the knee (nonarthroplasty). *J Am Acad Orthop Surg* 2009, 17:591–600.

89. Messier SP, Loeser RF, Mitchell MN et al.: Exercise and weight loss in obese older adults with knee osteoarthritis: A preliminary study. *J Am Geriatr Soc* 2000, 48:1062–1072.

90. Roddy E, Zhang W, Doherty M: Aerobic walking or strengthening exercise for osteoarthritis of the knee? A systematic review. *Ann Rheum Dis* 2005, 64:544–548.

91. Minor MA, Hewett JE, Webel RR, Anderson SK, Kay DR: Efficacy of physical conditioning exercise in patients with rheumatoid arthritis and osteoarthritis. *Arthritis Rheum* 1989, 32:1396–1405.

92. Kovar PA, Allegrante JP, MacKenzie CR, Peterson MG, Gutin B, Charlson ME: Supervised fitness walking in patients with osteoarthritis of the knee: A randomized, controlled trial. *Ann Intern Med* 1992, 116:529–534.

93. Sullivan T, Allegrante JP, Peterson MG, Kovar PA, MacKenzie CR: One-year followup of patients with osteoarthritis of the knee who participated in a program of supervised fitness walking and supportive patient education. *Arthritis Care Res* 1998, 11:228–233.

94. Thomas KS, Muir KR, Doherty M, Jones AC, O'Reilly SC, Bassey EJ: Home based exercise programme for knee pain and knee osteoarthritis: Randomised controlled trial. *BMJ* 2002, 325:752.

95. Ettinger WH, Jr., Burns R, Messier SP et al.: A randomized trial comparing aerobic exercise and resistance exercise with a health education program in older adults with knee osteoarthritis: The Fitness Arthritis and Seniors Trial (FAST). *JAMA* 1997, 277:25–31.

96. Caserotti P, Aagaard P, Larsen JB, Puggaard L: Explosive heavy-resistance training in old and very old adults: Changes in rapid muscle force, strength and power. *Scand J Med Sci Sports* 2008, 18:773–782.

97. Jan MH, Lin JJ, Liau JJ, Lin YF, Lin DH: Investigation of clinical effects of high- and low-resistance training for patients with knee osteoarthritis: A randomized controlled trial. *Phys Ther* 2008, 88:427–436.

98. King LK, Birmingham TB, Kean CO, Jones IC, Bryant DM, Giffin JR: Resistance training for medial compartment knee osteoarthritis and malalignment. *Med Sci Sports Exerc* 2008, 40:1376–1384.

99. Hunder GG: *Atlas of Rheumatology.* 4th edn. Philadelphia, PA: Current Medicine; 2005.

100. Buch M, Emery P: The aetiology and pathogenesis of rheumatoid arthritis. *Hosp Pharm* 2002, 9:5–10.

101. Scott DL, Pugner K, Kaarela K et al.: The links between joint damage and disability in rheumatoid arthritis. *Rheumatology* 2000, 39:122–132.

102. Sherrer YS, Bloch DA, Mitchell DM, Young DY, Fries JF: The development of disability in rheumatoid arthritis. *Arthritis Rheum* 1986, 29:494–500.

103. Wolfe F, Mitchell DM, Sibley JT et al.: The mortality of rheumatoid arthritis. *Arthritis Rheum* 1994, 37:481–494.

104. Erhardt CC, Mumford PA, Venables PJ, Maini RN: Factors predicting a poor life prognosis in rheumatoid arthritis: An eight year prospective study. *Ann Rheum Dis* 1989, 48:7–13.

105. Kitas GD, Erb N: Tackling ischaemic heart disease in rheumatoid arthritis. *Rheumatology (Oxford)* 2003, 42:607–613.

106. Gonzalez-Gay MA, Gonzalez-Juanatey C, Lopez-Diaz MJ et al.: HLA-DRB1 and persistent chronic inflammation contribute to cardiovascular events and cardiovascular mortality in patients with rheumatoid arthritis. *Arthritis Rheum* 2007, 57:125–132.

107. Panoulas VF, Nikas SN, Smith JP et al.: Lymphotoxin 252A>G polymorphism is common and associates with myocardial infarction in patients with rheumatoid arthritis. *Ann Rheum Dis* 2008, 67:1550–1556.

108. Panoulas VF, Stavropoulos-Kalinoglou A, Metsios GS et al.: Association of interleukin-6 (IL-6)-174G/C gene polymorphism with cardiovascular disease in patients with rheumatoid arthritis: The role of obesity and smoking. *Atherosclerosis* 2009, 204:178–183.

109. Mattey DL, Dawes PT, Nixon NB, Goh L, Banks MJ, Kitas GD: Increased levels of antibodies to cytokeratin 18 in patients with rheumatoid arthritis and ischaemic heart disease. *Ann Rheum Dis* 2004, 63:420–425.

110. Panoulas VF, Douglas KM, Milionis HJ et al.: Prevalence and associations of hypertension and its control in patients with rheumatoid arthritis. *Rheumatology (Oxford)* 2007, 46:1477–1482.

111. Toms TE, Panoulas VF, Douglas KM, Griffiths HR, Kitas GD: Lack of association between glucocorticoid use and presence of the metabolic syndrome in patients with rheumatoid arthritis: A cross-sectional study. *Arthritis Res Ther* 2008, 10:R145.

112. Stevens RJ, Douglas KM, Saratzis AN, Kitas GD: Inflammation and atherosclerosis in rheumatoid arthritis. *Expert Rev Mol Med* 2005, 7:1–24.

113. Gonzalez A, Kremers HM, Crowson CS et al.: Do cardiovascular risk factors confer the same risk for cardiovascular outcomes in rheumatoid arthritis patients as in non-rheumatoid arthritis patients? *Ann Rheum Dis* 2008, 67:64–69.

114. Metsios GS, Stavropoulos-Kalinoglou A, Panoulas VF et al.: New resting energy expenditure prediction equations for patients with rheumatoid arthritis. *Rheumatology (Oxford)* 2008, 47:500–506.

115. Roubenoff R, Roubenoff RA, Cannon JG et al.: Rheumatoid cachexia: Cytokine-driven hypermetabolism accompanying reduced body cell mass in chronic inflammation. *J Clin Invest* 1994, 93:2379–2386.

116. Stavropoulos-Kalinoglou A, Metsios GS, Koutedakis Y et al.: Redefining overweight and obesity in rheumatoid arthritis patients. *Ann Rheum Dis* 2007, 66:1316–1321.

117. Kremers HM, Nicola PJ, Crowson CS, Ballman KV, Gabriel SE: Prognostic importance of low body mass index in relation to cardiovascular mortality in rheumatoid arthritis. *Arthritis Rheum* 2004, 50:3450–3457.

118. Summers GD, Deighton CM, Rennie MJ, Booth AH: Rheumatoid cachexia: A clinical perspective. *Rheumatology (Oxford)* 2008, 47:1124–1131.

119. Morley JE, Thomas DR, Wilson MM: Cachexia: Pathophysiology and clinical relevance. *Am J Clin Nutr* 2006, 83:735–743.

120. Roubenoff R, Roubenoff RA, Ward LM, Holland SM, Hellmann DB: Rheumatoid cachexia: Depletion of lean body mass in rheumatoid arthritis. Possible association with tumor necrosis factor. *J Rheumatol* 1992, 19:1505–1510.

121. Giles JT, Ling SM, Ferrucci L et al.: Abnormal body composition phenotypes in older rheumatoid arthritis patients: Association with disease characteristics and pharmacotherapies. *Arthritis Rheum* 2008, 59:807–815.

122. Elkan AC, Engvall IL, Cederholm T, Hafstrom I: Rheumatoid cachexia, central obesity and malnutrition in patients with low-active rheumatoid arthritis: Feasibility of anthropometry, mini nutritional assessment and body composition techniques. *Eur J Nutr* 2009, 48:315–322.

123. Symmons D, Turner G, Webb R et al.: The prevalence of rheumatoid arthritis in the United Kingdom: New estimates for a new century. *Rheumatology (Oxford)* 2002, 41:793–800.

124. Saravana S, Gillott T: Ischaemic heart disease in rheumatoid arthritis patients. *Rheumatology (Oxford)* 2004, 43:113–114; author reply 114.

125. Gordon MM, Thomson EA, Madhok R, Capell HA: Can intervention modify adverse lifestyle variables in a rheumatoid population? Results of a pilot study. *Ann Rheum Dis* 2002, 61:66–69.

126. The Information Centre for Health and Social Care: Health Survey for England 2005 Latest Trends http://www.ic.nhs.uk/statistics-and-data-collections/health-and-lifestyles-related-surveys/health-survey-for-england/health-survey-for-england-2005-latest-trends. Accessed: December 10, 2010.

127. Naranjo A, Sokka T, Descalzo MA et al.: Cardiovascular disease in patients with rheumatoid arthritis: Results from the QUEST-RA study. *Arthritis Res Ther* 2008, 10:R30.

128. Armstrong DJ, McCausland EM, Quinn AD, Wright GD: Obesity and cardiovascular risk factors in rheumatoid arthritis. *Rheumatology (Oxford)* 2006, 45:782; author reply 782–783.

129. Zaninotto P, Wardle H, Stamatakis E, Mindell J, Head J: Forecasting obesity to 2010. Department of Health (UK); 2006.

130. Gordon MM, Capell HA, Madhok R: The use of the Internet as a resource for health information among patients attending a rheumatology clinic. *Rheumatology (Oxford)* 2002, 41:1402–1405.

131. Zonana-Nacach A, Santana-Sahagun E, Jimenez-Balderas FJ, Camargo-Coronel A: Prevalence and factors associated with metabolic syndrome in patients with rheumatoid arthritis and systemic lupus erythematosus. *J Clin Rheumatol* 2008, 14:74–77.

132. Voigt LF, Koepsell TD, Nelson JL, Dugowson CE, Daling JR: Smoking, obesity, alcohol consumption, and the risk of rheumatoid arthritis. *Epidemiology* 1994, 5:525–532.

133. Symmons DP, Bankhead CR, Harrison BJ et al.: Blood transfusion, smoking, and obesity as risk factors for the development of rheumatoid arthritis: Results from a primary care-based incident case-control study in Norfolk, England. *Arthritis Rheum* 1997, 40:1955–1961.

134. Symmons DP: Looking back: Rheumatoid arthritis—Aetiology, occurrence and mortality. *Rheumatology (Oxford)* 2005, 44 Suppl 4:iv14–iv17.

135. Cerhan JR, Saag KG, Criswell LA, Merlino LA, Mikuls TR: Blood transfusion, alcohol use, and anthropometric risk factors for rheumatoid arthritis in older women. *J Rheumatol* 2002, 29:246–254.

136. Bartfai T, Waalen J, Buxbaum JN: Adipose tissue as a modulator of clinical inflammation: Does obesity reduce the prevalence of rheumatoid arthritis? *J Rheumatol* 2007, 34:488–492.

137. Rodriguez LA, Tolosa LB, Ruigomez A, Johansson S, Wallander MA: Rheumatoid arthritis in UK primary care: Incidence and prior morbidity. *Scand J Rheumatol* 2009, 38:173–177.

138. Pedersen M, Jacobsen S, Klarlund M et al.: Environmental risk factors differ between rheumatoid arthritis with and without auto-antibodies against cyclic citrullinated peptides. *Arthritis Res Ther* 2006, 8:R133.

139. Stavropoulos-Kalinoglou A, Metsios GS, Koutedakis Y, Kitas GD: Obesity in rheumatoid arthritis. *Rheumatology (Oxford)* 2010, 50:450–462.

140. Westhoff G, Rau R, Zink A: Radiographic joint damage in early rheumatoid arthritis is highly dependent on body mass index. *Arthritis Rheum* 2007, 56:3575–3582.

141. van der Helm-van Mil AHM, van der Kooij SM, Allaart CF, Toes REM, Huizinga TWJ: A high body mass index has a protective effect on the amount of joint destruction in small joints in early rheumatoid arthritis. *Ann Rheum Dis* 2008, 67:769–774.

142. Kaufmann J, Kielstein V, Kilian S, Stein G, Hein G: Relation between body mass index and radiological progression in patients with rheumatoid arthritis. *J Rheumatol* 2003, 30:2350–2355.

143. Morgan SL, Anderson AM, Hood SM, Matthews PA, Lee JY, Alarcon GS: Nutrient intake patterns, body mass index, and vitamin levels in patients with rheumatoid arthritis. *Arthritis Care Res* 1997, 10:9–17.

144. Giles JT, Allison M, Bingham CO, 3rd, Scott WM, Jr., Bathon JM: Adiponectin is a mediator of the inverse association of adiposity with radiographic damage in rheumatoid arthritis. *Arthritis Rheum* 2009, 61:1248–1256.

145. Garcia-Poma A, Segami MI, Mora CS et al.: Obesity is independently associated with impaired quality of life in patients with rheumatoid arthritis. *Clin Rheumatol* 2007, 26:1831–1835.

146. Hollingworth P, Melsom RD, Scott JT: Measurement of radiographic joint space in the rheumatoid knee: Correlation with obesity, disease duration, and other factors. *Rheumatol Rehabil* 1982, 21:9–14.

147. Stavropoulos-Kalinoglou A, Metsios GS, Panoulas VF et al.: Underweight and obese states both associate with worse disease activity and physical function in patients with established rheumatoid arthritis. *Clin Rheumatol* 2009, 28:439–444.

148. Bray GA, Bellanger T: Epidemiology, trends, and morbidities of obesity and the metabolic syndrome. *Endocrine* 2006, 29:109–117.

149. Grundy SM, Brewer HB Jr., Cleeman JI, Smith SC Jr., Lenfant C: Definition of metabolic syndrome: Report of the National Heart, Lung, and Blood Institute/American Heart Association conference on scientific issues related to definition. *Circulation* 2004, 109:433–438.

150. Berg AH, Scherer PE: Adipose tissue, inflammation, and cardiovascular disease. *Circ Res* 2005, 96:939–949.

151. Stavropoulos-Kalinoglou A, Metsios GS, Panoulas VF et al.: Associations of obesity with modifiable risk factors for the development of cardiovascular disease in patients with rheumatoid arthritis. *Ann Rheum Dis* 2009, 68:242–245.

152. Kremers HM, Crowson CS, Therneau TM, Roger VL, Gabriel SE: High ten-year risk of cardiovascular disease in newly diagnosed rheumatoid arthritis patients: A population-based cohort study. *Arthritis Rheum* 2008, 58:2268–2274.

153. Wolfe F, Michaud K: The risk of myocardial infarction and pharmacologic and nonpharmacologic myocardial infarction predictors in rheumatoid arthritis: A cohort and nested case-control analysis. *Arthritis Rheum* 2008, 58:2612–2621.
154. Escalante A, Haas RW, del Rincon I: Paradoxical effect of body mass index on survival in rheumatoid arthritis: Role of comorbidity and systemic inflammation. *Arch Intern Med* 2005, 165:1624–1629.
155. Horwich TB, Fonarow GC: Reverse epidemiology beyond dialysis patients: Chronic heart failure, geriatrics, rheumatoid arthritis, COPD, and AIDS. *Semin Dial* 2007, 20:549–553.
156. Kalantar-Zadeh K, Horwich TB, Oreopoulos A et al.: Risk factor paradox in wasting diseases. *Curr Opin Clin Nutr Metab Care* 2007, 10:433–442.
157. World Health Organisation: Obesity: Preventing and managing the global epidemic. Report of a WHO Consultation. World Health Organisation Technical Report Series 2000:1–253.
158. World Health Organisation: Appropriate body-mass index for Asian populations and its implications for policy and intervention strategies. *Lancet* 2004, 363:157–163.
159. Nevill AM, Stewart AD, Olds T, Holder R: Are adult physiques geometrically similar? The dangers of allometric scaling using body mass power laws. *Am J Phys Anthropol* 2004, 124:177–182.
160. Stavropoulos-Kalinoglou A, Metsios GS, Smith JP, Panoulas VF, Douglas KMJ, Jamurtas AZ, Koutedakis Y, Kitas GD: What predicts obesity in patients with rheumatoid arthritis? An investigation of the interactions between lifestyle and inflammation. *Int J Obes (Lond)* 2009, 34:295–301.
161. Stavropoulos-Kalinoglou A, Metsios GS, Panoulas VF et al.: Cigarette smoking associates with body weight and muscle mass of patients with rheumatoid arthritis: A cross-sectional, observational study. *Arthritis Res Ther* 2008, 10:R59.
162. Filozof C, Pinilla MCF, Fernández-Cruz A: Smoking cessation and weight gain. *Obes Rev* 2004, 5:95–103.
163. Froom P, Melamed S, Benbassat J: Smoking cessation and weight gain. *J Fam Pract* 1998, 46:460–464.
164. Heitmann BL, Kondrup J, Engelhart M et al.: Changes in fat free mass in overweight patients with rheumatoid arthritis on a weight reducing regimen: A comparison of eight different body composition methods. *Int J Obes Relat Metab Disord* 1994, 18:812–819.
165. Engelhart M, Kondrup J, Hoie LH, Andersen V, Kristensen JH, Heitmann BL: Weight reduction in obese patients with rheumatoid arthritis, with preservation of body cell mass and improvement of physical fitness. *Clin Exp Rheumatol* 1996, 14:289–293.
166. Marcora S, Lemmey A, Maddison P: Dietary treatment of rheumatoid cachexia with beta-hydroxy-beta-methylbutyrate, glutamine and arginine: A randomised controlled trial. *Clin Nutr* 2005, 24:442–454.
167. Ekdahl C, Broman G: Muscle strength, endurance, and aerobic capacity in rheumatoid arthritis: A comparative study with healthy subjects. *Ann Rheum Dis* 1992, 51:35–40.
168. Scott DL, Wolman RL: Rest or exercise in inflammatory arthritis? *Br J Hosp Med* 1992, 48:445, 447.
169. Metsios GS, Stavropoulos-Kalinoglou A, Veldhuijzen van Zanten JJ et al.: Rheumatoid arthritis, cardiovascular disease and physical exercise: A systematic review. *Rheumatology (Oxford)* 2008, 47:239–248.
170. de Jong Z, Munneke M, Zwinderman AH et al.: Is a long-term high-intensity exercise program effective and safe in patients with rheumatoid arthritis? Results of a randomized controlled trial. *Arthritis Rheum* 2003, 48:2415–2424.
171. Marcora SM, Lemmey AB, Maddison PJ: Can progressive resistance training reverse cachexia in patients with rheumatoid arthritis? Results of a pilot study. *J Rheumatol* 2005, 32:1031–1039.

172. Lemmey AB, Marcora SM, Chester K, Wilson S, Casanova F, Maddison PJ: Effects of high-intensity resistance training in patients with rheumatoid arthritis: A randomized controlled trial. *Arthritis Rheum* 2009, 61:1726–1734.
173. Hakkinen A, Pakarinen A, Hannonen P et al.: Effects of prolonged combined strength and endurance training on physical fitness, body composition and serum hormones in women with rheumatoid arthritis and in healthy controls. *Clin Exp Rheumatol* 2005, 23:505–512.
174. Cooney JK, Law RJ, Matschke V et al.: Benefits of exercise in rheumatoid arthritis. *J Aging Res* 2011, Vol. 2011, Article 1D 681640, 14 pages, doi: 10.4061/2011/681640.
175. Cashman KD: Diet, nutrition, and bone health. *J Nutr* 2007, 137:2507S–2512S.
176. Dirks AJ, Leeuwenburgh C: Caloric restriction in humans: Potential pitfalls and health concerns. *Mech Ageing Dev* 2006, 127:1–7.
177. Ravussin E, Burnand B, Schutz Y, Jequier E: Energy expenditure before and during energy restriction in obese patients. *Am J Clin Nutr* 1985, 41:753–759.
178. Mingrone G, Greco AV, Giancaterini A, Scarfone A, Castagneto M, Pugeat M: Sex hormone-binding globulin levels and cardiovascular risk factors in morbidly obese subjects before and after weight reduction induced by diet or malabsorptive surgery. *Atherosclerosis* 2002, 161:455–462.

17 Beyond Subcutaneous Fat

Richard L. Seip, PhD

CONTENTS

The obesity epidemic is a public health concern in high-income countries and is dramatically rising in low- and middle-income countries [1]. The medical community has taken notice and, not unlike investigation of smoking in relation to cancer in the 1950s and 1960s, has conducted research to carefully document the perils of excess adiposity. Significant to this evolution is the realization that adipose tissue functions as an endocrine entity. In addition, as the awareness of the importance of the distribution of body fat is rising, methods to assess it in the clinic are being perfected, and utility defined.

INTRODUCTION

Obesity is a major risk factor for insulin resistance (IR), type 2 diabetes mellitus, and cardiovascular disease (CVD). But not every obese patient is insulin resistant or at high risk of diabetes mellitus and CVD [2]. There is a growing recognition that the increased health risks of obesity and metabolic syndrome are more strongly associated with central rather than total adiposity, with an excess in intra-abdominal adipose tissue (IAAT) and liver fat being the key determinants [2] (Figure 17.1). Despres has stated [3], "Although obesity is recognized as a health hazard that has reached epidemic proportions in affluent and emerging economies [1,4] the strength of its relationship with coronary heart disease (CHD) and related mortality … is variable and inconsistent [5]."

More important than *how much* fat a person stores is *where* he or she stores it, in what amounts, and whether the volume of excess energy to be stored threatens the capacity of the adipocytes to store it. Abdominal obesity is increasingly understood to play a major role in the pathogenesis of several metabolic and cardiovascular

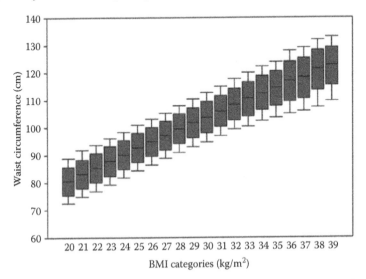

FIGURE 17.1 Waist and BMI are not interchangeable at the individual/patient level. (Reproduced from *J. Am. Coll. Cardiol.*, 57(19), Despres, J.-P., Excess visceral adipose tissue/ectopic fat the missing link in the obesity paradox? 1887–1889, Copyright 2011, with permission from Elsevier.)

medical problems including type 2 diabetes, hypertension, atherosclerosis, and coronary artery disease (CAD). Researchers and clinicians alike believe that clinical diagnosis of visceral adiposity may be more important than the current diagnosis of obesity using the body mass index (BMI). Abdominal obesity was recognized in 2006 as a core component of the metabolic syndrome according to the International Diabetes Federation (IDF) [6]. In patients with existing CAD, including those with normal and high BMI, central obesity, but not BMI, is directly associated with mortality [7] and increases the risk of stroke in people with no CVD history [8]. A new term, "adiposopathy," has been minted to describe a disease state associated with hypertrophied adipocytes in which adipose tissue endocrine and immune responses associate with metabolic disease [9–11]. Going farther, ectopic fat—that which is stored outside of ordinary adipose depots within cells in places like the liver or within or between muscles—may further exacerbate the risks [3,12]. It is clear that central adiposity is more strongly associated with these metabolic and cardiovascular problems than total adiposity [13–17]. Even within the normal range of BMI, accumulation of visceral fat remains an independent cardiovascular risk factor [18]. Evidence also points to major differences between the intra-abdominal visceral fat and the peripheral or subcutaneous fat in the pathogenesis of these medical problems, both in lean and obese individuals. Clearly, body shape and how regional adipose tissue handles and stores excess dietary energy have tremendous cardiometabolic implications. It is time to move on to better assessment tools.

CENTRAL ABDOMINAL OBESITY

Although waist circumference and BMI are strongly correlated at the population level, in clinical practice, clinicians should expect to find substantial individual variation in waist circumference among patients with similar BMI values [3]. Nevertheless, waist circumference should not replace the BMI in cardiology, because it has to be interpreted in the context of the BMI [3]. (Also, in some circumstances, as in predicting risk of venous thrombotic embolism risk, the predictive value of BMI is equivalent to that of waist girth [19]) (Figure 17.2). Even though two patients have exactly the same waist circumference value, they may have quite different BMI values. Consider two patients with waist circumference of 103 cm: Patient #1 has a BMI of 25 kg/m², whereas Patient #2 has a BMI of 30 kg/m². Had only the waist circumference been measured, the clinician would have missed tremendously important information: Patient #2 has a large waistline because he has overall obesity, whereas Patient #1 is not obese but clearly has an excess of abdominal fat. A large waist circumference was recently found to be particularly predictive of increased mortality in cardiac patients with presumably "normal" BMI values [7]. Waist circumference also independently predicts stroke [8]. These studies culminate 25 years of evidence, suggesting that clinicians give further attention to patients who have an exaggerated waistline for their BMI, particularly if this large waistline is accompanied by elevated triglyceride (TG) levels as a marker of excess visceral adipose tissue/ectopic liver fat deposition [3].

In contrast to excessive fat in the gluteofemoral regions, the accumulated fat in the intra-abdominal or visceral depots is strongly associated with obesity-related

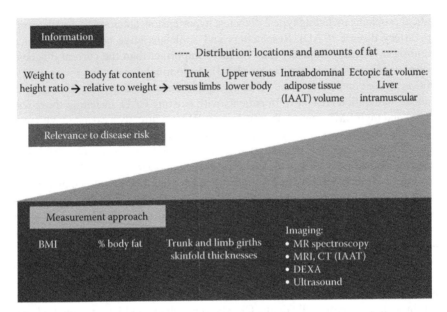

Information

----- Distribution: locations and amounts of fat -----

Weight to   Body fat content   Trunk   Upper versus   Intraabdominal   Ectopic fat volume:
height ratio → relative to weight → versus limbs   lower body   adipose tissue   Liver
                                                 (IAAT) volume   intramuscular

Relevance to disease risk

Measurement approach

                                             Imaging:
  BMI   % body fat   Trunk and limb girths   • MR spectroscopy
                             skinfold thicknesses   • MRI, CT (IAAT)
                                                 • DEXA
                                                 • Ultrasound

FIGURE 17.2 Clinical approaches to assessing adiposity. Simple measurements of girth, made with a measuring tape, can increase the clinician's knowledge about disease risks, supplementing the information about obesity status gained through BMI. Imaging methods can be used to quantify amounts of fat by depot.

complications [20]. In clinical practice, the waist circumference and waist-to-hip ratio (WHR) are the most commonly used anthropometric measures to diagnose abdominal obesity. These measures correlate with the total amount of visceral fat measured by abdominal CT scanning, and also with the risk factors for coronary heart disease such as hyperglycemia, hypertension, and dyslipidemia [21]. Analyses from the Nurses' Health Study and the Health Professionals Follow-up Study showed that the risk of diabetes increased in line with BMI and that obesity, especially abdominal obesity, increased the risk of subsequent diabetes by 10- to 11-fold [22,23]. In 2005, the Adult Treatment Panel III (ATP-III) of the National Cholesterol Education Program adopted "increased waist circumference" as a major component of the clinical diagnostic criteria of the metabolic syndrome, marked by waist circumference exceeding 102 cm (>40 in.) in men and 88 cm (>35 in.) in women [24].

RELATIONSHIP BETWEEN CENTRAL OBESITY AND CARDIOVASCULAR DISEASE

Waist measurement and waist-to-hip ratio: Vague wrote in 1956 [25] that android fat distribution (apple-shaped body) is related to increased risk of CVD and brought to light the idea that male pattern of fat distribution (as determined by WHR or waist circumference) is a powerful predictor of CAD. In the 1980s, studies showed that WHR can predict coronary heart disease in white men and women [26,27]. In the 1990s, several studies also showed similar strong association between WHR or visceral fat accumulation, as determined by abdominal CT scanning, and both carotid atherosclerosis [28,29] and angiographically documented CAD [15,20,27–38]. Just recently, all cause mortality was found to increase by 3% over 4.5 years for every centimeter of waist circumference in patients with coronary disease [39].

THIN-ON-THE-OUTSIDE, FAT-ON-THE-INSIDE

Surely, waist circumference and BMI together improve upon BMI alone as a means to expose central adiposity. But there is a large variation in IAAT, abdominal subcutaneous adipose tissue (ASAT), and intrahepatocyte lipid (IHCL) depots. A previously unidentified subphenotype has emerged that is not fully predicted by clinically obtained measurements of obesity such as BMI and waist and hip circumferences. This phenotype is called "thin-on-the-outside, fat-on-the-inside" (TOFI) [40].

VISCERAL ADIPOSITY

The viscera refer to the organs of the abdominal and pelvic cavities. Fat accumulation around and inside the intra-abdominal solid organs is called visceral or intra-abdominal fat. Portions of the visceral fat—mesenteric and omental adipose depots—are drained by the hepatic portal vein which delivers nutrient-rich blood to the liver. Retroperitoneal and subcutaneous abdominal depots are nonportal depots [41].

VISCERAL FAT

Progressive accumulation of intra-abdominal fat increases hepatic and adipose-tissue IR and metabolic abnormalities like glucose intolerance, low HDL cholesterol, elevated TGs, and hypertension [42–44] with IR as the fundamental etiology. A 7 year prospective study showed that the amount of visceral fat predicted the changes in glucose tolerance and fasting insulin, even in the absence of any change in total body weight or total body fat [45]. So there is a strong relationship between intra-abdominal fat accumulation and IR [46–48].

Three paradigms exist to explain the relationship between visceral fat and IR [49]. The portal/visceral paradigm proposes that visceral adiposity leads to fatty acid flux and inhibition of insulin action via the Randle hypothesis [50]. The second paradigm draws a parallel with the pathogenesis of the disease lipodystrophy (failure to develop adequate adipose tissue), which produces severe IR, diabetes, and ectopic storage of lipid in liver, skeletal muscle, and pancreatic islet cells. This explanation purports that obese persons display "acquired lipodystrophy"—that is, they shunt lipid into the liver, skeletal muscle, and probably the beta cells of the pancreas. The third paradigm is an endocrine explanation. It recognizes that adipose tissue secretes a variety of endocrine hormones such as leptin, interleukin-6 (IL-6), angiotensin II, and adiponectin. From this viewpoint, adipose tissue functions as an endocrine gland, secreting factors with effects on the metabolism of distant tissues [49]. Apart from adipocytes, macrophages residing in visceral adipose tissue produce proinflammatory cytokines like tumor necrosis factor-alpha (TNF-α) and IL-6 [51]. These paradigms form the working framework for understanding links between our current "obesogenic" environment and the risk of developing diabetes [49].

Lipid Metabolism and Visceral Adiposity

Visceral adiposity is associated with elevated serum levels of small-dense LDL-cholesterol particles, high apo-B [52], hypertriglyceridemia, and reduced HDL cholesterol [45,53]. In already dyslipidemic patients, intra-abdominal fat volume positively correlates with hepatic cholesterol synthesis [54].

Sex and Continent of Origin Effects

There are ethnogeographic and sex differences in the rate of accumulation and the amount of visceral fat, and also its relevance to metabolic disease. Men of South or East Asian or European ancestry seem to be the champions at accumulating visceral fat [55–60]. Universally men have greater IAAT than women [61–64], but the gender difference is weakest in African Americans [55,56,61,65,66]. Interestingly, visceral fat on the whole may be less atherogenic in African American women [67]; however, increments in VAT in African American women carry the same or greater disease risk than the same increments in men [62]. South Asians seem especially prone to metabolic disease, and for that reason, stricter cutoffs for waist circumference are proposed to limit intra-abdominal adiposity [60].

   Many other factors play a role in determining the volume of visceral fat including environmental factors, imbalance of sex hormones, in particular, serum free testosterone, growth hormone, IGF-1, insulin, excessive intake of sucrose and saturated fat, and lack of physical activity [68]. Age is also a major defining factor with older people having larger amounts of visceral fat than younger individuals [69].

Genetic Factors

The pattern of gene expression and secretory products in visceral fat is predicted to be more atherogenic compared to that in subcutaneous peripheral fat. Genetic research is promising though far from complete. Genetic loci determining propensity to store fat in the abdominal region have been identified [70]. Gene expression studies of visceral adipocytes have shown differences between patients with high and low visceral fat [71] and within obese patients whose blood TG and acyl-stimulating protein (ASP) levels differ [72]. Some genes of interest (and the proteins they encode) are *PPARG* (peroxisome proliferator–activated receptor gamma) and *SREBF1* (sterol regulatory element–binding transcription factor 1), which promote adipogenesis and lipid storage, and are associated with type 2 diabetes and possible adiposity; *ADIPOQ* and *ARL15*, which are associated with circulating levels of adiponectin; and *ADRB2* (β-2 adrenergic receptor) and *GPR74* (G-protein-coupled receptor 74) genes, which are associated with adipocyte lipolysis. Higher expression of genes in visceral compared to subcutaneous tissue may contribute to the ills associated with visceral adiposity. These include *AGT* (angiotensinogen), *PPARG*, *RETN* (resistin) [73,74], *LEP* (leptin), *ADIPOQ* (adiponectin) [75], TNF-α, and *IL6* [76]. Of note the Trp64Arg beta 3-adrenoceptor gene variant has been implicated in impaired weight loss in obese women [77]. The β-1, β-2, and β-3 adrenergic receptors are found in adipose tissue and are involved in sympathetic responses that regulate blood flow through adipose tissue and lipolysis which results in the release of fatty acids.

Assessment of Intra-Abdominal Adipose Tissue

Adipose tissue consists of adipocytes, macrophages, connective tissue, and blood vessels and technically is not the same as adipose fat, which refers to stored TGs. It is reasonable to subdivide body fat into at least three separate and measurable compartments, namely, subcutaneous, intramuscular, and visceral fat [78]. The gold standard methods for measuring visceral fat volume have been abdominal computed tomography (CT) (at L4–L5) and magnetic resonance imaging (MRI). Visceral fat, then, is approximated in CT and MRI images of abdominal transverse slices as the outline of the IAAT depot. The IAAT is that which is associated with the mesentery; omentum, surrounding the spleen; and pancreas. These methods have confirmed that abdominal body fat is localized mostly in the subcutaneous space and, to a smaller extent, in the visceral or intra-abdominal area (see, e.g., Ref. [48]). CT and MRI are not widely used clinically because of the limitations of cost and radiation exposure.

Anthropometric Measurement

Waist circumference and WHR are used more often in epidemiological studies to indirectly estimate the intra-abdominal fat volume. These measures correlate with IAAT volume measured by CT scanning, but they are less accurate [79] because of the uncertainty of the contributions of subcutaneous AT and IAAT. Circumference measures cost little and are easily used in large-scale studies. Compared to WHR, waist circumference is a better reflection of the intra-abdominal fat volume [80,81]. All factors considered, waist circumference is the easiest anthropometric measurement for health-care professionals to use in order to diagnose abdominal adiposity and to get at least a rough impression of the visceral fat volume [80].

Dual-Energy X-Ray Absorptiometry

Dual-energy x-ray absorptiometry (DEXA) was originally intended to examine bone mineral density but can accurately measure total body fat and regional fat distribution. DEXA is more accurate than anthropometric measures and more practical and cost effective than CT or MRI scans. The shortcoming of DEXA is that it cannot distinguish between subcutaneous and visceral abdominal fat depots, or between subcutaneous and intramuscular peripheral fat depots. Fat mass in the trunk region, as measured by DEXA, was shown to be a strong independent predictor of IR and dyslipidemia among postmenopausal women [82].

Abdominal Ultrasonography

Abdominal ultrasonographic imaging can be suitable for intra-abdominal fat measurement in research and clinical settings [83–85]. The lack of a universally followed protocol for positioning the ultrasound transducer and for timing the measurement in relation to respiratory cycle potentially hampers this technique [81]. Nevertheless, several studies found good correlation between intra-abdominal fat volume measured by abdominal ultrasound and abdominal CT scanning [68]. To be effective, measurements need to be performed at the end of quiet inspiration and by compressing the transducer against the abdomen to limit distortion of the abdominal cavity during scanning [86]. The distance between the peritoneum and the lumbar spine is used as measure of the intra-abdominal fat, and the distance is measured at three positions along the horizontal line between the highest point of iliac crest and the lower costal margin, and each measure should be repeated three times. The reproducibility of this technique is very good with coefficient of variability around 4%–5% [86] and a high correlation with visceral fat measurement in single CT slice at L4–L5 of $r = 0.82$ ($P < 0.001$). The association between intra-abdominal fat, measured ultrasonically using such a strict protocol, and the metabolic risk factors for CAD is more pronounced than the association between the latter and the waist circumference or WHR. Intra-abdominal fat measured by abdominal ultrasound associates with the metabolic risk factors just as intraabdominal fat (IAAF) measured by abdominal CT scanning [87]. Following this strict protocol makes it more possible to accurately measure visceral fat volume with ultrasound in clinical practice.

PERIPHERAL FAT DOES NO HARM

Peripheral fat mass (PFM), defined here as that which is deposited subcutaneously below the waist or on the arms, has poorly defined physiological roles beyond the traditional one of energy storage. Peripheral fat at worst is only a fraction as harmful as central fat and may be protective of normal energy metabolism based on the following. In several studies, PFM showed an independent negative correlation with glucose, atherogenic lipid, and metabolic syndrome components [88–93], arterial stiffness [94], and aortic calcification [95]. The different depots exhibit different influences on lipid metabolism, with central fat mass promoting and PFM counteracting atherogenicity. The lack of peripheral fat has been also associated with poorer insulin sensitivity [82,96], although a recent survey showed that absolute hip circumference was not protective against type 2 diabetes mellitus [97]. Whereas central fat accumulation is deleterious for cardiovascular risk in women, deposition of fat in the gluteofemoral regions possesses some degree of protection [82,88,98].

Hamdy et al. [68] suggested a possible active inhibitory influence of PFM that may overrule the atherogenic tendencies caused by high central fat mass. Alternatively, it may be that as long as peripheral adipose depots are expandable—that is, having adequate storage capacity in the form of existing adipocytes and proliferative ability of adipocytes—then fat storage in central, intra-abdominal, and ectopic depots is avoided, and the sparing of the central depots from having to process excess fatty acids averts adiposopathy [9].

Effects of selective removal of visceral or subcutaneous fat: It is interesting that bilateral surgical removal of subcutaneous inguinal fat mass in mice resulted in increased lipid accumulation in mesenteric fat, hyperinsulinemia, decreased insulin sensitivity, and increased TNF-α. These abnormalities were corrected after reimplantation of inguinal fat [99]. By the same token, surgical removal of visceral fat imparts metabolic benefits in animals including reversal of hepatic IR, prevention of age-related deterioration in peripheral and hepatic insulin action, decreased gene expression of TNF-α and leptin in subcutaneous adipose tissue [100], and delay in onset of diabetes [101]. In humans, surgical removal of large amount of abdominal subcutaneous fat by liposuction in a group of diabetic and nondiabetic individuals did not improve insulin sensitivity in muscles, liver, or adipose tissues and did not change plasma concentrations of circulating mediators of inflammation, including C-reactive protein, IL-6, and TNF-α profile [102]. It also did not change blood pressure, plasma glucose, and serum insulin or lipid profile [102].

BIOLOGICAL DIFFERENCES: VISCERAL VERSUS SUBCUTANEOUS BODY FAT

Biological differences include anatomical, cellular, molecular, physiological, clinical, and prognostic differences [103]. Anatomically, visceral fat is present mainly in the mesentery and omentum, and drains directly through the portal circulation to the liver (see Figure 17.3). Visceral compared to subcutaneous adipose tissue is more cellular, vascular, and innervated and contains a larger number of inflammatory and immune cells, has lesser preadipocyte-differentiating capacity, and contains a greater percentage of large adipocytes [103]. Adipocytes from the omentum are smaller than subcutaneous adipocytes and have lower lipoprotein lipase (LPL) activity [104]. Preadipocytes from abdominal subcutaneous, mesenteric, and omental sites differ in their ability to replicate (omental were slowest) and in their resistance to TNF-α-induced apoptosis (omental were least resistant) [105]. The propensity for adipocyte hypertrophy also differs by depot. In obese women, hyperplasia is predominant in the subcutaneous fat depot, whereas fat cell hypertrophy is observed both in the omental and subcutaneous compartments [106]. In men representing the entire spectrum of BMI, omental adipocyte size reached a plateau in the two upper tertiles of waist circumference, that is, from a waist circumference of 125 cm and above [107].

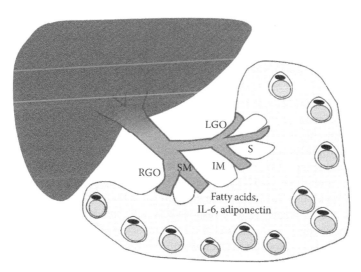

FIGURE 17.3 At rest, 75% of the liver blood supply derives from the hepatic portal vein which is fed by the left gastric omental (LGO), splenic (S), inferior mesenteric (IM), superior mesenteric (SM), and right gastric omental (RGO) veins. These vessels deliver FFAs and adipokines from the IAAT and intestinally absorbed glucose and fructose to the liver.

Men have larger adipocytes in all intra-abdominal depots compared to women [41]. Larger adipocytes may be closer to their maximal TG storage capacity, and IAAT may be more "adiposopathic" in men. Interestingly, there are sex and depot-specific differences in uptake of free fatty acid (FFA) [108]. Direct FFA uptake by subcutaneous adipose tissue is greater in women than men, whereas abdominal subcutaneous fat takes up FFAs more avidly than femoral fat in men, but not in women [108].

Of note some individuals display "benign obesity," characterized by high insulin sensitivity, low levels of ectopic fat (liver and muscle), and low-carotid-artery intima-media thickness compared to equally obese peers [109]. In a study comparing adipocyte size in "metabolically healthy" morbidly obese (low fasting insulin, low TG) to peers with metabolic syndrome, omental but not subcutaneous adipocyte size correlated with the degree of IR as measured by HOMA-IR (r = 0.73, P < 0.0005), and only omental, not subcutaneous, adipocyte size was an independent predictor of the presence or absence of hepatic fibrosis [110]. There are also differences in expression and secretion of adipose tissue–derived cytokines (adipokines, see Table 17.1) For example, compared to subcutaneous adipocyte adiponectin release, omental adipocyte adiponectin release is reduced to a greater extent in visceral obese women and better predicts obesity-associated metabolic abnormalities [115].

Intra-abdominal fat tissue (that associated with stomach, intestine, pancreas, spleen) is connected directly to the liver via the hepatic portal vein. Thus, the types and concentrations of factor(s) released by the IAAT can directly influence the metabolic activities of the hepatocytes and the inflammatory status of the liver lobules. In fact under typical resting conditions, the hepatic portal system contributes 75% of the blood flow to the liver, and the hepatic artery contributes 25% [116]. Abdominal fat, therefore, directly impacts hepatic FFA flux, increasing TG synthesis and decreasing hepatic insulin clearance [117,118].

In contrast, omental adipocytes display greater relative responsiveness to both adrenergic receptor- and postreceptor agonists compared to subcutaneous adipocytes. The mechanism for these differences remains unclear. There are two types of responses to catecholamine-stimulated lipolysis: a similar response from mesenteric and omental (portal) fat depots and from retroperitoneal and subcutaneous abdominal (nonportal) fat depots. Young women had higher lipolysis in nonportal than in portal adipose tissues. In the men, the reverse characteristics were found. These dissimilarities seem to be based on differences in beta-adrenergic responsiveness. Postmenopausal women showed no differences between depots. The differences in lipolytic responsiveness between these groups might be caused by sex steroid hormones [41]. In tissue obtained from women undergoing surgery, omental adipocytes display greater relative responsiveness to both adrenergic receptor- and postreceptor-acting agents compared with subcutaneous adipocytes. The mesenteric and omental depots respond to catecholamine-stimulated lipolysis differently from nonportal depots. At rest, men have higher lipolysis in the portal adipose tissues than in nonportal tissues probably due to beta-adrenergic responsiveness. The opposite was found for women [41]. As hard exercise stimulates catecholamine release [119], bouts of hard exercise may have greater potential to keep intra-abdominal fat stores at bay in men compared to women.

TABLE 17.1
Adipokines: Selected Factors Derived from Adipose Tissue with Special Reference to the Pathogenesis of IR

Adipokine	Site of Production	Levels in Obesity and NAFLD	Physiological Role	Role in IR Inflammation
Leptin	SAT > IAAT [11]	↑ In obesity	Prevents lipid accumulation in nonadipose tissues	Could modulate TNF-α production and macrophage activation
TNF-α	IAAT > SAT [11]	↑ In obesity; (note: not measurable in circulation)	Multifunctional cytokine with antiadipogenic properties; may limit adipose tissue expansion; promotes lipolysis and inhibits LPL through inhibition of LPL mRNA; can induce rapid release of leptin from adipose tissue [111]	Alters insulin sensitivity by triggering different key steps in the insulin signaling pathway [112]
IL-6	IAAT > SAT [11]	↑ In obesity	Inflammatory regulator; 35% of circulating levels derive from adipose tissue [113]	May induce hepatic CRP synthesis and may promote the onset of cardiovascular complications
Adiponectin	IAAT > SAT [11]	↓ In obesity; even lower in NAFLD	Antisteatotic, anti-inflammatory, antioxidative, and antiapoptotic effects [114]	Counteracts proinflammatory effects of TNF-α on the arterial wall and probably protects against the development of arteriosclerosis [112]; inhibits liver neoglucogenesis and promotes fatty acid oxidation in skeletal muscle [112]
AGT	IAAT > SAT [11]	↑ In obesity	Vascular tone and blood pressure regulation	Limited role; within adipose tissue, inhibits preadipocyte recruitment but promotes differentiation [11]

NONALCOHOLIC FATTY LIVER DISEASE

The incidence of nonalcoholic fatty liver disease (NAFLD) is burgeoning, rising in step with obesity. Ludwig et al. first used the term nonalcoholic steatohepatitis (NASH) in 1980 to describe histological liver disease observed in middle-aged patients in the absence of alcohol drinking history [120]. Nine of 10 patients were obese, and 25% had type 2 diabetes. Key features in biopsied liver tissue were moderate to severe steatosis (fatty droplets) with inflammation of liver lobules. Today NASH is part of the spectrum of NAFLD which includes simple fatty liver (steatosis, hepatocyte fat droplets of 1–3 μm diameter, mild lymphocytic infiltrate), NASH (fat droplets, 5–25 μm diameter causing ballooning of hepatocytes; inflammation), and NAFLD-associated fibrosis (extracellular deposition of type I and III collagen) and cirrhosis (replacement of liver tissue by fibrosis, scar tissue, and nodules) (Figure 17.4). Clinically relevant thresholds include >5% of liver volume as fat to define steatosis, and 30%, which is the cutoff for liver transplantation donors [121].

Grossly, steatosis causes organ enlargement and lightening in color [122]. This is due to the high lipid content, increasing the organ's volume and becoming visible to the unaided eye. On CT imaging, the increased fat component decreases the density of the liver tissue, making the image less bright. Typically the density of the spleen and liver is roughly equivalent. In steatosis, there is a difference between the density and brightness of the two organs, with the liver appearing darker [123]. On ultrasound, fat is more echogenic (capable of reflecting sound waves). The combination of liver steatosis being dark on CT and bright on ultrasound is sometimes known as the flip flop sign.

Historically NAFLD has affected 2%–24% of the general population, men more often than women, beginning around age 30, although NAFLD can be found in obese youth [124]. The Dallas Heart Study of free living adults, published in 2004,

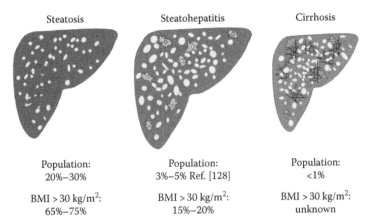

Steatosis	Steatohepatitis	Cirrhosis
Population: 20%–30%	Population: 3%–5% Ref. [128]	Population: <1%
BMI > 30 kg/m²: 65%–75%	BMI > 30 kg/m²: 15%–20%	BMI > 30 kg/m²: unknown

FIGURE 17.4 Spectrum of NAFLD and prevalences for severity estimated for the general population and in obese persons in the U.S. fat content >5% qualifies as steatosis. In steatohepatitis, inflammation is present and lymphocytes are increased. In cirrhosis, fibrosis is present and scar tissue has replaced damaged liver tissue. (Modified from Buechler, C. et al., *World J. Gastroenterol.*, 17(23), 2801, 2011.)

documented NAFLD in 34% of its participants [125]. African Americans have the lowest (24%), and Hispanic Americans have highest frequencies (45%) of NAFLD.

In morbidly obese persons (BMI > 35), up to 90% have NAFLD, with advanced disease in 9%–40% [126–130]. Currently the *presence* of NAFLD is related to dorso-cervical lipohypertrophy (buffalo hump) but no other subcutaneous depots [131]. The *severity* of NAFLD cannot be predicted by subcutaneous adiposity distribution [131].

FATTY LIVER

The prevalence of fatty liver in persons with BMI > 30 is estimated to be twice that of the general population [114]. Visceral adiposity is highly correlated with hepatic fat [3], and the idea that hepatic fat content, exemplified by NAFLD, is responsible for elevated CVD risk [132] has fully emerged. Suspected NAFLD in the 45–54 age group is a strong independent risk factor for cardiovascular death [133] and warrants further cardiovascular risk management guidelines. Assessment of hepatic fat content for CVD risk remains a research tool [134]. Leptin, adiponectin, TNF-α, retinol-binding protein 4 (RBP4) or fetuin-A may play a role in the development and progression of fatty liver disease [135].

What health dangers are associated with NAFLD? In its earliest stages, liver fat accumulation causes no overt symptoms, is reversible, and, by itself, is not necessarily damaging. In a series of 142 bariatric surgery patients, the prevalence of NAFLD was 70%, simple steatosis 23%, borderline nonalcoholic NASH 28%, and definitive NASH 18%. Type 2 diabetes mellitus and metabolic syndrome prevalences were 39% and 75%, respectively [136]. NAFLD is clearly associated with T2DM, which itself is debilitating, life shortening, and costly. Patients with NASH have severe hepatic, adipose tissue, and muscle IR versus healthy subjects without NASH [137]. T2DM and NASH together are associated with increased generation of ceramides, which are secondary messengers that mediate IR, cross the blood–brain barrier, and may be a mechanistic link to IR-mediated cognitive impairment [138]. Liver fibrosis and cirrhosis occur in 15%–25% of NASH cases over 10–20 years [139]. Finally, NASH may play a role in carcinogenesis, as the prevalence of hepatocellular carcinoma in NASH patients is 0%–2.8% over about 20 years [140] or ~10 times higher than the rate of 9.5/100,000 per year in the general U.S. population [116].

DEVELOPMENT OF NONALCOHOLIC LIVER DISEASE

How NAFLD develops is not well understood. Day and James first proposed a two-"hit" hypothesis in which dysregulation of fatty acid metabolism (lipotoxicity—the first insult) is followed by environmental or genetic perturbation causing hepatocyte necrosis [141]. Players in the second wave of insult are oxidative stress, adipocytokine imbalance, and upregulation of inflammatory mediators [139]. The first insult, dysregulation of fatty acid metabolism, occurs when the FFA supply from adipocytes and intestines exceeds the amount needed by the liver for mitochondrial oxidation, phospholipid synthesis, and cholesteryl ester synthesis. TG storage is increased. FFAs downregulate insulin receptor substrate 1 (IRS-1) signaling [142] (IRS-1, an intracellular substrate of the insulin receptor, is the effector of the insulin signal) contributing to IR. Hyperinsulinemia ensues. A newer "multihit" hypothesis stresses additional factors and a more complicated scheme [143].

Inflammation is considered to be a driving force behind NASH and the progression to fibrosis and subsequent cirrhosis [144]. Visceral adipose tissue is in a state of low grade inflammation in 75% of patients [145]. Visceral adipose tissue secretes more proinflammatory cytokines, including TNF-α, IL-6, and monocyte chemoattractant protein-1, compared to subcutaneous adipose tissue, possibly through recruitment of innate immune cells [144]. Inflammation of fat tissue is marked by the presence of macrophage crown-like structures [145]. Lymphocytes are found among IAAT, attracted by apoptotic (dying) adipocytes. Sickness of adipose tissue in susceptible patients has been named "adiposopathy" [9]. Adipose tissue may not be able to protect themselves from "lipotoxicity," the detrimental effect associated with excess fatty acid entry into cells. Cells protect themselves from these effects by either oxidizing the fatty acids or sequestering them as TAG within LDs [146]. When chronic energy supply overwhelms the adipocytes' capacity to store it, a condition exacerbated by inadequate adipocyte proliferation, apoptosis of individual adipocytes may occur [10,11,97]. This may not occur universally, and metabolically normal, benign obesity has been postulated [147].

Specific biomarkers for NASH do not exist. A prudent clinician may heed TG and liver enzyme levels in the obese. In bariatric surgery patients, TG and alanine transaminase (ALT) levels were strongly associated with advanced stages of NAFLD and NASH (P = 0.04) [93]. Blood TG levels >150 mg/dL increased the likelihood of NASH 3.4-fold, whereas circulating levels of TNF-α, leptin, and RBP4 did not identify NASH; however, adiponectin tended to be lower in NASH versus no NAFLD (P = 0.061) [93]. In other studies, low serum adiponectin was strongly correlated with NASH [148,149]. Systemic adiponectin is ordinarily about 20%–60% lower in NAFLD than healthy controls (reviewed in Ref. [114]). Impaired receptor-mediated signaling and transduction involving the adiponectin receptor AdipoR2 also contributes to the metabolic complications associated with hypoadiponectinemia in NAFLD [114].

PORTAL VEIN CONNECTION

It is important to realize the potential for visceral fat to contribute to steatosis and its progression. As mentioned earlier, the hepatic portal vein collects venous blood from the stomach, small intestine, pancreas, and spleen, and drains the omental and mesenteric adipose tissue depots associated with these organs. Under normal conditions, the liver receives 75% of its blood flow from the hepatic portal system and only 25% from the hepatic artery [150]. Thus, the inclination of IAAT to store TGs and release fatty acids directly affects liver. Also some adipokines and other factors are expressed to a different extent in IAAT compared to SAT (see Table 17.1).

IMAGING THE LIVER

Simple steatosis is detected by imaging studies, whereas the confirmation of NASH and its staging requires a liver biopsy. Because biopsy is invasive and involves risk, and sampling error limits its extrapolation to the entire liver mass, various noninvasive techniques have been developed, such as ultrasound, CT, magnetic resonance spectroscopy (MRS), and MRI-based methods. Landmark studies in the 1990s established the validity of localized proton MRS (1H MRS) to assess liver fat content. MRS-based methods can determine small amounts of fat accurately, whereas ultrasound and CT [151] provide only qualitative information about hepatic steatosis. Although used in clinical research, ultrasound is particularly challenging in obese patients due to impaired beam penetration and limited liver visualization. Thus, MRS is the preferred imaging method [152]. However, advances using MRI [153,154], MR elastography [155], and the use of approaches that combine quantifiable biochemical measurements and ultrasound imaging results may improve the recognition of NASH, in the absence of histological assessment by liver biopsy.

ARE WEIGHT GAIN, ABDOMINAL OBESITY, AND DEVELOPMENT OF FATTY LIVER A ONE-WAY STREET?

In the midst of the obesity epidemic, there is indeed some good news. Early-stage fatty liver, which is the most common form of NAFLD, is reversible. Strategies to enable and maintain weight loss are better known, countering the popular notion that nonsurgical weight loss is temporary. These strategies usually involve a social component and/or supervision by diet/exercise professionals.

How much reduction in visceral adipose tissue is required to induce favorable metabolic changes? One recent study showed that moderate reduction of visceral fat, as seen with short-term weight reduction programs, yields metabolic benefits on lipid profile, insulin sensitivity, and blood pressure similar to that observed after major weight reduction [156]. Interestingly, most of the fat loss during the first 2 weeks of caloric restriction and exercise is from the visceral fat.

DIET

Look AHEAD (Action for Health in Diabetes) studied >5000 overweight or obese individuals (60% females; mean age, 59 years) with type 2 diabetes mellitus. The average weight loss *across 4 years* among participants in the intensive lifestyle intervention arm of the study (−6.2%) exceeded that observed in the control arm of diabetes support and education (−0.9%, P < 0.001) [157]. Lifestyle intervention participants attended frequent group and individual sessions in support of behavioral change to increase moderate-intensity exercise progressively to 175 min/week, reduce caloric and saturated fat intake, and change macronutrient composition to improve glycemic control [158]. A substudy showed that a reduction in number of the largest of the abdominal (subcutaneous) fat cells drives the increase insulin sensitivity [159] possibly through increased adiponectin. (Large adipocytes secrete more adiponectin, and reduction in their size may maintain capacity for adiponectin secretion.) In another substudy, steatosis developed after 12 months in only 3% of the lifestyle intervention subjects compared to 26% of diabetes support and education participants [160].

Another trial [161] compared 2 years of lifestyle modification that included either a low-carbohydrate or a low-fat diet. Weight lost was ~11 kg (11%) at 1 year and 7 kg (7%) at 2 years with no major difference between the two methods except in HDL cholesterol, which was significantly higher in the low-carbohydrate group. The study concluded that successful long-term weight loss can be achieved with either a low-fat or low-carbohydrate diet when coupled with behavioral treatment, and that low-carbohydrate diet is associated with favorable changes in CVD risk factors at 2 years.

A third recent trial [162] confirmed that a diet that is high in protein content and lower in glycemic index was best for achieving a long-term weight maintenance and adherence after initial weight loss. The study enrolled 773 overweight adults from eight European countries who had lost at least 8% of their initial body weight with low-calorie diet. They were randomly assigned to one of five ad libitum diets to pre-vent weight regain over a 26-week period: a low-protein and low-glycemic-index diet, a low-protein and high-glycemic-index diet, a high-protein and low-glycemic-index diet, a high-protein and high-glycemic-index diet, or a control diet. Only the low-protein–high-glycemic-index diet was associated with subsequent significant weight regain. The study concluded that a modest increase in protein content and a modest reduction in the glycemic index led to maintenance of weight loss and less drop out.

Many other strategies fostering caloric restriction and physical activity can decrease visceral fat. These are too many to list. One example in African American and Hispanic patients showed that for every 10 g increase in soluble fiber eaten per day, visceral fat was reduced by 3.7% over 5 years [163].

EXERCISE

In free living people, physical activity is associated with smaller IAAT [164]. Active women have relatively small IAAT depots compared to other depots. In a study of 220 Caucasian women, IAAT was negatively related to physical activity [165]. When considering exercise programs, vigorous physical activity surpasses nonvigorous activity as a means to reduce IAAF. Regular moderate exercise (30 min of vigorous exercise two to four times a week) resulted in a 7.4% reduc-tion over 5 years [163]. Vigorous exercise was defined as that inducing sweating and heavy breathing. Omental adipocytes display greater relative responsiveness to both adrenergic receptor- and postreceptor-acting agents compared to subcu-taneous adipocytes [165]. The enhanced IAAT loss in response to more vigorous exercise may be attributed to the greater hormonal rises in high-intensity exercise versus low-intensity exercise. In regard to the exercise effects on IAAT, and aging, it may be that the increase in IAAT with aging is due, at least in part, to the steady decline in the pursuit of high-intensity (vigorous) exercise as we age, until the behavior is virtually absent.

DRUGS

Thiazolidinediones (TZDs) are PPARγ agonists that are used to treat IR in diabetes, and they can reduce visceral adiposity. In one study, pioglitazone not only resulted in weight gain but also lowered WHR and improved insulin sensitivity through selective increase in lower body fat without changing visceral fat [166]. These data suggest that PPARγ agonists selectively stimulate adipocyte proliferation, mostly in peripheral adipose tissue, and redistribute body fat. However, TZD therapy has fallen out of favor owing to the side effect of increased incidence of myocardial infarction with one drug in its class, rosiglitazone [167].

In patients with type 2 diabetes mellitus, tight diabetic control sometimes comes with a price: weight gain and hypoglycemia. Targeting body weight as an alternative model to targeting hemoglobin A(1c) is emerging as a viable and potentially cost-effective approach to diabetes management in clinical practice [168]. Treatment with sulfonylureas, insulin, and TZDs compromises body weight, but metformin reduces IR [169] and is weight neutral or may even reduce weight. A critical review of metformin studies shows that approximately half of studies in drug-naive type 2 diabetic patients demonstrated significant weight loss with metformin compared to baseline or comparator drugs, although pooled analyses suggest no significant effect versus placebo [170].

Combinations of medications that induce satiety and reduce food intake (e.g., glucagon-like peptide 1 analogues and amylin analogues) together with several weight-neutral medications (e.g., dipeptidyl peptidase-4 inhibitors and metformin) in proper combinations can help patients with type 2 diabetes to lose weight and maintain the weight loss [169]. The WhyWAIT (Weight Achievement and Intensive Treatment) program is a 12-week multidisciplinary program for weight control and intensive diabetes management specifically designed for application in routine diabetes practice [168]. The first 85 patients lost an average of 11.2 kg (25 lb) of body weight and 9.1 cm (3.6 in.) of waist circumference in the first 12 weeks. Liver transaminase levels were decreased, suggesting decreased hepatic fat [168].

BARIATRIC SURGERY

Dietary restriction for just a few days prior to gastric bypass and gastric banding is recommended by bariatric surgeons for its ability to shrink the size of the liver to make the surgery technically easier. Such restriction markedly reduces hepatic fat in NAFLD. Since the objective of bariatric surgery is to restrict calorie intake and absorption, the surgery leads to an expectation of dramatic overall body weight loss. The most widely practiced surgical weight loss approaches are gastric banding and gastric bypass. These interventions decrease excess body weight (the weight in excess of BMI = 25) by 50%–60% at 5 years [171] and reverse type 2 diabetes in 62%–83% of patients [172], but there are no data regarding NAFLD effects [171].

THERAPIES FOR NASH

Bearing in mind that there are no treatments for NASH approved by the American Association for the Study of Liver Diseases [173], the following serve as anecdotal reports.

Diet and physical activity: Simple steatosis is reversible. In a small study of obese patients with NAFLD, carbohydrate restriction (20 g/day) reduced liver TG content by 55% compared to 28% reduction with caloric restriction [174]. This difference points to a metabolic advantage of carbohydrate restriction. Excess carbohydrate consumption results in de novo synthesis of fatty acids. In people with NASH, this pathway is accelerated and accounts for up to 25% of the hepatic content [149]. Exercise intensity may be more important than duration or total volume of exercise to prevent NASH and fibrosis [175]. In a cross-sectional survey of 812 patients with NAFLD, vigorous exercise decreased the odds of finding NASH (OR 0.65), and doubling the amount of vigorous exercise decreased the odds of advanced fibrosis (OR 0.53) [175].

Drugs: The widely prescribed lipid-lowering agents like gemfibrozil and statins, in general, have shown minor improvements in NAFLD patients [140]. Unfortunately statins slightly exacerbate diabetes risk [176]. Metformin decreased steatosis in ob/ob mice, a leptin-deficient mouse model of steatosis and IR [177], as well as in patients [178]. In addition, NAFLD patients treated with the thiazolidinedione pioglitazone show improved hepatic steatosis [179].

OTHER ECTOPIC DEPOTS

The ectopic deposition of fat hypothesizes that a lack of sufficient adipocytes and/or limited capacity results in excess storage around tissues and organs such as liver, heart, and kidneys [49]. Other ectopic depots include skeletal muscle, thoracic, and pericardial fat. Research on the metabolic implications associated with variable size of these depots is in early stages, preventing clinical interpretation.

CONCLUSION

Research in obesity has incorporated adipose depot-specific studies and an adipocentric perspective. The pathophysiology of weight gain, explained in terms of intra-abdominal and ectopic fat deposition and the endocrinology of obesity, is leading to the development of more effective treatment tools. In order to use these new treatment tools effectively, clinicians must develop an understanding of the pathophysiology of excess weight and the metabolic role and vascular implications of visceral adiposity and ectopic fat in at-risk individuals. The result of this new understanding is the adaptation of both weight management and vascular-protective goals for therapy. *The new definition of obesity is based on the location and relative amounts of fat stored*, especially when the endocrine function and the metabolic risk are considered.

REFERENCES

1. Ford ES, Mokdad AH. Epidemiology of obesity in the Western Hemisphere. *J Clin Endocrinol Metab* 2008; 93/11 Suppl 1: S1–S8.
2. Despres JP, Lemieux I. Abdominal obesity and metabolic syndrome. *Nature* 2006; 444/7121: 881–887.
3. Despres JP. Excess visceral adipose tissue/ectopic fat the missing link in the obesity paradox? *J Am Coll Cardiol* 2011; 57(19): 1887–1889.
4. Poirier P, Giles TD, Bray GA, Hong Y, Stern JS, Pi-Sunyer FX et al. Obesity and cardiovascular disease: Pathophysiology, evaluation, and effect of weight loss: An update of the 1997 American Heart Association Scientific Statement on Obesity and Heart Disease from the Obesity Committee of the Council on Nutrition, Physical Activity, and Metabolism. *Circulation* 2006; 113/6: 898–918.

5. Bogers RP, Bemelmans WJ, Hoogenveen RT, Boshuizen HC, Woodward M, Knekt P et al. Association of overweight with increased risk of coronary heart disease partly independent of blood pressure and cholesterol levels: A meta-analysis of 21 cohort studies including more than 300 000 persons. *Arch Intern Med* 2007; 167/16: 1720–1728.

6. Alberti KG, Zimmet P, Shaw J. International Diabetes Federation: A consensus on type 2 diabetes prevention. *Diabet Med* 2007; 24/5: 451–463.

7. Coutinho T, Goel K, Correa de Sa D, Kragelund C, Kanaya AM, Zeller M et al. Central obesity and survival in subjects with coronary artery disease: A systematic review of the literature and collaborative analysis with individual subject data. *J Am Coll Cardiol* 2011; 57/19: 1877–1886.

8. Bodenant M, Kuulasmaa K, Wagner A, Kee F, Palmieri L, Ferrario MM et al. Measures of abdominal adiposity and the risk of stroke: The MOnica Risk, Genetics, Archiving and Monograph (MORGAM) Study. *Stroke* 2011; 42/10: 2872–2877.

9. Bays H, Dujovne CA. Adiposopathy is a more rational treatment target for metabolic disease than obesity alone. *Curr Atheroscler Rep* 2006; 8/2: 144–156.

10. Bays HE, Laferrere B, Dixon J, Aronne L, Gonzalez-Campoy JM, Apovian C et al. Adiposopathy and bariatric surgery: Is 'sick fat' a surgical disease? *Int J Clin Pract* 2009; 63/9: 1285–1300.

11. Bays H, Blonde L, Rosenson R. Adiposopathy: How do diet, exercise and weight loss drug therapies improve metabolic disease in overweight patients? *Expert Rev Cardiovasc Ther* 2006; 4/6: 871–895.

12. Goodpaster BH. Measuring body fat distribution and content in humans. *Curr Opin Clin Nutr Metab Care* 2002; 5/5: 481–487.

13. Zamboni M, Armellini F, Sheiban I, De MM, Todesco T, Bergamo-Andreis IA et al. Relation of body fat distribution in men and degree of coronary narrowings in coronary artery disease. *Am J Cardiol* 1992; 70/13: 1135–1138.

14. Bjorntorp P. Abdominal obesity and the development of noninsulin-dependent diabetes mellitus. *Diabetes Metab Rev* 1988; 4/6: 615–622.

15. Folsom AR, Kaye SA, Sellers TA, Hong CP, Cerhan JR, Potter JD et al. Body fat distribution and 5-year risk of death in older women. *JAMA* 1993; 269/4: 483–487.

16. Folsom AR, Prineas RJ, Kaye SA, Munger RG. Incidence of hypertension and stroke in relation to body fat distribution and other risk factors in older women. *Stroke* 1990; 21/5: 701–706.

17. Price GM, Uauy R, Breeze E, Bulpitt CJ, Fletcher AE. Weight, shape, and mortality risk in older persons: Elevated waist-hip ratio, not high body mass index, is associated with a greater risk of death. *Am J Clin Nutr* 2006; 84/2: 449–460.

18. National Institutes of Health. Clinical guidelines on the identification, evaluation, and treatment of overweight and obesity in adults—The evidence report. *Obes Res* 1998; 6 Suppl 2: 51S–209S.

19. Severinsen MT, Kristensen SR, Johnsen SP, Dethlefsen C, Tjonneland A, Overvad K. Anthropometry, body fat, and venous thromboembolism: A Danish follow-up study. *Circulation* 2009; 120/19: 1850–1857.

20. Rexrode KM, Carey VJ, Hennekens CH, Walters EE, Colditz GA, Stampfer MJ et al. Abdominal adiposity and coronary heart disease in women. *JAMA* 1998; 280/21: 1843–1848.

21. Fox CS, Massaro JM, Hoffmann U, Pou KM, Maurovich-Horvat P, Liu CY et al. Abdominal visceral and subcutaneous adipose tissue compartments: Association with metabolic risk factors in the Framingham Heart Study. *Circulation* 2007; 116/1: 39–48.

22. Field AE, Coakley EH, Must A, Spadano JL, Laird N, Dietz WH et al. Impact of overweight on the risk of developing common chronic diseases during a 10-year period. *Arch Intern Med* 2001; 161/13: 1581–1586.

23. Wang Y, Rimm EB, Stampfer MJ, Willett WC, Hu FB. Comparison of abdominal adiposity and overall obesity in predicting risk of type 2 diabetes among men. *Am J Clin Nutr* 2005; 81/3: 555–563.

24. Grundy SM, Cleeman JI, Daniels SR, Donato KA, Eckel RH, Franklin BA et al. Diagnosis and management of the metabolic syndrome: An American Heart Association/National Heart, Lung, and Blood Institute scientific statement. *Circulation* 2005; 112/17: 2735–2752.

25. Vague J. The degree of masculine differentiation of obesities: A factor determining predisposition to diabetes, atherosclerosis, gout, and uric calculous disease. *Am J Clin Nutr* 1956; 4/1: 20–34.

26. Larsson B, Seidell J, Svardsudd K, Welin L, Tibblin G, Wilhelmsen L et al. Obesity, adipose tissue distribution and health in men—The study of men born in 1913. *Appetite* 1989; 13/1: 37–44.

27. Lapidus L, Bengtsson C, Larsson B, Pennert K, Rybo E, Sjostrom L. Distribution of adipose tissue and risk of cardiovascular disease and death: A 12 year follow up of participants in the population study of women in Gothenburg, Sweden. *Br Med J (Clin Res Ed)* 1984; 289/6454: 1257–1261.

28. Bonora E, Tessari R, Micciolo R, Zenere M, Targher G, Padovani R et al. Intimal-medial thickness of the carotid artery in nondiabetic and NIDDM patients: Relationship with insulin resistance. *Diabetes Care* 1997; 20/4: 627–631.

29. Yamamoto M, Egusa G, Hara H, Yamakido M. Association of intraabdominal fat and carotid atherosclerosis in non-obese middle-aged men with normal glucose tolerance. *Int J Obes Relat Metab Disord* 1997; 21/10: 948–951.

30. Hartz A, Grubb B, Wild R, Van Nort JJ, Kuhn E, Freedman D et al. The association of waist hip ratio and angiographically determined coronary artery disease. *Int J Obes* 1990; 14/8: 657–665.

31. Hauner H, Stangl K, Schmatz C, Burger K, Blomer H, Pfeiffer EF. Body fat distribution in men with angiographically confirmed coronary artery disease. *Atherosclerosis* 1990; 85/2–3: 203–210.

32. Thompson CJ, Ryu JE, Craven TE, Kahl FR, Crouse JR, III. Central adipose distribution is related to coronary atherosclerosis. *Arterioscler Thromb* 1991; 11/2: 327–333.

33. Flynn MA, Codd MB, Gibney MJ, Keelan ET, Sugrue DD. Indices of obesity and body fat distribution in arteriographically defined coronary artery disease in men. *Ir J Med Sci* 1993; 162/12: 503–509.

34. Nakamura T, Tokunaga K, Shimomura I, Nishida M, Yoshida S, Kotani K et al. Contribution of visceral fat accumulation to the development of coronary artery disease in non-obese men. *Atherosclerosis* 1994; 107/2: 239–246.

35. Pouliot MC, Despres JP, Lemieux S, Moorjani S, Bouchard C, Tremblay A et al. Waist circumference and abdominal sagittal diameter: Best simple anthropometric indexes of abdominal visceral adipose tissue accumulation and related cardiovascular risk in men and women. *Am J Cardiol* 1994; 73/7: 460–468.

36. World Health Organization. Definition, diagnosis and classification of diabetes mellitus and its complications: Report of a WHO Consultation. Part I: Diagnosis and classification of diabetes mellitus. 1999. Geneva, Switzerland, World Health Organization.

37. Arad Y, Newstein D, Cadet F, Roth M, Guerci AD. Association of multiple risk factors and insulin resistance with increased prevalence of asymptomatic coronary artery disease by an electron-beam computed tomographic study. *Arterioscler Thromb Vasc Biol* 2001; 21/12: 2051–2058.

38. National Institutes of Health—National Heart LaBI. Clinical guidelines on the identification, evaluation, and treatment of overweight and obesity in adults. NIH Publication No. 98-4083. 2011. Bethesda, MD, U.S. Department of Health and Human Services.

39. Kanhai DA, Kappelle LJ, van der Graaf Y, Uiterwaal CS, Visseren FL. The risk of general and abdominal adiposity in the occurrence of new vascular events and mortality in patients with various manifestations of vascular disease. *Int J Obes (Lond)* 2011, doi: 10.20138/ijo 2011.115, epub ahead of print.

40. Thomas EL, Parkinson JR, Frost GS, Goldstone AP, Dore CJ, McCarthy JP et al. The missing risk: MRI and MRS phenotyping of abdominal adiposity and ectopic fat. *Obesity (Silver Spring)* 2011; 20/1: 76–78.

41. Rebuffe-Scrive M, Andersson B, Olbe L, Bjorntorp P. Metabolism of adipose tissue in intraabdominal depots of nonobese men and women. *Metabolism* 1989; 38/5: 453–458.

42. Reaven GM. Banting lecture 1988. Role of insulin resistance in human disease. *Diabetes* 1988; 37/12: 1595–1607.

43. Pascot A, Despres JP, Lemieux I, Almeras N, Bergeron J, Nadeau A et al. Deterioration of the metabolic risk profile in women. Respective contributions of impaired glucose tolerance and visceral fat accumulation. *Diabetes Care* 2001; 24/5: 902–908.

44. Pascot A, Despres JP, Lemieux I, Bergeron J, Nadeau A, Prud'homme D et al. Contribution of visceral obesity to the deterioration of the metabolic risk profile in men with impaired glucose tolerance. *Diabetologia* 2000; 43/9: 1126–1135.

45. Pouliot MC, Despres JP, Nadeau A, Moorjani S, Prud'homme D, Lupien PJ et al. Visceral obesity in men. Associations with glucose tolerance, plasma insulin, and lipoprotein levels. *Diabetes* 1992; 41/7: 826–834.

46. Walton C, Lees B, Crook D, Godsland IF, Stevenson JC. Relationships between insulin metabolism, serum lipid profile, body fat distribution and blood pressure in healthy men. *Atherosclerosis* 1995; 118/1: 35–43.

47. Kahn BB, Flier JS. Obesity and insulin resistance. *J Clin Invest* 2000; 106/4: 473–481.

48. Miyazaki Y, DeFronzo RA. Visceral fat dominant distribution in male type 2 diabetic patients is closely related to hepatic insulin resistance, irrespective of body type. *Cardiovasc Diabetol* 2009; 8: 44.

49. Heilbronn L, Smith SR, Ravussin E. Failure of fat cell proliferation, mitochondrial function and fat oxidation results in ectopic fat storage, insulin resistance and type II diabetes mellitus. *Int J Obes Relat Metab Disord* 2004; 28 Suppl 4: S12–S21.

50. Randle PJ, Garland PB, Hales CN, Newsholme EA. The glucose fatty-acid cycle. Its role in insulin sensitivity and the metabolic disturbances of diabetes mellitus. *Lancet* 1963; 1/7285: 785–789.

51. Bremer AA, Devaraj S, Afify A, Jialal I. Adipose tissue dysregulation in patients with metabolic syndrome. *J Clin Endocrinol Metab* 2011; 96 (11): E1782–E1788.

52. Despres JP. The insulin resistance-dyslipidemic syndrome of visceral obesity: Effect on patients' risk. *Obes Res* 1998; 6 Suppl 1: 8S–17S.

53. Despres JP, Moorjani S, Lupien PJ, Tremblay A, Nadeau A, Bouchard C. Regional distribution of body fat, plasma lipoproteins, and cardiovascular disease. *Arteriosclerosis* 1990; 10/4: 497–511.

54. Lupattelli G, Pirro M, Mannarino MR, Siepi D, Roscini AR, Schillaci G et al. Visceral fat positively correlates with cholesterol synthesis in dyslipidaemic patients. *Eur J Clin Invest* 2011; 42/2: 164–170.

55. Hill JO, Sidney S, Lewis CE, Tolan K, Scherzinger AL, Stamm ER. Racial differences in amounts of visceral adipose tissue in young adults: The CARDIA (Coronary Artery Risk Development in Young Adults) study. *Am J Clin Nutr* 1999; 69/3: 381–387.

56. Despres JP, Couillard C, Gagnon J, Bergeron J, Leon AS, Rao DC et al. Race, visceral adipose tissue, plasma lipids, and lipoprotein lipase activity in men and women: The Health, Risk Factors, Exercise Training, and Genetics (HERITAGE) family study. *Arterioscler Thromb Vasc Biol* 2000; 20/8: 1932–1938.

57. Hoffman DJ, Wang Z, Gallagher D, Heymsfield SB. Comparison of visceral adipose tissue mass in adult African Americans and whites. *Obes Res* 2005; 13/1: 66–74.

58. Lear SA, Humphries KH, Kohli S, Chockalingam A, Frohlich JJ, Birmingham CL. Visceral adipose tissue accumulation differs according to ethnic background: Results of the Multicultural Community Health Assessment Trial (M-CHAT). *Am J Clin Nutr* 2007; 86/2: 353–359.

59. Camhi SM, Bray GA, Bouchard C, Greenway FL, Johnson WD, Newton RL et al. The relationship of waist circumference and BMI to visceral, subcutaneous, and total body fat: Sex and race differences. *Obesity (Silver Spring)* 2011; 19/2: 402–408.

60. Misra A, Khurana L. Obesity-related non-communicable diseases: South Asians vs White Caucasians. *Int J Obes (Lond)* 2011; 35/2: 167–187.

61. Demerath EW, Sun SS, Rogers N, Lee M, Reed D, Choh AC et al. Anatomical patterning of visceral adipose tissue: Race, sex, and age variation. *Obesity (Silver Spring)* 2007; 15/12: 2984–2993.

62. Liu J, Fox CS, Hickson DA, May WD, Hairston KG, Carr JJ et al. Impact of abdominal visceral and subcutaneous adipose tissue on cardiometabolic risk factors: The Jackson Heart Study. *J Clin Endocrinol Metab* 2010; 95/12: 5419–5426.

63. Shah A, Hernandez A, Mathur D, Budoff MJ, Kanaya AM. Adipokines and body fat composition in South Asians: Results of the Metabolic Syndrome and Atherosclerosis in South Asians Living in America (MASALA) study. *Int J Obes (Lond)* 2011, doi: 10.20138/ijo 2011.167, epub ahead of print.

64. Kim S, Cho B, Lee H, Choi K, Hwang SS, Kim D et al. Distribution of abdominal visceral and subcutaneous adipose tissue and metabolic syndrome in a Korean population. *Diabetes Care* 2011; 34/2: 504–506.

65. Conway JM, Yanovski SZ, Avila NA, Hubbard VS. Visceral adipose tissue differences in black and white women. *Am J Clin Nutr* 1995; 61/4: 765–771.

66. Lovejoy JC, Smith SR, Rood JC. Comparison of regional fat distribution and health risk factors in middle-aged white and African American women: The Healthy Transitions Study. *Obes Res* 2001; 9/1: 10–16.

67. Hunter GR, Giger JN, Weaver M, Strickland OL, Zuckerman P, Taylor H. Fat distribution and cardiovascular disease risk in African-American women. *J Natl Black Nurses Assoc* 2000; 11/2: 7–11.

68. Hamdy O, Porramatikul S, Al-Ozairi E. Metabolic obesity: The paradox between visceral and subcutaneous fat. *Curr Diabetes Rev* 2006; 2/4: 367–373.

69. Kuk JL, Saunders TJ, Davidson LE, Ross R. Age-related changes in total and regional fat distribution. *Ageing Res Rev* 2009; 8/4: 339–348.

70. Perusse L, Rice T, Chagnon YC, Despres JP, Lemieux S, Roy S et al. A genome-wide scan for abdominal fat assessed by computed tomography in the Quebec Family Study. *Diabetes* 2001; 50/3: 614–621.

71. Kovsan J, Bluher M, Tarnovscki T, Kloting N, Kirshtein B, Madar L et al. Altered autophagy in human adipose tissues in obesity. *J Clin Endocrinol Metab* 2011; 96/2: E268–E277.

72. MacLaren RE, Cui W, Lu H, Simard S, Cianflone K. Association of adipocyte genes with ASP expression: A microarray analysis of subcutaneous and omental adipose tissue in morbidly obese subjects. *BMC Med Genomics* 2010; 3: 3.

73. Gabriely I, Barzilai N. Surgical removal of visceral adipose tissue: Effects on insulin action. *Curr Diabetes Rep* 2003; 3/3: 201–206.

74. Steppan CM, Bailey ST, Bhat S, Brown EJ, Banerjee RR, Wright CM et al. The hormone resistin links obesity to diabetes. *Nature* 2001; 409/6818: 307–312.

75. Hofmann C, Lorenz K, Braithwaite SS, Colca JR, Palazuk BJ, Hotamisligil GS et al. Altered gene expression for tumor necrosis factor-alpha and its receptors during drug and dietary modulation of insulin resistance. *Endocrinology* 1994; 134/1: 264–270.

76. Hotamisligil GS, Peraldi P, Budavari A, Ellis R, White MF, Spiegelman BM. IRS-1-mediated inhibition of insulin receptor tyrosine kinase activity in TNF-alpha- and obesity-induced insulin resistance. *Science* 1996; 271/5249: 665–668.

77. Tchernof A, Starling RD, Turner A, Shuldiner AR, Walston JD, Silver K et al. Impaired capacity to lose visceral adipose tissue during weight reduction in obese postmenopausal women with the Trp64Arg beta3-adrenoceptor gene variant. *Diabetes* 2000; 49/10: 1709–1713.

78. Chowdhury B, Sjostrom L, Alpsten M, Kostanty J, Kvist H, Lofgren R. A multicompartment body composition technique based on computerized tomography. *Int J Obes Relat Metab Disord* 1994; 18/4: 219–234.

79. van der Kooy K, Leenen R, Deurenberg P, Seidell JC, Westerterp KR, Hautvast JG. Changes in fat-free mass in obese subjects after weight loss: A comparison of body composition measures. *Int J Obes Relat Metab Disord* 1992; 16/9: 675–683.

80. Bosello O, Zamboni M, Armellini F, Zocca I, Bergamo Andreis IA, Smacchia C et al. Modifications of abdominal fat and hepatic insulin clearance during severe caloric restriction. *Ann Nutr Metab* 1990; 34/6: 359–365.

81. van der Kooy K, Seidell JC. Techniques for the measurement of visceral fat: A practical guide. *Int J Obes Relat Metab Disord* 1993; 17/4: 187–196.

82. Van Pelt RE, Evans EM, Schechtman KB, Ehsani AA, Kohrt WM. Contributions of total and regional fat mass to risk for cardiovascular disease in older women. *Am J Physiol Endocrinol Metab* 2002; 282/5: E1023–E1028.

83. Armellini F, Zamboni M, Rigo L, Robbi R, Todesco T, Castelli S et al. Measurements of intra-abdominal fat by ultrasound and computed tomography: Predictive equations in women. *Basic Life Sci* 1993; 60: 75–77.

84. Tornaghi G, Raiteri R, Pozzato C, Rispoli A, Bramani M, Cipolat M et al. Anthropometric or ultrasonic measurements in assessment of visceral fat? A comparative study. *Int J Obes Relat Metab Disord* 1994; 18/11: 771–775.

85. Vikram NK, Bhatt SP, Bhushan B, Luthra K, Misra A, Poddar PK et al. Associations of -308G/A polymorphism of tumor necrosis factor (TNF)-alpha gene and serum TNF-alpha levels with measures of obesity, intra-abdominal and subcutaneous abdominal fat, subclinical inflammation and insulin resistance in Asian Indians in north India. *Dis Markers* 2011; 31/1: 39–46.

86. Stolk RP, Wink O, Zelissen PM, Meijer R, van Gils AP, Grobbee DE. Validity and reproducibility of ultrasonography for the measurement of intra-abdominal adipose tissue. *Int J Obes Relat Metab Disord* 2001; 25/9: 1346–1351.

87. Armellini F, Zamboni M, Castelli S, Micciolo R, Mino A, Turcato E et al. Measured and predicted total and visceral adipose tissue in women: Correlations with metabolic parameters. *Int J Obes Relat Metab Disord* 1994; 18/9: 641–647.

88. Williams MJ, Hunter GR, Kekes-Szabo T, Snyder S, Treuth MS. Regional fat distribution in women and risk of cardiovascular disease. *Am J Clin Nutr* 1997; 65/3: 855–860.

89. Lissner L, Bjorkelund C, Heitmann BL, Seidell JC, Bengtsson C. Larger hip circumference independently predicts health and longevity in a Swedish female cohort. *Obes Res* 2001; 9/10: 644–646.

90. Seidell JC, Perusse L, Despres JP, Bouchard C. Waist and hip circumferences have independent and opposite effects on cardiovascular disease risk factors: The Quebec Family Study. *Am J Clin Nutr* 2001; 74/3: 315–321.

91. Aucouturier J, Meyer M, Thivel D, Taillardat M, Duche P. Effect of android to gynoid fat ratio on insulin resistance in obese youth. *Arch Pediatr Adolesc Med* 2009; 163/9: 826–831.

92. Faloia E, Tirabassi G, Canibus P, Boscaro M. Protective effect of leg fat against cardiovascular risk factors in obese premenopausal women. *Nutr Metab Cardiovasc Dis* 2009; 19/1: 39–44.

93. Pulzi FB, Cisternas R, Melo MR, Ribeiro CM, Malheiros CA, Salles JE. New clinical score to diagnose nonalcoholic steatohepatitis in obese patients. *Diabetol Metab Syndr* 2011; 3/1: 3.

94. Schouten F, Twisk JW, de Boer MR, Stehouwer CD, Serne EH, Smulders YM et al. Increases in central fat mass and decreases in peripheral fat mass are associated with accelerated arterial stiffening in healthy adults: The Amsterdam Growth and Health Longitudinal Study. *Am J Clin Nutr* 2011; 94/1: 40–48.

95. Tanko LB, Bagger YZ, Alexandersen P, Larsen PJ, Christiansen C. Central and peripheral fat mass have contrasting effect on the progression of aortic calcification in postmenopausal women. *Eur Heart J* 2003; 24/16: 1531–1537.

96. Raynaud E, Perez-Martin A, Brun JF, Fedou C, Mercier J. Insulin sensitivity measured with the minimal model is higher in moderately overweight women with predominantly lower body fat. *Horm Metab Res* 1999; 31/7: 415–417.

97. Bays HE, Fox KM, Grandy S. Anthropometric measurements and diabetes mellitus: Clues to the "pathogenic" and "protective" potential of adipose tissue. *Metab Syndr Relat Disord* 2010; 8/4: 307–315.

98. Terry RB, Stefanick ML, Haskell WL, Wood PD. Contributions of regional adipose tissue depots to plasma lipoprotein concentrations in overweight men and women: Possible protective effects of thigh fat. *Metabolism* 1991; 40/7: 733–740.

99. Ishikawa K, Takahashi K, Bujo H, Hashimoto N, Yagui K, Saito Y. Subcutaneous fat modulates insulin sensitivity in mice by regulating TNF-alpha expression in visceral fat. *Horm Metab Res* 2006; 38/10: 631–638.

100. Barzilai N, She L, Liu BQ, Vuguin P, Cohen P, Wang J et al. Surgical removal of visceral fat reverses hepatic insulin resistance. *Diabetes* 1999; 48/1: 94–98.

101. Gabriely I, Ma XH, Yang XM, Atzmon G, Rajala MW, Berg AH et al. Removal of visceral fat prevents insulin resistance and glucose intolerance of aging: An adipokine-mediated process? *Diabetes* 2002; 51/10: 2951–2958.

102. Klein S, Fontana L, Young VL, Coggan AR, Kilo C, Patterson BW et al. Absence of an effect of liposuction on insulin action and risk factors for coronary heart disease. *N Engl J Med* 2004; 350/25: 2549–2557.

103. Ibrahim MM. Subcutaneous and visceral adipose tissue: Structural and functional differences. *Obes Rev* 2010; 11/1: 11–18.

104. Ohman MK, Wright AP, Wickenheiser KJ, Luo W, Eitzman DT. Visceral adipose tissue and atherosclerosis. *Curr Vasc Pharmacol* 2009; 7/2: 169–179.

105. Tchkonia T, Giorgadze N, Pirtskhalava T, Thomou T, DePonte M, Koo A et al. Fat depot-specific characteristics are retained in strains derived from single human preadipocytes. *Diabetes* 2006; 55/9: 2571–2578.

106. Drolet R, Richard C, Sniderman AD, Mailloux J, Fortier M, Huot C et al. Hypertrophy and hyperplasia of abdominal adipose tissues in women. *Int J Obes (Lond)* 2008; 32/2: 283–291.

107. Boivin A, Brochu G, Marceau S, Marceau P, Hould FS, Tchernof A. Regional differences in adipose tissue metabolism in obese men. *Metabolism* 2007; 56/4: 533–540.

108. Shadid S, Koutsari C, Jensen MD. Direct free fatty acid uptake into human adipocytes in vivo: Relation to body fat distribution. *Diabetes* 2007; 56/5: 1369–1375.

109. Stefan N, Kantartzis K, Machann J, Schick F, Thamer C, Rittig K et al. Identification and characterization of metabolically benign obesity in humans. *Arch Intern Med* 2008; 168/15: 1609–1616.

110. O'Connell J, Lynch L, Cawood TJ, Kwasnik A, Nolan N, Geoghegan J et al. The relationship of omental and subcutaneous adipocyte size to metabolic disease in severe obesity. *PLoS One* 2010; 5/4: e9997.

111. Hube F, Hauner H. The role of TNF-α in human adipose tissue: Prevention of weight gain at the expense of insulin resistance? *Horm Metab Res* 1999; 31: 626–631.

112. Bastard JP, Maachi M, Lagathu C, Kim MJ, Caron M, Vidal H et al. Recent advances in the relationship between obesity, inflammation, and insulin resistance. *Eur Cytokine Netw* 2006; 17/1: 4–12.

113. Kim JH, Bachmann RA, Chen J. Interleukin-6 and insulin resistance. *Vitam Horm* 2009; 80: 613–633.

114. Buechler C, Wanninger J, Neumeier M. Adiponectin, a key adipokine in obesity related liver diseases. *World J Gastroenterol* 2011; 17/23: 2801–2811.

115. Drolet R, Belanger C, Fortier M, Huot C, Mailloux J, Legare D et al. Fat depot-specific impact of visceral obesity on adipocyte adiponectin release in women. *Obesity (Silver Spring)* 2009; 17/3: 424–430.

116. Reid AE. Nonalcoholic fatty liver disease. In: Feldman M, Friedman LS, Brandt LJ (eds). *Sleisenger and Fordtran's Gastrointestinal and Liver Disease: Pathophysiology, Diagnosis, Management.* Saunders Elsevier: Philadelphia, PA, 2011, pp. 1401–1411.

117. Arner P. Differences in lipolysis between human subcutaneous and omental adipose tissues. *Ann Med* 1995; 27/4: 435–438.

118. Jensen MD. Lipolysis: Contribution from regional fat. *Annu Rev Nutr* 1997; 17: 127–139.

119. Robertson D, Johnson GA, Robertson RM, Nies AS, Shand DG, Oates JA. Comparative assessment of stimuli that release neuronal and adrenomedullary catecholamines in man. *Circulation* 1979; 59/4: 637–643.

120. Ludwig J, Viggiano TR, McGill DB, Oh BJ. Nonalcoholic steatohepatitis: Mayo Clinic experiences with a hitherto unnamed disease. *Mayo Clin Proc* 1980; 55/7: 434–438.

121. Busuttil RW, Tanaka K. The utility of marginal donors in liver transplantation. *Liver Transpl* 2003; 9/7: 651–663.

122. Robbins SL, Kumar V, Coutran RS. *Pathologic Basis of Disease.* Elsevier: London, U.K., 2010.

123. Helms CA, Brant WE. *Fundamentals of Diagnostic Radiology.* Lippincott Williams & Wilkins: Philadelphia, PA, 2007.

124. Sagi R, Reif S, Neuman G, Webb M, Phillip M, Shalitin S. Nonalcoholic fatty liver disease in overweight children and adolescents. *Acta Paediatr* 2007; 96/8: 1209–1213.

125. Browning JD, Szczepaniak LS, Dobbins R, Nuremberg P, Horton JD, Cohen JC et al. Prevalence of hepatic steatosis in an urban population in the United States: Impact of ethnicity. *Hepatology* 2004; 40/6: 1387–1395.

126. Dixon JB, Bhathal PS, Hughes NR, O'Brien PE. Nonalcoholic fatty liver disease: Improvement in liver histological analysis with weight loss. *Hepatology* 2004; 39/6: 1647–1654.

127. Hsiao TJ, Chen JC, Wang JD. Insulin resistance and ferritin as major determinants of nonalcoholic fatty liver disease in apparently healthy obese patients. *Int J Obes Relat Metab Disord* 2004; 28/1: 167–172.

128. Boza C, Riquelme A, Ibanez L, Duarte I, Norero E, Viviani P et al. Predictors of nonalcoholic steatohepatitis (NASH) in obese patients undergoing gastric bypass. *Obes Surg* 2005; 15/8: 1148–1153.

129. Scheen AJ, Luyckx FH, Desaive C, Lefebvre PJ. Severe/extreme obesity: A medical disease requiring a surgical treatment? *Acta Clin Belg* 1999; 54/3: 154–161.

130. Gholam PM, Flancbaum L, Machan JT, Charney DA, Kotler DP. Nonalcoholic fatty liver disease in severely obese subjects. *Am J Gastroenterol* 2007; 102/2: 399–408.

131. Cheung O, Kapoor A, Puri P, Sistrun S, Luketic VA, Sargeant CC et al. The impact of fat distribution on the severity of nonalcoholic fatty liver disease and metabolic syndrome. *Hepatology* 2007; 46/4: 1091–1100.

132. Klein S. Abdominal adiposity: An emerging marker. Introduction. *Clin Cornerstone* 2008; 9/1: 8–10.

133. Dunn W, Xu R, Wingard DL, Rogers C, Angulo P, Younossi ZM et al. Suspected nonalcoholic fatty liver disease and mortality risk in a population-based cohort study. *Am J Gastroenterol* 2008; 103/9: 2263–2271.

134. Frimel TN, Deivanayagam S, Bashir A, O'Connor R, Klein S. Assessment of intrahepatic triglyceride content using magnetic resonance spectroscopy. *J Cardiometab Syndr* 2007; 2/2: 136–138.

135. Tonjes A, Bluher M, Stumvoll M. Retinol-binding protein 4 and new adipocytokines in nonalcoholic fatty liver disease. *Curr Pharm Des* 2010; 16/17: 1921–1928.

136. Kashyap SR, Diab DL, Baker AR, Yerian L, Bajaj H, Gray-McGuire C et al. Triglyceride levels and not adipokine concentrations are closely related to severity of nonalcoholic fatty liver disease in an obesity surgery cohort. *Obesity (Silver Spring)* 2009; 17/9: 1696–1701.

137. Lomonaco R, Ortiz-Lopez C, Orsak B, Finch J, Webb A, Bril F et al. Role of ethnicity in overweight and obese patients with nonalcoholic steatohepatitis. *Hepatology* 2011; 54/3: 837–845.

138. de la Monte SM, Longato L, Tong M, Wands JR. Insulin resistance and neurodegeneration: Roles of obesity, type 2 diabetes mellitus and non-alcoholic steatohepatitis. *Curr Opin Investig Drugs* 2009; 10/10: 1049–1060.

139. Della CC, Alisi A, Iorio R, Alterio A, Nobili V. Expert opinion on current therapies for nonalcoholic fatty liver disease. *Expert Opin Pharmacother* 2011; 12/12: 1901–1911.

140. Starley BQ, Calcagno CJ, Harrison SA. Nonalcoholic fatty liver disease and hepatocellular carcinoma: A weighty connection. *Hepatology* 2010; 51/5: 1820–1832.

141. Day CP, James OF. Steatohepatitis: A tale of two "hits"? *Gastroenterology* 1998; 114/4: 842–845.

142. Sun XJ, Miralpeix M, Myers MG, Jr., Glasheen EM, Backer JM, Kahn CR et al. Expression and function of IRS-1 in insulin signal transmission. *J Biol Chem* 1992; 267/31: 22662–22672.

143. Polyzos SA, Kountouras J, Zavos C. Nonalcoholic fatty liver disease: The pathogenetic roles of insulin resistance and adipocytokines. *Curr Mol Med* 2009; 9/3: 299–314.

144. Harmon RC, Tiniakos DG, Argo CK. Inflammation in nonalcoholic steatohepatitis. *Expert Rev Gastroenterol Hepatol* 2011; 5/2: 189–200.

145. Farb MG, Bigornia S, Mott M, Tanriverdi K, Morin KM, Freedman JE et al. Reduced adipose tissue inflammation represents an intermediate cardiometabolic phenotype in obesity. *J Am Coll Cardiol* 2011; 58/3: 232–237.

146. Greenberg AS, Coleman RA, Kraemer FB, McManaman JL, Obin MS, Puri V et al. The role of lipid droplets in metabolic disease in rodents and humans. *J Clin Invest* 2011; 121/6: 2102–2110.

147. Pataky Z, Bobbioni-Harsch E, Golay A. Open questions about metabolically normal obesity. *Int J Obes (Lond)* 2010; 34 Suppl 2: S18–S23.

148. Baranova A, Gowder SJ, Schlauch K, Elariny H, Collantes R, Afendy A et al. Gene expression of leptin, resistin, and adiponectin in the white adipose tissue of obese patients with non-alcoholic fatty liver disease and insulin resistance. *Obes Surg* 2006; 16/9: 1118–1125.

149. Donnelly KL, Smith CI, Schwarzenberg SJ, Jessurun J, Boldt MD, Parks EJ. Sources of fatty acids stored in liver and secreted via lipoproteins in patients with nonalcoholic fatty liver disease. *J Clin Invest* 2005; 115/5: 1343–1351.

150. Shah VH, Kamath PS. Portal hypertension and gastrointestinal bleeding. In: Feldman M, Friedman LS, Brandt LJ (eds). *Sleisenger and Fordtran's Gastrointestinal and Liver Disease: Pathophysiology, Diagnosis, Management*. Saunders Elsevier: Philadelphia, PA, 2010.

151. Reeder SB, Sirlin CB. Quantification of liver fat with magnetic resonance imaging. *Magn Reson Imaging Clin N Am* 2010; 18/3: 337–357, ix.

152. Springer F, Machann J, Claussen CD, Schick F, Schwenzer NF. Liver fat content determined by magnetic resonance imaging and spectroscopy. *World J Gastroenterol* 2010; 16/13: 1560–1566.

153. Hines CD, Frydrychowicz A, Hamilton G, Tudorascu DL, Vigen KK, Yu H et al. T(1) independent, T(2) (*) corrected chemical shift based fat-water separation with multipeak fat spectral modeling is an accurate and precise measure of hepatic steatosis. *J Magn Reson Imaging* 2011; 33/4: 873–881.

154. d'Assignies G, Kauffmann C, Boulanger Y, Bilodeau M, Vilgrain V, Soulez G et al. Simultaneous assessment of liver volume and whole liver fat content: A step towards one-stop shop preoperative MRI protocol. *Eur Radiol* 2011; 21/2: 301–309.

155. MacDougall JD, Ward GR, Sale DG, Sutton JR. Biochemical adaptation of human skeletal muscle to heavy resistance training and immobilization. *J Appl Physiol* 1977; 43/4: 700–703.

156. Brochu M, Tchernof A, Turner AN, Ades PA, Poehlman ET. Is there a threshold of visceral fat loss that improves the metabolic profile in obese postmenopausal women? *Metab* 2003; 52/5: 599–604.

157. Wing RR. Long-term effects of a lifestyle intervention on weight and cardiovascular risk factors in individuals with type 2 diabetes mellitus: Four-year results of the Look AHEAD trial. *Arch Intern Med* 2010; 170/17: 1566–1575.

158. Wadden TA, West DS, Delahanty L, Jakicic J, Rejeski J, Williamson D et al. The Look AHEAD study: A description of the lifestyle intervention and the evidence supporting it. *Obesity (Silver Spring)* 2006; 14/5: 737–752.

159. Pasarica M, Tchoukalova YD, Heilbronn LK, Fang X, Albu JB, Kelley DE et al. Differential effect of weight loss on adipocyte size subfractions in patients with type 2 diabetes. *Obesity (Silver Spring)* 2009; 17/10: 1976–1978.

160. Lazo M, Solga SF, Horska A, Bonekamp S, Diehl AM, Brancati FL et al. Effect of a 12-month intensive lifestyle intervention on hepatic steatosis in adults with type 2 diabetes. *Diabetes Care* 2010; 33/10: 2156–2163.

161. Foster GD, Wyatt HR, Hill JO, Makris AP, Rosenbaum DL, Brill C et al. Weight and metabolic outcomes after 2 years on a low-carbohydrate versus low-fat diet: A randomized trial. *Ann Intern Med* 2010; 153/3: 147–157.

162. Larsen TM, Dalskov SM, van BM, Jebb SA, Papadaki A, Pfeiffer AF et al. Diets with high or low protein content and glycemic index for weight-loss maintenance. *N Engl J Med* 2010; 363/22: 2102–2113.

163. Hairston KG, Vitolins MZ, Norris JM, Anderson AM, Hanley AJ, Wagenknecht LE. Lifestyle factors and 5-year abdominal fat accumulation in a minority cohort: The IRAS Family Study. *Obesity (Silver Spring)* 2011; 20/2: 421–427.

164. Hunter GR, Kekes-Szabo T, Treuth MS, Williams MJ, Goran M, Pichon C. Intraabdominal adipose tissue, physical activity and cardiovascular risk in pre- and postmenopausal women. *Int J Obes Relat Metab Disord* 1996; 20/9: 860–865.

165. Tchernof A, Belanger C, Morisset AS, Richard C, Mailloux J, Laberge P et al. Regional differences in adipose tissue metabolism in women: Minor effect of obesity and body fat distribution. *Diabetes* 2006; 55/5: 1353–1360.

166. Shadid S, Jensen MD. Effects of pioglitazone versus diet and exercise on metabolic health and fat distribution in upper body obesity. *Diabetes Care* 2003; 26/11: 3148–3152.

167. Nissen SE, Wolski K. Effect of rosiglitazone on the risk of myocardial infarction and death from cardiovascular causes. *N Engl J Med* 2007; 356/24: 2457–2471.

168. Hamdy O, Carver C. The Why WAIT program: Improving clinical outcomes through weight management in type 2 diabetes. *Curr Diabetes Rep* 2008; 8/5: 413–420.

169. Mitri J, Hamdy O. Diabetes medications and body weight. *Expert Opin Drug Saf* 2009; 8/5: 573–584.

170. Golay A. Metformin and body weight. *Int J Obes (Lond)* 2008; 32/1: 61–72.

171. O'Brien PE. Bariatric surgery: Mechanisms, indications and outcomes. *J Gastroenterol Hepatol* 2010; 25/8: 1358–1365.

172. Meijer RI, van Wagensveld BA, Siegert CE, Eringa EC, Serne EH, Smulders YM. Bariatric surgery as a novel treatment for type 2 diabetes mellitus: A systematic review. *Arch Surg* 2011; 146/6: 744–750.

173. Sanyal AJ, Brunt EM, Kleiner DE, Kowdley KV, Chalasani N, Lavine JE et al. Endpoints and clinical trial design for nonalcoholic steatohepatitis. *Hepatology* 2011; 54/1: 344–353.

174. Browning JD, Baker JA, Rogers T, Davis J, Satapati S, Burgess SC. Short-term weight loss and hepatic triglyceride reduction: Evidence of a metabolic advantage with dietary carbohydrate restriction. *Am J Clin Nutr* 2011; 93/5: 1048–1052.

175. Kistler KD, Brunt EM, Clark JM, Diehl AM, Sallis JF, Schwimmer JB. Physical activity recommendations, exercise intensity, and histological severity of nonalcoholic fatty liver disease. *Am J Gastroenterol* 2011; 106/3: 460–468.

176. Sattar N, Preiss D, Murray HM, Welsh P, Buckley BM, de Craen AJ et al. Statins and risk of incident diabetes: A collaborative meta-analysis of randomised statin trials. *Lancet* 2010; 375/9716: 735–742.

177. Lin HZ, Yang SQ, Chuckaree C, Kuhajda F, Ronnet G, Diehl AM. Metformin reverses fatty liver disease in obese, leptin-deficient mice. *Nat Med* 2000; 6/9: 998–1003.

178. Bugianesi E, Gentilcore E, Manini R, Natale S, Vanni E, Villanova N et al. A randomized controlled trial of metformin versus vitamin E or prescriptive diet in nonalcoholic fatty liver disease. *Am J Gastroenterol* 2005; 100/5: 1082–1090.

179. Promrat K, Lutchman G, Uwaifo GI, Freedman RJ, Soza A, Heller T et al. A pilot study of pioglitazone treatment for nonalcoholic steatohepatitis. *Hepatology* 2004; 39/1: 188–196.

Index

Printed and bound by CPI Group (UK) Ltd, Croydon, CR0 4YY

21/10/2024

01777105-0015